Advanced Research in Ophthalmology

Advanced Research in Ophthalmology

Editor: Ryan Loren

FOSTER ACADEMICS

www.fosteracademics.com

www.fosteracademics.com

FOSTER ACADEMICS

Cataloging-in-Publication Data

Advanced research in ophthalmology / edited by Ryan Loren.
p. cm.
Includes bibliographical references and index.
ISBN 978-1-63242-524-9
1. Ophthalmology--Research. 2. Eye--Diseases. I. Loren, Ryan.
RE14 .A38 2018
617.7--dc23

Foster Academics,
118-35 Queens Blvd., Suite 400,
Forest Hills, NY 11375, USA

ISBN 978-1-63242-524-9 (Hardback)

Printed and bound in China.

Contents

Preface ... IX

Chapter 1 **Development and Validation of the Self-Acceptance Scale for Persons with Early Blindness: The SAS-EB** ... 1
Fabiane Frota da Rocha Morgado, Angela Nogueira Neves Betanho Campana, Maria da Consolação Gomes Cunha Fernandes Tavares

Chapter 2 **Gene Profiling of Postnatal *Mfrp*^{rd6} Mutant Eyes Reveals Differential Accumulation of *Prss56*, Visual Cycle and Phototransduction mRNAs** ... 10
Ramani Soundararajan, Jungyeon Won, Timothy M. Stearns, Jeremy R. Charette, Wanda L. Hicks, Gayle B. Collin, Jürgen K. Naggert, Mark P. Krebs, Patsy M. Nishina

Chapter 3 **Geometrical Custom Modeling of Human Cornea In Vivo and its use for the Diagnosis of Corneal Ectasia** ... 23
Francisco Cavas-Martínez, Daniel G. Fernández-Pacheco, Ernesto De la Cruz-Sánchez, José Nieto Martínez, Francisco J. Fernández Cañavate, Alfredo Vega-Estrada, Ana B. Plaza-Puche, Jorge L. Alió

Chapter 4 **The Concordance of Care for Age Related Macular Degeneration with the Chronic Care Model: A Multi-Centered Cross-Sectional Study** ... 35
Stefan Markun, Elisabeth Brändle, Avraham Dishy, Thomas Rosemann, Anja Frei

Chapter 5 **Acute Increase of Children's Conjunctivitis Clinic Visits by Asian Dust Storms Exposure - A Spatiotemporal Study in Taipei, Taiwan** ... 43
Lung-Chang Chien, Yi-Jen Lien, Chiang-Hsin Yang, Hwa-Lung Yu

Chapter 6 **Analysis of Fundus Shape in Highly Myopic Eyes by using Curvature Maps Constructed from Optical Coherence Tomography** ... 53
Masahiro Miyake, Kenji Yamashiro, Yumiko Akagi-Kurashige, Akio Oishi, Akitaka Tsujikawa, Masanori Hangai, Nagahisa Yoshimura

Chapter 7 **Regulation of Nitric Oxide Production by δ-Opioid Receptors during Glaucomatous Injury** ... 62
Shahid Husain, Yasir Abdul, Sudha Singh, Anis Ahmad, Mahvash Husain

Chapter 8 **Whole Exome Analysis Identifies Frequent *CNGA1* Mutations in Japanese Population with Autosomal Recessive Retinitis Pigmentosa** ... 73
Satoshi Katagiri, Masakazu Akahori, Yuri Sergeev, Kazutoshi Yoshitake, Kazuho Ikeo, Masaaki Furuno, Takaaki Hayashi, Mineo Kondo, Shinji Ueno, Kazushige Tsunoda, Kei Shinoda, Kazuki Kuniyoshi, Yohinori Tsurusaki, Naomichi Matsumoto, Hiroshi Tsuneoka, Takeshi Iwata

Chapter 9 **Arginase 2 Deficiency Prevents Oxidative Stress and Limits Hyperoxia-Induced Retinal Vascular Degeneration** ... 82
Jutamas Suwanpradid, Modesto Rojas, M. Ali Behzadian, R. William Caldwell, Ruth B. Caldwell

Chapter 10 **Rhegmatogenous Retinal Detachment Surgery in Elderly People over 70 Years Old: Visual Acuity, Quality of Life, and Cost-Utility Values** ... 92
Yingyan Ma, Xiaohua Ying, Haidong Zou, Xiaocheng Xu, Haiyun Liu, Lin Bai, Xun Xu, Xi Zhang

Chapter 11 **Angiogenic Potential of Vitreous from Proliferative Diabetic Retinopathy and Eales' Disease Patients** ... 100
Ponnalagu Murugeswari, Dhananjay Shukla, Ramasamy Kim, Perumalsamy Namperumalsamy, Alan W. Stitt, Veerappan Muthukkaruppan

Chapter 12 **Looking the Cow in the Eye: Deletion in the *NID1* Gene is Associated with Recessive Inherited Cataract in Romagnola Cattle** ... 108
Leonardo Murgiano, Vidhya Jagannathan, Valerio Calderoni, Monika Joechler, Arcangelo Gentile, Cord Drögemüller

Chapter 13 **The Whole Macular Choroidal Thickness in Subjects with Primary Open Angle Glaucoma** ... 118
Shunsuke Nakakura, Minami Yamamoto, Etsuko Terao, Toshihiko Nagasawa, Hitoshi Tabuchi, Yoshiaki Kiuchi

Chapter 14 **Neuroprotection of a Novel Cyclopeptide C*HSDGIC* from the Cyclization of PACAP (1-5) in Cellular and Rodent Models of Retinal Ganglion Cell Apoptosis** ... 127
Huanhuan Cheng, Yong Ding, Rongjie Yu, Jiansu Chen, Chunyun Wu

Chapter 15 **Outcomes in Cochrane Systematic Reviews Addressing Four Common Eye Conditions: An Evaluation of Completeness and Comparability** ... 138
Ian J. Saldanha, Kay Dickersin, Xue Wang, Tianjing Li

Chapter 16 **Characterization of a New Epidemic Necrotic Pyoderma in Fur Animals and its Association with *Arcanobacterium phocae* Infection** ... 148
Heli Nordgren, Kirsi Aaltonen, Tarja Sironen, Paula M. Kinnunen, Ilkka Kivistö , Mirja Raunio- Saarnisto, Anna-Maria Moisander-Jylhä , Johanna Korpela, Ulla-Maija Kokkonen, Udo Hetzel, Antti Sukura, Olli Vapalahti

Chapter 17 **Low Birth Weight is a Risk Factor for Severe Retinopathy of Prematurity Depending on Gestational Age** ... 156
Pia Lundgren, Anna Kistner, Eva M. Andersson, Ingrid Hansen Pupp, Gerd Holmström, David Ley, Aimon Niklasson, Lois E. H. Smith, Carolyn Wu, Ann Hellström, Chatarina Löfqvist

Chapter 18 **Exploring Combinations of Auditory and Visual Stimuli for Gaze-Independent Brain-Computer Interfaces** ... 164
Xingwei An, Johannes Höhne, Dong Ming, Benjamin Blankertz

Chapter 19 **Systemic Adverse Events after Intravitreal Bevacizumab versus Ranibizumab for Age-Related Macular Degeneration** ... 178
Wei Wang, Xiulan Zhang

Chapter 20 **Grasping without Sight: Insights from the Congenitally Blind** ... 186
Kayla D. Stone, Claudia L. R. Gonzalez

Chapter 21 ***In Vitro* and *In Vivo* Models of *Staphylococcus aureus* Endophthalmitis Implicate Specific Nutrients in Ocular Infection**......194
Ama Sadaka, Kelli Palmer, Takashi Suzuki, Michael S. Gilmore

Chapter 22 **Assessment of Choroidal Thickness in Healthy and Glaucomatous Eyes using Swept Source Optical Coherence Tomography**......208
Chunwei Zhang, Andrew J. Tatham, Felipe A. Medeiros, Linda M. Zangwill, Zhiyong Yang, Robert N. Weinreb

Chapter 23 **Diabetes, Glucose Metabolism, and Glaucoma: The 2005-2008 National Health and Nutrition Examination Survey**......220
Di Zhao, Juhee Cho, Myung Hun Kim, David Friedman, Eliseo Guallar

Permissions

List of Contributors

Index

Preface

This book has been an outcome of determined endeavour from a group of educationists in the field. The primary objective was to involve a broad spectrum of professionals from diverse cultural background involved in the field for developing new researches. The book not only targets students but also scholars pursuing higher research for further enhancement of the theoretical and practical applications of the subject.

The branch of medicine which studies eye related diseases and their treatment is known as ophthalmology. Some of the subspecialties of ophthalmology which deal with particular eye problems are anterior segment surgery, cataracts, cornea, ocular oncology, uveitis, refractive surgery and neuro-ophthalmology. Ophthalmology is a field of medicine that has undergone rapid development over the past few decades. This book strives to provide a fair idea about this discipline and to help develop a better understanding of the latest advances within this field. It is meant for students who are looking for an elaborate reference text on ophthalmology.

It was an honour to edit such a profound book and also a challenging task to compile and examine all the relevant data for accuracy and originality. I wish to acknowledge the efforts of the contributors for submitting such brilliant and diverse chapters in the field and for endlessly working for the completion of the book. Last, but not the least; I thank my family for being a constant source of support in all my research endeavours.

Editor

Development and Validation of the Self-Acceptance Scale for Persons with Early Blindness: The SAS-EB

Fabiane Frota da Rocha Morgado[1]*, Angela Nogueira Neves Betanho Campana[2], Maria da Consolação Gomes Cunha Fernandes Tavares[1]

1 Department of Physical Education, University of Campinas, Campinas, São Paulo, Brazil, 2 Sagrado Coração University, Bauru, São Paulo, Brazil

Abstract

Investigations of self-acceptance are critical to understanding the development and maintenance of psychological health. However, valid and reliable instruments for measuring self-acceptance in persons with early blindness have yet to be developed. The current research describes three studies designed to develop and validate the Self-acceptance Scale for Persons with Early Blindness (SAS-EB). In Study 1, we developed the initial item pool. Thirty-three items were generated, based on data from specialized literature and from 2 focus groups. Items were organized in a three-factor structure, theoretically predicted for SAS-EB - (1) body acceptance, (2) self-protection from social stigmas, and (3) feeling and believing in one's capacities. In Study 2, information obtained from a panel of 9 experts and 22 persons with early blindness representing the target population was used to refine the initial item pool, generating a new pool of 27 items. In Study 3, 318 persons with early blindness (141 women and 177 men), between 18 and 60 years of age (M = 37.74 years, SD = 12.37) answered the new pool of 27 items. After the elimination of 9 items using confirmatory factor analysis, we confirmed the theoretical three-factor structure of the SAS-EB. Study 3 also provided support for the scale's internal consistency and construct validity. Finally, the psychometric properties of the SAS-EB, its utility, and its limitations are discussed along with considerations for future research.

Editor: Yong Liu, National Laboratory of Pattern Recognition, China

Funding: This work was supported by the FAPESP (2010/50684-5). The funders had no role in study design, data collection and analysis, decision to publish, or preparation of the manuscript.

Competing Interests: The authors have declared that no competing interests exist.

* Email: fabi.frm@hotmail.com

Introduction

Self-acceptance is an important concept in understanding the development of psychological health [1-2-3]. It is defined as an individual's acceptance of all of his/her attributes, positive or negative. Self-acceptance enables an individual to appropriately evaluate his/her efficient and inefficient features and accept any negative aspects as parts of their personality [4-5].

Three main attitudes are markedly inherent in self-acceptance. The first is "*body acceptance*", defined by Tilka [6] (p. 59) as "expressing comfort with and love for the body, despite not being completely satisfied with all aspects of the body". Another important attitude is "*self-protection from negative judgments from others*", which consists in a lack of concern that others are judging oneself negatively [7-8]. The third attitude focuses on "*feeling and believing in one's capacities*", which includes recognizing, appreciating and developing positives thoughts and feelings about one's capacities and realizations [9-10].

Self-acceptance has been positively associated with different positive aspects of mental health, such as high self-esteem, interpersonal satisfaction and affect regulation [1-11]. Given its features, self-acceptance allows the individual to experience a healthy relationship with the self, contributing to the development of a positive body image [12-13-14]. In contrast, self-acceptance has been negatively associated with different psychopathologies, such as depression and anxiety [15-16]. Additionally, a lack of self-acceptance is considered as a principal contributor to the development and maintenance of eating disorders and obesity [17-18] and may contribute to the emergence of a negative body image [13].

In individuals with a disability, self-acceptance has been hypothesized to be a particularly important construct. It is considered to be a crucial psychological advantage, especially because it enables individuals to view themselves positively, to accept limitations stemming from the disability, and to be better equipped to cope with the disability and to establish healthy practices [19]. Lack of self-acceptance is characterized by feelings of worthlessness, inadequacy, depression, self-blame and self-hatred, which block motivation, inhibit positive behaviors, and cause difficulties in rehabilitation and adjustment [20-21]. Despite the importance of this concept, no measurement scales are available to assess self-acceptance in people with early blindness.

Early visual deprivation may hinder emotional and psychological development, as well as personality organization. The psychological adjustment of these individuals in a seeing world may be more egocentric, especially if their environment is deficient in interpersonal interaction, which contributes to the complexities of personality development, impacting self-acceptance [22-23]. In addition, reports have been published on the presence of eating disorders in persons with early onset blindness [24-25-26-27-28-29-30-31]. A possible explanation for the development of these disorders may be the presence of low levels of self-acceptance. However, so far, this has not been well explored.

The Self-Acceptance Questionnaire (SAQ) [32] is the only available instrument specifically adapted for individuals in China to assess self-acceptance in individuals with visual impairment. Although the psychometric properties of the SAQ are adequate, this instrument is not specifically suited to persons with early blindness. The lack of an appropriate scale to assess self-acceptance in people with early blindness limits the advancement of studies in this field, hampering the development of efficient interventions for prevention and therapy. Measuring self-acceptance for sample groups of individuals with early blindness is important in order to help identify people at risk for a lack of self-acceptance. Thus, there is a great need for the development and validation of a specific scale for these persons.

The aim of this study was to create and evaluate the psychometric properties of the new Self-acceptance Scale for Persons with Early Blindness (SAS-EB). Building on the large body of research on scale development [33-34-35-36], the present paper describes three studies: (1) item generation, (2) scale refinement, and (3) confirmatory factor analysis, reliability and construct validity. This study was approved by an institutional review board (Research Ethics Committee of the Campinas State University - Rep. 187/2010).

Study 1: Item Generation

The purpose of Study 1 was to develop the SAS-EB items. The initial item pool generation was created and selected on the basis of two information sources: data acquired from the specialized literature and from focus groups including participants with early blindness. Consistent with previous theory and research on self-acceptance [6-7-8-10], we hypothesized that the SAS-EB would consist of three factors: (1) body acceptance, (2) self-protection from negative judgments from others, and (3) feeling and believing in one's capacities.

Methods

Participants. There were 11 participants with early-onset blindness (5 men and 6 women, mean age = 34.8, SD = 7.3 years, range 26–48 years) conveniently recruited from the Benjamin Constant Institute, located in Rio de Janeiro, Brazil. We considered blind subjects, participants who were self-reported to have vision scores of less than 3/60 in their best eye, with the best optical correction, i.e., those who are able to see only 3 meters ahead, when a person with normal vision could see up to 60 meters [37]. Early blindness occurs in individuals who had lost their vision in early childhood (range: birth-8 years of age). The present definition of early blindness is consistent with a number of prior studies [38-39-40], but differs from some, which consider early blindness to be loss of vision before the age of 1 [41] or between the ages of 1.4–13 years [42]. In order to be eligible to participate in this study, participants must: (1) have reported a diagnosis of early blindness, with no other clinical conditions, (2) be ≥18 years of age, and (3) have agreed to freely participate in the research.

Procedure. Two focus groups were conducted. The first included six women, while the second group consisted of five men. Men and women were separated in order to achieve greater homogeneity among the participants. Prior to the group formation, information about the purpose of the study and confidentiality were provided and informed written consent was obtained. No compensation was offered.

Each focus group session lasted 90–120 min and was led by two moderators with prior experience in conducting focus group. Moderators sat around an oval table with the participants, one on each side of the table. The main moderator led the discussion and the second moderator intermittently introduced questions of interest regarding the understanding of self-acceptance.

Moderators asked different questions related to self-acceptance, structured on the three factors we hypothesized to constitute the construct. As examples of moderate issues, we proposed: a) to the first factor - Comment on the relationship that you establish with your body – is it positive, is it negative, is it irrelevant? Does the blindness interfere with your relationship to your own body? Do you like to take care of yourself? How is the care of the body in the absence of vision? b) to the second factor - How does society view a person who cannot see? Is the opinion of others important to you? Does the opinion of others interfere with your feelings about yourself? c) to the third factor - What is needed for you to develop and maintain feelings and beliefs of capability? What would increase your love for yourself? Are the opinions of people who are blind valued? These questions were previously established. However, during the focus group, other questions emerged and the moderators had the freedom to go beyond those previously established. The participants gave their opinions of the issues, disagreed amongst themselves, agreed, discussed controversial issues, and, in short, intensely participated in the discussions. Moderators avoided giving any opinion, leading the group so as not to interfere with the view of the participants, thus avoiding bias.

The sessions also had an observer, who made important notes about the attitudes of the participants, as well as a qualified professional who audio/video-recorded the discussions, with the participants' permission. The discussion material was literally transcribed. Qualitative data from the focus group were analyzed thematically with the content analysis [43].

Results

The first study provided the initial item pool generation. There were 33 items generated from the specialized literature and from two focus groups. Items were rated on a 5-point Likert scale (1 = *never*, 2 = *seldom*, 3 = *sometimes*, 4 = *often*, 5 = *always*) and were distributed in the three initially hypothesized factors (Table S1 in File S1).

The first factor, labeled *body acceptance*, was central to the participants' conceptualization of self-acceptance. Congruent with a previous study [44], participants in this study reported that, even without visual experience since an early age, satisfaction with appearance, body care, body love, and the value attributed to one's body are inherent attributes of self-acceptance. Thus, 14 items were generated to compose this factor and assess the expression of love, care and satisfaction with the body.

The second factor was changed. In our initial hypothesis, it had been labeled *self-protection from negative judgments from others*, which consisted in evaluating the ability of the individual to accept themselves without the worry of being negatively evaluated by others. However, after an analysis of the discussions from the two focus groups and in accordance with studies of Brittain [45], Hughes [46], Lobianco and Sheppard-Jones [47], Sahin and Akyol [48], Tripp [49], and Watson [50], we found that for individuals with disabilities, an important source of negative judgment comes from social stigmas. Stigma is an attribute that others perceive to be deeply discrediting [51-52]. In disabled persons, stigma usually demonstrates discrimination, avoidance, social exclusion [49], invalidation, and disfigurement [46]. Stigmas associated with disability may have a negative impact on self-acceptance [20]. Therefore, the second factor is now termed *self-protection from social stigmas*, and comprises 5 items, which assess the subjects' ability to accept themselves without worry about negative judgments from others related to social stigma.

The third factor, labeled *feeling and believing in one's capacities*, assesses the positive thoughts and feelings about the capacities of the individual related to daily life with early blindness. These thoughts and feelings were considered critical to the development and maintenance of self-acceptance in the participants. This factor is composed of 14 items. We hypothesized that all of the individual items from all three categories would be capable assessors of the self-acceptance of persons with early blindness.

As a result, we constructed an initial version of the SAS-EB, which will be subsequently refined over the course of following studies.

Study 2: Scale Refinement

The aim of Study 2 was to assess the theoretical quality of the first version of the SAS-EB. We assessed the content validity of the new scale by consulting both a panel of experts and persons with early blindness representing the target population.

Methods

Participants. A panel of nine independent Ph.D. - level scientists with expertise in self-acceptance, visual impairment or scale development research reviewed the preliminary version of the SAS-EB. This panel included three self-acceptance specialists, three professors who had experience in research on visual impairment, one professor who had experience in research on both visual impairment and self-acceptance, and two experts who had published several scale development-related articles.

A group of 22 participants with early blindness, 10 women and 12 men, aged 29 to 48 years ($M = 34.2$, $SD = 7.2$), recruited from the Benjamin Constant Institute and from the Association for the Blind of Juiz de Fora, Minas Gerais, Brazil, with varying levels of education (range: elementary - higher education) and different social traits (living in the boarding system in the Association for the Blind of Juiz de Fora ($n = 14$), Braille teacher ($n = 4$), and Braille reviewer ($n = 4$) of the Benjamin Constant Institute), agreed to assess the preliminary version of the SAS-EB, in the "pretest" procedure [35]. The criteria for participant inclusion were: (1) diagnosis of early blindness, with no other clinical conditions, (2) aged ≥18 years, and (3) agreed to freely participate in the research.

Instruments. The **Content Validity Form** was a specific judgment report created especially for this purpose. We asked the participants to judge how relevant they thought the content of each item was to assess self-acceptance. They might rate relevance to be high (+1 = appropriate item), moderate (0 = rewrite item), or low (-1 = delete item). In addition, we invited the experts to comment on individual items as they saw fit, and to make notation of new items that they would recommend, helping us to maximize the content validity of the SAS-EB.

Procedures. All participants provided written informed consent to participate in the study. No compensation was offered. The participants assessed item relevance, clarity, conciseness, and redundancy [33]. The ratio of content validity criterion was 0.70[36]. Items considered to be of low relevance for at least 70% of the judges were eliminated. Items considered to be of moderate relevance for at least 70% of the judges were rewritten. Items considered problematic regarding these aspects by at least 70% of the experts were eliminated and those considered partly problematic by at least 70% of the experts were rewritten.

After the expert review, a second and adjusted version of the scale was submitted to the pretest. Three pretests were performed. In the first, seven subjects with early blindness were individually invited to participate in the study and all agreed to participate. Then, in a reserved and silent room, the researcher read the scale for each participant, individually, asking him/her to answer items by "thinking aloud". At the same time, according to the responses of the participant, the researcher completed a judgment report that had been specially developed for this stage of the study. In this report, we evaluated: (1) the understanding of item content by the participants, and (2) the level of difficulty in answering the items. All questions asked of the participants in relation to item content and the difficulty in answering the questions were recorded for later analysis. In the second pretest, seven other subjects with early blindness were invited to participate in the study and all gave their consent. The procedures were the same as in the first pretest; however, a new judgment measure was used to assess the reformulated scale from the first pretest. In this new report, we also evaluated: (1) the understanding of the content of the items by the participants, and (2) the level of difficulty in answering the questions. Finally, in the last pretest, eight other representatives of the target population agreed to participate in the study. This pretest was different from the previously administered test. We evaluated whether or not the aural application of the scale, appropriately reproduced via electronic equipment, would be effectively understood. The aurally applied scale could facilitate and homogenize the data collection procedure. Then, beyond the researcher reading the scale to the participants, a previously recorded, standardized reading could be used for all study subjects. Participants were asked which method between the two (reading or audio) they felt more comfortable answering. The answers were recorded for later analysis. Data analysis of the pretest was given qualitatively, i.e., by the subjective evaluation of the researcher.

Results

Study 2 provided the SAS-EB content validity through the opinions of both experts and representatives of the target population. The experts review resulted in the rewording of 21 items, the deletion of 7 items that were considered of low relevance in content or were redundant, and the inclusion of 1 item, leaving a total of 27 items (*body acceptance* = 11 items, *self-protection from social stigmas* = 4 items, and *feeling and believing in one's capacities* = 12 items). These 27 items formed the second and adjusted version of the SAS-EB, which was used in the subsequent pretest.

The first pretest indicated that 6 items were difficult for the participants to understand. As a result, the content of these items was rewritten, and a third and refined version of the SAS-EB was directed for a second pretest. In the second pretest, the participants were able to understand all of the item content and they had no difficulty answering the questions from the scale. In the last pretest, the third and refined version of scale (Table S2 in File S1) was applied with an audio CD and received the approval of the majority ($n = 7$) of participants. Therefore, this scale was aurally applied in the following procedures.

Study 3: Confirmatory Factor Analyses, Reliability and Construct Validity

The main goals of Study 3 were to perform Confirmatory Factor Analyses (CFA) to test the three-factor model of the SAS-

EB that was hypothesized in Study 1 and refined in Study 2 and to assess the SAS-EB internal reliability and construct validity.

In relation to convergent validity, we hypothesized that, consistent with previous theory and research about self-acceptance [5-20-53-54-55-56-57], the SAS-EB factors would be positively related to certain components, e.g., body satisfaction, visual impairment acceptance, level of education, and intensity of physical activity. Conversely, they would be negatively related to both intensity of perceived social stigma and BMI. These relationships were examined in the present study.

Concerning discriminant validity, research suggests that self-acceptance may encompass several different distinct criteria groups. For example, professional status includes variables for being in or out of the job market [55-58], marital status can be with or without a romantic partner [59], the sex variable encompasses men and women [5-60], age can be young or old [5], and BMI variables include normal weight, overweight or underweight [57]. Based on this evidence, we also hypothesized that the SAS-EB could differ significantly with varying group criteria.

Methods

Participants. In Study 3, 339 individuals with early blindness were invited. Twenty-one individuals refused to participate (12 male, 9 female, 25 to 35 years old). The new sample included 318 individuals (141 women and 177 men), between 18 and 60 years of age ($M = 37.74$ years, $SD = 12.37$). The average self-reported weight was 69.14 kg ($SD = 13.80$ kg), height was 1.62 m ($SD = .09$ m), and average self-reported body mass index (BMI) was 26.05 kg/m^2 ($SD = 4.5$). Our sample size exceeded the number of participants needed (270) for a case-to-parameter ratio of 10:1, in order to examine the model fit and to conduct all planned analyses [33-34].

The most common cause of early blindness was congenital glaucoma ($n = 99$, 31.1%), followed by undetermined causes ($n = 46$, 14.5%), retinitis pigmentosa ($n = 27$, 8.5%), retinopathy of prematurity ($n = 26$, 8.2%), optic nerve atrophy ($n = 23$, 7.2%), congenital cataract ($n = 17$, 5.3%) and other ($n = 80$, 25.2%). Most of the participants described themselves as single ($n = 118$, 37.1%), employed ($n = 170$, 53.5%), having completed a basic education ($n = 104$, 32.7%) and as not routinely engaging in exercise ($n = 203$, 63.8%).

Participants were recruited from three distinct regions of Brazil: Midwest, Southeast and Northeast. Selection of participants occurred both in centers specializing in the care of people with visual impairments, including educational institutions and public philanthropic institutions, and at cultural and scientific events in which the primary audience was composed of people with visual impairments - Blind Encounter Brazil (Rio de Janeiro and Fortaleza) and the XV Brazilian Meeting of DOSVOX users (Rio de Janeiro).

Instruments. Self-acceptance Scale for Persons with Early Blindness (SAS-EB): The scale used was the same developed in Study 1 and refined in Study 2.

Demographic questionnaire: The questionnaire was developed specifically for this study. Participants were asked about their age, weight, height, level of education, intensity of physical activity, professional status, and marital status. They were also asked about their level of body satisfaction (*Regarding your body, you are: (1) dissatisfied, (2) somewhat satisfied, (3) indifferent, (4) very satisfied, (5) completely satisfied*), visual impairment acceptance (*Do you accept your blind condition? The response options were: (1) never, (2) seldom, (3) sometimes, (4) often, and (5) always*), and intensity of perceived social stigma (*When you go out into the street, at work, at school, or in your family, have you experienced any kind of social stigma regarding your blindness? The answer options were rated on a 5-point scale ranging from (1) never to (5) always*).

Procedure. The researcher individually invited all participants. We included participants who self-reported early blindness, with no other clinical conditions, who freely agreed to participate in the study, and who were between 18 and 60 years old. Participants who: (1) did not precisely report the age at which they became blind, (2) did not precisely declare their visual condition (low vision or blindness), (3) reported having acquired blindness after 8 years of age, or (4) reported having low vision were excluded. All participants included in the study ($n = 318$) were informed about the research procedures and provided written informed consent. No compensation was offered.

After agreeing to participate in the study, the volunteer was individually led to a quiet, reserved room. The scale instructions were then played on an audio recording. The researcher took note of all answers for later analysis. Each volunteer took approximately 20 minutes to answer the survey. The LISREL system [61] and SPSS software were used for statistical analyses.

Results

Confirmatory Factor Analyses. Using the LISREL system, we conducted the CFA on the 27 item responses testing for the hypothesized three-factor model of SAS-EB. The unweighted least square method of estimation was used because of the lack of multivariate normality of our data. The *listwise* deletion criterion was adopted for missing data. GFI (Goodness-of-fit)>.90, AGFI (Adjusted Goodness-of-Fit)>.90, NNFI (Non-normed Fit)>.90, CFI (Comparative Fit)>.90, X^2/df (Standardized Chi-square) <3, and RMSEA (Root Mean Square Error of Approximation) <.08 indices evaluated the model fit. Items were considered for deletion if they produced scores that had factor loadings ≤.35 [36].

As result, the hypothesized three-factor model did not provide an adequate fit to the data (χ^2/df = 2.21, RMSEA = .062, GFI = .94, AGFI = .93, NNFI = .96, CFI = .96). The GFI and AGFI statistics were below (<.95 for both) cutoffs for good fit. Items 11 ($\lambda = .24$) and 21 ($\lambda = .21$) had low factor loading and were eliminated. Once these items were eliminated, the model provided a good fit to the data (χ^2/df = 2.13, RMSEA = .060, GFI = .96, AGFI = .95, NNFI = .97, CFI = .98). However, items 2, 7, 8, 25 and 27 had the lowest factor loading ($\lambda = .34$, $\lambda = .31$, $\lambda = .35$, $\lambda = .33$, and $\lambda = .35$, respectively) and showed large associated residuals (.88,.89,.87,.87,.85, respectively), therefore, we consequently eliminated them. After this elimination, we decided to also eliminate items 4 and 18 because of their high positive residuals (≥ ±2.58). Finally, a better model fit was achieved (χ^2/df = 1.86, RMSEA = .052, GFI = .97, AGFI = .96, NNFI = .98, CFI = .99). Subsequently, after the elimination of the nine items, we confirmed the factor structure of the SAS-EB three-factor model. The SAS-EB now has 18 items: first factor = 6 items, second factor = 4 items and third factor = 8 items. Items 9, 10, 13, 16, 20, 22, 24, and 26 had reverse scores (Table 1).

Reliability and Construct validity. To determine the internal consistency of the SAS-EB scores, we used Cronbach's alpha and examined item total and inter-item correlations. Alpha values greater than or equal to.6 suggest acceptable reliability for exploratory studies [34]. Item-total correlations between.30 and.70 and a mean inter-item correlation greater than.20 indicate adequate reliability [34-62]. In this study, all three factors showed moderate reliability indices: the first factor ($\alpha = .70$), second factor ($\alpha = .69$), and third factor ($\alpha = .74$). Item-total correlations ranged between.31 and.62 and mean inter-item correlation ranged

Table 1. Item-factor loadings and descriptive statistics of SAS-EB item scores in Study 3.

Items		M	SD	λ	θ
	First Factor: Body acceptance				
BA1	Do you like your body the way it is? [*Você gosta de seu corpo como ele é?*]	4.06	1.14	.63	.59
BA3	Do you like your appearance, for example, your hair, your face, the way you dress? [*Você gosta de sua aparência, por exemplo, seu cabelo, seu rosto, seu modo de vestir?*]	4.23	.95	.54	.70
BA14	Do you like yourself the way you are? [*Você gosta do jeito que você é?*]	4.31	.93	.76	.41
BA15	Do you take care of your appearance, for instance, your hair, your skin, and your clothes? [*Você cuida de sua aparência, por exemplo, de seu cabelo, sua pele, seu vestuário?*]	4.44	.81	.40	.84
BA17	Do you recognize your good qualities? [*Você reconhece suas qualidades?*]	4.19	.92	.39	.84
BA19	Do you think you are physically attractive? [*Você se considera fisicamente atraente?*]	3.29	1.12	.46	.78
	Second Factor: Self-protection from social stigmas				
SP13	Do you worry about negative attitudes from society regarding your blindness? [*Você se incomoda com algumas atitudes negativas da sociedade a respeito de sua condição de cego?*]	3.34	1.31	.46	.78
SP20	Do you get annoyed with prejudiced opinions of your blindness? [*Você se incomoda com opiniões preconceituosas a respeito de sua cegueira?*]	2.84	1.45	.52	.72
SP22	When you observe some kind of prejudice related with your blindness, do you feel yourself to be less of a person? [*Quando você observa algum tipo de preconceito social em relação a sua cegueira, você se sente inferior às outras pessoas?*]	2.02	1.23	.72	.48
SP26	Do you worry about preposterous questions about your blindness? [*Você se incomoda com perguntas inadequadas sobre sua cegueira?*]	2.22	1.36	.43	.81
	Third Factor: Feeling and believing in one's capacities				
FB5	Do you think that you are capable of deciding what is best for you? [*Você se considera capaz de decidir o que é melhor para você?*]	4.50	.76	.43	.81
FB6	Are you highly positive about your life? [*Você é muito positivo em relação a sua vida?*]	4.31	.87	.54	.54
FB9	Does blindness cause difficulties in your social interactions? [*Ser cego lhe dificulta se relacionar com outras pessoas?*]	2.35	1.2	.51	.73
FB10	Does blindness hinder you from taking part in your favorite activities? [*Sua cegueira lhe atrapalha a fazer coisas que você gosta?*]	2.33	1.07	.54	.71
FB12	Do you feel that you are capable of overcoming your day-to-day difficulties? [*Você se sente capaz de superar as dificuldades que possam existir no seu dia-a-dia?*]	4.32	.83	.57	.66
FB16	Does being blind have negative effect on your romantic relationships? [*Ser cego lhe dificulta ter um relacionamento amoroso?*]	2.05	1.26	.55	.69
FB23	Are your opinions highly respected in the places you give them, for example, in your work, school, and home? [*Suas opiniões são muito respeitadas nos lugares que você frequenta, por exemplo, trabalho, escola, lar?*]	3.61	.94	.36	.87
FB24	Does blindness hinder you from doing the things you have to do? [*Sua cegueira lhe atrapalha a fazer coisas que você necessita fazer?*]	2.48	.99	.55	.69

Note. BA = body acceptance, SP = self-protection from social stigmas, FB = feeling and believing in one's capacities, M = mean, SD = standard deviation, λ = item-factor loading, θ = error term.
Brazilian Portuguese original version of the items are given in brackets.

between.28 and.26, providing additional evidence of internal reliability (Table 2).

To determine convergent validity, we used Spearman's correlations between each of the three factors of the SAS-EB and body satisfaction, visual impairment acceptance, level of education, intensity of physical activity, intensity of perceived social stigma, and BMI variables (Table 2). As hypothesized, higher scores of the SAS-EB were associated with higher body satisfaction: first factor ($r_s = .52, p < .01$), second factor ($r_s = .21, p < .01$), and third factor ($r_s = .32, p < .01$). For visual impairment acceptance, our results were also as predicted. We found positive and significant associations for the first factor ($r_s = .33, p < .01$), second factor ($r_s = .25, p < .01$), and third factor ($r_s = .32, p < .01$). Additional evidence of convergent validity was shown for the second and third factors. The second factor showed a significant, negative correlation with intensity of perceived social stigma ($r_s = -.15, p < .01$), confirming our previous hypotheses. The third factor also revealed a significant, negative correlation with intensity of perceived social stigma ($r_s = -.14, p < .05$), and a significant, positive correlation with level of education ($r_s = .13, p < .05$), and intensity of physical activity ($r_s = .245, p < .01$). Contrary to what we initially hypothesized, BMI did not correlate with any of the factors. However, the correlations that were found indicate satisfactory parameters of convergent validity for the three factors of SAS-EB.

To determine discriminant validity, the Mann-Whitney test was conducted to evaluate differences in SAS-EB factor scores concerning different group criteria, e.g., working ($n = 170$) and unemployed ($n = 148$), with a romantic partner ($n = 164$) and without a romantic partner ($n = 154$), men ($n = 177$) and women ($n = 141$), younger, 18–39 years old, ($n = 176$) and older, 40–60 years old, ($n = 142$), and normal weight ($n = 126$) and overweight or underweight ($n = 192$). Our results showed discriminant validity for the second and third factor. The *self-protection from social*

Table 2. Item total and mean interitem correlations, alphas, and Spearman's correlations among the measures of Study 3 (N = 318).

Factors	Items	Item-total (r)	Mean interitem (r)	α	Body satisfaction (rho)	Visual impairment acceptance (rho)	LevelEduc. (rho)	Intensity physical activity (rho)	Intensity perceived social stigma(rho)	BMI(rho)
	BA1	.48								
	BA3	.52								
Body	BA14	.62	.28	.70	.52**	.33**	−.01	.18	−.63	−.03
acceptance	BA15	.31								
	BA17	.34								
	BA19	.42								
Self-	SP13	.51								
protection	SP20	.54								
from social	SP22	.41	.36	.69	.21**	.25**	.06	.18	−.15**	−.02
stigmas	SP26	.42								
	FB5	.34								
	FB6	.42								
Feeling and	FB9	.42								
believing in	FB10	.5	.27	.74	.32**	.32**	.13*	.24**	−.14*	.01
oneself	FB12	.47								
capacities	FB16	.54								
	FB23	.32								
	FB24	.47								

** Correlation is significant at.01 (2-tailed)
* Correlation is significant at.05 (2-tailed)
P<0,001
rho = Spearman's correlation.

stigmas factor significantly discriminated groups with and without a romantic partner (participants with a partner had higher mean ranks than those without partner, $p<.05$), and men and women (men had higher mean ranks than women, $p=.001$). The *feeling and believing in one's capacities* factor significantly discriminated groups by employment status (subjects in the job market had higher mean ranks than subjects outside, $p<.05$) and by age (younger participants had higher mean ranks than those who were older, $p=.05$). No factor discriminated between BMI groups, contradicting our previous hypotheses. The second and third factors showed evidence of discriminant validity.

General Discussion

The present study was designed to develop a reliable and valid measure of self-acceptance for use with samples from Brazil with early blindness. Results of the three studies suggest that the SAS-EB is reliable and valid for measuring self-acceptance in this portion of the population. In Study 1, we initially developed the three-factor self-acceptance model (*body acceptance*, *self-protection from social stigmas,* and *feeling and believing in one's capacities).* The initial item pool included 33 items carefully drawn to be easily understood by the target population and to represent the hypothesized three factors. The first factor was created to assess the level of love, care and satisfaction with oneself, including one's own body and bodily appearance. The second factor was structured to assess the organization of the individuals' protection cognitive filter, qualifying them to reject negative information about their blindness derived from social stigmas. The third factor was organized to assess the feelings and beliefs of one's capacities to face everyday situations identified by participants as important to the development and maintenance of self-acceptance.

In Study 2, we confirmed the content validity of the SAS-EB. After a review by nine experts in self-acceptance, visual impairment, or scale development research, a total of 27 items were retained from the initial pool of 33 items. As a result of the three pretests given to 22 representatives of the target population, minor adjustments were made in the wording of 6 items. One important aspect of this study was that it tested and approved the application of the new scale in an audio format, adapting it specifically to our sample with blindness. The audio version of the SAS-EB is an improvement over the previous study [32], because it makes the instrument easier to administer to large sample groups of blind individuals, making homogeneous conditions of application and data collection feasible.

In Study 3, a psychometric investigation of the SAS-EB indicated that it shows satisfactory evidence of factorial validity, internal reliability and construct validity. Results of the CFA revealed that the data fit the hypothesized three-factor model well, with item scores showing suitable loadings (range $\lambda=.36-\lambda=.76$) on the intended factors. However, to better fit the model, it was necessary to reduce the number of items, retaining 18 of the initial 27 initial. Despite the brevity of the scale, the three factors were comprised of a number of indicators that exceeded the minimum number required of three item scales [36]. Moreover, the SAS-EB three-factor model with 18 items provided a quick and comprehensive assessment of self-acceptance in persons with early blindness.

The internal reliability of SAS-EB was moderate (range $\alpha=.69$–$.74$). This result is close to that reported in a previous study on scale development of self-acceptance with sighted people ($\alpha=.72$) [4], but it differs from other similar previous investigations ($\alpha=.42$ [63]; $\alpha=.85$ [14]; $\alpha=.83$ [32]). The modest alpha coefficients found in this study likely reflect the small number of indicators per factor and the fact that items were chosen to represent a multifaceted construct, such as self-acceptance. Although moderate, alpha values seem acceptable given that the scale presented appropriate values of item total and mean inter-item correlation, supporting the internal consistency of the scale.

In relation to convergent validity, the results indicated that the greater self-acceptance was related to higher levels of body satisfaction and visual impairment acceptance, confirming previous research [20-53-54]. Further evidence of convergent validity was also found. Consistent with prior research examining the impact of perceived social stigma on psychological correlates of obese Americans [57], the *self-protection from social stigmas* factor correlated modestly and negatively with the intensity of perceived social stigma, showing that the perception of social stigmas has a deleterious effect on the self-protection of people with early blindness. Similarly, the *feeling and believing in one's capacities* factor correlated modestly and negatively with the intensity of perceived social stigma, clarifying that the perception of social stigmas also has a negative effect on the feelings and beliefs of self-capacities in individuals with early blindness. In addition, greater scores for *feeling and believing in one's capacities* were modestly related to higher levels of education, as found by Balon *et al.* [55], and intensity of physical activity, as found by Crone, Smith and Gough [56], highlighting that both education about and practice of regular physical activity are important elements to increase levels of self-acceptance in persons who are blind from an early age. Taken together, these findings confirm the construct validity of the SAS-EB.

When investigating discriminant validity, this study showed satisfactory results for *self-protection from social stigmas* and *feeling and believing in one's capacities*, but not for the *body acceptance* factor. Consistent with prior research, the second factor significantly discriminated criteria groups related to marital status [59] and to sex [5-60]. The third factor significantly discriminated criteria groups related to professional status [55-58] and age [5]. Given that these criteria groups should theoretically discriminate, this study provided support to confirm the discriminant validity of the second and third factors of the SAS-EB. A possible explanation for the lack of discriminant validity for the first factor may be the fact that specific criteria groups related to *body acceptance*, such as internalization of the thin ideal and self-esteem [64], were not evaluated. Future research could investigate the ability of the *body acceptance* factor to successfully differentiate between the two groups mentioned. However, the biggest challenge would be to find appropriate ways to evaluate these variables in the population of the visually impaired.

Carr and Friedman [57] highlighted that higher BMI scores are associated with lower levels of self-acceptance. Accordingly, a significant negative correlation was expected between BMI and factors of the SAS-EB and that the factors of the new scale would be able to differentiate between groups with different measures of BMI. Curiously, contradicting our previously formed hypothesis, the findings found no convergent or discriminant validity regarding the measure of BMI. Two hypotheses may be formulated to explain this finding. The first is that BMI was self-reported, which may have affected the quality of collected measurements of weight and height. In accordance with Gardner, Jappe and Gardner [65], self-reporting weight and height can be a problem, because individuals often overestimate height and underestimate weight, making this measure somewhat inaccurate. In addition, numerous variables affect self-reporting, including sex, age, race/ethnicity, marital status, income, and activity level. The second and more probable hypothesis is that self-acceptance for individuals with early blindness would be independent of body size and weight. It would have to be an unconditional acceptance of oneself, allowing individuals who are blind from an early age to develop and maintain high levels of self-acceptance, even when their appearance does not conform to societal ideals of attractiveness. However, future work in this area should use real measurements of weight and height, examining the relationship between the SAS-EB and BMI.

The present scale offers advantage over the only existing scale for the assessment of self-acceptance in individuals with visual impairment (SAQ), particularly, because it was created and validated specifically for people who were blind at an early age (birth-8 years of age), respecting and appraising the peculiar emotional and psychological characteristics of this population. However, it is worth highlighting that the age limits for the establishment of early blindness are controversial in the literature and this fact can hinder the wide application of the SAS-EB. In this sense, we suggest future studies that investigate the validity of the SAS-EB in groups of blind subjects of different ages, making it possible to know if the new scale is associated with the age of the onset of blindness.

Despite its contributions, the limitations of this study also need to be addressed. The first relates to self-reported weight and height used in study 3. The inaccuracy of self-estimates and inaccuracy in individual perception may have affected the validity of the results, since reported BMI does not allow for the confirmation of convergent or discriminant validity. However, some authors have defended the use of self-reported weight and height as actual predictor of these measures, for the reason that the discrepancies between actual and self-reported measure were sufficiently small to allow using self-estimates in place of measurements [65-66]. In addition, Study 3 recruited a peculiar population - numerous and hard to reach - marking it difficult to achieve ideal conditions for data collection (access to laboratories with scale and stadiometer), requiring that the measurements of weight and height were quick, thus self-reported. Future studies could examine these factors.

The second limitation was the lack of the use of a validated scale to assess the main variable used to check the convergent validity for body satisfaction. Although there is a valid and reliable Brazilian measure for body satisfaction in blind people (Three-Dimensional Body Rating Scale (3BRS) [67]), it was validated for congenitally blind women, and would not be suitable for men or for people who became blind after the age of five, as in the case of some members of this sample. Similarly, another limitation was that no validated scale was used to assess the acceptance of the visual impairment variable for convergent validity. However, in this instance, no specific Brazilian scale was found for this type of measure.

Finally, one additional limitation relates to the inability of scale to provide information on normal or abnormal levels of self-acceptance, failing to derive a standard for Brazil. As a result, this study is limited in its application. Therefore, new and more sophisticated analyses should be performed to establish the norm for people with early blindness in the Brazil.

Despite these limitations, the evidence presented in this preliminary and exploratory study suggests that the SAS-EB may serve as a useful tool in future research related to self-acceptance in persons with early blindness in Brazil. In general, results from the three studies demonstrated that the SAS-EB produced scores that were reliable, with evidence supporting multiple facets of construct validity for the factors intended to measure *body acceptance*, *self-protection from social stigmas,* and *feeling and believing in one's capacities*. However, future research is needed to provide additional evidence regarding the psychometric properties of the SAS-EB.

Supporting Information

File S1 Supporting tables. Table S1, The initial item pool (thirty-three items) generated in Study 1. Table S2, The item pool refined in Study 2 after content validity (panel of experts and pretest).

Acknowledgments

The authors would like to thank all experts who shared their time and opinions, all participants, and the Blind Centers, which helped us to accomplish this research.

Author Contributions

Conceived and designed the experiments: FFRM ANNBC MCGCFT. Performed the experiments: FFRM. Analyzed the data: FFRM ANNBC. Contributed reagents/materials/analysis tools: FFRM ANNBC MCGCFT. Wrote the paper: FFRM.

References

1. Williams JC, Lynn SJ (2011) Acceptance: an historical and conceptual review. Imagin Cogn Pers 30: 5–56.
2. Ryff CD, Singer BH (1996) Psychological well-being: meaning, measurement, and implications for psychotherapy research. Psychother Psychosom 65: 14–23.
3. Ryff CD, Singer BH (2008) Know thyself and become what you are: a eudaimonic approach to psychological well-being. J Happiness Stud 9: 13–39.
4. Chamberlain JM, Haaga DAF (2001) Unconditional self-acceptance and psychological health. J Ration Emot Cogn Behav Ther 19: 163–176.
5. Ceyhan A, Ceyhan E (2011) Investigation of university students' self-acceptance and learned resourcefulness: a longitudinal study. High Educ 61: 649–661.
6. Tylka TL (2011) Positive Psychology perspectives on body image. In: Cash, TF.; Smolak, L. Body image: a handbook of science, practice, and prevention. New York: Guilford press.
7. Carson SH, Langer EJ (2006) Mindfulness and self-acceptance. J Ration Emot Cogn Behav Ther 24: 29–43.
8. Sheerer ET (1949) An analysis of the relationship between acceptance of and respect for self and acceptance of and respect for others in ten counseling cases. J Consult Psychol 13: 169–175.
9. APA (American Psychological Association) (2010) Dictionary of Psychology por American Psychological Association. São Paulo: Artmed Editora.
10. Ghahramani MH, Besharat MA, Naghipour B (2011) An examination of the relationship between perfectionism and self-esteem in a sample of student athletes. Social and Behavioral Sciences 30: 1265–1271.
11. Macinnes DL (2006) Self-esteem and self-acceptance: an examination into their elationship and their effect on psychological health. J Psychiatr Ment Health Nurs 13: 483–489.
12. Besteiro MPV, Franco CP, Morales LG, Sagardoy RC, Mateos AGL (2009) La razón y la emoción: integración de las intervenciones cognitivoconductuales y experenciales en el tratamiento de los trastornos de alimentación de larga evolución. Nutr Hosp 24: 614–617.
13. Smith-Jackson T, Reel JJ, Thackeray R (2011) Coping with "Bad Body Image Days": Strategies from first-year young adult college women. Body Image 8: 335–342.
14. Potocka A, Turczyn-Jabłońska K, Kieć-Świerczyńska M (2008) Self-image and quality of life of dermatology patients. Int J Occup Med Environ Health 21: 309–317.
15. Jimenez SS, Niles BL, Park CL (2010) A mindfulness model of affect regulation and depressive symptoms: Positive emotions, mood regulation expectancies, and self-acceptance as regulatory mechanisms. Pers Individ Dif 49: 645–650.
16. Singh S, Tanu (2011) Personal Influences in Depression among Female Adolescents. Journal of the Indian Academy of Applied Psychology 37: 40–46.
17. McClintock JM, Evans IM (2001) The underlying psychopathology of eating disorders and social phobia: a structural equation analysis. Eat Behav 2: 247–261.
18. Espíndola CR, Blay SL (2009) Anorexia nervosa treatment from the patient perspective: A metasynthesis of qualitative studies. Annals of Clinica l Psychiatry 21: 38–48.

19. Farber RS (2000) Mothers with disabilities: in their own voice. Am J Occup Ther 54: 260–268.
20. Brillhart B (1986) Predictors of self-acceptance. Rehabil Nurs 11: 8–12.
21. Grayson M (1950) The concept of acceptance in physical rehabilitation. Mil Surg 107: 221–226.
22. Cole NJ, Taboroff LH (1954) The psychological problems of the congenitally blind child. Am J Orthopsychiatry 25: 627–643.
23. Sandler AM, Hobson RP (2001) On engaging with people in early childhood: the case of congenital blindness. Clin Child Psychol Psychiatry 6: 205–222.
24. Fernández-Aranda F, Crespo JM, Jiménez-Murcia S, Krug I, Vallejo-Ruiloba J (2006) Blindness and bulimia nervosa: a description of a case report and its treatment. Int J Eat Disord 39: 263–265.
25. McFarlane AC (1989) Blindness and anorexia nervosa. Can J Psychiatry 34: 431–433.
26. Sharp CW (1993) Anorexia nervosa and depression in a woman blind since the age of nine months. Can J Psychiatry 38: 469–471.
27. Touyz S, O'Sullivan B, Gertler R, Beumont P (1988) Anorexia nervosa in a woman totally blind since birth. Br J Psychiatry 153: 248–250.
28. Vandereycken W (1986) Anorexia nervosa and visual impairment. Compr Psychiatry 27: 545–548.
29. Yager J, Hatton CA, Ma L (1986) Anorexia nervosa in a woman totally blind since the age of two. Br J Psychiatry 149: 506–509.
30. Ostojic MS, Hansen AMJ (2012) Sociocultural Factors in the Development of Bulimia Nervosa in a Blind Woman: A Case Report. Int J Eat Disord 00: 1–5.
31. Thomas JJ, Weigel TJ, Lawton RK, Levendusky PG, Becker AE (2012) Cognitive -Behavioral Treatment of Body Image Disturbance in a Congenitally Blind Patient with Anorexia Nervosa. Am J Psychiatry, 169: 16–20.
32. Zhang X, Wang A (2011) Development of a psychosocial adaptation questionnaire for Chinese patients with visual impairments. J Clin Nur 20: 2822–2829.
33. DeVellis RF (2003) Scale development: theory and applications. Newbury Park CA: Sage Publications.
34. Nunnally JC (1967) Psychometric theory. New York: McGraw Hill.
35. Clark LA, Watson D (1995) Constructing validity: basic issues in objective scale development. Psychol Assess 7: 309–319.
36. Hair JF, Black WC, Babin BJ, Anderson RE, Tatham RL (2009) Análise Multivariada de Dados. S.Paulo: Bookman.
37. Thylefors B, Négrel AD, Pararajasegaram R, Dadzie KY (1995) Global data on blindness. Bull World Health Org 73: 15–21.
38. Bedny M, Konkle T, Pelphrev K, Saxe R, Pascual-Leone A (2010) Sensitive period for a multimodal response in human visual motion area MT/MST. Curr Biol 20: 1900–1906.
39. Bedny M, Pascual-Leone A, Dravida S, Saxe R (2012) A sensitive period for language in the visual cortex: Distinct patterns of plasticity in congenitally versus late blind adults. Brain Lang 122: 162–170.
40. Ruotolo F, Ruggiero G, Vinciguerra M, Iachini T (2012) Sequential vs simultaneous encoding of spatial information: a comparison between the blind and the sighted. Acta Psychol 139: 382–389.
41. Jiang J, Zhu W, Shi F, Liu Y, Qin W, et al. (2009) Thick visual cortex in the early blind. J of Neurosci 29: 2205–2211.
42. Wan CY, Wood AG, Reutens DC, Wilson SJ (2010) Congenital blindness leads to enhanced vibrotactile perception. Neuropsychologia 48: 631–635.
43. Bardin L (1977) Análise de conteúdo. Lisboa: Edições 70.
44. Kaplan-Myrth N (2000) Alice without a looking glass: blind people and body image. Anthropol Med 7: 277–299.
45. Brittain I (2004) Perceptions of disability and their impact upon involvement in sport for people with disabilities at all levels. Journal of Sport and Social Issues; 28: 429–452.
46. Hughes B (1999) The constitution of impairment: modernity and the aesthetic of oppression. Disabil Soc 14: 155–172.
47. Lobianco AF, Sheppard-Jones K (2007) Perceptions of disability as related to medical and social factors. J Appl Soc Psychol 37: 1–13.
48. Sahin H, Akyol AD (2010) Evaluation of nursing and medical students' attitudes towards people with disabilities. J Clin Nur 19: 2271–2279.
49. Tripp S (1997) What contribution, if any, can social construction theories make to understanding the experience of disabling conditions? Journal of Orthopedic Nursing 1: 17–20.
50. Watson N (2002) Well, I know this is going to sound very strange to you, but I don't see myself as a disabled person: identity and disability. Disabil Soc 17: 509–527.
51. Goffman E (1963) Stigma: Notes on the Management of Spoiled Identity. Engelwood Cliffs, NJ: Prentice-Hall.
52. Wood N, Ward S (2010) Stigma, secrets, and the human condition: seeking to remedy alienation in postsecret's digitally mediated environment. Symbolic Interaction 33: 578–602.
53. Pearson A, Follette V, Hayes SC (2012) A pilot study of Acceptance and Commitment Therapy (ACT) as a workshop intervention for body image, Cogn Behav Pract. 19: 181–197.
54. Tager D, Good GE, Morrinson JB (2006) Our bodies, ourselves revisited: male body image and psychological well-Being. Int J Mens Health 5: 228–237.
55. Balon YE, Then KL, Rankin JA, Talk F (2008) Looking beyond the biophysical realm to optimize health: results of a survey of psychological well-being in adults with congenital cardiac disease. Cardiol Young 18: 494–501.
56. Crone D, Smith A, Gough B (2005) 'I feel totally at one, totally alive and totally happy': a psycho-social explanation of the physical activity and mental health relationship. Health Education Research 20: 600–611.
57. Carr D, Friedman MA (2005) Is obesity stigmatizing? body weight, perceived discrimination, and psychological well-being in the United States. *Journal of* Health and Social Behavior 46: 244–259.
58. Strauser DR, Lustig DC, Ciftci A (2008) Psychological well-being: its relation to work personality, vocational identity, and career thoughts. J Psychol 142: 21–35.
59. Eastman D (1958) Self acceptance and marital happiness. J Consult Psychol 22: 95–99.
60. Ahrens CJC, Ryff CD (2006) Multiple Roles and Well-being: Sociodemographic and Psychological Moderators. Sex Roles 55: 801–815.
61. Jöreskog K, Sörbom D (1999) Prelis 2: User's reference guide. Chicago: Scientific Software International.
62. Munro BH (2001) Statistical methods for health care research. 4th ed. Philadelphia: Lippincott.
63. Ryff CD, Keyes CLM (1995) The Structure of Psychological well-being revisited. J Pers Soc Psychol 69: 719–727.
64. Forbes GB, Doroszewicz K, Card K, Adams-Curtis L (2004) Association of the thin body ideal, ambivalent sexism, and self-esteem with body acceptance and the preferred body size of college women in Poland and the United States. Sex Roles 50: 331–345.
65. Gardner RM, Jappe LM, Gardner L (2009) Development and Validation of a New Figural Drawing Scale for Body-Image Assessment: The BIAS-BD. J Clin Psychol 65: 113–122.
66. Bowman RL, DeLucia JL (1992) Accuracy of self-reported weight: A meta-analysis. Behavior Therapy 23: 637–655.
67. Morgado FFR, Ferreira MEC, Campana ANNB, Rigby AS, Tavares MCGCF (2013) Initial evidence of the reliability and validity of a Three-dimensional Body Rating Scale for the congenitally blind. Percept Mot Skills 116: 91–105.

2

Gene Profiling of Postnatal *Mfrp*^{rd6} Mutant Eyes Reveals Differential Accumulation of *Prss56*, Visual Cycle and Phototransduction mRNAs

Ramani Soundararajan[1], Jungyeon Won[2], Timothy M. Stearns[1], Jeremy R. Charette[1], Wanda L. Hicks[1], Gayle B. Collin[1], Jürgen K. Naggert[1], Mark P. Krebs[1], Patsy M. Nishina[1]*

1 The Jackson Laboratory, Bar Harbor, Maine, United States of America, **2** National Disaster Management Institute, Seoul, Korea

Abstract

Mutations in the membrane frizzled-related protein (*MFRP/Mfrp*) gene, specifically expressed in the retinal pigment epithelium (RPE) and ciliary body, cause nanophthalmia or posterior microphthalmia with retinitis pigmentosa in humans, and photoreceptor degeneration in mice. To better understand MFRP function, microarray analysis was performed on eyes of homozygous *Mfrp*^{rd6} and C57BL/6J mice at postnatal days (P) 0 and P14, prior to photoreceptor loss. Data analysis revealed no changes at P0 but significant differences in RPE and retina-specific transcripts at P14, suggesting a postnatal influence of the *Mfrp*^{rd6} allele. A subset of these transcripts was validated by quantitative real-time PCR (qRT-PCR). In *Mfrp*^{rd6} eyes, a significant 1.5- to 2.0-fold decrease was observed among transcripts of genes linked to retinal degeneration, including those involved in visual cycle (*Rpe65, Lrat, Rgr*), phototransduction (*Pde6a, Guca1b, Rgs9*), and photoreceptor disc morphogenesis (*Rpgrip1* and *Fscn2*). Levels of RPE65 were significantly decreased by 2.0-fold. Transcripts of *Prss56*, a gene associated with angle-closure glaucoma, posterior microphthalmia and myopia, were increased in *Mfrp*^{rd6} eyes by 17-fold. Validation by qRT-PCR indicated a 3.5-, 14- and 70-fold accumulation of *Prss56* transcripts relative to controls at P7, P14 and P21, respectively. This trend was not observed in other RPE or photoreceptor mutant mouse models with similar disease progression, suggesting that *Prss56* upregulation is a specific attribute of the disruption of *Mfrp*. *Prss56* and *Glul in situ* hybridization directly identified Müller glia in the inner nuclear layer as the cell type expressing *Prss56*. In summary, the *Mfrp*^{rd6} allele causes significant postnatal changes in transcript and protein levels in the retina and RPE. The link between *Mfrp* deficiency and *Prss56* up-regulation, together with the genetic association of human *MFRP* or *PRSS56* variants and ocular size, raises the possibility that these genes are part of a regulatory network influencing postnatal posterior eye development.

Editor: Knut Stieger, Justus-Liebig-University Giessen, Germany

Funding: This research was supported by the National Institutes of Health (NIH) grant EY011996 awarded to P.M.N. and National Institutes of Health Cancer Center Support (CORE) grant 5P30CA034196 to The Jackson Laboratory. The funders had no role in study design, data collection and analysis, decision to publish, or preparation of the manuscript.

Competing Interests: The authors have declared that no competing interests exist.

* Email: patsy.nishina@jax.org

Introduction

MFRP mutations in humans are associated with nanophthalmia or posterior microphthalmia with autosomal recessive retinitis pigmentosa (RP), characterized by retinal spots, foveoschisis and optic nerve head drusen [1–6]. A homozygous mutation of *Mfrp* in mice recapitulates central features of the human disease, including retinal spots and a slowly progressing retinal degeneration [7–9]. The *MFRP/Mfrp* disease phenotype is variable in humans [1–6] and mice [9,10], suggesting an influence of allelic effects and/or genetic modifiers in both species. The common attributes of the human and mouse phenotypes, and the similar genetic modification on disease phenotype make *Mfrp* mutant mice attractive for delineating the mechanism(s) that underlie *MFRP/Mfrp*-associated ocular disease and its genetic variability, which are poorly understood.

Within the eye, MFRP is exclusively localized to the apical surface of the retinal pigment epithelium (RPE) and the ciliary body epithelium [11–13]. The protein has been suggested to play a role in the normal development as well as maintenance of photoreceptor outer segments (OS) [12]. MFRP is a type II transmembrane protein and contains multiple domains, including an N-terminal cytoplasmic domain, a transmembrane domain, two extracellular cubulin (CUB) domains, a low-density lipoprotein domain (LDLa) and a C-terminal cysteine-rich domain (CRD) [8,14]. Complement C1q tumor necrosis factor–related protein 5 (C1QTNF5, also known as CTRP5) is expressed from the same dicistronic transcript as *Mfrp* [8,11,15]. Dicistronic messages often function in common pathways [16]. Therefore, it is notable that MFRP and C1QTNF5 co-localize in the posterior eye [8,11,15] and have been shown to interact directly by two-hybrid and biochemical studies [11]. The functional consequence of this interaction, however, is unknown, and other potentially interacting partners of MFRP remain to be identified.

To obtain insight into the functional role of MFRP in the RPE and retina during normal eye development and disease, gene-profiling studies were carried out in *Mfrp*^{rd6} and wildtype postnatal eyes. Microarray analysis revealed a moderate decrease in phototransduction, visual cycle, and gene transcripts associated with retinal degeneration in *Mfrp*^{rd6} mutants. Most interestingly, an increased temporal expression of *Prss56*, a gene linked to posterior microphthalmia [17] and associated with ocular growth defects in myopia [18,19] was observed. *Prss56* upregulation appeared to be specific to *Mfrp*^{rd6} mice, as it was not observed in other retinal degeneration models with similar disease progression. Broadly, our findings delineate a potential role of MFRP in postnatal development and/or maintenance of the posterior eye, and provide evidence that MFRP and PRSS56 participate in the same functional pathway.

Materials and Methods

Ethics Statement

Protocols using mice in this study were approved by The Jackson Laboratory Institutional Animal Care and Use Committee (Animal Welfare Assurance Number: A3268-01) in accordance with the "Guide for the Care and Use of Experimental Animals" established by the National Institutes of Health (NIH) (1996, Revised 2011).

Animals

Mouse strains utilized in this study, B6.C3Ga-*Mfrp*^{rd6}/J (*Mfrp*^{rd6}) and C57BL/6J were bred and maintained in a vivarium with a 12 hour light and 12 hour dark cycle in the Research Animal Facility at The Jackson Laboratory. Autoclaved NIH31 diet (6% fat) and HCl acidified water (pH 2.8–3.2) were provided *ad libitum*.

Gene Profiling

GeneChip Mouse Genome 430 v2.0 array (Affymetrix) was performed at The Jackson Laboratory Gene Expression Analysis Service (GES). Total RNA from *Mfrp*^{rd6} and C57BL/6J eyes at P0 and P14 (three biological replicates per group) was extracted with Trizol (Life Technologies, Carlsbad, CA, USA) according to the manufacturer's instructions. Two µg of total RNA was used for cDNA synthesis with the One-Cycle Target Labeling cDNA Synthesis Kit (Affymetrix, Santa Clara, CA, USA) and fragmented cRNA was synthesized using the GeneChip IVT Labeling kit (Affymetrix, Santa Clara, CA, USA) according to the manufacturer's protocol (GeneChip Expression analysis Technical manual, Affymetrix 1999–2004). Following cRNA fragmentation, 15 µg of cRNA were hybridized on a GeneChip Mouse Genome 430 v2.0 array at 45°C for 16 h and the microarray was scanned using the GeneChip Scanner 3000 (Affymetrix, Santa Clara, CA, USA). Average signal intensities for each probe set within the arrays were calculated by and exported from Affymetrix's Expression Console (Version 1.2) software using the RMA method, which incorporates convolution background correction, sketch-quantile normalization, and summarization based on a multi-array model fit using the median polish algorithm to generate gene expression data. For this experiment, six pairwise comparisons were used to statistically resolve gene expression differences between sample groups using the R/maanova analysis package. Specifically, differentially accumulated transcripts were detected by using Fs, a modified F-statistic incorporating shrinkage estimate of variance components from within R/maanova. Statistical significance levels of the pairwise comparisons were calculated by permutation analysis (1000 permutations) and adjusted for multiple testing using the false discovery rate (FDR) q-value threshold of 0.05. For each probe set, the raw intensities for all probes were log2-transformed. The log2-transformed intensities were quantile-normalized and a volcano plot was generated for each of the six pairwise comparisons. Differentially accumulated transcripts were classified into various biological pathways using the Ingenuity Pathway Analysis Systems software (Ingenuity Systems, Qiagen, Valencia, CA, USA). Microarray data (MIAME compliant) were submitted to the Gene expression Omnibus (GEO) database (http://www.ncbi.nlm.noh.gov/geo) under GEO Accession Number GSE53411 (http://www.ncbi.nlm.nih.gov/geo/info/linking.html).

Ingenuity Pathway Analysis

Ingenuity pathway analysis software (IPA; Ingenuity Systems, www.ingenuity.com, Summer 2013 release, Qiagen, Valencia, CA, USA) was used to identify potential networks affected by the disruption of *Mfrp* across one dataset (*Mfrp*^{rd6} versus C57BL/6J at P14). The dataset was derived from differential gene expression analysis resulting from the comparison of mRNA from whole eye tissue samples of *Mfrp*^{rd6} versus C57BL/6J mice. Data uploaded into IPA consisted of Affymetrix Mouse Gene 430 2.0 probe sets as identifiers. Each identifier was mapped to its corresponding object in the IPA knowledge base (Summer 2013 release). Expression results were limited to genes having a q-value <0.05. Gene networks were algorithmically generated based on their connectivity to the uploaded data set. Networks pertaining to phototransduction and visual pathways were retained, and expression and significance values were overlaid onto networks of interest so as to identify differential patterns of up- and down-regulated genes. In each network, molecules are represented as nodes, and the biological relationship between two nodes is represented as an edge (line). All edges are supported by at least one reference from the literature, from a textbook, or from canonical information stored in the IPA Knowledge Base. The intensity of the node color indicates the degree of up- (red) or down- (green) regulation with regards to all expression values in the dataset. Nodes are displayed using various shapes that represent the functional class of the gene product; these are defined in the figure legends. Edges are displayed with various labels that describe the nature of the relationship between the nodes (e.g., P for phosphorylation, T for transcription).

Isolation of RPE and Retina

Mice were sacrificed by carbon dioxide asphyxiation and enucleated eyes were placed in chilled phosphate buffered saline (PBS). The connective tissue, muscles and conjunctiva were carefully removed using iris scissors. A circumferential incision was made below the level of ciliary body and the anterior segment consisting of cornea, lens, iris and ciliary body was discarded. The neural retina was peeled from the RPE layer using surgical forceps and the remaining posterior eyecup consisting of the sclera, choroid and RPE was flash frozen in liquid nitrogen and stored at −70°C.

Quantitative Real time PCR

Eyes were collected at different time points (P7, P14 and P21). Total RNA was extracted from whole eyes, retina, and RPE cells using Trizol reagent (Life Technologies, Carlsbad, CA, USA) combined with the RNeasy kit (Qiagen, Valencia, CA, USA) as per manufacturer's instructions. Genomic DNA contamination of RNA was prevented by on-column treatment with DNase I (Qiagen, Valencia, CA, USA) according to the manufacturer's instructions (Qiagen, Valencia, CA, USA). One µg of total RNA was reverse transcribed using the Retroscript kit (Ambion, Life Technologies, Carlsbad, CA, USA). Quantitative real-time PCR (qRT-PCR) was performed with the SYBR Green Master Mix

(Life Technologies, Carlsbad, CA, USA) and gene-specific primers using the ViiA7 Real Time PCR Cycler (Life Technologies, Carlsbad, CA, USA). Appropriate controls including no RT control was included in the assay to rule out genomic DNA contamination of the cDNA samples. A relative fold change in gene transcript was calculated using ViiA7 software V1.2.2 (Life Technologies), applying the comparative CT method ($\Delta\Delta C_T$) and was quantified using $2^{-\Delta\Delta C_T}$ with β-actin as an internal calibrator. Melting curve analysis was performed to validate accurate amplification of the target gene. The primers used for qRT-PCR were designed using mouse qPrimerDepot (mouseprimerdepot.nci.nih.gov). The primers spanned exon-exon borders that overlapped intron(s) (Table 1).

Western blot analysis

Whole eyes were dissected from C57BL/6J and *Mfrp*^{rd6} mice and placed in ice-cold PBS. The anterior portion of the eye including cornea, lens and ciliary body was excised. The neural retina was gently peeled from the underlying RPE layer, and the RPE layer including the choroid and sclera was flash frozen in liquid nitrogen and stored at −70°C. For preparation of tissue lysates, the aggregate RPE sample was combined with 100 µl of 1× SDS Laemmli sample buffer (Bio-Rad Laboratories, Hercules, CA, USA) containing 5% β-mercaptoethanol, and sonicated three times for 5 min using a probe sonicator 3000 Ultrasonic Liquid Processor (Misonix Incorporated, Farmingdale, NY, USA) and stored in a −70°C freezer. The protein samples were suspended using a vortex mixer. Proteins were resolved by SDS-PAGE using a 10% Tris-glycine gel, (Bio-Rad Laboratories, Hercules, CA, USA) and transferred onto nitrocellulose (Bio-Rad Laboratories, Hercules, CA, USA) by semi-dry electroblotting using the Trans Blot Turbo Transfer System (Bio-Rad Laboratories, Hercules, CA, USA) according to the manufacturer's instructions. The membrane was washed briefly in PBS and blocked with Odyssey blocking buffer, (927–40000; LI-COR Biosciences, Lincoln, NB, USA) for 1 h at room temperature and subsequently incubated with anti-RPE65 antibody (ab13826; Abcam, Cambridge, MA, USA) at 1:1000 dilution, overnight at 4°C. After four 5-min washes in 1× TBS containing 0.05% Tween20 (TBST), the blots were incubated with secondary antibodies, anti-mouse IRDye 700DX conjugated antibody (KFA011; Rockland Immunochemicals Inc, Gilbertsville, PA, USA) in blocking buffer for 45 min. Following four washes for 5 min in 1× TBST, the blots were scanned using the Odyssey Infrared Imaging system (LI-COR Biosciences, Lincoln, Nebraska, USA) at 700 nm. Blots were stripped and incubated with mouse β-actin antibody (A5441; Sigma, St. Louis, MO, USA) at a 1:10,000 dilution overnight at 4°C and processed as previously described. Odyssey Infrared Imaging System software 3.0 was used to quantify the protein bands using a standard curve after normalizing with the β-actin control. The normalized, relative change in protein concentration was expressed in arbitrary units.

In situ hybridization

Eye tissue from P14 C57BL/6J and homozygous *Mfrp*^{rd6} mice was freshly harvested and fixed in 4% paraformaldehyde for 24 h at 4°C, immersed in 70% ethanol, dehydrated and embedded in paraffin blocks [12]. Five µm sections were cut and 3–4 sections were placed on positively charged glass slides (Milennium 2000 superfrost Adhesive slides, StatLab, McCkiney, TX, USA), which were then baked at 60°C for 1 h and stored at −20°C prior to *in situ* hybridization. We performed *in situ* hybridization using both the QuantiGene ViewRNA ISH Tissue 1-Plex and 2-Plex assay according to the manufacturer's instructions (Affymetrix, Santa Clara, CA, USA). Briefly, PFA- fixed paraffin-embedded tissues were baked, dewaxed using xylene for 5 min with gentle agitation, twice, followed by two ethanol washes for 5 min each. A hydrophobic barrier was drawn on the glass slide using a template and the samples were heated at 90–95°C for 10 min, followed by protease treatment at 40°C using a Thermobrite Controlled Temperature Slide Processing System (Abbott Laboratories, Abbott Park, IL, USA) for 10 min. Both heat and protease treatments were optimized for the eye tissue and to allow probe to access the specific RNA by unmasking the RNA. Mouse *Prss56* Type 1 (FastRed) probe set (VB1-15207) and Mouse Glul Type 6 probe (FastBlue) set (VB6-16850) were custom designed (Affymetrix, Santa Clara, CA, USA) for target hybridization. Each probe set contained 20 oligonucleotide pairs that were specific for *Prss56* or *Glul* and had a binding site for TYPE-specific sequences for signal amplification. Samples were incubated with *Prss56* probe and/or *Glul* probe or no probe control at 40°C for 3 h using the slide processer. For signal amplification, a series of sequential hybridization steps were carried out using bDNA technology and signals were detected by addition of Fast Red substrate and/or Fast Blue substrate to the tissue section as per manufacturer's instructions (Affymetrix, Santa Clara, CA, USA). Target RNA was detected at specific sites within the tissue by chromogenic substrate deposition, which was visualized by using an SP5 confocal

Table 1. Primers for qRT-PCR.

Gene	Forward primer (5′ to 3′)	Reverse primer (5′ to 3′)	Amplicon size (bp)
Prss56	GTTTGACCCGCAGACTTTTC	ACCCTGGGGAAGGCAAAT	100
Rpe65	GATGGCTTGAAACGATCACTG	GATCCCTCCACTGAAAGCAG	90
Lrat	CTAATCCCAAGACAGCCGAA	TATGGCTCTCGGATCAGTCC	103
Rgr	AGGTACAGGAGGGCATAGGG	TACCGGTTCATGGAGCAGA	110
Rgs9	GTTCTGCATGTCCTTCACCA	GAATTCATCCAGGGTCCAGA	107
Fscn2	TTCATCCTGATTGGCTGAG	AACTCTTCGACCTGGAGCAA	107
Guca1b	CCAGGAAGTCAATGGTGTTG	GTTCAAGCGCTTCTTCAAGG	107
Pde6a	GCCACCTTGCTCTGTACCT	CATGATGCTGGAGCAGACAC	105
Rpgrip1	GAATCAGCTCCACGTTCTCC	CATCCAAAGTTGAAAAGCCTG	99
Actb	CCAGTTCGCCATGGATGACGATAT	GTCAGGATACCTCTCTTGCTCTG	207

microscope (Leica Microsystems Inc, Buffalo Grove, IL, USA) and fluorescent microscopy (Leica Microsystems Inc). Nuclei were visualized with Vectashield mounting medium with DAPI (4′,6-Diamidino-2-Phenylindole, Dihydrochloride) (H1200, Vector Laboratories Inc, Burlingam, CA, USA). For FastRed substrate, we imaged using Cy3 filter and for FastBlue substrate, we imaged using the Cy5 filter. Images were processed using the Image J software (NIH, Bethesda, MA, USA) and Adobe Photoshop CS6 (Adobe Systems Incorporated, San Jose, CA, USA) was used to create final images.

Histological analysis and Immunofluorescence

The procedure for histological assays was previously described [20]. Briefly, the mice were euthanized by carbon dioxide asphyxiation. The harvested whole eyes were placed in either 4% paraformaldehyde or ice-cold acetic acid/methanol solution overnight followed by paraffin embedding using standard protocol. Eyes were cut into 6 µm sections, stained using Hematoxylin & Eosin, and visualized by light microscopy. For Immunofluorescence, PFA fixed sections were used. Deparaffinized sections were incubated with Mouse anti-Glutamine monoclonal antibody (MAB302, Chemicon) at a dilution of 1:200 overnight at 4°C. Glutamine synthetase was fluorescently labeled using Donkey Anti-mouse Alexa 488 (A21202, Life technology) at a dilution of 1:200 at RT for 1 h and visualized by fluorescent microscopy (Leica Microsystems Inc).

Statistical Analysis

In this study, GraphPad Prism Version 5 software was used for statistical analyses. Student's t-test was used to calculate statistical significance (p-value) between two groups. P-values <0.05 were considered statistically significant.

Results

Microarray analysis of *Mfrp*^{rd6} mutant mice relative to controls

In *Mfrp*^{rd6} mutant mice, the earliest phenotypic changes, observed at P14, are disorganization and shortening of OSs [7,12]. The absence of MFRP in *Mfrp*^{rd6} RPE cells appears to cause the OSs to develop abnormally, and, combined with the observed *in vivo* impairment of RPE phagocytosis [12] leads in turn to progressive retinal degeneration. MFRP, therefore, plays a central role in the normal function of RPE, which is essential for photoreceptor maintenance. To determine the functional role of MFRP in the eye, gene expression profiling of homozygous *Mfrp*^{rd6} and C57BL/6J eyes was carried out at P0 and P14. Strain C57BL/6J served as control, as the *Mfrp*^{rd6} allele has been introgressed for more than seven generations on this background and genome-wide single nucleotide polymorphism analysis indicates at least 95% shared identity between B6.C3Ga-*Mfrprd6*/J and C57BL/6J [10].

Gene expression analysis was performed using the Affymetrix Mouse 430v2 microarray. Volcano plots were generated to graphically represent differentially accumulated gene transcripts at a significance level of $q<0.05$ using six pairwise analyses. Comparison of *Mfrp*^{rd6} and C57BL/6J samples at the P0 time point did not yield any significant differences in transcript levels, indicating that the effects of *Mfrp* mutation occur postnatally (Fig. 1A). In contrast, comparison at the P14 time point resulted in 2,454 differentially expressed probe sets (Fig. 1B). Not surprisingly, comparison of the P0 and P14 time points in *Mfrp*^{rd6} mice yielded 28,452 significant differentially accumulated probe sets (Fig. 1C), and a similar result was obtained in C57BL/6J mice (Fig. S1A). Further analysis of differential accumulated gene transcripts between the two strains (*Mfrp*^{rd6} and C57BL/6J) irrespective of the time point yielded a relatively small set of significantly accumulated probe sets (Fig. S1B). By contrast, the comparison of the difference in time point (P0 vs P14) irrespective of the strain difference yielded a relatively large set of significant differentially accumulated probe sets (Fig. S1C). Taken together, this analysis suggests that these probe sets likely change as a consequence of ocular development between P0 and P14.

We generated Venn diagram by comparing all the three sets of data, B6 P14 vs B6 P0, *rd6/rd6* P14 vs *rd6/rd6* P0 and *rd6/rd6* P0 vs *rd6/rd6* P14 to determine overlapping and unique genes in each set of comparison (Fig. S2). In *rd6/rd6* P14 vs B6 P14 comparison, there were 108 unique set of genes (Fig. S2). When we compared all the three groups, there were 1709 overlapping genes (Fig. S2). B6 P14 vs B6 P0 and *rd6/rd6* P14 vs B6 P0 yielded 260 overlapping genes (Fig. S2). Comparison of *rd6/rd6* P14 vs *rd6/rd6* P0 and *rd6/rd6* P0 yielded 377 overlapping genes (Fig. S2).

Differentially accumulated probe sets in *Mfrp*^{rd6} mutant mice at P14

We further analyzed the differentially accumulated probe sets at P14 in *Mfrp*^{rd6} mutants relative to controls. Heatmaps were generated for both up- and down-regulated probe sets in *Mfrp*^{rd6} mutants. The heatmap color scale corresponds to the fluorescence (log-2, normalized) intensity level of the probe sets, where light blue represents a low level of hybridization to the probe set and dark blue a high level. Upregulated probe sets (5) with a relative fold change >5.0 are listed (Figure S3A). Heatmaps of the down-regulated probe sets at relative fold changes −2.0 to −5.0 include 17 probe sets (Fig. S3B). Heatmaps of downregulated genes at relative fold change −1.5 to −2.0 include 118 probe sets (Fig. S3C).

Ingenuity pathway analysis

To determine the molecular networks and biological pathways affected in *Mfrp*^{rd6} mutant eye at the P14 time point, we examined the microarray data by Ingenuity Pathway Analysis (IPA). The top five canonical IPA pathways that were altered significantly in *Mfrp*^{rd6} mutant eyes were B cell development, allograft rejection signaling, autoimmune thyroid disease signaling, phototransduction, cytotoxic T lymphocyte-mediated apoptosis of target cells, and visual cycle. The genes identified in these pathways and results of statistical tests are given in Table S1. Of particular interest are the phototransduction and visual cycle genes that were perturbed in *Mfrp*^{rd6} mutant eyes. The *Mfrp*^{rd6} allele, which is a loss of function mutation leading to the absence of MFRP protein from the RPE [8], is likely to have a direct effect on RPE cell function/maintenance. In accordance with this effect, visual cycle gene transcripts expressed in the RPE, including *Rpe65* and *Lrat*, were decreased significantly in *Mfrp*^{rd6} mice (Fig. 2, A, B). Transcripts of *Rgr*, which encode a visual cycle protein found in both RPE and Müller cells, were also significantly decreased (Fig. 2B). The *Mfrp*^{rd6} mutation also affected retina-specific transcript levels, as evidenced by a significant relative fold change (RFC) of −1.2 to −2.0 in transcripts expressed in photoreceptor cells (Fig. 2, A, B). These included transcripts from genes specifically expressed in rod cells (*Rho*, *Gnb1* and *Gnb5*; Fig. 2A), cone cells (*Opn1sw*, *Gnat2*, *Gnb3* and *Gnb5*; Fig. 2B), or in both rods and cones (*Rgs9*, *Rgs9bp*, *Prkaca*, *Pde6a*, *Pde6b*, *Guca1a and Guca1b*; Fig. 2, A, B). Transcripts encoded by genes implicated in maintaining photoreceptor OS morphology, *Fscn2* and *Rpgrip1*, were also significantly decreased in the *Mfrp*^{rd6} mutant (Fig. 2, A, B),

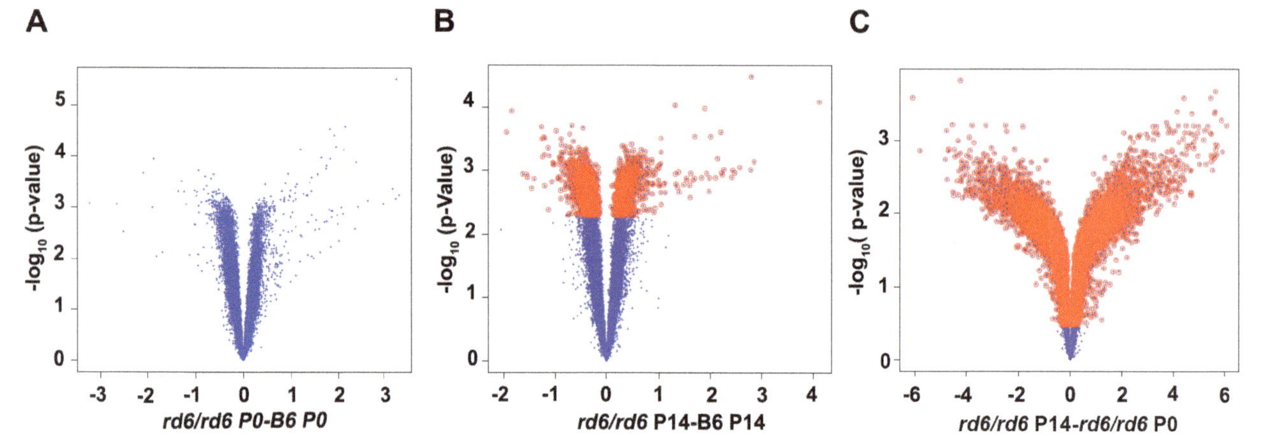

Figure 1. Volcano plots showing the relationship between fold change (represented as mean A − mean B) and the level of significance (represented by the *Fs* permutated *p*-value). Differentially expressed probe sets (q<0.05 shown in red across all fold change levels) at and fold change greater than 2 are depicted in volcano plots in three pairwise comparisons. (A) *rd6/rd6* (*Mfrp*^{rd6}/*Mfrp*^{rd6}) P0 vs B6 (C57BL/6J) P0, (B) *rd6/rd6* P14 vs B6 P14 and (C) *rd6/rd6* P14 vs *rd6/rd6* P0.

consistent with the early OS disorganization that is observed in this mutant.

Selective analysis of our microarray data, examining 250 genes listed in the IPA retinal degeneration (RD) pathway, identified additional transcripts that were differentially regulated in *Mfrp*^{rd6} mutants compared to B6 controls at P14. Forty RD pathway gene transcripts were significantly decreased in *Mfrp*^{rd6} eyes, with an RFC from −1.15 to −2.39 (Table S2). These include the *C1qtnf5* and *Mertk* transcripts, which are known to be decreased in *Mfrp*^{rd6} mice [12]. A further 9 RD pathway gene transcripts were significantly increased in *Mfrp*^{rd6} eyes (Table S3), while the remaining 201 failed to show significant change and therefore were not considered further. As RD pathway genes are typically expressed in the retina or RPE, these results suggest that the *Mfrp*^{rd6} mutation broadly decreases retina- and RPE-specific transcripts in the posterior eye.

Validation of differentially accumulated transcripts by qRT-PCR

To validate the microarray data, qRT-PCR analysis was performed on whole eyes from *Mfrp*^{rd6} mutants and C57BL/6J mice. Transcripts that were significantly increased in the microarray analysis are listed in (Table 2). Transcripts that were significantly decreased in the microarray analysis (Table 3),

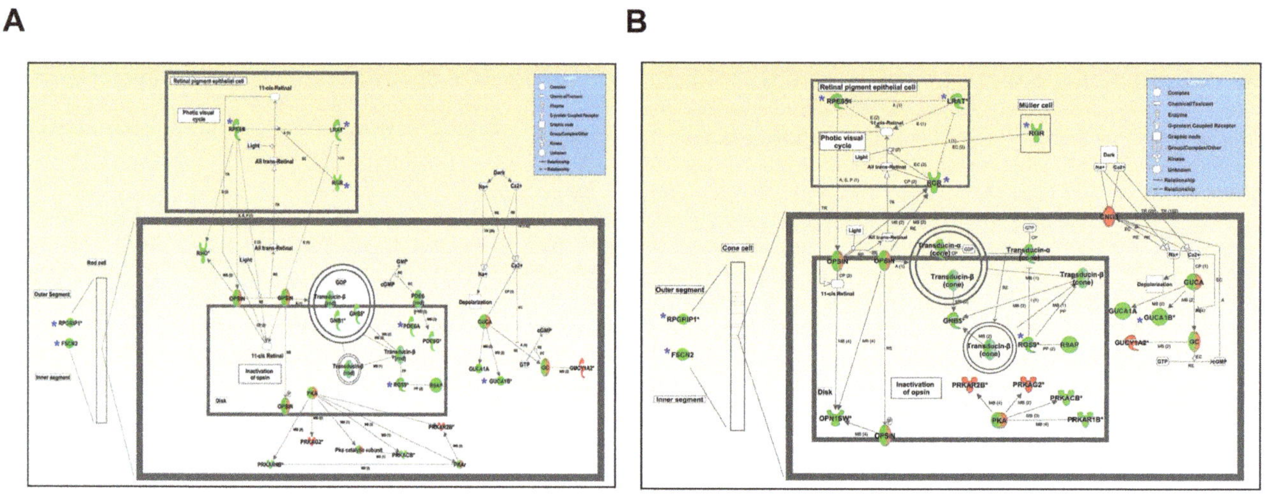

Figure 2. Ingenuity pathway analysis identified Visual Cycle and Phototransduction pathways to be downregulated genes in homozygous *Mfrp*^{rd6} mutant mice. (A) Genes in the visual cycle (RPE) and phototransduction pathway (rod photoreceptors) are represented in this panel. The asterisk represents the visual cycle genes (*Rpe65, Lrat and Rgr*), phototransduction pathway genes (*Rgs9, Guca1b, Pde6a*) and genes encoding structural components of the rod-cells (*Rpgrip1* and *Fscn2*) that were validated by qRT-PCR. (B) Genes in the visual cycle (RPE) and phototransduction pathway (cone photoreceptors) are represented in this panel. The asterisk represents the visual cycle genes (*Rpe65, Lrat* and *Rgr*), Müller glia cell expressed gene (*Rgr*), phototransduction pathway genes (*Rgs9* and *Guca1b*), and genes encoding structural components of the cone cells (*RpGrip1* and *Fscn2*) that were validated by qRT-PCR. The molecules associated with the symbols are as depicted in the inset. The solid and dashed lines represent direct or indirect interactions, respectively, between the genes. The arrow indicates interaction between genes. A = Activation, B = Binding, E = Expression (includes metabolism/synthesis for chemicals), I (Inhibition), PP (Protein-Protein binding), P (Phosphorylation/ Dephosphorylation), RB (Regulation of binding), MB (Group/complex Membership).

Table 2. Transcripts that are upregulated in *Mfrp*^{rd6}/*Mfrp*^{rd6} mutant relative to B6 control at P14.

Affymetrix Probe Set ID	Gene Symbol	Gene Name	Fold change	FDR	13_Rd6_ P14	14_Rd6_ P14	15_Rd6_ P14	7_B6_ P14	8_B6_ P14	9_B6_ P14	Validated by qRT-PCR	Location	Family
1429647_at	Prss56	protease, serine 56	17.31	0.047	8.87	9.68	10.18	5.64	5.38	5.37	Yes	Cytoplasm	peptidase
1418199_at	Hemgn	hemogen	7.21	0.047	6.3	8.05	6.45	3.98	3.86	4.41	No	Nuclear	other
1425324_x_at	Igh-6	Immunoglobulin heavy chain 6	5.37	0.047	7.61	8.56	7.37	5.32	5.11	5.83	No	Membrane/ Secreted	other
1449077_at	Ahsp	alpha hemoglobin stabilizing protein	4.79	0.047	9.26	10.42	8.9	6.76	7.2	7.84	No	Cytoplasm	other
1442459_at	Adamts19	a disintegrin-like and metallopeptidase (reprolysin type) with thrombospondin type 1 motif, 19	4.59	0.047	5.91	6.17	6.97	4.18	4.16	4.11	Yes	Extracellular matrix	other
1418989_at	Ctse	Cathepsin E	3.79	0.047	7.71	7.79	7.2	5.27	5.35	5.97	No	Endosome	other
1417714_x_at	Hba-a1/a2	Hemoglobin alpha adult chain 1/chain 2	3.22	0.047	12.56	13.37	12.41	10.63	11.32	11.33	No	Cytoplasm	other
1419014_at	Rhag	Rhesus blood group-associated A glycoprotein	3.16	0.047	4.93	5.87	4.73	3.09	3.47	3.99	No	Membrane	other
1451675_a_at	Alas2	aminolevulinic acid synthase 2, erythroid	3.06	0.047	8.47	8.87	7.76	6.62	7.26	6.37	No	Mitochondria matrix	other
1416193_at	Car1	carbonic anhydrase 1	2.9	0.047	5.77	7.18	6.1	4.61	4.72	5.11	No	Cytoplasm	enzyme
1423016_a_at	Gypa	glycophorin A	2.57	0.047	4.92	5.83	4.03	3.31	3.62	3.77	No	Membrane	other

The number in the column heading (Table 2) represents the mouse identity used in the microarray analysis.

Table 3. Transcripts that are downregulated in *Mfrp*^{rd6}/*Mfrp*^{rd6} mutant relative to B6 control at P14.

Affymetrix Probe Set ID	Gene Symbol	Gene Name	Fold change	FDR	13_Rd6_ P14	14_Rd6_ P14	15_Rd6_ P14	7_B6_ P14	8_B6_ P14	9_B6_ P14	Validated by qRT-PCR	Location	Family
1420511_at	*Prph2*	Peripherin 2	−4.18	0.0605	6.32	6.37	11.56	12.05	6.57	11.82	No	Plasma Membrane	transmembrane receptor
1420578_at	*Optc*	Opticin	−2.40	0.0407	7.02	6.78	7.33	8.24	8.29	8.38	No	Extracellular Space	other
1418818_at	*Aqp5*	Aquaporin 5	−2.2	0.0407	9	8.88	8.84	9	8.88	8.84	No	Extracellular Space	transporter
1421345_at	*Lrat*	lecithin retinol acyltransferase (phosphatidylcholine–retinol O-acyltransferase)	−1.82	0.0407	7.72	7.81	8.16	8.97	8.74	8.58	Yes	Cytoplasm	enzyme
1450197_at	*Rpe65*	retinal pigment epithelium-specific protein 65kDa	−1.81	0.0407	9.80	9.61	9.62	10.56	10.57	10.47	Yes	Cytoplasm	enzyme
1425441_at	*Guca1b*	guanylate cyclase activator 1B (retina)	−1.73	0.0407	8.41	8.36	8.30	9.09	9.14	9.20	Yes	Cytoplasm	other
1422832_at	*Rgr*	retinal G protein coupled receptor	−1.62	0.0407	10.52	10.51	10.50	11.20	11.25	11.17	Yes	Plasma Membrane	G-protein coupled receptor
1450415_at	*Pde6a*	phosphodiesterase 6A, cGMP-specific, rod, alpha	−1.55	0.0407	9.12	9.20	9.20	9.61	10.17	9.64	Yes	Plasma Membrane	enzyme
1431357_a_at	*Rpgrip1*	retinitis pigmentosa GTPase regulator interacting protein 1	−1.54	0.0407	9.01	9.15	9.24	9.77	9.82	9.67	Yes	Extracellular Space	other
1440605_at	*Fscn2*	fascin homolog 2, actin-bundling protein, retinal (Strongylocentrotus purpuratus)	−1.52	0.0418	8.39	8.33	7.86	8.71	8.95	8.74	Yes	Cytoplasm	other
1421061_at	*Guca1a*	guanylate cyclase activator 1A (retina)	−1.43	0.0407	10.54	10.47	10.20	10.98	10.93	10.84	Yes	Cytoplasm	other

The number in the column heading (Table 3) represents the mouse identity used in the microarray analysis.

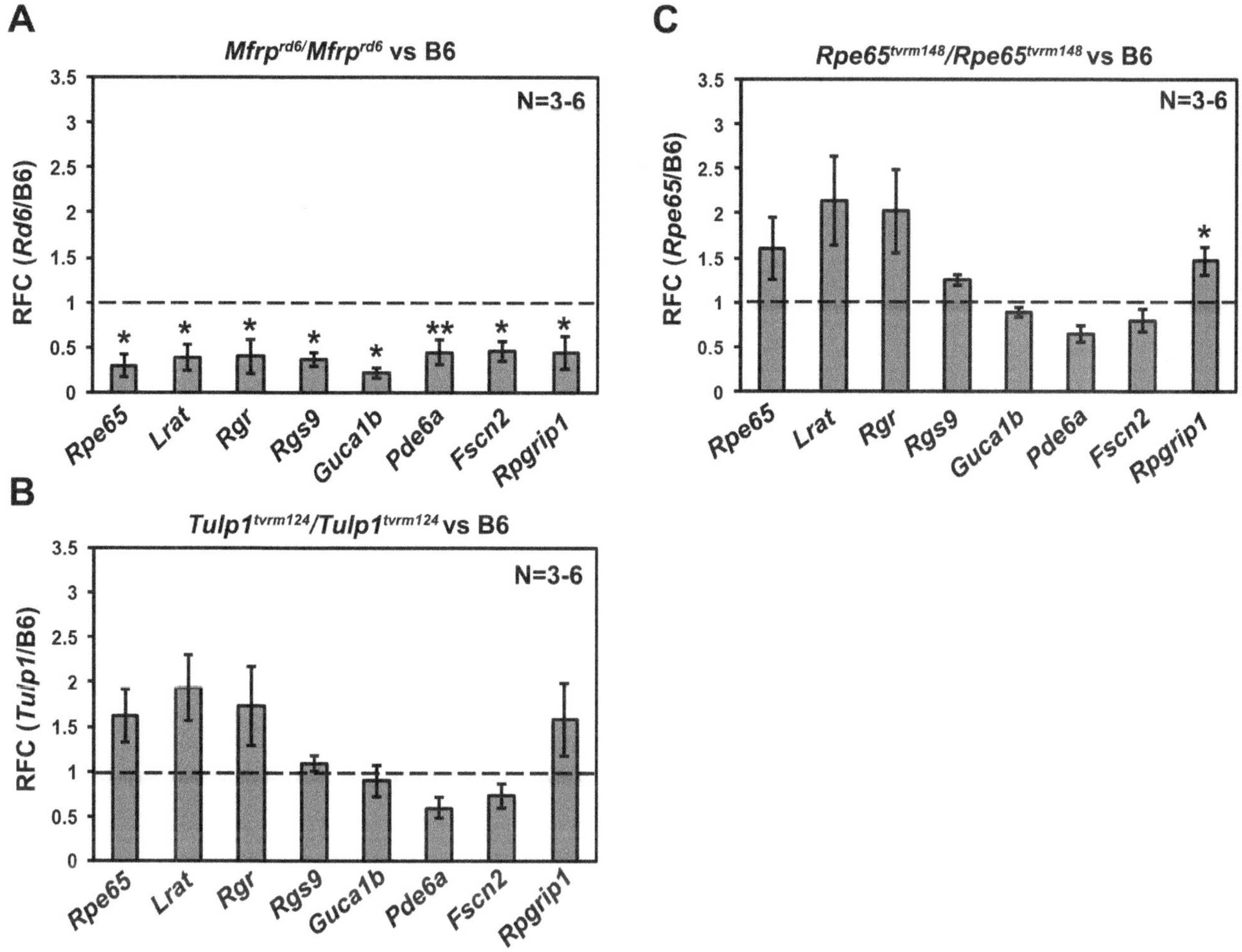

Figure 3. qRT-PCR analysis of RPE and retinal- specific genes in homozygous ***Mfrp***^{rd6}**,** ***Tulp1***^{tvrm124} ***and Rpe65***^{tvrm148} **mutants.** (A) In homozygous *Mfrp*^{rd6} mutant mice, the transcripts in the visual cycle (*Rpe65, Lrat* and *Rgr*), phototransduction pathway (*Rgs9, GuCa1b, Pde6a*) and structural components of rods and cones (*Fscn2* and *RpGrip1*) were significantly decreased relative to the wild-type control (B6/J), validating the microarray results. (B) qRT-PCR analysis in *Tulp1*^{tvrm124}/*Tulp1*^{tvrm124} mutants at P14 revealed no significant change in any of the transcripts tested. (C) In *Rpe65*^{tvrm148}/*Rpe65*^{tvrm148} mutants, there was only a significant increase in *RpGrip1* from transcripts tested, relative to wild-type (B6/J) controls. The data are expressed as relative fold change (RFC) after normalizing to the wild-type control. RFC was calculated using $\Delta\Delta C_T$ method after internal calibration to β-Actin control. Each value represents RFC ± S.E.M. * $P<0.05$ and ** $P<0.001$ relative to controls. N = 3–6 per group.

including those encoding components of the visual cycle (*Rpe65, Lrat, Rgr*), phototransduction pathway (*Rgs9, Pde6a, Guca1b*), and involved in disc morphogenesis (*Fscn2, Rpgrip1*), were also reduced as determined by qRT-PCR (Fig. 3A). However, some of the changes in transcripts including *Prph2* (−4.1795, *q* value = 0.06), *Optc* (−2.395, $q<0.05$), *Aqp5* (−2.197, $q<0.05$) (Table 3) were not validated by qRT-PCR. The failure to validate these transcripts was unlikely to be caused by assay limitations. Amplification primers were targeted to exon-exon junctions to amplify only processed RNA (Table 1); a PCR product of the correct size was verified; the PCR efficiency of the primers for genes of interest and calibrator was the same; C_T values in control and *Mfrp*^{rd6} mutant samples, indicated robust target amplification in both; and melting curve analysis confirmed the presence of a single amplified product. However, the lack of verification may be due the difference in samples used for the microarray and the qRT-PCR analyses, to the low abundance of some transcripts, or in some cases the differences were not significant (e.g. *Prph2*, which is highly expressed in the retina, had a FDR of 0.0605).

Quantitative Real Time PCR analysis of visual and phototransduction genes in *Tulp1* and *Rpe65* mutants

To determine if the decrease in the transcript levels of visual and phototransduction genes in the *Mfrp*^{rd6} mutant was a non-specific effect of the disease process that occurs during retinal degeneration, we examined the levels of visual cycle and phototransduction pathway transcripts in two unrelated retinal degeneration models with mutations in the retina-specific gene, *Tulp1* or the RPE-specific gene, *Rpe65*. Homozygous *Tulp1* (*Tulp1*^{tvrm124}) mutant mice model early onset retinal degeneration and have characteristically shorter OSs at P14 [21], comparable to those observed in *Mfrp*^{rd6} mutants. Homozygous null mutation of *Rpe65* (*Rpe65*^{tvrm148}) results in slow retinal degeneration and disorganized OS discs at P14 [22], as observed in *Mfrp*^{rd6} mice. These three retinal degeneration models show a similar extent of photoreceptor degeneration at P14 (Fig. S4). We reasoned that if the decrease in visual and photoreceptor transcripts observed *in Mfrp*^{rd6} mutants were due to non-specific, secondary effects of OS shortening or disorganization, a similar reduction of visual cycle and phototransduction pathway gene transcripts would also be observed. No significant decrease in either visual cycle or phototransduction pathway transcripts were found in either *Tulp1* (Fig. 3B) or *Rpe65* mutant mice (Fig. 3C), suggesting that the observed effects are specific to *Mfrp* disruption.

Western blot analysis of RPE65 protein in *Mfrp^{rd6}* eyes

The parallel decrease in retina- and RPE-specific transcripts revealed by transcript analysis raised the possibility that the *Mfrp^{rd6}* mutation might diminish retinal health by reducing the levels of RPE visual cycle proteins, which are critical for photoreceptor maintenance [23]. To test this possibility, we examined levels of the *Rpe65* gene product RPE65, a 65 kDa RPE-specific isomerohydrolase that is essential for producing 11-*cis* retinal from all-*trans*-retinyl esters in the visual cycle [23,24]. Western blot analysis of RPE/choroid/sclera lysates revealed decreased levels of RPE65 protein in *Mfrp^{rd6}* mice compared to C57BL/6J controls (Fig. 4A). An *Rpe65* mutant (*Rpe65^{tvrm124}*/*Rpe65^{tvrm124}*) was used to control for antibody specificity. No RPE65 protein was detected in lysates from the *Rpe65* mutant mice, whereas a 65 kDa protein was detected in all other samples (Fig. 4A), thus confirming that the detected band is RPE65. Quantitation of the blot indicated a significant 2.0-fold decrease of RPE65 in the *Mfrp^{rd6}* mutant eyes (Fig. 4B).

Increased *Prss56* transcript levels in *Mfrp^{rd6}* eyes

Microarray analysis revealed a number of transcripts that accumulated at higher levels in *Mfrp^{rd6}* mutant mice compared to wild-type controls. The highest change (17-fold) was observed in

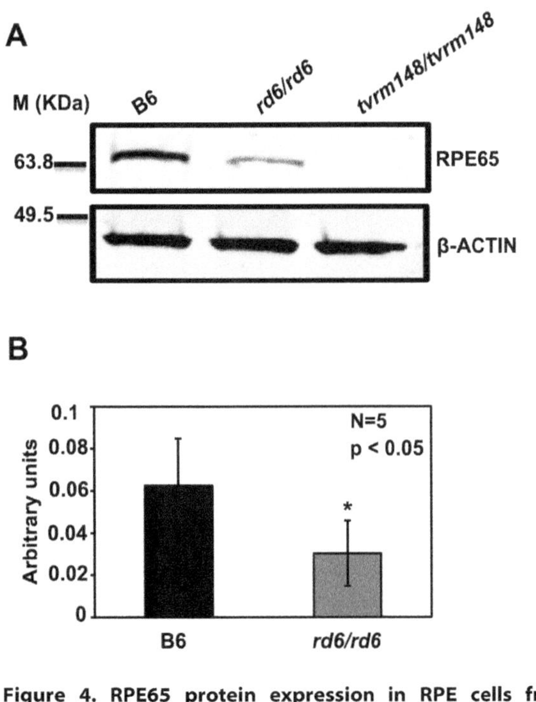

Figure 4. RPE65 protein expression in RPE cells from B6 (C57BL/6J) and homozygous *Mfrp^{rd6}* mice. (A) Western blot analysis of RPE65 protein extracted from RPE cells of B6 (C57BL/6J) and homozygous *Mfrp^{rd6}* mice. There was a 2.0-fold decrease in RPE65 protein in *Mfrp^{rd6}*/*Mfrp^{rd6}* (Lane 2) relative to the B6 control (Lane 1), whereas in *Rpe65^{tvrm148}*/*Rpe65^{tvrm148}* mutant, RPE65 protein was undetected (Lane 3). β-Actin loading confirms equal protein loading in all lanes (1–3). (B) Quantitation of RPE65 protein in RPE cells of B6 (C57BL/6J) and *Mfrp^{rd6}*/*Mfrp^{rd6}* mice. Student's T test was used to calculate statistical significance (* $P<0.05$ relative to B6 control).

Prss56, a gene encoding a serine protease (Table 2). Other transcripts involved in hematological (*Hemgn*, *Ahsp*, *Alas2*, *Hba-a1/2*, *Gypa*, *Rhag* and *Car1*) and immune (*Ctse* and *Ighm*) function, were also upregulated (Table 1). However, despite being of sufficient abundance for detection by qRT-PCR, significant differences between wild type and *Mfrp^{rd6}* mutants in the latter transcripts were not validated upon further testing.

PRSS56/*Prss56* variants in human and mouse are associated with defects in ocular growth [17–19,25], a process that is also affected by human *MFRP* mutations [1–6]. Therefore, we focused on characterizing *Prss56* expression in greater detail. Microarray data indicated no difference in *Prss56* transcript accumulation between *Mfrp^{rd6}* mice and controls at P0, suggesting that the increase in *Prss56* expression occurs during postnatal development of the *Mfrp^{rd6}* eye. To assess the temporal variation of *Prss56* expression in the postnatal period, qRT-PCR was performed at three different time points (Fig. 5A). At P7, there was a 3.5-fold increase in *Prss56* transcript, which increased to 14-fold at P14 and 70-fold at P21 (Fig. 5A). Thus, the *Mfrp^{rd6}* mutation causes a progressive accumulation of *Prss56* transcript throughout postnatal development.

To test whether the increase in *Prss56* expression was a specific attribute of *Mfrp^{rd6}* mutant mice, we also examined *Prss56* transcript levels by qRT-PCR in wild type and the *Tulp1* and *Rpe65* mutants. In P14 *Tulp1* mutant mice, there was no significant change in *Prss56* transcript (Fig. 5B), whereas in the *Rpe65* mutant, there was a significant decrease (Fig. 5B). These results suggest that *Prss56* upregulation is specific to homozygous *Mfrp^{rd6}* mice. Lastly, we also determined the wildtype level of *Prss56* at P7, P14 and P21 (Fig. 5C). The wildtype level of *Prss56* decreased from P7 to P21 (Fig. 5C). While there was a significant decrease in *Prss56* transcript from P7 to P21, the difference from P7 to P14 was not statistically different (Fig. 5C).

Cellular localization of *Prss56* and *Glul* in *Mfrp^{rd6}*

In the absence of an antibody that could reliably detect murine PRSS56, *in situ* hybridization was used to determine the cellular localization of the *Prss56* transcript. In the no probe control, no *Prss56* transcript was observed (data not shown). In the wild-type control at P14, confocal microscopy revealed a few cells in the retinal inner nuclear layer (INL) that showed expression of *Prss56* transcript (Fig. 6A, upper panel). By contrast, in *Mfrp^{rd6}* eyes at P14, intense specific staining of the transcript was observed in the INL (Fig. 6A, lower panel). This increased staining further validates both the microarray and qRT-PCR results of increased *Prss56* transcripts in *Mfrp^{rd6}* mutant eyes relative to controls.

Further we performed 2-plex *in situ* hybridization using both *Prss56* type 1 probe and *Glul* type 6 probe on the same eye sections. The co-localization of the *Prss56* probe to the same cell bodies expressing *Glul* within the INL of retina in wildtype control (Fig. 6B, upper panel) and *Mfrp^{rd6}* (Fig. 6B, lower panel) directly identified Müller cells as specifically expressing *Prss56*.

We also stained eye sections with an antibody to glutamine synthetase, which specifically marks Müller glial cells in the INL. Comparable positive antibody staining of Müller cells was observed in the retinas of both wild type and *Mfrp^{rd6}* mice, with a cell body staining pattern in the INL very similar to that observed by *in situ* hybridization of *Prss56* transcripts (Fig. 6C, upper and lower panels). Taken together, these results suggest that Müller cells in the INL express the *Prss56* transcript and are primarily responsible for the observed upregulation of the *Prss56* gene in *Mfrp^{rd6}* mice.

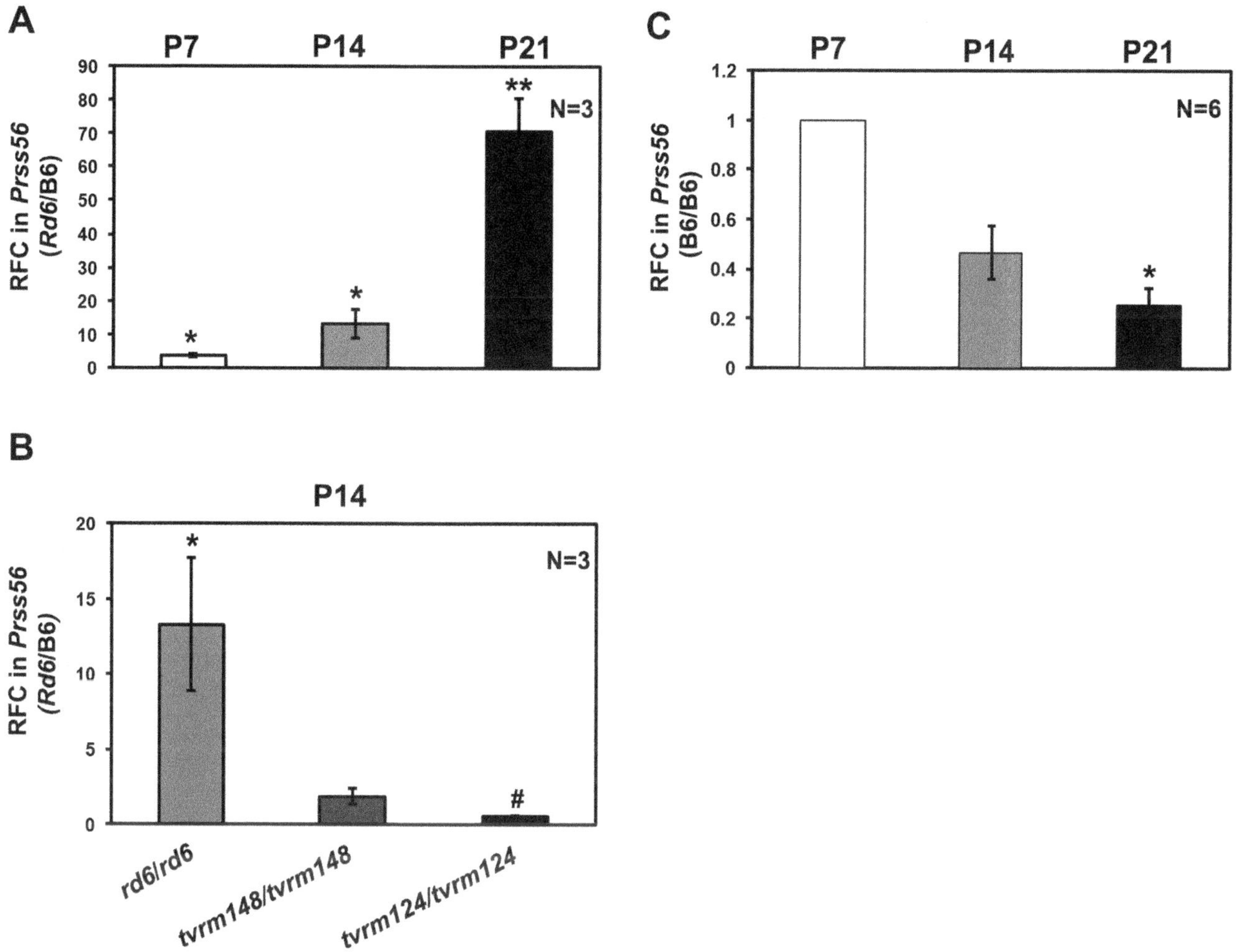

Figure 5. Independent qRT-PCR validation of genes that were differentially expressed in *Mfrp^rd6^/Mfrp^rd6^* mutants by array analysis. The upregulated gene *Prss56* was evaluated at three different time points. (A) At P7, there was a 3.5-fold increase in *Prss56* transcript and it increased to 14-fold by P14, followed by a further 70-fold increase in *Prss56* transcript in $Mfrp^{rd6}/Mfrp^{rd6}$ mutants at P21. (B) At P14, when compared to the $Mfrp^{rd6}/Mfrp^{rd6}$ mutant, in $Tulp1^{tvrm124}/Tulp1^{tvrm124}$ mutants, there was no significant change in *Prss56* transcript, whereas in $Rpe65^{tvrm148}/Rpe65^{tvrm148}$ mutants, there was a significant decrease. (C) Wildtype levels of *Prss56* transcript revealed a significant decrease between P7 and P21 timpoints, whereas the decrease from P7 to P14 was not statistically significant. Data are expressed as relative fold change (RFC) in the *Prss56* transcript after normalizing to the wild-type control (B6). RFC was calculated by the $\Delta\Delta C_T$ method using β-actin as an internal calibrator. Each value represents RFC ± S.E.M. * $P<0.05$ and ** $P<0.001$ relative to controls. N = 3 per group.

Discussion

Mouse models of retinal degeneration, in which the causative gene has been identified, are important tools for translational vision research [21], as they allow for in-depth study of cellular and molecular changes during development and disease progression. Such studies are especially important when the underlying function of the disrupted protein and molecular basis of the disease or pathology is unknown. Mutations in human *MFRP* [1–6] and mouse *Mfrp* [7–9] lead to retinal degeneration in both species and have been associated with a decrease in axial length in humans. Although nanophthalmia in *Mfrp* mutants has not been observed, posterior microphthalmia has yet to be assessed. The localization of MFRP to the RPE cell and ciliary body, suggests a potential role in posterior eye homeostasis, however, its function is unclear, and the molecular mechanisms by which mutations of this protein cause disease pathology are unknown. The microarray and validation studies of ocular transcripts in the mouse $Mfrp^{rd6}$ mutant described in the present study provide new insights into MFRP function.

Reduced accumulation of retina- and RPE-specific gene transcripts

Microarray analysis identified a modest but significant postnatal decrease in a large number of retina- and RPE-specific gene transcripts in P14 $Mfrp^{rd6}$ mutant eyes, prior to the degenerative decline in ONL thickness that is associated with photoreceptor cell loss [12]. This result indicates an effect of the mutation beyond the RPE where *Mfrp* is expressed. In our study, the decreased accumulation of posterior eye transcripts was a distinct feature of $Mfrp^{rd6}$ mice, as qRT-PCR analysis of the *Tulp1* [26] and *Rpe65* [21] mutant models at P14 revealed no significant change in selected visual cycle and phototransduction pathway transcripts that were decreased in $Mfrp^{rd6}$ mutants. Importantly, our *Tulp1* and *Rpe65* mutant models exhibit a similar time course of retinal degeneration as $Mfrp^{rd6}$ and show similar OS shortening and

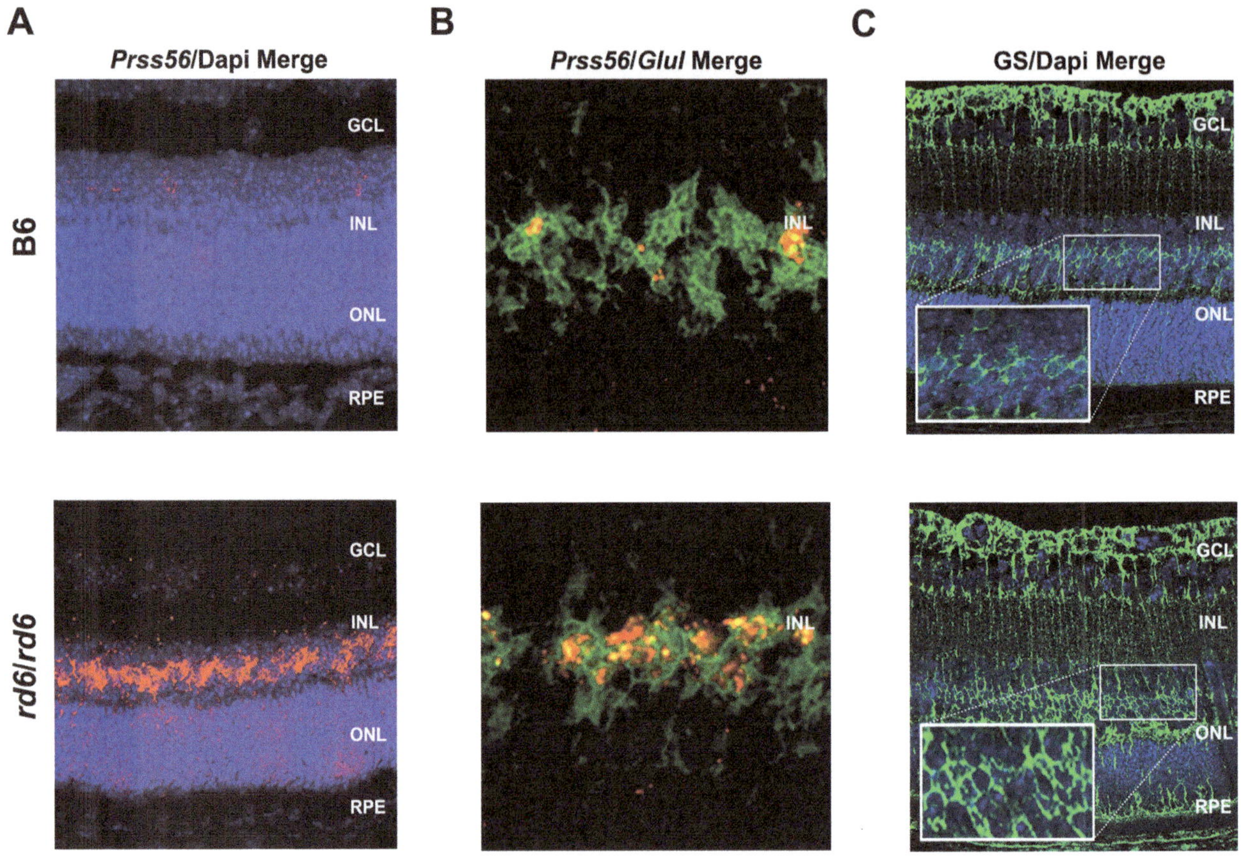

Figure 6. Cellular localization of *Prss56 and Glul* in B6 (C57BL/6J) and *Mfrp*^{rd6}/*Mfrp*^{rd6} mice. (A) By *in situ* hybridization, in B6 (C57BL/6J) controls at P14, we observed *Prss56* transcript in only very few cells of the inner nuclear layer (INL) of the retina (top panel), whereas in *Mfrp*^{rd6}/*Mfrp*^{rd6} mutants, an intense staining of *Prss56* transcript was observed in INL of the retina (bottom panel). (B) By 2-plex *in situ* hybridization, in B6 controls, we observed co-localization of *Prss56* (red) and *Glul* (pseudo colored green) transcripts in only a few cell body of the (INL) of the retina (top panel), whereas in *Mfrp*^{rd6}/*Mfrp*^{rd6}, strong co-localization of *Prss56* and *Glul* transcripts in the cell body of the INL of the retina was observed (bottom panel). (C) Glutamine synthetase (GS) staining of Müller cells. In both C57BL/6J (B6) and *Mfrp*^{rd6}/*Mfrp*^{rd6} mice, Müller cells marked with glutamine synthetase showed a similar localization pattern (inset, top and bottom panels) as observed for *Prss56 in situ* hybridization staining, suggesting that Müller cells in the INL of retina express *Prss56* transcripts at P14.

disorganization at P14 without a change in ONL thickness. Decreased accumulation of phototransduction pathway transcripts has been documented in other retinal degeneration models [27–29]. However, these studies may not be directly comparable to ours, since the disease models were analyzed at ages when ONL thickness was significantly decreased [27,28] or photoreceptor outer segments were absent [29]. Gene profiling of additional models with a disease progression closely similar to that of *Mfrp*^{rd6} may be required to assess whether the decreased accumulation of visual cycle and phototransduction pathway transcripts is a truly distinguishing characteristic of the *Mfrp*^{rd6} mutation. Nevertheless, the microarray and qRT-PCR data on *Mfrp*^{rd6} and other retinal degeneration mutants suggest a broad and possibly unique role for MFRP protein in postnatal development of the RPE and retina.

A potential explanation for the widespread but modest reduction of visual cycle and phototransduction transcripts in *Mfrp*^{rd6} mutants is a defect in the postnatal development of the retina and RPE. The CUB domains, found in MFRP, are prevalent in genes that are developmentally regulated [30]. The CRD domain in MFRP has a high homology to the Frizzled family of proteins, which are normally involved in Wnt signaling and are important in RPE development [31,32]. Finally, human mutations in *MFRP* have been associated with nanophthalmia or posterior microphthalmia with shortening of the posterior segment of the eye [1–6], an expected consequence of reduced retinal and RPE development.

Although no one has actually assessed RPE development in *Mfrp* mutants, apical microvilli defects have been reported [12]. It is interesting to note that during normal eye development, there is a specific and strong increase in *Rpe65* transcription that coincides with the extension of RPE microvilli and the increase in the photoreceptor OS length (reviewed in [24]). Thus, the decrease in *Rpe65* transcript observed in *Mfrp*^{rd6} mice may contribute to the decrease in OS length and organization [12]. Moreover, in *Mfrp*^{rd6} mutants, the significant decrease in transcripts of *Fscn2*, encoding a protein involved in outer segment morphogenesis, may contribute to the failure to elaborate OS and to the disorganization of OS, followed by photoreceptor degeneration similar to that observed in the *Fscn2* haploinsufficient mouse model [33]. In summary, although we do not know currently how MFRP mediates its effects on the visual cycle and phototransduction genes, it is likely that the observed reductions play a role in the pathogenesis of the disease induced by disruptions in *Mfrp*.

Mfrp and *Prss56*, features of a common pathway?

In this study, we have demonstrated significant upregulation of the retina-specific *Prss56* transcript in *Mfrp*^{rd6} eyes. Increased expression was observed during postnatal eye development in Müller cells of *Mfrp*^{rd6} mutants, but not in other similarly affected retinal degeneration models, suggesting that *Prss56* upregulation is unique to *Mfrp* disruption. *Prss56* encodes a trypsin-like serine protease [34] of unknown function and substrate specificity in the eye. Interestingly, *PRSS56/Prss56* mutations are associated with autosomal recessive posterior microphthalmia in humans and mice [17,25,35]. Moreover, two different genome-wide association studies (GWAS) involving multi-ethnic cohorts identified *Prss56* as significantly associated with refractive errors and myopia [18,19] that relate to a change in axial length. *MFRP* mutations in humans are also associated with posterior microphthalmia characterized by abnormal posterior segment size leading to hyperopia [2] and cause recessive nanophthalmos [36]. Studies on the postnatal progression of refractive error in nanophthalmos patients having mutations in MFRP suggest a role of MFRP protein in embryonic ocular growth and postnatal emmetropization [36]. As both PRSS56 and MFRP variants affect axial length and potentially the process of emmetropization, it is plausible that they may function through a common biological pathway, yet to be determined.

Like other serine proteases [37], PRSS56 may either directly or indirectly be involved in extracellular matrix (ECM) processing, degradation and remodeling, as suggested previously [17]. Accordingly, upregulation of *Prss56* expression in *Mfrp*^{rd6} mutants may promote ECM remodeling. Matrix metalloproteinases are also thought to play an important role in eye development and disease [38]. Consistent with enhanced metalloproteinase activity, IPA analysis of microarray data revealed a significant decrease in *Timp3* transcripts (Table S2), which encode tissue inhibitor of metalloproteinase-3, and a significant increase in *Adamts19* (Table 1) transcripts, which encode a disintegrin and metalloproteinase with thrombospondin motif family member. Taken together, these findings suggest that altered ECM processing may contribute to the progressive loss of photoreceptor cells in the *Mfrp*^{rd6} mutant, as observed in other mouse retinal degeneration models [39].

In conclusion, the present study suggests a broad role of MFRP in determining retinal and RPE transcript levels during postnatal development. Most importantly, the upregulation of *Prss56* expression in *Mfrp*^{rd6} Müller cells suggests a possible interaction between *Mfrp* and *Prss56* in posterior eye maintenance and development during this period. Future studies would be directed toward understanding how MFRP influences transcript accumulation in the postnatal RPE and retina, and also address how MFRP and PRSS56 interact.

Supporting Information

Figure S1 Volcano plots showing the relationship between fold change (represented as mean A-mean B) and the level of significance (represented by the Fs permutated p-value). Differentially expressed probe sets ($q<0.05$ shown in red across all fold change levels) at and fold change greater than 2 are depicted in volcano plots in three pairwise comparisons. (A) B6 (C57BL/6J) P14 vs B6 (C57BL/6J) P0, (B) B6 (C57BL/6J) P14; *rd6/rd6* (*Mfrp*^{rd6}) P14 vs B6 (C57BL/6J) P0; *rd6/rd6* (*Mfrp*^{rd6})P0 and (C) *rd6/rd6* (*Mfrp*^{rd6}) P0; *rd6/rd6* (*Mfrp*^{rd6}) P14 vs B6 (C57BL/6J) P0; B6 (C57BL/6J) P14.

Figure S2 Venn diagram depicting the overlapping and unique genes in the three data sets. *rd6/rd6* (*Mfrp*^{rd6}) P14 vs B6 (C57BL/6J) P14; *rd6/rd6* (*Mfrp*^{rd6}) P14 vs *rd6/rd6* (*Mfrp*^{rd6})P0 and B6 (C57BL/6J) P14 vs B6 (C57BL/6J) P0.

Figure S3 Heat maps of differentially expressed genes in *Mfrp*$^{rd6/rd6}$ mice in comparison to age matched WT controls. (A) Upregulated genes in *rd6/rd6* (*Mfrp*^{rd6}) P14 vs B6 (C57BL/6J) P14, RFC>5.0, $q<0.05$ (B) Downregulated genes in *rd6/rd6* (*Mfrp*^{rd6}) P14 vs B6 (C57BL/6J) P14, RFC <-2.0, $q<0.05$ (C) Downregulated genes in *rd6/rd6* (*Mfrp*^{rd6}) P14 vs B6 (C57BL/6J) P14, RFC <-1.5 to -2.0, $q<0.05$. Asterisk denotes the genes that were validated by qRT-PCR analysis.

Figure S4 Outer segment degeneration at P14 in *Mfrp*$^{rd6/rd6}$, *Tulp1*$^{tvrm124/tvrm124}$, *Rpe65*$^{tvrm148/tvrm148}$ mice compared to age matched controls visualized by light microscopy. Retinal sections at p14 were obtained from B6 (A), *Tulp1*$^{tvrm124/tvrm124}$ (B) *Mfrp*$^{rd6/rd6}$ (C) and *Rpe65*$^{tvrm148/tvrm148}$ (D) and stained with hematoxylin & eosin. GC, gangalion cell layer; INL, inner nuclear layer; ONL, outer nuclear layer; OS, outer segments. Magnification: 20 x.

Table S1 Canonical pathways identified in *Mfrp*^{rd6} mice.

Table S2 Transcripts in retinal degeneration pathway that is downregulated in *Mfrp*^{rd6} mutant mice at P14.

Table S3 Transcripts in retinal degeneration pathway that is up-regulated in *Mfrp*^{rd6} mutant mice at P14.

Acknowledgments

We thank Dr. Gregory Cox and Dr. Saidas Nair for critical review of the manuscript. We also thank Mark Lessard and Dr. Jim Denegre for their expert assistance with the confocal microscopy studies and the Gene Expression Services at The Jackson Laboratory for conducting the Affymetrix array study.

Author Contributions

Conceived and designed the experiments: RS JW MPK PMN. Performed the experiments: RS JW MPK JC WLH GBC. Analyzed the data: RS JW TMS MPK PMN. Wrote the paper: RS MPK JKN PMN.

References

1. Sundin OH, Leppert GS, Silva ED, Yang JM, Dharmaraj S, et al. (2005) Extreme hyperopia is the result of null mutations in MFRP, which encodes a Frizzled-related protein. Proc Natl Acad Sci U S A 102: 9553–9558.
2. Ayala-Ramirez R, Graue-Wiechers F, Robredo V, Amato-Almanza M, Horta-Diez I, et al. (2006) A new autosomal recessive syndrome consisting of posterior microphthalmos, retinitis pigmentosa, foveoschisis, and optic disc drusen is caused by a MFRP gene mutation. Mol Vis 12: 1483–1489.
3. Crespi J, Buil JA, Bassaganyas F, Vela-Segarra JI, Diaz-Cascajosa J, et al. (2008) A novel mutation confirms MFRP as the gene causing the syndrome of nanophthalmos-renititis pigmentosa-foveoschisis-optic disk drusen. Am J Ophthalmol 146: 323–328.
4. Zenteno JC, Buentello-Volante B, Quiroz-Gonzalez MA, Quiroz-Reyes MA (2009) Compound heterozygosity for a novel and a recurrent MFRP gene

mutation in a family with the nanophthalmos-retinitis pigmentosa complex. Mol Vis 15: 1794–1798.
5. Mukhopadhyay R, Sergouniotis PI, Mackay DS, Day AC, Wright G, et al. (2010) A detailed phenotypic assessment of individuals affected by MFRP-related oculopathy. Mol Vis 16: 540–548.
6. Neri A, Leaci R, Zenteno JC, Casubolo C, Delfini E, et al. (2012) Membrane frizzled-related protein gene-related ophthalmological syndrome: 30-month follow-up of a sporadic case and review of genotype-phenotype correlation in the literature. Mol Vis 18: 2623–2632.
7. Hawes NL, Chang B, Hageman GS, Nusinowitz S, Nishina PM, et al. (2000) Retinal degeneration 6 (rd6): a new mouse model for human retinitis punctata albescens. Invest Ophthalmol Vis Sci 41: 3149–3157.
8. Kameya S, Hawes NL, Chang B, Heckenlively JR, Naggert JK, et al. (2002) Mfrp, a gene encoding a frizzled related protein, is mutated in the mouse retinal degeneration 6. Hum Mol Genet 11: 1879–1886.
9. Fogerty J, Besharse JC (2011) 174delG mutation in mouse MFRP causes photoreceptor degeneration and RPE atrophy. Invest Ophthalmol Vis Sci 52: 7256–7266.
10. Won J, Charette JR, Philip VM, Stearns TM, Zhang W, et al. (2014) Genetic modifier loci of mouse Mfrp(rd6) identified by quantitative trait locus analysis. Exp Eye Res 118: 30–35.
11. Mandal MN, Vasireddy V, Jablonski MM, Wang X, Heckenlively JR, et al. (2006) Spatial and temporal expression of MFRP and its interaction with CTRP5. Invest Ophthalmol Vis Sci 47: 5514–5521.
12. Won J, Smith RS, Peachey NS, Wu J, Hicks WL, et al. (2008) Membrane frizzled-related protein is necessary for the normal development and maintenance of photoreceptor outer segments. Vis Neurosci 25: 563–574.
13. Dinculescu A, Estreicher J, Zenteno JC, Aleman TS, Schwartz SB, et al. (2012) Gene therapy for retinitis pigmentosa caused by MFRP mutations: human phenotype and preliminary proof of concept. Hum Gene Ther 23: 367–376.
14. Katoh M (2001) Molecular cloning and characterization of MFRP, a novel gene encoding a membrane-type Frizzled-related protein. Biochem Biophys Res Commun 282: 116–123.
15. Hayward C, Shu X, Cideciyan AV, Lennon A, Barran P, et al. (2003) Mutation in a short-chain collagen gene, CTRP5, results in extracellular deposit formation in late-onset retinal degeneration: a genetic model for age-related macular degeneration. Hum Mol Genet 12: 2657–2667.
16. Liu H, Jang JK, Graham J, Nycz K, McKim KS (2000) Two genes required for meiotic recombination in Drosophila are expressed from a dicistronic message. Genetics 154: 1735–1746.
17. Nair KS, Hmani-Aifa M, Ali Z, Kearney AL, Ben Salem S, et al. (2011) Alteration of the serine protease PRSS56 causes angle-closure glaucoma in mice and posterior microphthalmia in humans and mice. Nat Genet 43: 579–584.
18. Verhoeven VJ, Hysi PG, Wojciechowski R, Fan Q, Guggenheim JA, et al. (2013) Genome-wide meta-analyses of multiancestry cohorts identify multiple new susceptibility loci for refractive error and myopia. Nat Genet 45: 314–318.
19. Kiefer AK, Tung JY, Do CB, Hinds DA, Mountain JL, et al. (2013) Genome-wide analysis points to roles for extracellular matrix remodeling, the visual cycle, and neuronal development in myopia. PLoS Genet 9: e1003299.
20. Lee Y, Kameya S, Cox GA, Hsu J, Hicks W, et al. (2005) Ocular abnormalities in Large(myd) and Large(vls) mice, spontaneous models for muscle, eye, and brain diseases. Mol Cell Neurosci 30: 160–172.
21. Won J, Shi LY, Hicks W, Wang J, Naggert JK, et al. (2012) Translational vision research models program. Adv Exp Med Biol 723: 391–397.
22. Won J, Shi LY, Hicks W, Wang J, Hurd R, et al. (2011) Mouse model resources for vision research. J Ophthalmol 2011: 391384.
23. Redmond TM, Yu S, Lee E, Bok D, Hamasaki D, et al. (1998) Rpe65 is necessary for production of 11-cis-vitamin A in the retinal visual cycle. Nat Genet 20: 344–351.
24. Cai X, Conley SM, Naash MI (2009) RPE65: role in the visual cycle, human retinal disease, and gene therapy. Ophthalmic Genet 30: 57–62.
25. Gal A, Rau I, El Matri L, Kreienkamp HJ, Fehr S, et al. (2011) Autosomal-recessive posterior microphthalmos is caused by mutations in PRSS56, a gene encoding a trypsin-like serine protease. Am J Hum Genet 88: 382–390.
26. Ikeda S, Shiva N, Ikeda A, Smith RS, Nusinowitz S, et al. (2000) Retinal degeneration but not obesity is observed in null mutants of the tubby-like protein 1 gene. Hum Mol Genet 9: 155–163.
27. Hackam AS, Strom R, Liu D, Qian J, Wang C, et al. (2004) Identification of gene expression changes associated with the progression of retinal degeneration in the rd1 mouse. Invest Ophthalmol Vis Sci 45: 2929–2942.
28. Cheng CL, Molday RS (2013) Changes in gene expression associated with retinal degeneration in the rd3 mouse. Mol Vis 19: 955–969.
29. Sharma YV, Cojocaru RI, Ritter LM, Khattree N, Brooks M, et al. (2012) Protective gene expression changes elicited by an inherited defect in photoreceptor structure. PloS one 7: e31371.
30. Bork P, Beckmann G (1993) The CUB domain. A widespread module in developmentally regulated proteins. J Mol Biol 231: 539–545.
31. Fujimura N, Taketo MM, Mori M, Korinek V, Kozmik Z (2009) Spatial and temporal regulation of Wnt/beta-catenin signaling is essential for development of the retinal pigment epithelium. Dev Biol 334: 31–45.
32. Bharti K, Gasper M, Ou J, Brucato M, Clore-Gronenborn K, et al. (2012) A regulatory loop involving PAX6, MITF, and WNT signaling controls retinal pigment epithelium development. PLoS Genet 8: e1002757.
33. Yokokura S, Wada Y, Nakai S, Sato H, Yao R, et al. (2005) Targeted disruption of FSCN2 gene induces retinopathy in mice. Invest Ophthalmol Vis Sci 46: 2905–2915.
34. Ross J, Jiang H, Kanost MR, Wang Y (2003) Serine proteases and their homologs in the Drosophila melanogaster genome: an initial analysis of sequence conservation and phylogenetic relationships. Gene 304: 117–131.
35. Said MB, Chouchene E, Salem SB, Daoud K, Largueche L, et al. (2013) Posterior microphthalmia and nanophthalmia in Tunisia caused by a founder c.1059_1066insC mutation of the PRSS56 gene. Gene 528: 288–294.
36. Sundin OH, Dharmaraj S, Bhutto IA, Hasegawa T, McLeod DS, et al. (2008) Developmental basis of nanophthalmos: MFRP Is required for both prenatal ocular growth and postnatal emmetropization. Ophthalmic Genet 29: 1–9.
37. Mott JD, Werb Z (2004) Regulation of matrix biology by matrix metalloproteinases. Curr Opin Cell Biol 16: 558–564.
38. Wride MA, Geatrell J, Guggenheim JA (2006) Proteases in eye development and disease. Birth Defects Res C Embryo Today 78: 90–105.
39. Al-Ubaidi MR, Naash MI, Conley SM (2013) A perspective on the role of the extracellular matrix in progressive retinal degenerative disorders. Invest Ophthalmol Vis Sci 54: 8119–8124.

Geometrical Custom Modeling of Human Cornea In Vivo and Its Use for the Diagnosis of Corneal Ectasia

Francisco Cavas-Martínez[1]*, Daniel G. Fernández-Pacheco[1], Ernesto De la Cruz-Sánchez[2], José Nieto Martínez[1], Francisco J. Fernández Cañavate[1], Alfredo Vega-Estrada[3], Ana B. Plaza-Puche[3], Jorge L. Alió[3]

1 Department of Graphical Expression, Technical University of Cartagena, Cartagena, Spain, **2** Department of Physical Activity and Sport, University of Murcia, Murcia, Spain, **3** Vissum Corporación Oftalmológica, Alicante, Spain

Abstract

Aim: To establish a new procedure for 3D geometric reconstruction of the human cornea to obtain a solid model that represents a personalized and in vivo morphology of both the anterior and posterior corneal surfaces. This model is later analyzed to obtain geometric variables enabling the characterization of the corneal geometry and establishing a new clinical diagnostic criterion in order to distinguish between healthy corneas and corneas with keratoconus.

Method: The method for the geometric reconstruction of the cornea consists of the following steps: capture and preprocessing of the spatial point clouds provided by the Sirius topographer that represent both anterior and posterior corneal surfaces, reconstruction of the corneal geometric surfaces and generation of the solid model. Later, geometric variables are extracted from the model obtained and statistically analyzed to detect deformations of the cornea.

Results: The variables that achieved the best results in the diagnosis of keratoconus were anterior corneal surface area (ROC area: 0.847, $p<0.000$, std. error: 0.038, 95% CI: 0.777 to 0.925), posterior corneal surface area (ROC area: 0.807, $p<0.000$, std. error: 0.042, 95% CI: 0,726 to 0,889), anterior apex deviation (ROC area: 0.735, $p<0.000$, std. error: 0.053, 95% CI: 0.630 to 0.840) and posterior apex deviation (ROC area: 0.891, $p<0.000$, std. error: 0.039, 95% CI: 0.8146 to 0.9672).

Conclusion: Geometric modeling enables accurate characterization of the human cornea. Also, from a clinical point of view, the procedure described has established a new approach for the study of eye-related diseases.

Editor: Alexander V. Ljubimov, Cedars-Sinai Medical Center; UCLA School of Medicine, United States of America

Funding: The authors have no support or funding to report.

Competing Interests: Three authors are researchers employed by Vissum Corporacion S.L. These three authors do not have any competing interest or financial disclosure interest in this collaborative research.

* Email: francisco.cavas@upct.es

Introduction

Characterization of corneal topography is critical for the assessment of vision quality and for several clinical applications including the diagnosis and management of corneal diseases [1–3], the planning of refractive surgery [4–5], and the construction of corneal numerical models [6].

At present, several non-invasive technologies that do not require the use of anesthesia or contact with the cornea have been developed for the comprehensive characterization of corneal topography. These include Scheimpflug photography [7], a combination of scanning-slit and Placido-disc technologies [8], very-high-frequency ultrasonography [9], and optical coherence tomography [10–12]. Scheimpflug photography–based systems allow the study and characterization of both anterior and posterior corneal surfaces [13–14]. Different studies have validated the consistency of the measurements obtained with this technique, using different commercially available devices [15–16]. The combination of accurate Scheimpflug photography analysis for corneal characterization with classical Placido-disc technology [17] has been recently developed, with the aim of maintaining the benefits of the Scheimpflug technology and optimizing the measurements of the anterior corneal curvature. This combined technology has been shown to provide highly consistent anterior and posterior corneal curvature measurements [18–20]. These data allow the human cornea to be modeled in order to detect corneal ectatic disorders, such as keratoconus.

Modeling of the human cornea can be approached by two different strategies: i) using a generic model which is valid to reproduce and extract results that can be applied to the whole population, or ii) creating a personalized model that allows the particular case of a specific patient to be studied. Both types of models have been reported in the literature [21–22] using a corneal geometry approach consisting of a base or regular surface (B) and a residue (R), which represents the local and global irregularities of the corneal topography with respect to the regular base model (B). Other authors simulate the human cornea using finite-elements models [23–27]. However, the reconstructions performed until now have the following problems:

a) The low density of data from the posterior corneal surface provided by the ophthalmological devices makes it difficult to obtain a full 3D reconstruction of the human cornea [28–29].
b) Most of the mathematical models used in the approaches are based on the Zernike polynomial, which has problems that have been widely discussed in the literature [30–32]. Some authors try to solve this issue using first a coarse adjustment by means of the Zernike polynomial and secondly a fine adjustment based on a lineal combination of radial basis Gaussian functions [33]. However, this method does not properly represent the corneal geometry when it has high irregularity levels due to corneal ectatic disorders, both on anterior and posterior surfaces.

For all the above-mentioned reasons, this paper proposes a procedure for the geometric reconstruction of the human cornea which allows a 3D solid model to be obtained which reproduces the actual and personalized morphology of both the anterior and posterior surfaces of the cornea. Once the 3D model has been created, several geometric variables are defined from the model, obtaining a personalized characterization of the corneal topography. The study of these variables allows a new clinical diagnostic criterion to be established which enables healthy corneas to be distinguished from corneas with keratoconus, in which the deformation of the cornea directly affects several of the geometric variables studied.

Methods

Participants

A total of 131 subjects (aged 36.03±13.41 years old) volunteered to participate in this study. Participants were recruited in Vissum Alicante (Vissum Corporation, Alicante, Spain). The subjects were informed in detail about the procedures.

All subjects were divided into two different groups according to the presence or absence of keratoconus:

1) The first group did not present any ocular pathology and consisted of 90 healthy eyes of 90 patients with an age range of between 7 and 66 years old. Participants with any ocular or corneal pathology, or those whose eyes had undergone any previous procedure, were excluded.
2) The second group of eyes with ocular pathology consisted of 41 clinically diagnosed keratoconic eyes of 41 patients, with an age range of between 14 and 65. Rabinowitz criterion was used for clinical diagnosis of keratoconus, which considers the presence of a localized corneal topography curving and/or the presence of an asymmetric bow tie with or without topographical angulated principal meridians. Moreover, we also considered any microscopic keratoconic sign [34–36]: stromal thinning, Fleischer ring, Vogt striae, anterior corneal scars in the corneal stroma or protrusion apex. Exclusion for this group was considered when there was any previous eye surgery or any other eye disease. The severity of the disease in this group was rated according to the Amsler-Krumeich classification [36–38].

Only one eye per patient was included in both groups, following a numerical sequence (dichotomous sequence 0 and 1) created by computer software in order to avoid interference potential correlations that could exist between the eyes of the same person.

This study was approved by the Vissum Corporacion Oftalmologica's Clinical Research Ethics Committee, and was performed in accordance with the ethical standards laid down in the 1964 Declaration of Helsinki. Written informed consent was obtained after explaining the nature of the procedure prior to surgery in all cases.

Measurement protocol

Eye exam. All eyes selected underwent a thorough and comprehensive eye and vision examination which included uncorrected distance visual acuity (UDVA), corrected distance visual acuity (CDVA), manifest refraction, Goldmann tonometry, biometry (IOLMaster, Carl Zeiss Meditec AG) and corneal topographic analysis with Sirius System (CSO, Florence, Italy). All measurements were performed by the same experienced examiner. With respect to the corneal topographic analysis, three consecutive measurements were performed to calculate the average values for posterior analysis.

The Sirius topographer is an ophthalmic instrument that uses a rotating Scheimpflug camera [39] with a Placido disc [14] to obtain the corneal topography. In a few seconds it captures and processes 25 image sections made with the Scheimpflug camera and the image of 22 rings of a Placido disc projected onto the cornea. The device has a second chamber to control the correct alignment of the system with the eye for data acquisition. The corneal topographer has a good level of consistency for taking measurements [16] of sagital and tangential curvature of both faces of the corneal refractive power, points of the anterior and posterior corneal surface, corneal pachymetry and estimations of other biometric structures above, such as the anterior chamber depth segment. Data registration for the present study was performed with the Phoenix (Phoenix, CSO, Florence, Italy) software.

Geometrical modeling. The method proposed in this article for the geometric reconstruction of the cornea consists of the following steps:

i) Preparation of the point cloud. The proposed reconstruction process is based on the generation of a surface from the geometry that a point cloud presents in a coordinate system for a three-dimensional space, usually in Cartesian coordinate format. This technique of geometric reconstruction is not new in the field of biomedical engineering, having already been successfully used in the reconstruction of other parts of the body [40–41].

The point cloud reconstruction of the geometry of the anterior and posterior surfaces of the cornea was obtained by the Sirius corneal topographer. However, this device has a low density of data in the geographical area of the cornea known as the 'peripheral zone' (radius 4 mm to 5.5 mm) and in the limbo (6 mm radius), due to the time taken for rotation and data collection. This suboptimal performance of the device is caused by the presence of intrinsic patient factors in the measurement process, such as the stability of the tear film, or an obstruction of the visual field by tabs or inadequate eyelid opening at the moment of the data collection. This led to the development of a method for geometric reconstruction that comprises the corneal surface from its geometric center ($r = 0$ mm) to the beginning of the so-called peripheral zone ($r = 4$ mm), which is mainly justified by the following two reasons:

- Geometric principle. The Sirius corneal topographer permits the collection of all the points that make up the geometry of the cornea in the region defined for reconstruction ($r = 0$ to 4 mm). Specifically, 10752 spatial points corresponding to both anterior and posterior corneal surfaces (5376 for each one)

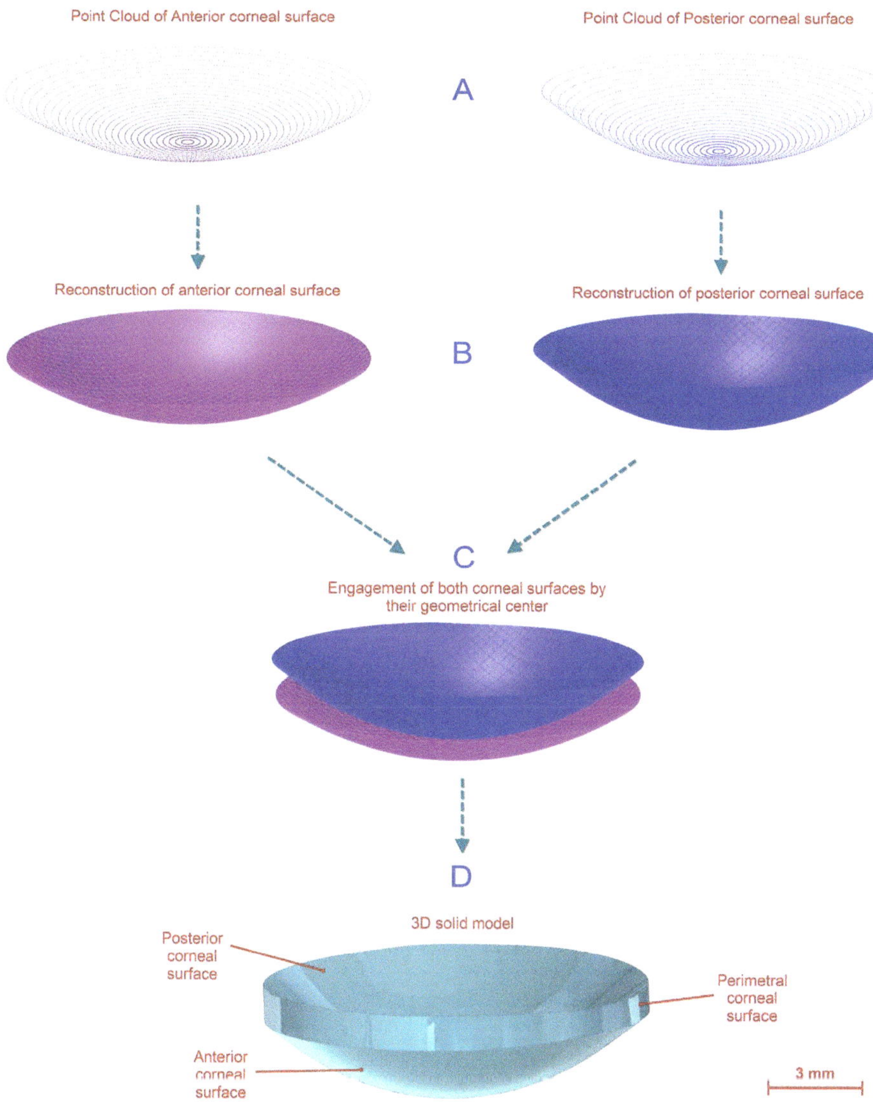

Figure 1. Scheme of the 3D geometric reconstruction procedure of the cornea.

were obtained for each patient of the population under study, including both healthy and diseased cases.

- Clinical principle. The corneal surface defined for the study (r = 0 to 4 mm) is considered to have more information on corneal morphology for both healthy and diseased eyes. This region includes both the central area (r = 0 to 2 mm), which corresponds to the more spherical area with more visual impact and accounts for 25% of keratoconus cases, and the paracentral area (r = 2 to 4 mm), which corresponds to the area where the cornea begins to flatten and accounts for 72% of keratoconus cases [42]. In total, the region targeted for the geometric reconstruction (r = 0 to 4 mm) presents levels of irregularity in corneal morphology for both anterior and posterior surfaces which encompasses 97% of keratoconus cases.

The Sirius corneal topographer can provide raw data of the spatial points that conform both anterior and posterior corneal surfaces, indicating the coordinates (X, Y, Z) of every scanned point. This data is the most reliable information to be used due to it has not been processed by any software algorithm or manipulated [17]. For this reason the raw data provided by the topographer was used in this study.

Due to the Sirius topographer only providing spatial points data in Cartesian format for the anterior corneal surface (not for the posterior surface), it was necessary to export data in polar format to obtain data from both corneal surfaces. This data was given as a CSV table where every row represented a circle in the map and every column represented a semi-meridian, giving 256 points for each radius. This way, each i-th row sampled a map on a circle of i*0.2 mm radius, and each j-th column sampled a map on a semi-meridian in the direction of j*360/256°, so each Z value of the matrix [i, j] represented the point P (i*0.2, j*360/256°) in polar coordinates. In order to perform these calculations, exported data were further formatted in Cartesian coordinates by an algorithm programmed using Matlab software (Fig. 1-A).

ii) Geometric Surface Reconstruction. The point cloud representing the corneal geometry was imported by the surface reconstruction software Rhinoceros v5.0. This uses a mathematical model to generate surfaces based on non-uniform rational

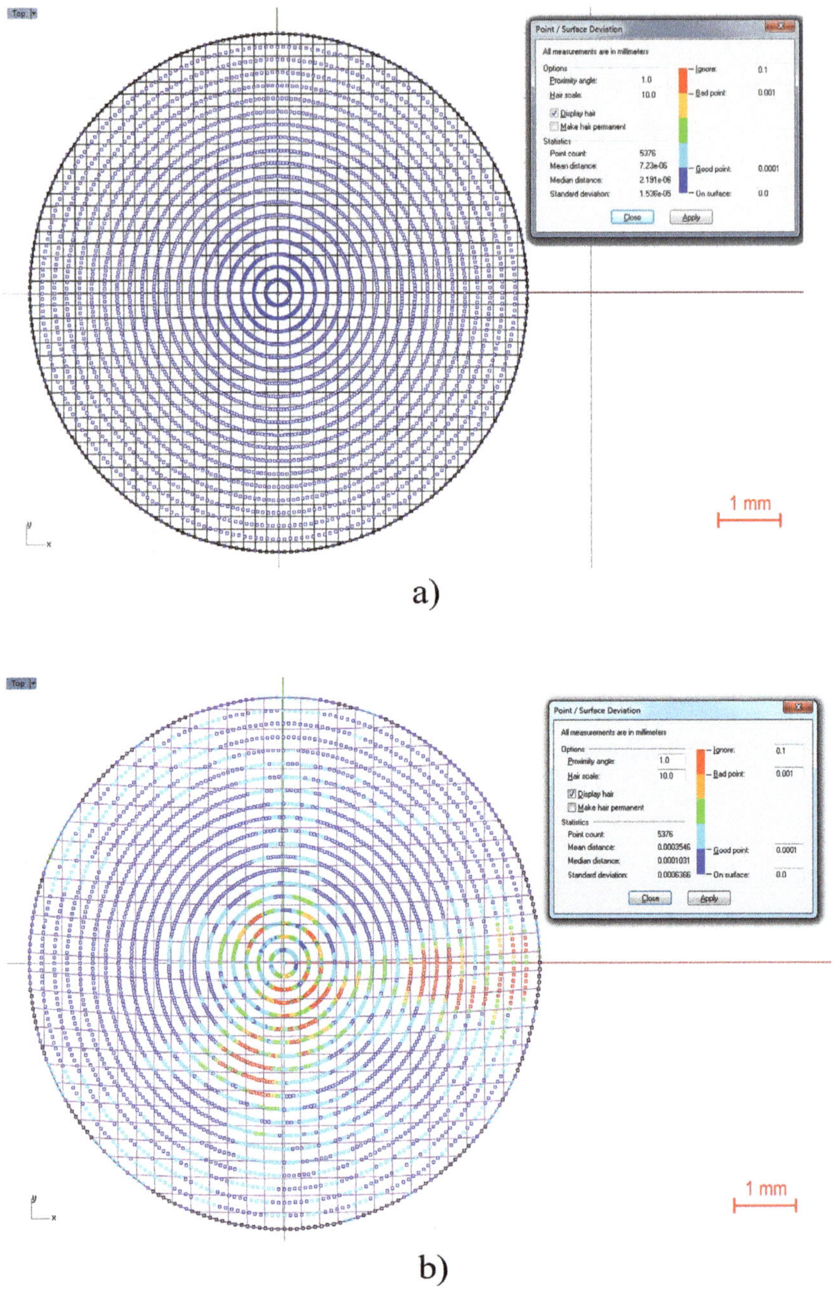

Figure 2. Analysis of the point-surface deviation for the anterior surface reconstruction of: a) a healthy cornea, b) a cornea with advanced keratoconus.

B-spline (NURBS) [43]. The surface generated from these spatial points is characterized by two parametric directions u and v. Besides, these types of surface are invariant under affine or perspective transformations, providing the flexibility to design a wide variety of surfaces with low memory consumption when compared to other methods.

The surface that best fits the point cloud was generated with the Rhinoceros's patch surface function (Fig. 1-B), a reconstruction software option that fits a surface through given curves, meshes, point objects, and point clouds [44]. For this research, this function tried to minimize the nominal distance between the 3D point cloud and the solution surface. For this objective, the function was configured by setting the sample point spacing at 256 (number of points for each data ring), the surface span planes at 255 for both u and v directions (the maximum number of span planes that the software permitted), and the stiffness of the solution surface at 10^{-3} [mm]. This last parameter provides information on how much the best fit plane can be deformed in order to match the input points. This deviation can be calculated later by the software, providing a mean value of the distance error for the solution surface. This can be seen in Figure 2a, where the top view of the point cloud for the anterior surface of a healthy cornea is represented and a mean distance error of $7.23\times10^{-6}\pm 1.536\times10^{-5}$ [mm] (mean $\pm$ standard deviation) is obtained. Figure 2b shows the deviation error for the anterior surface of a cornea with advanced keratoconus, obtaining in this case a mean

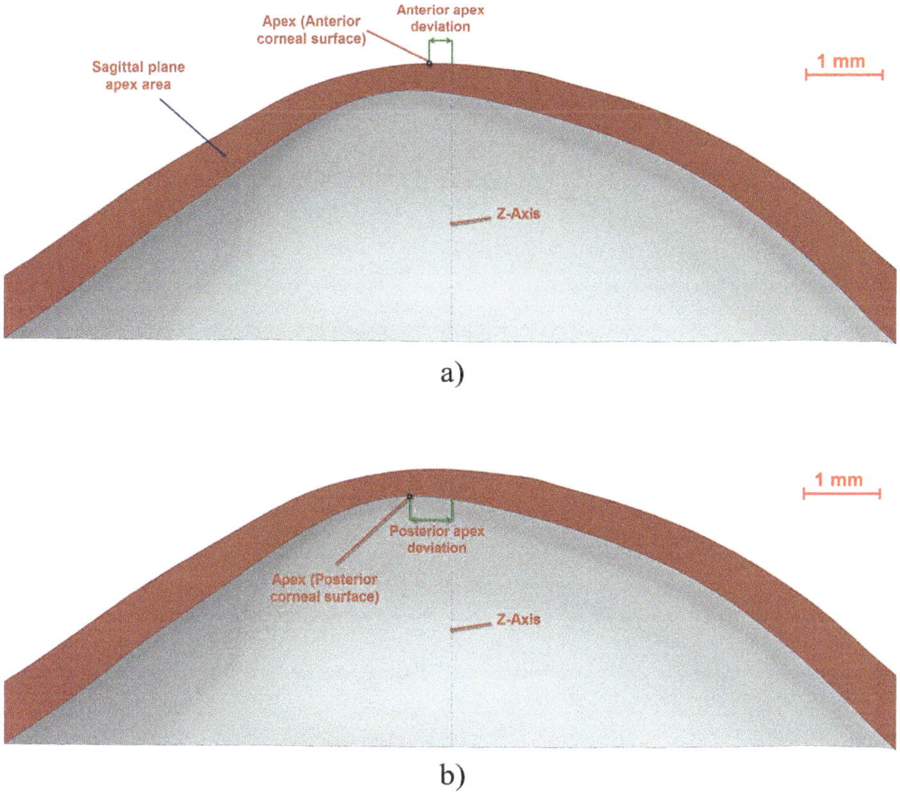

Figure 3. Sagittal plane of the cornea: a) passing through anterior apex and the Z-axis, b) passing through posterior apex and the Z-axis.

distance error of $3.54\times10^{-4}\pm6.36\times10^{-4}$ [mm] (mean ± standard deviation). In both figures the same good/bad threshold values have been configured: 10^{-3} [mm] for bad points (in red) and 10^{-4} [mm] for good points (in blue). These figures show how the points are distributed in perfect circular rings from r = 0 mm to r = 4 mm in steps of 0.2 mm. This is because, as previously mentioned, the Sirius device gives the 3D points in polar coordinates, and once converted into Cartesian format, they are distributed in a circular map.

Using this procedure, anterior and posterior cornea surfaces with radius 4 mm were generated, and engaged by their geometrical center and Z axis (Fig. 1-C). Both surfaces and the perimetric surface (bonding surface between both sides in the Z-axis direction) were then joined to form a single surface.

iii) Solid Modeling. The resulting surface was imported using the solid modeling software SolidWorks v2012, which allowed the generation of the solid model that is representative of the custom and actual geometry of each cornea (Fig. 1-D). Taking into account all previously mentioned aspects about the data to be used for the model reconstruction, it is important to clarify that the solid models were reconstructed up to a 4 mm radius. Any case in which the data provided by the Sirius topographer had some point left until the 4 mm radius was discarded from this study.

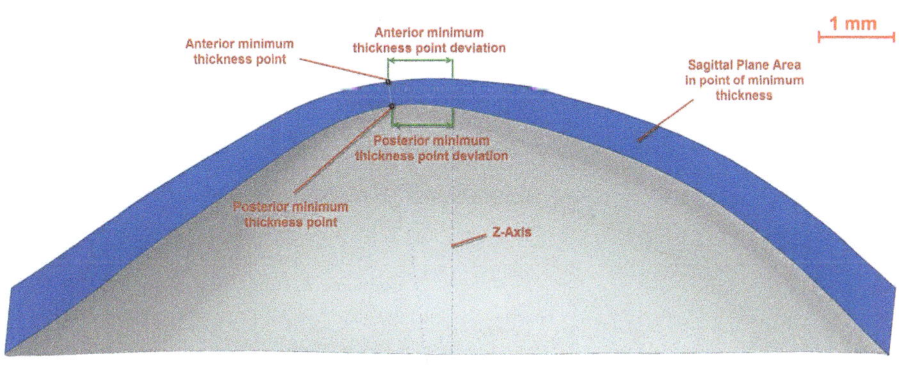

Figure 4. Sagittal plane of the cornea passing through the Z axis and minimum thickness points of both corneal surfaces.

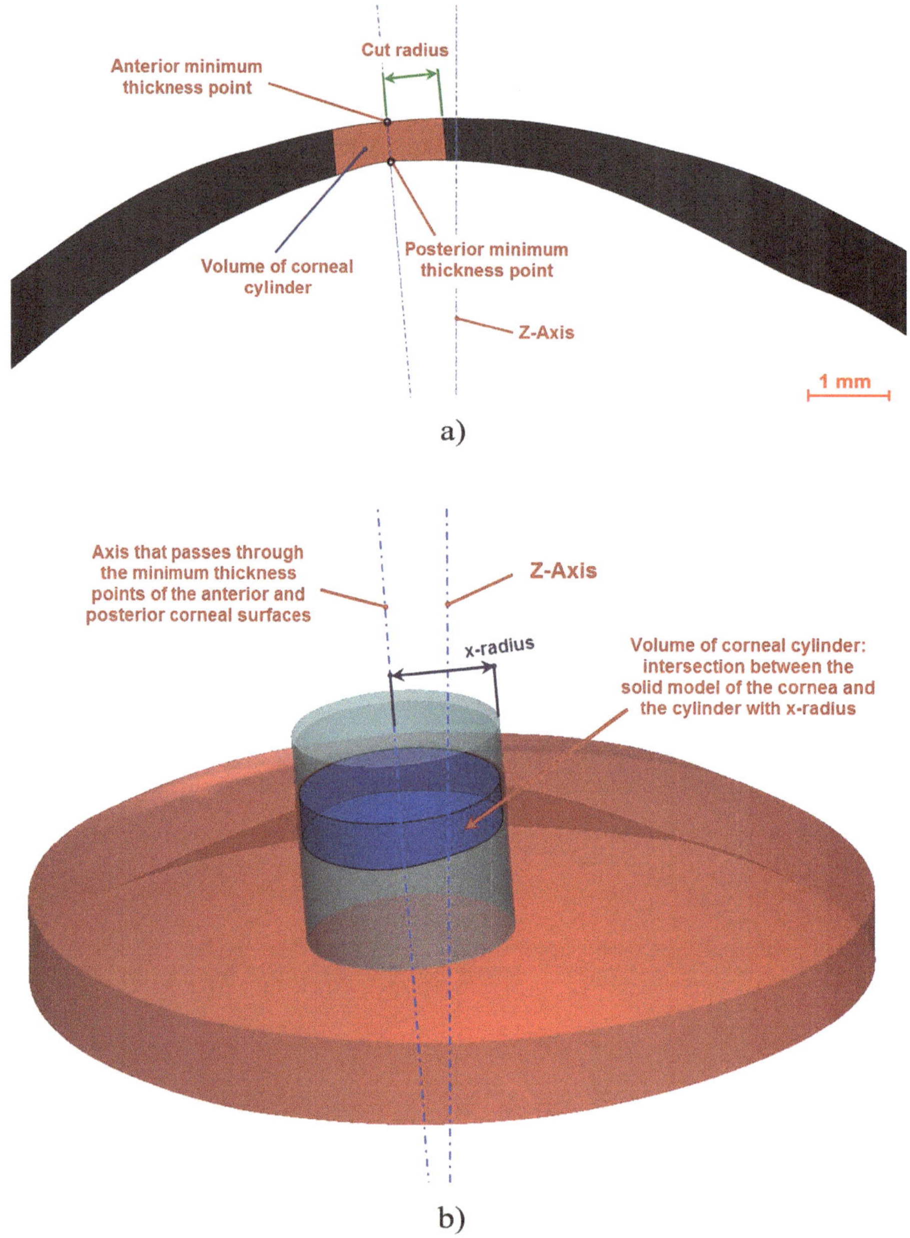

Figure 5. Volume of corneal cylinder with a determined radius: a) 2D view of the cylinder and its parameters, b) 3D view of the intersection between the solid model of the cornea and the cylinder.

iv) Definition of geometric variables. From the solid model obtained, the following geometric variables were defined:

- Total corneal volume [mm^3] (Fig. 1-D): volume limited by front, back and peripheral surfaces of the solid model generated.
- Anterior corneal surface area [mm^2] (Fig. 1-D): area of the front/exterior surface.
- Posterior corneal surface area [mm^2] (Fig. 1-D): area of the rear/interior surface.
- Total corneal surface area [mm^2] (Fig. 1-D): sum of anterior, posterior and perimetral corneal surface areas of the solid model generated.
- Sagittal plane apex area [mm^2] (Fig. 3a): area of the cornea within the sagittal plane passing through the Z axis and the highest point (apex) of the anterior corneal surface.
- Anterior and posterior apex deviation [mm] (Figs. 3a and 3b): average distance from the Z axis to the highest point (apex) of the anterior/posterior corneal surfaces.
- Sagittal plane area in minimum thickness points (maximum curvature) [mm] (Fig. 4): area of the cornea within the sagittal plane passing through the Z axis and the minimum thickness points (maximum curvature) of the anterior and posterior corneal surfaces.
- Anterior and posterior minimum thickness point deviation (maximum curvature) [mm] (Fig. 4): average distance in the XY plane from the Z axis to the minimum thickness points

Table 1. Descriptive values (mean and 95% CI) and differences between normal and keratoconus corneal variables modeled.

Measurement	Normal Group, n = 90	Keratoconus Group, n = 41	
	Mean (95% CI)	Mean (95% CI)	p (statistical test)
Total corneal volume [mm^3]	25.81 (25.47–26.14)	23.42 (22.81–24.03)	0.000 (Mann–Whitney)
Anterior corneal surface area [mm^2]	43.08 (43.04–43.11)	43.39 (43.30–43.40)	0.000 (Mann–Whitney)
Posterior corneal surface area [mm^2]	44.24 (44.18–44.30)	44.73 (44.57–44.89)	0.000 (Mann–Whitney)
Total corneal surface area [mm^2]	103.93 (103.67–104.20)	103.59 (103.13–104.05)	0.169 (Mann–Whitney)
Sagittal plane apex area [mm^2]	4.33 (4.27–4.39)	3.90 (3.80–4.00)	0.000 (Mann–Whitney)
Sagittal Plane Area in minimum thickness points [mm^2]	4.32 (4.26–4.38)	3.88 (3.78–3.99)	0.000 (t-test)
Anterior apex deviation [mm]	0.0003 (0.0001–0.0006)	0.0083 (0.0048–0.0118)	0.000 (Mann–Whitney)
Posterior apex deviation [mm]	0.0768 (0.063–0.0905)	0.1886 (0.1587–0.2185)	0.000 (Mann–Whitney)
Center of mass X [mm]	0.044 (0.0409–0.0478)	0.0415 (0.0331–0.0499)	0.341 (t-test)
Center of mass Y [mm]	0.034 (0.0304–0.0375)	0.0364 (0.0279–0.0449)	0.964 (Mann–Whitney)
Net deviation from center of mass XY [mm]	0.0577 (0.0538–0.0616)	0.0606 (0.0517–0.0694)	0.132 (t-test)
Center of mass Z [mm]	0.771 (0.766–0.776)	0.785 (0.771–0.800)	0.156 (Mann–Whitney)
Anterior minimum thickness point deviation [mm]	0.864 (0.812–0.917)	1.031 (0.901–1.161)	0.010 (Mann–Whitney)
Posterior minimun thickness point deviation [mm]	0.800 (0.749–0.851)	0.958 (0.835–1.081)	0.009 (Mann–Whitney)

(maximum curvature) of the anterior/posterior corneal surfaces.

- Center of mass coordinates X, Y, Z of the solid [mm].
- Net Deviation from the center of mass in XY [mm]: projective XY Modulus of the center of mass.
- Volume of corneal cylinder with r-x [mm^3]: volume of the intersection in 3D (see Fig. 5b) between the solid model of the cornea generated and a cylinder with x radius whose axis passes through the minimum thickness points (maximum curvature) of the anterior and posterior corneal surfaces (see Fig. 5a). Radiuses adopted for this study were 0.5, 1, 1.5 and 2 mm.

Statistical analysis

Data engagement scores were confirmed by means of the Kolmogorov–Smirnov test. According to this analysis, a Student's t-test or U-Mann Whitney Wilcoxon test for unpaired data was performed (depending on normality), in order to describe differences between normal and keratoconus groups in all the measurements proposed. An additional Kruskal-Wallis test was used to compare differences between groups according to disease stages (Amsler– Krumeich grading system). Pairwise comparisons were performed using Dunn's procedure with a Bonferroni correction for multiple comparisons. Finally, a ROC curve analysis was performed in order to obtain the accuracy of the different measurements. An area of 1 represents the most accurate test, while an area of 0.5 represents a worthless test. The closer the curve follows, the left-hand border, and then, the top borders of the ROC space, the more accurate the test is. So this is an estimation of the ability of these measurements to identify more true positives while minimizing the number of false positives. All the statistical analyses mentioned were performed using Graphpad Prism 6 and SPSS 17.0 software.

Results

From the total of 131 patients, this study included a total of 90 healthy eyes (persons aged from 7 to 66 years old) and 41 eyes (persons aged from 14 to 66 years old) with keratoconus diagnosis in several grades (51.2% in stage I, 36.6% in stage II, 12.2% in the most extreme stages, III and IV).

Most of the modeled variables showed differences between normal and keratoconus diagnosed eyes, as seen in table 1: total corneal volume is greater in normal eyes ($p<0.000$), anterior and posterior corneal surface areas are smaller in the healthy subjects ($p<0.000$). This pattern of difference can be seen for most of variables studied: normal eyes have a greater sagittal plane apex area and a greater sagittal plane area in minimum thickness points ($p<0.000$), whereas anterior and posterior apex deviations are greater in keratoconus eyes ($p<0.000$) and also in anterior and posterior minimum thickness point deviation ($p<0.01$). The eyes' center of mass is not a good predictor of differences between

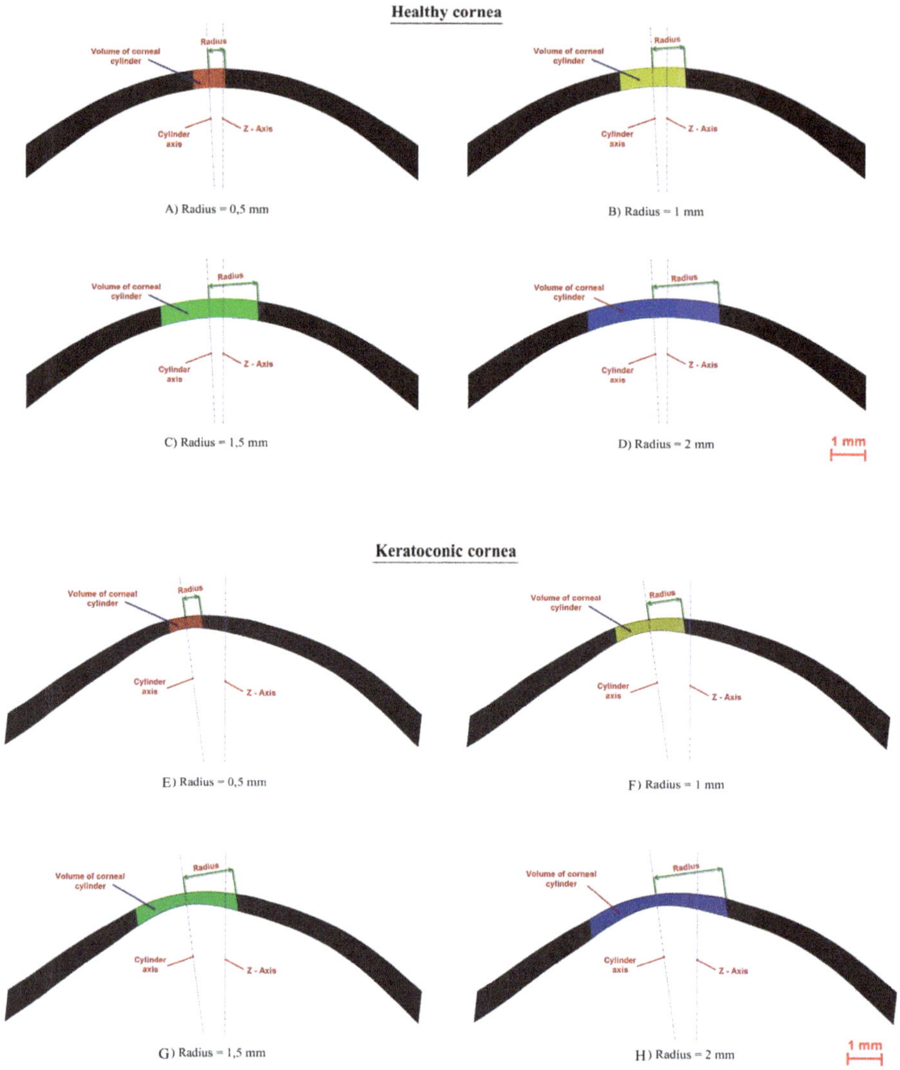

Figure 6. Schematic representation of the difference in the volume of corneal cylinder with radius 0.5, 1.0, 1.5 and 2.0 between a normal cornea (A–D) and a cornea with keratoconus (E–H).

normal and keratoconus eyes, and there is no statistical difference in x, y and z, or in net deviation from the center of mass in x, y. Also, the total corneal area modeled does not show differences between groups.

Additionally, figure 6 shows the differences between normal and keratoconus groups in the volumes of corneal cylinder modelled using different radius (maximum bending in 0.5, 1.0, 1.5 and 2.0 mm from the axis that passes through the minimum thickness points). Please note the differences between a normal eye

Table 2. Differences between the normal group (Figs. 7a–d) versus the keratoconus group (Figs. 7e–h) in the volume of corneal cylinder with radius 0.5, 1.0, 1.5 and 2.0 mm (mean and standard deviation; U-Mann-Whitney-Wilcoxon test).

Volume of corneal cylinder (mm^3) with Radius×(mm)	Normal Group, n = 90 (figs. 7a–d)	Keratoconus Group, n = 41 (figs. 7e–h)		
	Mean±SD	**Mean±SD**	**z**	**p**
r = 0.5	0.46±0.29	0.35±0.041	-8.280	0.000
r = 1	1.71±0.11	1.46±0.15	-7.980	0.000
r = 1.5	3.91±0.24	3.33±0.50	-7.650	0.000
r = 2	7.10±0.44	6.26±0.57	-7.211	0.000

Table 3. Comparison between groups of the outcomes modeled; Kruskall-Wallis test (with p values) and effect size, (ES)[1].

	Normal	I Stage	II Stage	III–IV Stage	p (Krskall-Wallis test)
Total corneal volume [mm^3]	26.00 [21.37–29.50]	23,88 [19,82–26.66]	23,32 [19,09–27,60]	19,78 [16,97–22,60]	0.000
(ES)	-	1,19	1,42	3,35	
Anterior corneal surface area [mm^2]	43,07 [42,73–43,38]	43,27 [42,89–43,58]	43,46 [43,14–44,12]	44,10 [43,86–44,35]	0.000
(ES)	-	−1,18	−1,70	-4,85	
Posterior corneal surface area [mm^2]	44,25 [43,49–44,90]	44,55 [43,93–45,07]	44,85 [44,21–45,90]	45,75 [45,72–45,78]	0.000
(ES)	-	−0,99	−1,54	-4,18	
Total corneal surface area [mm^2]	103,94 [100,69–106,15]	103.59 [100,91–104–75]	103,71 [99,97–106,18]	103,58 [101,68–105,48]	0.185
(ES)	-	0,28	0,18	0,28	
Sagittal plane apex area [mm^2]	4,34 [3,58–5,00]	3,94 [3,28–4,50]	3,91 [3,19–4,48]	3,35 [3,00–3,70]	0.000
(ES)	-	1,30	1,37	3,25	
Sagittal Plane Area in minimum thickness points [mm^2]	4,35 [3,57–5,01]	3,94 [3,28–4,50]	3,92 [3,03–4,48]	3,34 [2,99–3,69]	0.000
(ES)	-	1,33	1,28	3,29	
Anterior apex deviation [mm]	0,000 [0,000–0,007]	0,003 [0,000–0,016]	0,008 [0,000–0,041]	0,029 [0,014–0,044]	0.000
(ES)	-	−1,12	−1,41	-5,93	
Posterior apex deviation [mm]	0,068 [0,024–0,650]	0,164 [0,054–0,339]	0,198 [0,032–0,453]	0,132 [0,054–0,209]	0.000
(ES)	-	−1,25	−1,44	-0,97	
Center of mass X [mm]	0,044 [0,009–0,089]	0,042 [0,002–0,083]	0,030 [0,006–0,083]	0,059 [0,002–0,116]	0.184
(ES)	-	0,12	0,79	−0,82	
Center of mass Y [mm]	0,032 [0,000–0,095]	0,036 [0,005–0,084]	0,021 [0,008–0,281]	0,065 [0,001–0,129]	0.187
(ES)	-	−0,22	0,37	−1,67	
Net deviation from center of mass XY [mm]	0,056 [0,009–0,108]	0,059 [0,031–0,105]	0,042 [0,014–0,281]	0,123 [0,116–0,129]	0.006
(ES)	-	−0,16	0,48	-3,25	
Center of mass Z [mm]	0,770 [0,708–0,813]	0,771 [0,730–0,795]	0,799 [0,709–0,864]	0,839 [0,809–0,869]	0.013
(ES)	-	−0,04	−1,02	−2,55	
Anterior minimum thickness point deviation [mm]	0,839 [0,438–2,171]	1,050 [0,558–2,051]	1,084 [0,527–3,107]	0,391 [0,233–0,549]	0.001
(ES)	-	−0,71	−0,69	1,72	
Posterior minimum thickness point deviation [mm]	0,771 [0,375–2,059]	0,953 [0,536–1,924]	0,996 [0,444–2,941]	0,358 [0,197–0,519]	0.000
(ES)	-	−0,65	−0,67	1,66	

Sample was stratified according to the Amsler– Krumeich grading system according to the severity of the disease.
[1]Comparing each stage of the disease versus normal eyes, effects size was estimated as follows: $d=(\overline{X}_1-\overline{X}_n)/\sigma$, calculating $\overline{X}_1$ for the normal eyes group, $\overline{X}_n$ for each stage of the keratoconus group, and σ being a pooled standard deviation of compared data.

(Figs. 6a–d) versus one with keratoconus (Figs. 6e–h). Statistical differences were found for all these geometric variables, enabling the differentiation of keratoconus eyes (see table 2).

The outcomes according to keratoconus severity are shown in Table 3, where comparisons are established according to the severity of the disease following the Amsler–Krumeich grading system. Only total corneal surface area and center of mass in x and y are not suitable for differentiating between groups, with the other geometrical variables being statistically significant between stages (from $p<0.000$ to $p<0.013$). For center of mass in z and net deviation from the center of mass in xy, it can be observed that III and IV stages are well differentiated from the other groups, as

Table 4. ROC analysis of sensitivity versus 1-specificity in the disease diagnosis for proposed measurements.

Measurement	Area	Accuracy ratio	p
Total corneal volume [mm^3]	0.153	−0.694	1.000
Anterior corneal surface area [mm^2]	0.847	0.694	0.000
Posterior corneal surface area [mm^2]	0.807	0.614	0.000
Total corneal surface area [mm^2]	0.430	−0.14	0.171
Sagittal plane apex area [mm^2]	0.135	−0.73	0.000
Sagittal Plane Area in minimum thickness points [mm^2]	0.139	−0.722	0.000
Anterior apex deviation [mm]	0.735	0.47	0.000
Posterior apex deviation [mm]	0.891	0.782	0.000
Center of mass X [mm]	0.444	−0.112	0.168
Center of mass Y [mm]	0.485	−0.03	0.911
Net deviation from center of mass XY [mm]	0.503	0.006	0.821
Center of mass Z [mm]	0.567	0.134	0.159
Anterior minimum thickness point deviation [mm]	0.632	0.264	0.010
Posterior minimun thickness point deviation [mm]	0.634	0.268	0.009

post-hoc analysis reveals (Dunn's method and Bonferroni correction for multiple comparisons). Note that the calculated effects size for each disease stage (versus normal group) allows quantifying the degree of change, greater for stages III and IV in most of the variables, becoming more evident with the progress of the disease.

The predictive value of the variables modeled was established through a ROC analysis (see Table 4). Four variables with an area under the curve of over 0.7 were found (see figure 7): anterior corneal surface area (area: 0.847, $p<0.000$, std. error: 0.038, 95% CI: 0.777 to 0.925), the cut-off value obtained was 43.11 mm^2, with an associated sensitivity and specificity of 89% and 57% respectively; posterior corneal surface area (area: 0.807, $p<0.000$, std. error: 0.042, 95% CI: 0,726 to 0,889), the cut-off value obtained was 44.2 mm^2, with an associated sensitivity and specificity of 91% and 44% respectively; anterior apex deviation (area: 0.735, $p<0.000$, std. error: 0.053, 95% CI: 0.630 to 0.840), the cut-off value obtained was 0.0015 mm, with an associated sensitivity and specificity of 71.4% and 91.6% respectively; finally, posterior apex deviation (area: 0.891, $p<0.000$, std. error: 0.039, 95% CI: 0.8146 to 0.9672), the cut-off value obtained was 0.0855 mm, with an associated sensitivity and specificity of 91.1% and 72.9% respectively.

Discussion

This paper proposes a procedure for 3D geometric reconstruction of the human cornea aiming to obtain a solid model that represents a personalized and in vivo morphology of both the anterior and posterior corneal surfaces. This method has been applied with success in both healthy and keratoconic corneas. In order to obtain a personalized characterization of the corneal topography several geometric variables are calculated from the 3D model, enabling to establish a new clinical diagnostic criterion for

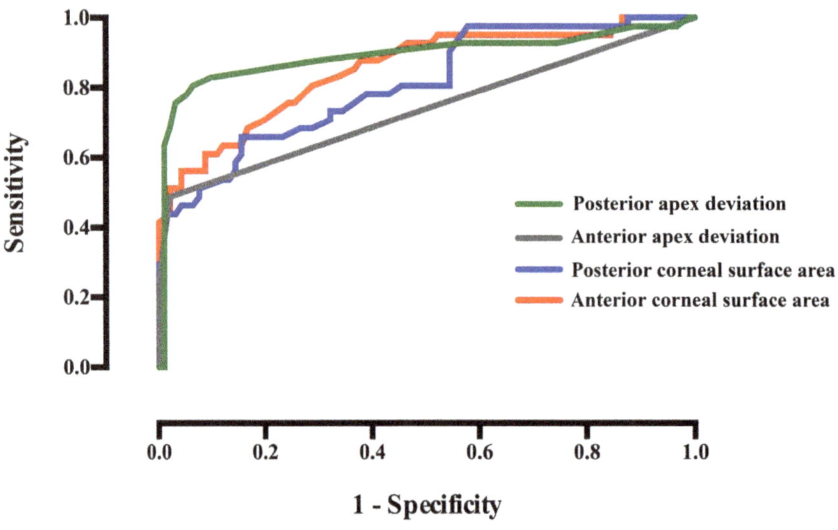

Figure 7. ROC curve modeling the sensitivity versus 1-specificity for variables diagnosing the existence of keratoconus disease (plotted only selected variables with area under the curve over 0.7).

the differentiation of healthy corneas from corneas with keratoconus.

Some studies have proposed novel methods for geometric modeling of human body parts using a 3D point cloud [40,41,45]. However, to the authors knowledge there is no information about the development of this procedure in human corneal modeling. Other authors have reconstructed the corneal surface using approximations to a basic geometry (sphere, ellipsoid) plus a residue representative of the irregularities with respect to the base geometry [21–22].

However, these procedures are based on the development of the Zernike polynomials, which have problems that have been widely discussed in the literature [30–32]. Some authors try to solve this issue using first a coarse adjustment by means of the Zernike polynomial and secondly a fine adjustment based on a lineal combination of radial basis Gaussian functions [33]. However, this method does not properly represent the corneal geometry when it has high irregularity levels due to ectasia related disorders, both on anterior and posterior surfaces. In contrast, the method proposed in this article provides a reliable solid model that reproduces the geometry of both corneal surfaces, both in keratoconic and healthy corneas, with minimum deviation errors for both surfaces (see figure 2).

Furthermore, current corneal topographers only provide a low data density from the posterior corneal surface, which makes it difficult to obtain a full 3D reconstruction of the human cornea [28–29]. For this reason, the criteria applied in this study establishes a method of reconstruction of the corneal region from its geometric center ($r = 0$ mm) to the beginning of the peripheral zone ($r = 4$ mm). This criterion is based on two main reasons: i) a geometric one, due to a total of 10752 spatial points representing the geometry of both anterior and posterior corneal surfaces obtained from the SIRIUS; and ii) a clinical one, due to this region comprising 97% of keratoconus cases [42].

A second objective of this work is the characterization of the corneal morphology as a new technique for the clinical diagnosis of keratoconus. There are some studies where the keratoconic eye is diagnosed by studying certain intrinsic geometric parameters directly provided by corneal topographers [3,46–47]. However, in this study we propose new geometric variables extracted from a solid model and representative of the corneal geometry that allow the irregularities in the corneal morphology to be characterized as a new diagnostic technique using a non-invasive clinical approach.

In this sense, the variables that achieved the best results in the diagnosis of the disease were anterior corneal surface area (ROC area: 0.847, $p<0.000$, std. error: 0.038, 95% CI: 0.777 to 0.925), posterior corneal surface area (ROC area: 0.807, $p<0.000$, std. error: 0.042, 95% CI: 0,726 to 0,889), anterior apex deviation (ROC area: 0.735, $p<0.000$, std. error: 0.053, 95% CI: 0.630 to 0.840) and posterior apex deviation (ROC area: 0.891, $p<0.000$, std. error: 0.039, 95% CI: 0.8146 to 0.9672). Nevertheless, there are other relevant statistical differences between healthy and diseased eyes, and most of variables studied differ between groups (as seen in table 1), making it possible to differentiate healthy corneas from those patients diagnosed with keratoconus. Thus, geometric modeling enables accurate characterization of the human cornea. In addition, from a clinical point of view, the procedure described has established a new approach for the study of eye-related diseases.

Author Contributions

Conceived and designed the experiments: FCM DGFP EDCS AVE ABPP JLA. Performed the experiments: AVE ABPP JLA. Analyzed the data: FCM DGFP EDCS. Contributed reagents/materials/analysis tools: FCM DGFP EDCS JNM FJFC. Contributed to the writing of the manuscript: FCM DGFP EDCS AVE ABPP JLA.

References

1. Levy D, Hutchings H, Rouland JF, Guell J, Burillon C, et al. (2004) Videokeratographic anomalies in familial keratoconus. Ophthalmology 111: 867–874.
2. Vryghem JC, Devogelaere T, Stodulka P (2010) Efficacy, safety, and flap dimensions of a new femtosecond laser for laser in situ keratomileusis. Journal of Cataract and Refractive Surgery 36: 442–448.
3. Ambrósio R Jr, Caiado AL, Guerra FP, Louzada R, Roy AS, et al. (2011) Novel pachymetric parameters based on corneal tomography for diagnosing keratoconus. J Refract Surg 27: 753–758.
4. Alessio G, Boscia F, La Tegola MG, Sborgia C (2001) Topography-driven excimer laser for the retreatment of decentralized myopic photorefractive keratectomy. Ophthalmology 108: 1695–1703.
5. Ribeiro FJ, Castanheira-Dinis A, Dias JM (2012) Personalized Pseudophakic Model for Refractive Assessment. PLoS ONE 7: e46780.
6. Elsheikh A, Wang D (2007) Numerical modelling of corneal biomechanical behaviour. Comput Methods Biomech Biomed Engin 10: 85–95.
7. Dubbelman M, Sicam VA, Van der Heijde GL (2006) The shape of the anterior and posterior surface of the aging human cornea. Vision Res 46: 993–1001.
8. Maldonado MJ, Nieto JC, Diez-Cuenca M, Piñero DP (2006) Repeatability and reproducibility of posterior corneal curvature measurements by combined scanning-slit and placido-disc topography after LASIK. Ophthalmology 113: 1918–1926.
9. Rondeau MJ, Barcsay G, Silverman RH, Reinstein DZ, Krishnamurthy R, et al. (2004) Very high frequency ultrasound biometry of the anterior and posterior chamber diameter. J Refract Surg 20: 454–464.
10. Ang M, Chong W, Huang H, Tay WT, Wong TY, et al. (2013) Comparison of Anterior Segment Optical Tomography Parameters Measured Using a Semi-Automatic Software to Standard Clinical Instruments. PLoS ONE 8: e65559.
11. Kang JJ, Allemann N, Vajaranant T, de la Cruz J, Cortina MS (2013) Anterior Segment Optical Coherence Tomography for the Quantitative Evaluation of the Anterior Segment Following Boston Keratoprosthesis. PLoS ONE 8: e70673.
12. Wang X, Dong J, Wang X, Wu Q (2013) IOL Tilt and Decentration Estimation from 3 Dimensional Reconstruction of OCT Image. PLoS ONE 8: e59109.
13. Belin MW, Khachikian SS (2009) An introduction to understanding elevation-based topography: how elevation data are displayed - a review. Clin Experiment Ophthalmol 37: 14–29.
14. Piñero DP (2013) Technologies for Anatomical and Geometric Characterization of the Corneal Structure and Anterior Segment: A Review. Semin Ophthalmol.
15. Piñero DP, Saenz Gonzalez C, Alio JL (2009) Intraobserver and interobserver repeatability of curvature and aberrometric measurements of the posterior corneal surface in normal eyes using Scheimpflug photography. J Cataract Refract Surg 35: 113–120.
16. Wang Q, Savini G, Hoffer KJ, Xu Z, Feng Y, et al. (2012) A Comprehensive Assessment of the Precision and Agreement of Anterior Corneal Power Measurements Obtained Using 8 Different Devices. PLoS ONE 7: e45607.
17. Ramos-López D, Martinez-Finkelshtein A, Castro-Luna GM, Piñero D, Alio JL (2011) Placido-based indices of corneal irregularity. Optom Vis Sci 88: 1220–1231.
18. Savini G, Carbonelli M, Barboni P, Hoffer KJ (2011) Repeatability of automatic measurements performed by a dual Scheimpflug analyzer in unoperated and post-refractive surgery eyes. J Cataract Refract Surg 37: 302–309.
19. Montalbán R, Piñero DP, Javaloy J, Alio JL (2012) Intrasubject repeatability of corneal morphology measurements obtained with a new Scheimpflug photography-based system. J Cataract Refract Surg 38: 971–977.
20. Bao F, Chen H, Yu Y, Yu J, Zhou S, et al. (2013) Evaluation of the Shape Symmetry of Bilateral Normal Corneas in a Chinese Population. PLoS ONE 8: e73412.
21. Navarro R, Gonzalez L, Hernandez JL (2006) Optics of the average normal cornea from general and canonical representations of its surface topography. J Opt Soc Am A Opt Image Sci Vis 23: 219–232.
22. Alastrue V, Calvo B, Pena E, Doblare M (2006) Biomechanical modeling of refractive corneal surgery. J Biomech Eng 128: 150–160.
23. Pandolfi A, Fotia G, Manganiello F (2009) Finite element simulations of laser refractive corneal surgery. Eng Comput-Germany 25: 15–24.
24. Roy AS, Dupps WJ Jr (2011) Patient-specific modeling of corneal refractive surgery outcomes and inverse estimation of elastic property changes. J Biomech Eng 133: 011002.
25. Han Z, Sui X, Zhou D, Zhou C, Ren Q (2013) Biomechanical and refractive behaviors of keratoconic cornea based on three-dimensional anisotropic hyperelastic models. J Refract Surg 29: 282–290.

26. Studer HP, Riedwyl H, Amstutz CA, Hanson JV, Buchler P (2013) Patient-specific finite-element simulation of the human cornea: a clinical validation study on cataract surgery. J Biomech 46: 751–758.
27. Sánchez P, Moutsouris K, Pandolfi A (2014) Biomechanical and optical behavior of human corneas before and after photorefractive keratectomy. J Cataract Refract Surg 40: 905–917.
28. Auvinet E, Meunier J, Ong J, Durr G, Gilca M, et al. (2012) Methodology for the construction and comparison of 3D models of the human cornea. Conf Proc IEEE Eng Med Biol Soc 2012: 5302–5305.
29. Zheng S, Ying J, Wang B, Xie Z, Huang X, et al. (2013) Three-dimensional model for human anterior corneal surface. J Biomed Opt 18: 065002.
30. Smolek MK, Klyce SD (2003) Zernike polynomial fitting fails to represent all visually significant corneal aberrations. Invest Ophthalmol Vis Sci 44: 4676–4681.
31. Klyce SD, Karon MD, Smolek MK (2004) Advantages and disadvantages of the Zernike expansion for representing wave aberration of the normal and aberrated eye. J Refract Surg 20: S537–541.
32. Ares M, Royo S (2006) Comparison of cubic B-spline and Zernike-fitting techniques in complex wavefront reconstruction. Appl Opt 45: 6954–6964.
33. Martinez-Finkelshtein A, Lopez DR, Castro GM, Alio JL (2011) Adaptive cornea modeling from keratometric data. Invest Ophthalmol Vis Sci 52: 4963–4970.
34. Rabinowitz YS, McDonnell PJ (1989) Computer-assisted corneal topography in keratoconus. Refract Corneal Surg 5: 400–408.
35. Rabinowitz YS (1998) Keratoconus. Surv Ophthalmol 42: 297–319.
36. Piñero DP, Alio JL, Aleson A, Escaf Vergara M, Miranda M (2010) Corneal volume, pachymetry, and correlation of anterior and posterior corneal shape in subclinical and different stages of clinical keratoconus. J Cataract Refract Surg 36: 814–825.
37. Alio JL, Shabayek MH (2006) Corneal higher order aberrations: a method to grade keratoconus. J Refract Surg 22: 539–545.
38. Vega-Estrada A, Alio JL, Brenner LF, Javaloy J, Plaza Puche AB, et al. (2013) Outcome analysis of intracorneal ring segments for the treatment of keratoconus based on visual, refractive, and aberrometric impairment. Am J Ophthalmol 155: 575–584 e571.
39. Merklinger HM (1993) Focusing the View Camera: A Scientific Way to Focus the View Camera and Estimate Depth of Field. Canada: MacNab Print.
40. Ding S, Ye Y, Tu J, Subic A (2010) Region-based geometric modelling of human airways and arterial vessels. Comput Med Imaging Graph 34: 114–121.
41. Duan CY, Lü HB, Hu JZ (2012) In vivo study on three-dimensional structure of lumbar facet joints based on computer-assisted medical image processing method. Yiyong Shengwu Lixue/Journal of Medical Biomechanics 27: 159–165.
42. Wilson SE, Lin DT, Klyce SD (1991) Corneal topography of keratoconus. Cornea 10: 2–8.
43. Piegl L, Tiller W (1997) The NURBS Book: U.S. Government Printing Office.
44. Cheng RKC (2014) Inside Rhinoceros 5. USA: Cengage Learning. 656 p.
45. Reiffel AJ, Kafka C, Hernandez KA, Popa S, Perez JL, et al. (2013) High-Fidelity Tissue Engineering of Patient-Specific Auricles for Reconstruction of Pediatric Microtia and Other Auricular Deformities. PLoS ONE 8: e56506.
46. Montalban R, Alio JL, Javaloy J, Piñero DP (2013a) Intrasubject repeatability in keratoconus-eye measurements obtained with a new Scheimpflug photography-based system. J Cataract Refract Surg 39: 211–218.
47. Montalban R, Alio JL, Javaloy J, Piñero DP (2013b) Comparative analysis of the relationship between anterior and posterior corneal shape analyzed by Scheimpflug photography in normal and keratoconus eyes. Graefes Arch Clin Exp Ophthalmol 251: 1547–1555.

4

The Concordance of Care for Age Related Macular Degeneration with the Chronic Care Model: A Multi-Centered Cross-Sectional Study

Stefan Markun[1]*, Elisabeth Brändle[1], Avraham Dishy[2], Thomas Rosemann[1], Anja Frei[1,3]

1 Institute of General Practice and Health Service Research, University of Zurich, University Hospital of Zurich, Zurich, Switzerland, **2** Department of Ophthalmology, Cantonal Hospital Aarau, Aarau, Switzerland, **3** Institute of Social and Preventive Medicine, University of Zurich, Zurich, Switzerland

Abstract

Aims: The aim of the study was to assess the concordance of care for age related macular degeneration with the evidence-based framework for care for chronic medical conditions known as the chronic care model. Furthermore we aimed to identify factors associated with the concordance of care with the chronic care model.

Methods: Multi-centered cross-sectional study. 169 patients beginning medical treatment for age related macular degeneration were recruited and analyzed. Patients completed the Patient Assessment of Chronic Illness Care (PACIC) questionnaire, reflecting accordance to the chronic care model from a patient's perspective, the National Eye Institute Visual Functioning Questionnaire-25 (NEI-VFQ-25) and Patient Health Questionnaire (PHQ-9). Visual acuity and chronic medical conditions were assessed. Nonparametric tests and correlation analyses were performed, also multivariable regression analysis.

Results: The median PACIC summary score was 2.4 (interquartile range 1.75 to 3.25), the lowest PACIC subscale score was "follow-up/coordination" with a median of 1.8 (interquartile range 1.00 to 2.60). In multivariable regression analysis the presence of diabetes type 2 was strongly associated with low PACIC scores (coefficient = −0.85, p = 0.007).

Conclusion: Generally, care for patients with age related macular degeneration by ophthalmologists is in moderate concordance with the chronic care model. Concerning follow-up and coordination of health service, large improvements are possible. Future research should answer the question how healthcare delivery can be improved effecting relevant benefits to patients with AMD.

Editor: Tammy Clifford, Canadian Agency for Drugs and Technologies in Health, Canada

Funding: This trial was supported by the non-commercial foundation "Zukunft Hausarzt, Zürcher Stiftung zur Förderung der Hausarztmedizin", Zürich (www.zukunfthausarzt.ch). The funders had no role in study design, data collection and analysis, decision to publish, or preparation of the manuscript.

Competing Interests: The authors have declared that no competing interests exist.

* Email: stefan.markun@usz.ch

Introduction

Health care in general is being challenged by the unprecedented increase in chronic conditions. [1,2] The need to react to this epidemiological transition has led to initiatives, targeting to improve care for chronic conditions. [3] The chronic care model (CCM) developed by Wagner and colleagues is an evidence-based multifaceted recommendation package, targeting to improve care in different categories that are regarded as determinants for adequate care of chronic conditions. [4–6] These categories are organization of healthcare, clinical information systems, delivery-system design, decision support, self-management support and community resources. The CCM is supported by the WHO and has gained widespread acceptance because interventions enhancing the concordance with the CCM effectively improved relevant outcomes in chronic diseases such as diabetes, osteoarthritis or depression. [7–9] A validated tool to measure the concordance of care with the CCM from the patient's perspective has been developed [10].

Age related macular degeneration (AMD) is a chronic condition with severe potential impact on diseased patients. In AMD, visual loss is for the greatest part triggered by the growth of abnormal blood vessels in proximity of the retina. These abnormal blood vessels cause leakage of blood constituents with consecutive anatomic disruption, cell death and ultimately loss of central vision. The growth of new blood vessels including the consequences on visual function, however, can be effectively antagonized by therapies targeting the vascular endothelial growth factor

A (VEGF-A). [11] These therapies are applied by periodic intravitreal injections. Current treatment strategies aim to administer injections in phases of disease activity notable by sudden deteriorations of visual function. [12,13] This individualized and patient-centered approach potentially reduces unnecessary injections, however, it requires health services to provide a thorough follow-up management. Furthermore patients need to be adequately informed and empowered as they take great responsibility by self-monitoring their disease. This is especially important in stages of presumed disease inactivity, when re-occurrence of neovascularizations should prompt immediate re-uptake of an anti-VEGF-A therapy capable of slowing down or even avert permanent visual loss. Such features of healthcare delivery are represented in the CCM, which is therefore relevant in AMD on both the caregivers' and the patients' levels. Whether care for AMD is in concordance with the CCM, however, is currently unknown.

The aim of this study was to assess if and to what extent care for patients with AMD is in concordance with the CCM in Swiss ophthalmology clinics (1). Furthermore we aimed to identify factors that determine the concordance of care with the CCM (2).

Materials and Methods

Study design

This is a cross-sectional study, based on the baseline data gathered for the randomized trial "The chronic care for age-related macular degeneration study" (CHARMED). The study has been registered at Current Controlled Trials (ISRCTN32507927), the study protocol is publically available. [14] In brief about 20 ophthalmologists from 20 leading ophthalmology clinics in Switzerland providing therapy for patients with AMD were invited to participate in the study by a formal letter. Participating ophthalmologists where trained to gather outcome measures in a standardized format. Also in every participating clinic chronic care coaches where trained to deliver chronic care and conduct structured interviews for outcome measurements. According to the trial's power calculation 352 patients where intended to be recruited, however, recruiting was stopped after 20 months when the number of newly recruited patients per month reached zero.

Ethics statement

Ethics committee approval was obtained (ethics committee of the Canton Zurich, KEK-ZH-NR: 2010-04391/1). The study was performed adhering to the tenets of the Declaration of Helsinki and according to Good Clinical Practice Guidelines.

Patients

Patients were recruited consecutively from April 1 2011 until January 28 2013 by the participating ophthalmologists during clinical visits.

To be eligible for inclusion, patients were required to meet the following inclusion criteria: Diagnosis of wet AMD, age above 50 years, eligible for antiangiogenic drug therapy and visual acuity of at least 20 letters in the assessment with the Early Treatment Diabetic Retinopathy Study (ETDRS) chart. Written informed consent in the study participation was obtained before any study related procedures were taken. Exclusion criteria were former invasive medical treatment for AMD, severe general illness (i.e. advanced malignant tumors or dementia), severe psychological illness and insufficient German or French language skills.

Measures and data collection

Data collection was performed directly after written informed consent was obtained. A questionnaire was filled in by the ophthalmologists containing the following measures retrieved at the recruitment visit: Visual acuity (using ETDRS charts, standardized measurements were assured by conducting a visit with a teaching session at each ophthalmology clinic); central retinal thickness by optical coherence tomography; specific comorbidities such as hypertension, diabetes type 2, diabetic retinopathy, coronary artery disease, congestive heart failure, stroke or transient ischemic attack, asthma or chronic obstructive lung disease and neoplasms; family anamnesis of wet AMD; smoking status; current medication; estimation of the patients compliance on a four-point scale (range from 1 = very good to 4 = very bad).

A second questionnaire was given to the patients at the recruiting visit to fill in and return directly to the University of Zurich using a readily stamped and accordingly addressed envelope. The questionnaire was self-administered and contained the Patient Assessment of Chronic Illness Care (PACIC) as a measure for concordance of care with the CCM, [10] the PHQ-9 questionnaire as a measure for depression [15] and questions about socio-demographic data and health service utilization.

The PACIC is a validated self-administered instrument that measures the concordance of care with the CCM from the patient's perspective. According to the key-elements of the CCM the PACIC is organized containing five essential categories of chronic care asked in 20 individual items. In specific these categories are patient activation, delivery system design/decision support, goal setting/tailoring, problem solving/contextual counselling and follow-up/coordination. Each of the individual items are scored on a five point Likert-scale ranging from "almost never" (= 1, corresponding to poorest concordance with the CCM) to "almost always" (= 5, corresponding to highest concordance with the CCM). The PACIC summary score is the mean score of the 20 individual items and gives an overall rating of the concordance with the CCM. Five subscales are defined that allow estimations of the CCM concordance with the respective essential categories of chronic care. Such as the CCM, the PACIC itself has shown to be associated with favorable outcomes in chronic conditions. [16] The PACIC summary score was our predefined primary outcome.

The Patient Health Questionnaire (PHQ-9) is a self-administered tool that allows rapid screening for depression and rating severity that recently has showed consistency in patients with visual impairment. [17,18] The PHQ-9 was introduced in the measurements as a confounder control, because depression is known to be highly prevalent among patients with AMD and might influence outcomes of the CHARMED randomized trial (not discussed in this article) [19].

In a face-to-face or telephone interview with the patients the trained chronic care coaches operated the National Eye Institute Visual Functioning Questionnaire-25 (NEI-VFQ-25) in the interviewer administered format. [20] The NEI-VFQ-25 is a validated measure of the visual disability specific quality of life and functioning, it consists of 25 vision-targeted questions that generate 11 subscales of vision related health and functioning [21,22].

Patients and ophthalmologists' answers remained concealed from each other; the University of Zurich had no access to the patients' personal informations ensuring anonymity.

Statistical analysis

Continuous variables are presented as means and standard deviations or medians and interquartile ranges if not otherwise

Table 1. Demographical and social characteristics of study patients, smoking status and patient compliance from the ophthalmologist's perspective; table n = 169.

Variable	*Category*	*n*	*percent*
Gender	Male	62	36.7
	Female	107	63.3
	Missing information	0	0.0
Age	<60 years old	3	1.8
	60–69 years old	33	19.5
	70–79 years old	69	40.8
	80–89 years old	58	34.3
	≥90 years old	6	3.6
	Missing information	0	0.0
Living situation	Living with partner or family	103	60.9
	Living alone	53	31.4
	Missing information	13	7.7
Working situation	Still working	12	7.1
	Retired	144	85.2
	Missing information	13	7.7
Education years completed	≤6 years	2	1.2
	7 to 9 years	41	24.3
	10 to 12 years	56	33.1
	≥13 years	56	33.1
	Missing information	14	8.3
Smoking status	Current smoker	26	15.4
	Former smoker	49	29.0
	Never smoker	94	55.6
	Missing information	0	0.0
Compliance	Very good	96	56.8
	Rather good	69	40.8
	Rather bad	3	1.8
	Very bad	1	0.6
	Missing information	0	0

declared; categorical data is presented as frequencies and percentages. Bivariate association between the PACIC summary score and continuous variables were conducted using Spearman correlations, between PACIC summary score and categorical variables using Mann-Whitney-U Test and Kruskal-Wallis Test (more than two groups). Potential determinants of the PACIC summary score were investigated by multivariable regression model. We included all variables in the model that showed both a significant bivariate relationship with the PACIC summary score on a 5% level and could be interpreted in terms of content as potential determinants. We further controlled for the cluster-effect of clinics, thus taking into account that patient observations are not independent, i.e. observations in one cluster tend to be more similar to each other than to individuals in the rest of the sample. A two-sided alpha of 0.05 was set as level of significance for all comparisons. Missing data were left as missing, for the construction of the PACIC summary score one missing item (out of 20) was allowed. Analyses were calculated using the software SPSS version 21.0 and STATA version 12.

Results

Ophthalmologist characteristics

Twelve different ophthalmologists from twelve different clinics could be recruited for the study. Amongst the clinics, three different categories of organization type were found: Three clinics were single handed practices (median number of patients recruited = 7, range 2–12), five clinics were group practices (median number of patients recruited = 5, range 1–18), four were clinics run within hospitals (median number of patients recruited = 25, range 11–54).

Patient characteristics and clinical measures

In total, 169 patients were enrolled in the study. 21 (12.4%) patients were recruited in single handed practices, 32 (18.9%) in group practices and 116 (68.6%) in clinics run within hospitals. 107 (63.3%) of the patients were female, the mean age was 76.7 (±8.0) years. The average of total education years absolved was 12.0 (±3.4). In all patients, treatment with ranibizumab was started. Further characteristics are shown in Table 1.

Table 2. Vision-specific variables of study patients: visual acuity was assessed with the Early Treatment Diabetic Retinopathy Study (ETDRS) Chart; disability was assessed with the National Eye Institute Visual Functioning Questionnaire-25 (NEI-VFQ-25), range 0 to 100 (0 represents worst, 100 represents best possible visual functioning); table n = 169.

Variable	*Category*	*Mean*	*Standard deviation*	*n*	*Percent*
ETDRS Visual acuity better eye	Total ETDRS letters correct	74.1	14.9		
	<31 ETRDS letters correct			4	2.4
	31–50 ETRDS letters correct			9	5.3
	51–70 ETRDS letters correct			30	17.8
	>70 ETRDS letters correct			118	69.8
	Missing information			8	4.7
ETDRS Visual acuity worse eye	Total ETDRS letters correct	52.6	18.9		
	<31 ETRDS letters correct			18	10.7
	31–50 ETRDS letters correct			48	28.4
	51–70 ETRDS letters correct			68	40.2
	>70 ETRDS letters correct			27	16.0
	Missing information			8	4.7
NEI-VFQ-25 subscales*	General health	54.6	19.5		
	General vision	67.0	13.6		
	Ocular pain	90.0	15.8		
	Near activities	76.4	20.6		
	Distant activities	79.9	19.9		
	Social functioning	94.0	14.2		
	Mental health	78.7	18.7		
	Role difficulties	82.1	24.6		
	Dependency	93.8	17.0		
	Driving	68.8	33.9		
	Color vision	96.2	13.8		
	Peripheral vision	88.7	18.9		

*) Missing information for all items ranged from 6 to 8, except for "Driving" which was unanswered in 83 cases.

The mean number (± standard deviation) of correctly identified ETDRS letters was 74.1 (±14.9) with the better eye and 52.6 (±18.9) with the worse eye. The mean (± standard deviation) NEI-VFQ-25 composite score was 83.8 (±12.4). The mean general health rating (not component of the composite score) was 54.6 (±19.5). Detailed vision-specific information is given in Table 2.

In 111 (65.7%) of the patients at least one co-occurring chronic medical condition was present. 99 (58.6%) of the patients had cardiovascular comorbidities. The median number of ophthalmologist consultations within one year was 2 (interquartile range 1 to 3), the median number of GP consultations was 3 (interquartile range 1 to 6). 37 (21.9%) patients had at least one hospitalization during the last year, 27 (16.0%) had emergency hospitalizations. Data about comorbidities and healthcare utilization is displayed in Table 3.

PACIC scores

The median PACIC summary score was 2.4 (interquartile range 1.75 to 3.25). There were substantial differences between the different PACIC subscale scores. The subscale score "follow-up/coordination" resulted lowest with a median subscale score of 1.8 (interquartile range 1.00 to 2.60), corresponding with an average rating of the items in the PACIC questionnaire somewhat lower than "generally not". The highest subscale score was "delivery system design/decision support" with a median subscale score of 3.7 (interquartile range 2.33 to 4.67), corresponding with an average rating of the items in the PACIC questionnaire between "sometimes" and "most of the time". Details about the distribution of the PACIC summary score and subscale results are displayed in Table 4 and Figure 1.

Bivariate associations with PACIC summary score

The PACIC summary score was not significantly associated with the practice organization type (single handed, group practices and ambulatory clinics in hospitals: independent sample Kruskal-Wallis Test $p = 0.187$). No significant associations with the PACIC summary score were found for patients' socio-demographic characteristics, smoking status or physician-reported compliance. Also no significant association with the PACIC summary score was found for the number of comorbidities and for the PHQ-9. The presence of diabetes type 2 was significantly associated with lower PACIC scores (median [interquartile range] PACIC summary score of group with diabetes type 2 = 1.5 [1.11 to 2.13]), group without diabetes type 2 = 2.7 [1.83 to 3.28]; Mann Whitney U Test $p = 0.002$). Also the presence of coronary artery disease was significantly associated with lower PACIC scores (median [interquartile range] PACIC summary score of group with coronary artery disease = 2.0 [1.37 to 2.89]), group without coronary artery disease = 2.7 [1.80 to 3.30]; Mann Whitney U Test $p = 0.037$). No

Table 3. Comorbidity and Health Service Utilization; table n = 169.

Variable	*Category*	*n*	*percent*
Number of comorbidities	0 comorbidities	58	34.3
	1 comorbidity	60	35.5
	2 comorbidities	34	20.1
	3 comorbidities	10	5.9
	≥4 comorbidities	6	3.6
	Missing information	1	0.6
Specific comorbidities	Hypertension	92	54.4
	Diabetes type 2	14	8.3
	Diabetic retinopathy	0	0.0
	Coronary artery disease	29	17.2
	Congestive heart failure	8	4.7
	Stroke/TIA[1)]	14	8.3
	Asthma/COPD[2)]	16	9.5
	Neoplasm	11	6.5
Depression according to PHQ-9[3)]	No depression	116	68.6
	Mild depression	32	18.9
	Moderate major depression	3	1.8
	Severe major depression	2	1.2
	Missing information	16	9.5
Number of ophthalmologist consultations last year	1–2 consultations	87	51.5
	3–4 consultations	38	22.5
	5–6 consultations	14	8.3
	≥7 consultations	8	4.7
	Missing information	22	13.0
Number of GP[4)] consultations last year	0–2 consultations	65	38.5
	3–4 consultations	36	21.3
	5–6 consultations	23	13.6
	≥7 consultations	31	18.3
	Missing information	14	8.3
Number of days in hospital last year	0 days	117	69.2
	1–3 days	8	4.7
	4–10 days	18	10.7
	≥11 days	11	6.5
	Missing information	15	8.9

[1)]TIA = Transient ischemic attack;
[2)]COPD = Chronic obstructive pulmonary disease;
[3)]PHQ-9 = Patient Health Questionnaire-9;
[4)]GP = General practitioner.

vision-specific variable showed association with the PACIC summary score.

Multivariate associations with PACIC summary score

For the multivariable regression model we considered the comorbidity diabetes type 2 and coronary artery disease (both significant in bivariate analysis), gender and age (potential confounders) and visual acuity of the better eye (as an indicator for the severity of visual loss). The model was controlled for the cluster-effect originating from the different study clinics.

After application of the model, the only significant determinant of the PACIC summary score was diabetes type 2 (coefficient = −0.85, $p = 0.007$). Coronary artery disease closely missed significance (coefficient = −0.44, $p = 0.059$), the other variables showed no association (Table 5).

Discussion

The CCM is an evidence-based template for the care for patients with chronic illnesses. We aimed to measure the concordance of care with the CCM in patients treated for AMD. We found that patients perceived moderate overall concordance with the CCM, especially low concordance was found in the "follow-up/coordination" subscale score.

A broad spectrum of different types of ophthalmology clinics participated in the study. Interestingly the PACIC summary score

Table 4. Patient Assessment of Chronic Illness Care (PACIC) scores; range 1 to 5, 1 corresponds to poorest concordance with the Chronic Care Model (CCM), 5 corresponds to highest concordance with the CCM; for the construction of the PACIC summary score one missing item was allowed.

PACIC Scores	*Valid n*	*Median*	*Interquartile range*
Summary score[1)]	131	2.4	1.75 to 3.25
Subscale "Patient activation"	141	3.0	1.67 to 4.67
Subscale "Delivery system design/decision support"	133	3.7	2.33 to 4.67
Subscale "Goal setting/tailoring"	138	2.2	1.30 to 3.40
Subscale "Problem solving/contextual counselling"	138	2.0	1.19 to 3.81
Subscale "Follow-up/coordination"	139	1.8	1.00 to 2.60

[1)]For calculation of PACIC summary score one missing item (out of twenty) in the questionnaire was allowed.

showed no significant association with the organization type of the clinics. Although relevant structural differences between hospital-run ophthalmology clinics and single handed ophthalmology practices must be assumed, those differences did not affect the concordance with the CCM from the patients perspective.

According to the inclusion and exclusion criteria, patients that just newly qualified for antiangiogenic therapy were recruited in this study. The sample is thus representative for AMD patients at the beginning of their chronic care situation. The relatively intact ETDRS visual acuity and the high NEI-VFQ-25 scores showed that these patients are mostly in early stages of the disease and have therefore the highest potential to benefit from preventive interventions enabled by successful healthcare delivery.

PACIC scores we identified, however, were modest. The subscale score "follow-up/coordination" was particularly low also in comparison to PACIC scores from research done in other chronic conditions such as diabetes, osteoarthritis or inflammatory bowel disease. [23–25] In AMD, however, a low concordance of follow-up organization with the CCM is especially undesirable because successful follow-up is regarded to be critical for outcomes. [26] It remains, however, debatable whether the PACIC subscales truly represent the different domains of the CCM, because of the high internal consistency of the total PACIC score itself [10,27].

Furthermore, we found specific comorbidities to be associated with low PACIC scores in ophthalmological care. In the case of

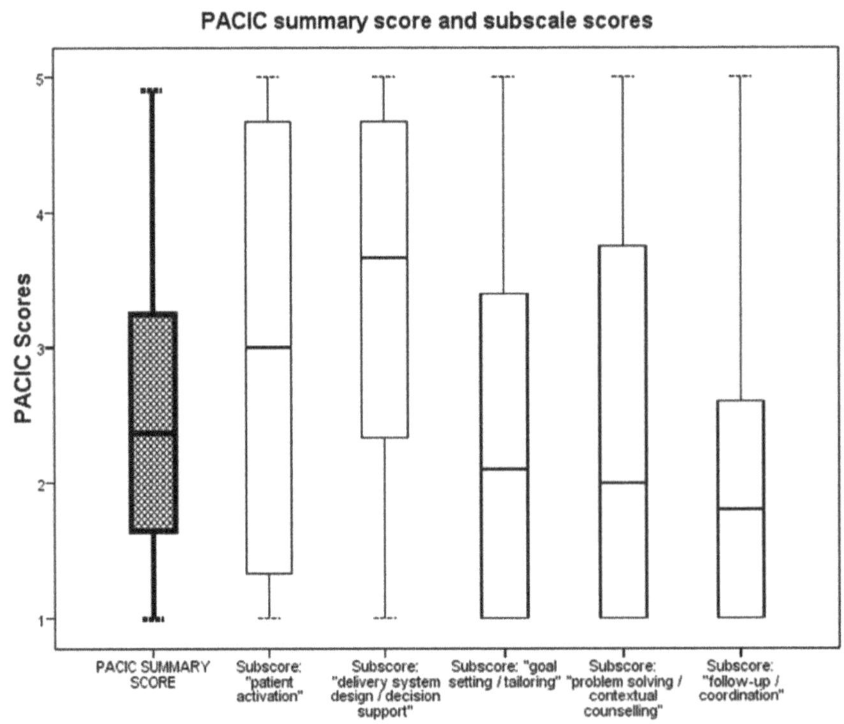

Figure 1. Distribution of PACIC summary score and subscale scores. PACIC scores are represented in boxplots. The PACIC summary score is displayed on the left, other boxplots are the respective PACIC subscale scores. The lower and the upper margin of the box indicate the 25th and 75th percentile respectively. The bar inside the box indicates the median. Whiskers extend to the most extreme data point within 1.5 times the interquartile range.

Table 5. Adjusted Regression Coefficients (95%CI) for the Patient Assessment of Chronic Illness Care (PACIC) summary score (n = 126)[1)].

Variable	*Category*	*Adjusted Regression Coefficient (95%CI)*
Gender	Male	Ref
	Female	−0.06 (−0.41 to 0.29)
Age	Years	0.01 (−0.02 to 0.03)
Visual acuity of better eye	ETDRS	0.008 (−0.004 to 0.02)
Diabetes Type 2	Absent	Ref
	Present	−0.85 (−1.47 to −0.24)*
Coronary artery disease	Absent	Ref
	Present	−0.44 (−0.91; 0.02)†

1)Multivariable regression model adjusted for all determinants in column and additionally controlled for the cluster-effect originating from the different study clinics (n = 126 patients with complete determinant and PACIC data); there was a significant cluster-effect resulting in an intra-class correlation coefficient (ICC) of 9.1% (p = 0.027).
*p = 0.007.
†p = 0.059.

diabetes type 2 this is troublesome because patients with both AMD and diabetes are in the highest need for successful chronic care as their visual acuity is endangered by two treatable chronic conditions simultaneously. With our data we cannot explain this finding of co-occurring conditions being associated with decreased PACIC scores. A possible explanation for this finding could be that ophthalmologists feel less responsible for care for multimorbid patients since they assume that the GP coordinates the care for them.

Limitations

Undoubtedly, the implementation of the different important elements of chronic care is a dynamic process requiring several contacts of healthcare professionals with the individual patient. Patients in our sample, however, were newly entering a chronic care situation for AMD. The PACIC results we obtained might therefore be representative for patients in an early stage of chronic care implementation, thus showing the gaps that still need to be filled. This might especially apply to our results in the "follow-up/coordination" subscale. Only 131 of 169 patients provided enough data to allow calculation of the PACIC summary score. A greater number of cases would have provided more power to detect significant results. Also, we cannot exclude bias from selective answering; we assume, however, that patients dissatisfied with their healthcare would be less motivated to answer the questionnaire, thus causing bias towards false high PACIC scores. PACIC scores in our study would thus tend to be overestimated, the potential for enhancements even greater. Finally, the PACIC score reflects the patient perspective of chronic illness care only, leaving the healthcare provider's perspective unclear.

Conclusion

Generally, care for patients with age related macular degeneration by ophthalmologists is in moderate concordance with the chronic care model. Concerning follow-up and coordination of health service, large improvements are possible, for example with follow-up calls by health service professionals (in order to prevent loss of follow-up during inactive stage of the disease) or with coordination of health service between primary care and specialized ophthalmologic care (in order to allocate responsibilities and avoid under- or overtreatment especially if additional chronic diseases as diabetes exist). Future research should answer the question how healthcare delivery can be improved effecting relevant benefits to patients with AMD.

Acknowledgments

The authors thank Oliver Senn, PhD for statistical assistance.

Author Contributions

Conceived and designed the experiments: TR AF. Performed the experiments: SM AF. Analyzed the data: SM EB AF. Contributed reagents/materials/analysis tools: AF. Contributed to the writing of the manuscript: SM EB AD TR AF. Interpretation of data: SM EB AD TR AF.

References

1. Lochner KA, Cox CS (2013) Prevalence of multiple chronic conditions among Medicare beneficiaries, United States, 2010. Prev Chronic Dis 10: E61.
2. Thorpe KE, Ogden LL, Galactionova K (2010) Chronic conditions account for rise in Medicare spending from 1987 to 2006. Health Aff (Millwood) 29: 718–724.
3. Tsai AC, Morton SC, Mangione CM, Keeler EB (2005) A meta-analysis of interventions to improve care for chronic illnesses. Am J Manag Care 11: 478–488.
4. Wagner EH (1998) Chronic disease management: what will it take to improve care for chronic illness? Eff Clin Pract 1: 2–4.
5. Wagner EH, Austin BT, Davis C, Hindmarsh M, Schaefer J, et al. (2001) Improving chronic illness care: translating evidence into action. Health Aff (Millwood) 20: 64–78.
6. Epping-Jordan JE, Pruitt SD, Bengoa R, Wagner EH (2004) Improving the quality of health care for chronic conditions. Qual Saf Health Care 13: 299–305.
7. Stellefson M, Dipnarine K, Stopka C (2013) The chronic care model and diabetes management in US primary care settings: a systematic review. Prev Chronic Dis 10: E26.
8. Rosemann T, Joos S, Laux G, Gensichen J, Szecsenyi J (2007) Case management of arthritis patients in primary care: a cluster-randomized controlled trial. Arthritis Rheum 57: 1390–1397.
9. Gensichen J, von Korff M, Peitz M, Muth C, Beyer M, et al. (2009) Case management for depression by health care assistants in small primary care practices: a cluster randomized trial. Ann Intern Med 151: 369–378.

10. Glasgow RE, Wagner EH, Schaefer J, Mahoney LD, Reid RJ, et al. (2005) Development and validation of the Patient Assessment of Chronic Illness Care (PACIC). Med Care 43: 436–444.
11. Vedula SS, Krzystolik MG (2008) Antiangiogenic therapy with anti-vascular endothelial growth factor modalities for neovascular age-related macular degeneration. Cochrane Database Syst Rev: CD005139.
12. Chakravarthy U, Williams M, Group AG (2013) The Royal College of Ophthalmologists Guidelines on AMD: Executive Summary. Eye (Lond) 27: 1429–1431.
13. Brand CS (2012) Management of retinal vascular diseases: a patient-centric approach. Eye (Lond) 26 Suppl 2: S1–16.
14. Frei A, Woitzek K, Wang M, Held U, Rosemann T (2011) The chronic care for age-related macular degeneration study (CHARMED): study protocol for a randomized controlled trial. Trials 12: 221.
15. Lowe B, Kroenke K, Herzog W, Grafe K (2004) Measuring depression outcome with a brief self-report instrument: sensitivity to change of the Patient Health Questionnaire (PHQ-9). J Affect Disord 81: 61–66.
16. Schmittdiel J, Mosen DM, Glasgow RE, Hibbard J, Remmers C, et al. (2008) Patient Assessment of Chronic Illness Care (PACIC) and improved patient-centered outcomes for chronic conditions. J Gen Intern Med 23: 77–80.
17. Lamoureux EL, Tee HW, Pesudovs K, Pallant JF, Keeffe JE, et al. (2009) Can clinicians use the PHQ-9 to assess depression in people with vision loss? Optom Vis Sci 86: 139–145.
18. Kroenke K, Spitzer RL, Williams JB (2001) The PHQ-9: validity of a brief depression severity measure. J Gen Intern Med 16: 606–613.
19. Brody BL, Gamst AC, Williams RA, Smith AR, Lau PW, et al. (2001) Depression, visual acuity, comorbidity, and disability associated with age-related macular degeneration. Ophthalmology 108: 1893–1900; discussion 1900–1891.
20. Mangione CM, Lee PP, Gutierrez PR, Spritzer K, Berry S, et al. (2001) Development of the 25-item National Eye Institute Visual Function Questionnaire. Arch Ophthalmol 119: 1050–1058.
21. Revicki DA, Rentz AM, Harnam N, Thomas VS, Lanzetta P (2010) Reliability and validity of the National Eye Institute Visual Function Questionnaire-25 in patients with age-related macular degeneration. Invest Ophthalmol Vis Sci 51: 712–717.
22. Mangione CM (2000) The National Eye Institute 25-Item Visual Function Questionnaire (VFQ-25) - Version 2000. Available: http://www.nei.nih.gov/resources/visionfunction/manual_cm2000.pdf. Accessed 2013 Nov 6.
23. Rosemann T, Laux G, Droesemeyer S, Gensichen J, Szecsenyi J (2007) Evaluation of a culturally adapted German version of the Patient Assessment of Chronic Illness Care (PACIC 5A) questionnaire in a sample of osteoarthritis patients. J Eval Clin Pract 13: 806–813.
24. Frei A, Herzog S, Woitzek K, Held U, Senn O, et al. (2012) Characteristics of poorly controlled Type 2 diabetes patients in Swiss primary care. Cardiovasc Diabetol 11: 70.
25. Randell RL, Long MD, Martin CF, Sandler RS, Chen W, et al. (2013) Patient perception of chronic illness care in a large inflammatory bowel disease cohort. Inflammatory bowel diseases 19: 1428–1433.
26. Rasmussen A, Bloch SB, Fuchs J, Hansen LH, Larsen M, et al. (2013) A 4-Year Longitudinal Study of 555 Patients Treated with Ranibizumab for Neovascular Age-related Macular Degeneration. Ophthalmology 120: 2630–2636.
27. Gugiu C, Coryn CL, Applegate B (2010) Structure and measurement properties of the Patient Assessment of Chronic Illness Care instrument. J Eval Clin Pract 16: 509–516.

5

Acute Increase of Children's Conjunctivitis Clinic Visits by Asian Dust Storms Exposure - A Spatiotemporal Study in Taipei, Taiwan

Lung-Chang Chien[1], Yi-Jen Lien[2], Chiang-Hsin Yang[3], Hwa-Lung Yu[2]*

1 Division of Biostatistics, University of Texas School of Public Health at San Antonio Regional Campus, San Antonio, Texas, United States of America, **2** Department of Bioenvironmental Systems Engineering, National Taiwan University, Taipei, Taiwan, **3** Department of Health Care Management, National Taipei University of Nursing and Health Sciences, Taipei, Taiwan

Abstract

Adverse health impacts of Asian dust storms (ADS) have been widely investigated and discussed in respiratory disease, but no study has examined the association between ADS events and their impact on eye diseases, especially in children. The impact of ADS events on the incidence of children's conjunctivitis is examined by analyzing the data from children's clinic visits registered in the 41 districts of Taipei area in Taiwan during the period 2002–2007. The structural additive regression modeling approach was used to assess the association between ADS events and clinic visits for conjunctivitis in children with consideration of day-of-the-week effects, temperature, and air quality levels. This study identifies an acute increase in the relative rate for children's conjunctivitis clinic visits during ADS periods with 1.48% (95% CI = 0.79, 2.17) for preschool children (aged <6 years old) and 9.48% (95% CI = 9.03, 9.93) for schoolchildren (aged ≥ 6 years old), respectively. The relative rates during post-ADS periods were still statistically significant, but much lower than those during ADS periods. The spatial analysis presents geographic heterogeneity of children's conjunctivitis clinic visits where higher relative rates were more likely observed in the most populated districts Compared to previous ADS studies related to respiratory diseases, our results reveals significantly acute impacts on children's conjunctivitis during ADS periods, and much influence on schoolchildren. Vulnerable areas were also identified in high density population.

Editor: Chen-Wei Pan, Medical College of Soochow University, China

Funding: This research and data collection was supported by funds from the National Science Council of Taiwan (NSC101-2628-E-002-017-MY3 and NSC101-2628-E-002-003) and the Environmental Protection Department of the New Taipei City Government (Taiwan). The funders had no role in study design, data collection and analysis, decision to publish, or preparation of the manuscript.

Competing Interests: The authors have declared that no competing interests exist.

* Email: hlyu@ntu.edu.tw

Introduction

Asian dust storm (ADS) events, severe wide-spread disasters that spawn from Mongolia and North China, cause many diseases including respiratory diseases, cardiovascular diseases, asthma, chronic obstructive pulmonary disease, pneumonia, and stroke. The health outcomes of these diseases range from death to various stages of illness that may require hospital admissions, emergency room visits, and clinic visits [1–7]. ADS events diversely impact human health primarily due to a rapid elevation of concentrated levels of air pollutants over a large scale area in a short period of time [8]. Inhalation of air pollutants during these storms has been implicated as the leading cause of adverse health effects. However, eye exposure to direct contact with air pollutants during these storms and the subsequent development of conjunctivitis has rarely been discussed.

The eyes are particularly vulnerable and highly sensitive to direct contact with air pollutants due to the dense neuronal innervations on the ocular surface [9]. For eye-related diseases which are highly correlated with exposure to air pollutants, conjunctivitis is the most significant Conjunctivitis, defined as an irritation or an inflammation of the conjunctiva, usually elicits symptoms of eye irritation and itching. Previous research has established an association between the development of conjunctivitis and the ambient levels of outdoor air pollution or airborne allergens, such as fungal spores and pollen grains [10–12]. Indoor air pollution, such as the cooking smoke from the combustion of biomass (e.g., charcoal, wood, and dung), has also been investigated as a causal agent in the development of conjunctivitis and other eye diseases [13]. ADS events are characterized by extremely high concentrations of air pollutants and allergens compared to the concentrations of these same pollutants and allergens during general periods. Thus, the development of conjunctivitis as a result of exposure during ADS events would be highly likely [14]. However, epidemiological research on the ADS effects to eye health is still rare,, and has not yielded any significant findings [15].

Children, in particular, are very susceptible to the adverse effects of airborne exposures because their immune systems are not as fully developed as those of adults [16]. Previous studies focused on the adverse effects of air pollution on children's health in terms of both short-term [17–21] and long-term exposure [22–24], These pediatrics researches have been centered on investigating pulmonary and lung dysfunction, asthma and respiratory symptoms, and pneumonias, especially for the case of the studies regarding to the influence of ADS events In addition, findings regarding the health impact of ADS events are commonly uncertain because of limited health observations [25]. In the other words, previous ADS and children's health studies have seldom focused on conjunctivitis and analyzed large scale populations of children observed over long periods of time and at varied locations [26]. Due to the availability of nationwide health insurance data in Taiwan, it allows the population-based analysis to reveal the epidemiological linkages between ADS events and the diseases of concern, e.g. conjunctivitis [27,28].

The main purpose of this study was to investigate the spatiotemporal influence of ADS events on the development of conjunctivitis in children by using a large, population-based database taken from daily clinic visits registered in hospitals and clinics in Northern Taiwan from 2002–2007. Specifically, three main questions were addressed: (1) whether there is an increase in children's clinic visits for conjunctivitis during ADS events and for one week after the storm; (2) whether preschool children are more vulnerable than school children to the impact of ADS events as they relate to the development of conjunctivitis; and (3) whether geographic location plays a role in the impact of ADS events on children's conjunctivitis clinic visits.

Materials and Methods

Ethic statement: The data were obtained from National Health Research Institute of Taiwan (NHRI). All of the data request should be approved by IRB of NHRI. The approval number of this study is NHIRD-102-097. Due to concerns regarding personal confidentiality, all individually identifiable health information (e.g., personal identification or hospital identification number) is encrypted prior to release.

Children's clinic visit data

This study retrieve the children's clinic visit data from Taiwan's National Health Insurance (NHI) database which covers the claim data of over 99.6% of the inhabitants of the entire Taiwan, including both emergency and ambulatory visits for various diseases and diagnosis. The database uses International Classification of Diseases, Ninth Revision, Clinical Modification (ICD-9-CM) classification codes to record cause-specific data. Due to concerns regarding personal confidentiality, all individually identifiable health information (e.g., personal identification or hospital identification number) is encrypted prior to release from Bureau of NHI. This study retrieved patients aged ≤14 years with recorded conjunctival disorders (ICD-9: 372). Because children older than 6 years old in Taiwan receive compulsory education, this population was categorized into a preschool group for <6 years-old and a schoolchildren group aged ≥6 years old. This population-based data also contained space-time information for any clinic and hospital visits of children with the diagnosis of conjunctivitis in Taipei City and New Taipei City from 2002–2007. These visits included both ambulatory and emergency room encounters.

Study Area

Taipei has more than six million citizens within an area of approximately 2324.37 km^2. Taipei is best described as a geographic location in Northern Taiwan that contains two administrative regions, Taipei City and New Taipei City. Among them, New Taipei City surrounds Taipei City. The northern boundary is the coastline for to the Taiwan Straits and the Pacific Ocean. This northern coastline border offers no geographic barrier to ADS events that sweep in from the north. In addition, Taipei City has a characteristic basin type of topography that is geographically bounded by three different Mountains to the north, the west, and the southeast. The basin topography reduces air diffusion and increases air pollutant concentrations. According to insurance administrative divisions, a total of 41 districts are contained in the study area with 12 districts for Taipei City and 29 districts for New Taipei City, as shown in Figure 1.

Asian dust storm and air pollution data

A total of 30 ADS events occurring from 2002–2007 were identified by the Taiwan Environmental Protection Agency (TWEPA), during a total of 90 days (Table 1). The TWEPA defines the criteria to determine the incidence of a ADS event, including performing a dust storm track nowcasting along with Taiwan Central Weather Bureau, interpreting remote sensing data, and observing the PM_{10} level at the four ADS indicator stations, i.e., Matsu, Wanli, Guanyin, and Yilan. If forecasting results reveal a high probability that ADS events are headed toward Taiwan, the TWEPA will issue warnings when at least one of the four indicator stations measure PM_{10} concentrations > 100 $\mu g/m^3$ [29]. For the analyses purposes the study period from 2002 to 2007 was divided into three sub-periods. First, the time period of the actual ADS event (Table 1) is defined as the ADS period. Second, the time period up to and including 7 days after an ADS event has ended is defined as the post-ADS period. Third, all the other days in the study period are defined as the other period. In addition to the ADS data, PM_{10} concentrations have been regularly monitored at TWEPA stations across Taiwan since 1994. Both the PM_{10} concentrations and temperature measurements used in our analysis were based on the daily observations at the Jhongshan monitoring station located in the most populated area of Taipei City (see Figure 1).

Statistical Modeling Analysis

We analyzed the spatiotemporal pattern of children's conjunctivitis clinic visits in the 41 study districts from 2002 to 2007 using a structured additive regression (STAR) model. The count data for clinic visits followed a Poisson distribution, and can be modeled via a Poisson model framework taking into account both linear and nonlinear explanatory variables, i.e.,

$$Y_{dt}|\mu_{dt} \sim \text{Poisson}(\mu_{dt})$$

Y_{ct} is the number of children's conjunctivitis clinic visits in district d (d = 1, 2,..., 41) at day t (t = 1, 2,..., 2191).

$$\log(\mu_{dt}) = \text{intercept} + X'\beta + Z'\gamma + f(TP) + f(T) + f_{spat}(d) + \log(POP),$$

where μ_{dt} is the expected value of Y_{dt}. The β is a vector of categorical fixed effects $X = [I_{MON}, I_{TUE}, I_{WED}, I_{THUR}, I_{FRI}, I_{SAT}, I_{ADS}, I_{POST\text{-}ADS}]'$ corresponding to six dummy variables for day-of-the-week (DOW) from Monday to Saturday plus two dummy

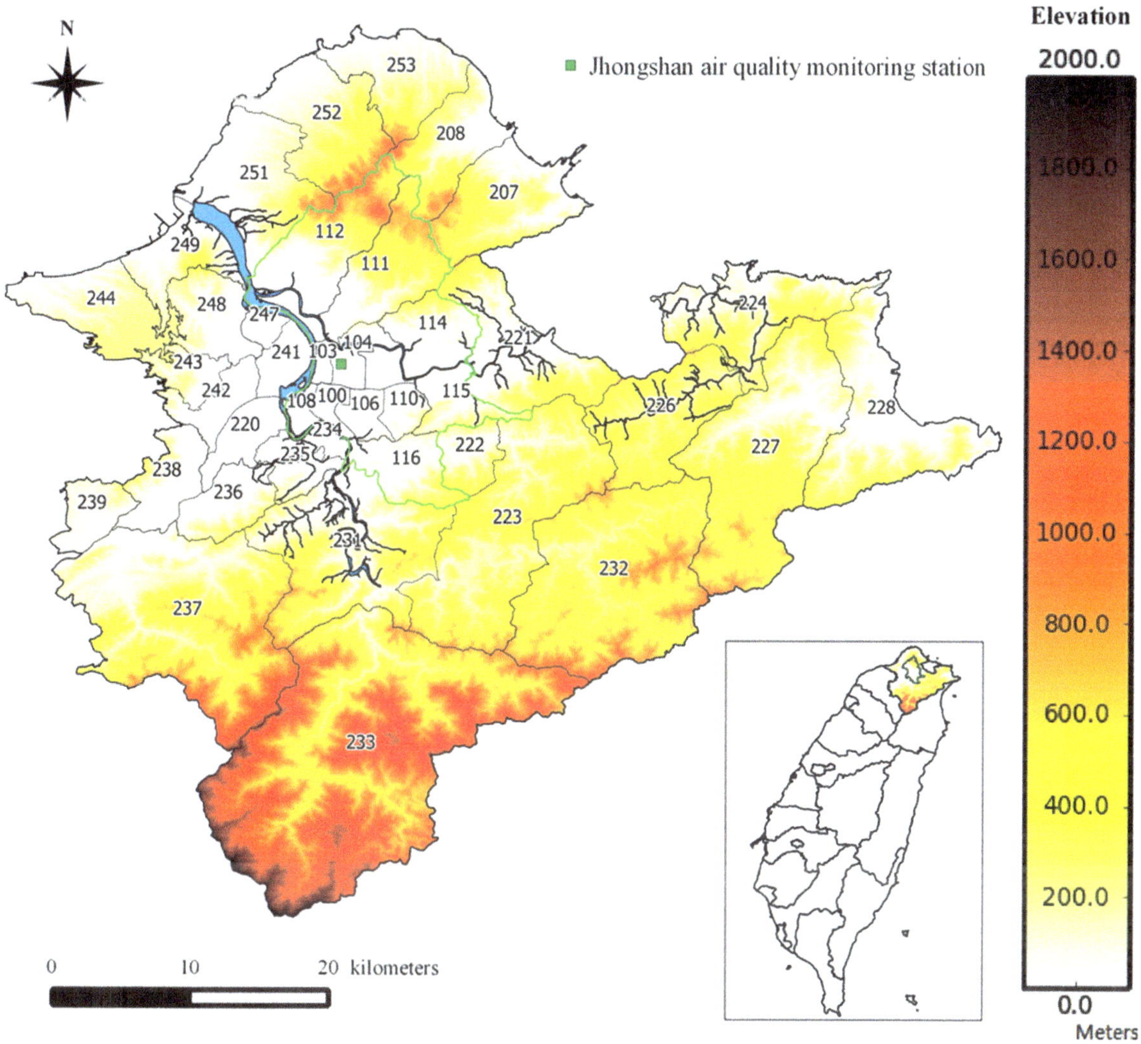

Zip code	District name	Zip code	District name	Zip code	District name	Zip code	District name	Zip code	District name
100	Jhongjheng	112	Beitou	222	Shenkeng	233	Wulai	242	Sinjhuang
103	Datong	114	Neihu	223	Shihding	234	Yonghe	243	Taishan
104	Jhongshan	115	Nangang	224	Rueifang	235	Jhonghe	244	Linkou
105	Songshan	116	Wunshan	226	Pingsi	236	Tucheng	247	Lujhou
106	Daan	207	Wanli	227	Shuangsi	237	Sansia	248	Wugu
108	Wanhua	208	Jinshan	228	Gongliao	238	Shulin	249	Bali
110	Sinyi	220	Banciao	231	Sindian	239	Yingge	251	Danshui
111	Shilin	221	Sijhih	232	Pinglin	241	Sanchong	252	Sanjhih
								253	Shihmen

Figure 1. Map of Taipei City (surrounded by green boundaries) and New Taipei City, along with the map of their geographical locations in the Taiwan Island. The district names are denoted by their zip codes with the names shown at the table below. The Jhongshan air quality monitoring station is highlighted by a green square.

variables for the ADS period and post-ADS period. Theoretically, DOW variables are mainly used to adjust for short-term temporal autoregressive correlations. From a practical standpoint, we are able to investigate the peak number of children's conjunctivitis clinic visits within one week of an ADS event which reflects a special attribute of medical service in Taiwan. Two ADS variables can be used to evaluate the impact of ADS on children's conjunctivitis clinic visit during the ADS period and the post-ADS period compared to other period. The γ is the vector of continuous confounders Z, which contains at least one of five air pollutants (CO, NO_x, O_3, PM_{10}, and SO_2). Two nonlinear smoothing functions for calendar time T and for daily mean temperature TP applied a B-spline with a second order random walk penalty [30,31] to adjust for long-term temporal trends and the effects of weather. The spatial function $f_{spat}(d)$ is defined by a structured spatial effect using the Markov random fields [32] with a normally distributed conditional autoregressive prior:

$$f_{spat}(d')|d \neq d' \sim N(\Sigma_{d' \in \Theta_d} f_{spat}(d')/N_d, \sigma_d^2/N_d),$$

Table 1. Dust storm events in Taiwan, 2002–2007.

Year	Date	# of events	# of days
2002	2/11-2/12, 3/6-3/9, 3/23-3/24, 3/31-4/1, 4/8-4/15, 4/17-4/19	6	21
2003	2/18-2/19, 2/23-2/25, 3/6-3/9, 3/25-3/30, 4/25-4/28	5	19
2004	1/1-1/4, 1/13-1/14, 1/21-1/22, 1/24-1/25, 2/6-2/12, 2/14-2/16, 2/26-2/27, 3/3-3/7, 4/2-4/4	9	30
2005	3/18-3/19, 11/29-11/30, 12/21-12/22	3	6
2006	3/19-3/20, 3/29-3/30, 4/20-4/21	3	6
2007	1/28-1/29, 4/2-4/3, 4/17-4/18, 12/30-12/31	4	8

where the denominator N_d in both the mean and the variance is the number of neighboring districts adjacent to district d, and θ_d is a subset of neighbors of district d. The variance σ^2_d and unknown smoothing parameters are estimated simultaneously with hyperpriors following an inverse Gamma distribution IG(0.001, 0.001). Last, the term log(POP) is the offset defined by the logarithm of the district-level population of children approximated by multiplying the proportion of children in Taipei by the total population of each district.

The STAR model's estimates are calculated according to an empirical Bayes influence that utilizes a restricted maximum likelihood method. This is a surrogate of the maximum likelihood method designed to avoid the loss of degrees of freedom and to prevent biasing estimated coefficients toward zero [33,34]. Model selection for choosing the best combinations of air pollutants utilized the Akaike Information Criterion (AIC) [35]. Specifically, seven one-pollutant models were fitted for selecting significant positive estimated coefficients of air pollutants. Then, several two-pollutant and three-pollutant models were fitted retaining the significant air pollutants from one-pollutant models. Only the models with positively significant air pollutants were included in the selection to determine the final model according to the smallest AIC separately for preschool children and schoolchildren. In these models, the estimated coefficient of this fixed effect can be explained by the percentage change in the relative rate (RR) of children's conjunctivitis clinic visits compared to the reference level. The spatial function can be interpreted by the RR in district 'd' compared with the mean value for the population as a whole and accounting for spatial autocorrelations by taking a logarithm of it [36]. The spatial effect in each district has a posterior distribution which can be used to generate a 95% credible interval (CI) in order to determine the significance of each spatial estimate according to the 95% posterior probability. For a more meaningful presentation, the spatial effect can be categorized into: (1) a strictly positive effect if 95% of the posterior distribution is above one; (2) a strictly negative effect if 95% of the posterior distribution is below one; (3) a non-significant effect if 95% of the posterior distribution contains one. Maps for the estimated spatial effects with corresponding 95% posterior probability were constructed to highlight the spatial pattern of children's conjunctivitis clinic visits. Data were cleaned and managed by using SAS v9.3 software (SAS Institute Inc., Cary, NC), and the spatiotemporal data analyses were accomplished by the BayesX v2.01 software package [37].

Results

Figure 2 depicts the crude rate of daily children's conjunctivitis clinic visits among the 41 districts in Taipei, clearly demonstrating that the crude clinic visit rate was not uniformly distributed across the study area. By city, the crude rate per 100,000 children in Taipei City ranged from 47.98 to 266.28, but there was a wider range from 0.72 to 400.89 in New Taipei City, which means that the geographic disparity of children's conjunctivitis morbidity there may be larger than that in Taipei City. Table 2 documents that the daily average measurements of O_3 and PM_{10} were elevated during the ADS period. Their averages decreased during the post-ADS period, but were still higher than levels during other period. The other air pollutants had decreased average measurements from the other period through the ADS period, but these were increased during the post-ADS period.

Figure 3 gives ranked values of AIC for the fit and complexity of the selected models. It suggests that among those 31 models, the AIC was when more air pollutants were included, and the smallest AIC appeared in the five-pollutant models. Models shown in red dots in Figure 3 were not considered because they had non-significant or significantly negative estimates even if they had a smaller AIC. Therefore, the four-pollutant model NO_x+O_3+PM_{10}+SO_2 for preschool children and the two-pollutant model NOx+O3 for schoolchildren were finally determined as the best final models.

Table 3 displays the percentage change of RR for children's conjunctivitis clinic visits, suggesting: (1) Compared to Sunday, a relatively higher percentage of RR increase for preschool children's and schoolchildren's conjunctivitis clinic visits was more likely happened on a Monday, a Wednesday, and a Saturday; (2) schoolchildren had a higher increased percentage change in RR than preschool children for conjunctivitis clinic visits during ADS periods; (3) a lasting positive impact (i.e., an increased percentage change of RR) during post-ADS periods was noted in schoolchildren; and (4) both NO_2 and O_3 were significantly and positively associated with children's conjunctivitis clinic visits. Specifically, the strongest DOW effect appeared on Monday for preschool children with a 47.90% (95% CI = 47.33, 48.47) elevated RR and on Saturday for schoolchildren with a 29.20% (95% CI = 28.67, 29.72) elevated RR, compared to Sunday, a day on which the clinics are closed. During the ADS period, the RR significantly increased 1.48% (95% CI = 0.79, 2.17) for preschool children's conjunctivitis clinic visits, while the percentage increased over 6-fold to 9.48% (95% CI = 9.03, 9.93) for schoolchildren. This impact did not extend through the post-ADS period for preschool children and the effect showed a negative decline with a −2.16% (95% CI = −2.68, −1.63) RR. However, schoolchildren were still significantly affected during the post-ADS period with a 2.32% (95% CI = 1.98, 2.66) elevation in the RR for conjunctivitis clinic visits. Moreover, air pollutants, NO_x and O_3, also had a stronger influence on conjunctivitis clinic visits for schoolchildren than for preschool children. Interestingly, O_3 had a stronger impact than NO_x for both groups.

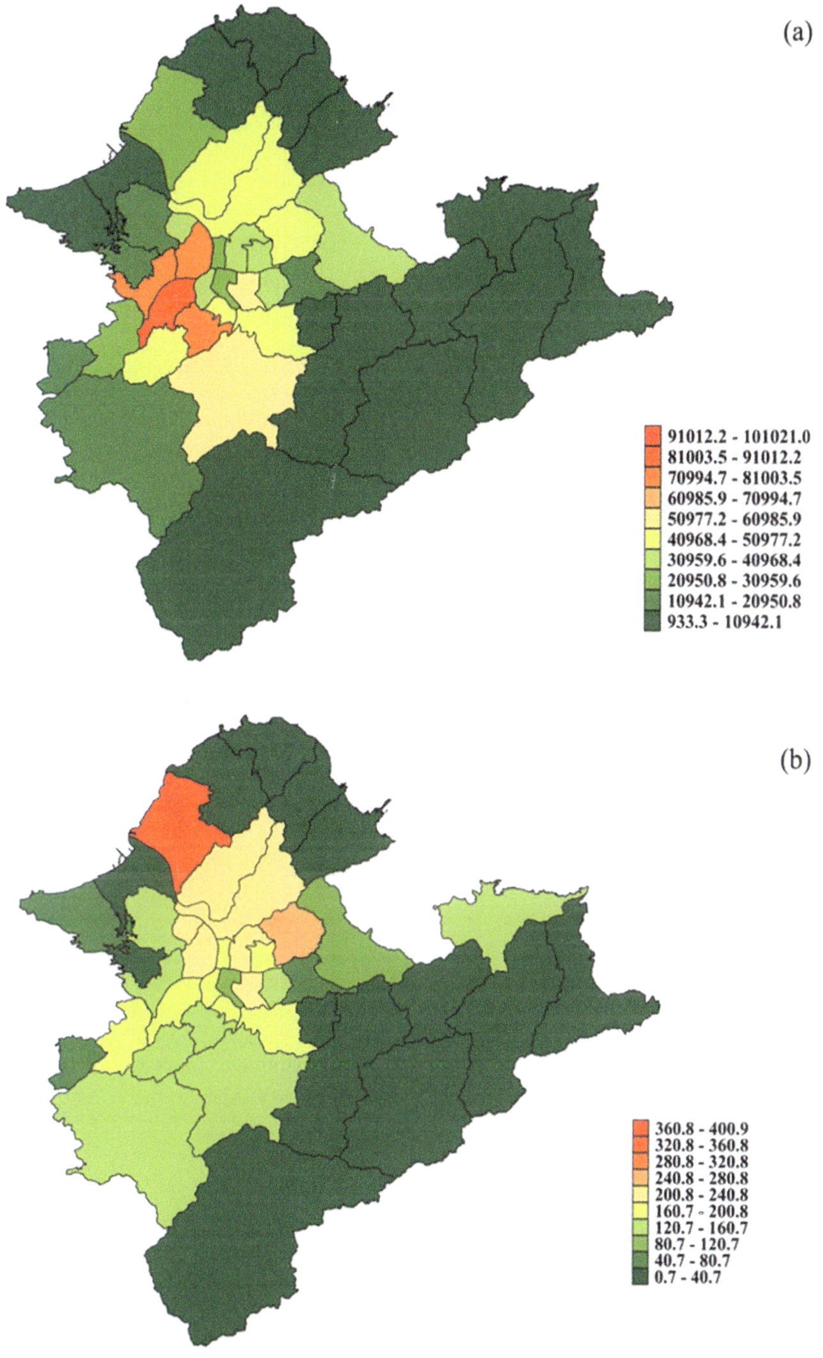

Figure 2. Maps of (a) spatial distribution of the average children population and (b) crude daily children's conjunctivitis clinic visit rate per 100,000 children population in Taipei, 2002–2007.

The influences of time and temperature on children's conjunctivitis clinic visits demonstrated a greater RR during summers when the temperature was hotter (see Figure 4). In particular, in preschool children there was a consistent significantly positive association between conjunctivitis clinic visits and temperature, especially when the temperature increased from 23.92°C to 26.19°C. The greatest RR = 1.18 (95% CI = 1.12, 1.25) appeared at an extremely hot temperature (33.76°C). For schoolchildren, a significant RR >1 for conjunctivitis clinic visits happened between temperatures of 21.80°C to 26.61°C, and the greatest RR of 1.11 (95% CI = 1.07, 1.16) occurred at a temperature of 24.84°C.

Figure 5 depicts the distribution of spatial effects attributed to children's conjunctivitis clinic visits across 41 districts. It suggests that the significant RR >1, appeared in the more populated areas which included 11 of the 12 districts in Taipei City and 16 of the 29 districts in New Taipei City. Districts near the mountains in the southwest and the coastlines in the north exhibited a significant RR<1. The two maps of 95% posterior probability in the two children's groups were almost identical, except for the Nangang

Table 2. Average measurement of air pollutants during ADS periods, post-ADS periods and Other periods in Taipei, Taiwan, 2002–2007.

Air pollutant	ADS period		Post-ADS period		Other period		P-value††
	Mean	Std†	Mean	Std†	Mean	Std	
CO (ppm)	0.82	0.30	1.01	0.33	0.88	0.32	<.0001
NO_x (ppb)	45.50	17.43	60.10	23.38	49.77	19.51	<.0001
O_3 (ppb)	25.13	7.40	20.60	8.00	18.99	8.29	<.0001
PM_{10} ($\mu g/m^3$)	81.11	35.41	63.04	25.44	53.32	22.51	<.0001
SO_2 (ppb)	3.91	2.03	4.17	2.28	4.35	2.08	<.0001

†Std = standard deviation.
††P-value was determined by the ANOVA test with null hypothesis H_0: $\mu_{ADS} = \mu_{post\text{-}ADS} = \mu_{other}$.

District. Moreover, out of all the 27 districts with a significantly elevated RR, the average RR was 2.70 for preschool children and 3.80 for schoolchildren. The Danshui District displayed the strongest spatial effect contributing to conjunctivitis clinic visits for both children's groups. Comparisons between the two children's groups reveal that 25 of the 41 districts had larger RRs for schoolchildren's conjunctivitis clinic visits than for preschool children's conjunctivitis clinic visits. Of these districts, 11 were in Taipei City and 14 were in New Taipei City.

Discussion

As extreme weather events, ADS bring a higher concentration of air pollutants to Taiwan, and lead to increased risk of disease incidence and hospitalizations. This risk has been documented to be heterogeneous across space and time [38]. Previous studies emphasized the ADS impact on upper respiratory tract diseases, pneumonia and cardiovascular diseases [4,5,39]. Thus far, no significant finding related to the impact of ADS on the development of conjunctivitis had been documented [15]. This may have been due to inadequate sample sizes and the lack of inclusion of spatiotemporal associations leading to insufficient power and possible biases [15]. This research reveals the statistically significant associations between ADS exposure and children's eye health. Based on the large Taiwan National Health Insurance dataset, this study has a lower risk of containing biased estimates resulting from sampling limitations. In addition, spatial and temporal autocorrelations relating to health outcomes are also controlled in this analysis. Therefore, this study reliably provides objective findings based on a large sample size that also covers a broad geographic area during the defined study period and utilizes a well-established statistical modeling approach.

In this study, we found a significant association between ADS exposure and conjunctivitis in both preschool children and schoolchildren. Previous findings showed a similar association between ADS exposure and respiratory diseases in children [26–28]. Importantly, this study notes that increased impacts of children's conjunctivitis occurred during ADS periods; while increased impacts of children's respiratory illnesses occurred during post-ADS periods [26–28]. Moreover, during the ADS period, schoolchildren had a 6.41 times higher percentage of RR for conjunctivitis clinic visits than preschool children. Previous research has shown that the increase of PM concentration outdoors during ADS events is significantly higher than the increase of PM concentration indoors [40]. While the prevalent seasons for ADS events, winter and spring, overlap the two academic semesters, there is not an ADS-related class suspension policy in Taiwan. As a result, schoolchildren have a higher chance of outdoor exposures during ADS events, going to and from school, than preschool children. Schoolchildren may also have more outdoor activities than preschool children. This exposure most likely explains a greater increase in the conjunctivitis clinic visit rates for schoolchildren. The influence of schoolchildren and preschool children had opposite directions during post-ADS period where schoolchildren still positively affected by ADS with an increased RR% (2.32%) while preschool children's RR% became negative (−2.16%). This situation may be explained by the distinct behavior patterns between the two groups of children. Schoolchildren, as compared to preschool children, have a greater opportunity for ADS exposures during and after the ADS events because they experience more outdoor activities. The negative RR% in preschool children could be interpreted by a protective mentality of parents who feel uncertainty about when the ADS finishes, and may bring children outside to look for eye doctors

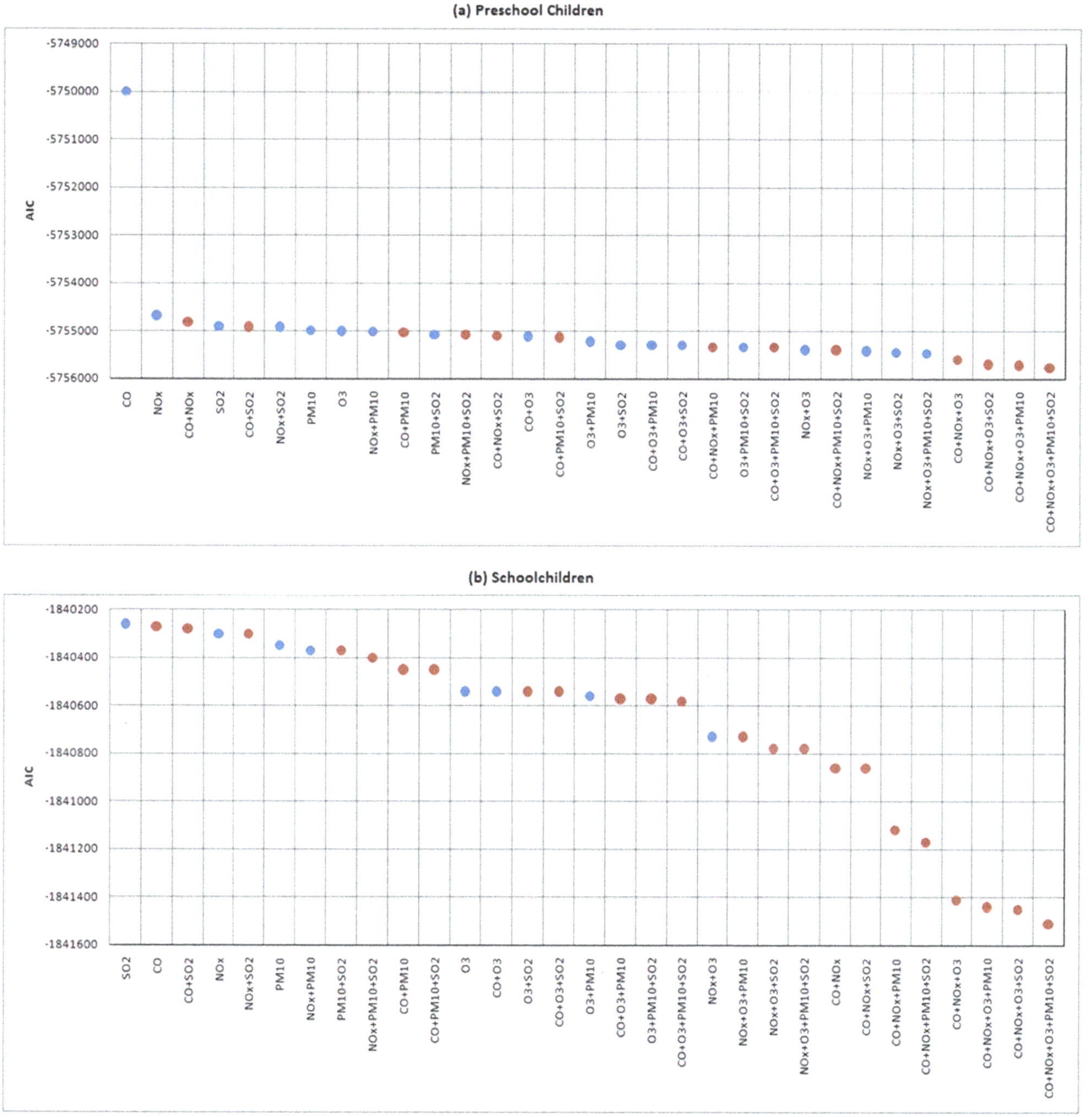

Figure 3. The model selection for (a) preschool children and (b) schoolchildren, where blue dots represent models with all significantly positive estimates for air pollutants, and red dots represent models with at least one non-significant or significantly negative estimate for air pollutants. Our final models were only considered among blue dots.

instead of directly using medicines which can be bought from pharmacy stores without prescriptions.

In order to delineate the health impact of ADS events in regards to conjunctivitis, the short-term and long-term temporal patterns of conjunctivitis clinic visit rates were also analyzed. Among them, the day-of-week pattern is an important confounding factor for clinic visits, and this is true for other diseases as shown in previous studies [26,27]. In Taiwan, major medical services in both hospitals and clinics are closed from Saturday afternoon until Monday morning. Therefore, there is a strong incentive to visit clinics on Saturday (before the weekend effect) and Monday (after the weekend effect). The day-of-the-week clinic visit pattern observed in this study is quite consistent with the medical care-seeking pattern that has resulted under the current national health care delivery system in Taiwan. Moreover, the highly elevated relative rates on Monday essentially accounts for those patients unable to seek medical treatments from Saturday through Sunday. In the case of children, who are incapable of accessing clinic care independently and are dependent on a parent's working schedule which allows for only nighttime availability, this may be especially true. In addition, while the implementation of NHI in Taiwan increases the accessibility of medical services with relatively low co-

Table 3. Percentage change of relative rate in children's conjunctivitis clinic visits.

	Preschool children		Schoolchildren	
Variable	**%**	**95% CI**	**%**	**95% CI**
Day-of-week†				
Monday	47.90	(47.33, 48.47)	26.75	(26.41, 27.10)
Tuesday	6.91	(6.44, 7.38)	−7.13	(−7.41, −6.84)
Wednesday	14.43	(13.95, 14.92)	26.82	(26.48, 27.17)
Thursday	3.18	(2.72, 3.63)	−13.23	(−13.50, −12.96)
Friday	6.42	(5.96, 6.89)	4.17	(3.87, 4.47)
Saturday	29.20	(28.67, 29.72)	74.70	(74.29, 75.12)
ADS episode†				
ADS period	1.48	(0.79, 2.17)	9.48	(9.03, 9.93)
Post-ADS period	−2.16	(−2.68, −1.63)	2.32	(1.98, 2.66)
Air pollutant (interquartile range)††				
NO_x (22.16 ppb)	1.63	(1.34, 1.92)	3.49	(3.34, 3.66)
O_3 (11.22 ppb)	3.26	(2.93, 3.59)	6.21	(6.02, 6.40)
PM_{10} (29.88 μg/m^3)	0.42	(0.10, 0.74)	–	–
SO_2 (2.63 ppb)	1.19	(0.87, 1.51)	–	–

†The reference level of day-of-week and ADS episode are Sunday and the other days, respectively.
††The estimate was presented by the increase percentage of relative rate for an interquartile range change in air pollutants, calculated from [exp(interquartile range×estimated coefficient)−1]×100%.

payments, prescription medications can only be issued for a three day period [41]. After three days, the patient must see the physician again to obtain more medication if necessary. This prescription regulation may induce higher clinic visit rates on Wednesdays as noted in this study and in previous studies [27].

This study reveals a geographic heterogeneity for conjunctivitis incidence as verified by studying the documented clinic visits. Notably, there is a decreasing trend in relative rates from the northwestern coastal districts to the urban areas. In particular, the Danshui District has a greater RR than its surrounding coastal districts, i.e., the Sanjhih District, Shihmen District, Jinshan District, Wanli District, and Bali District. This result can be attributed to the imbalance of medical resources in the area. Though the northwestern coastal districts are noted for their

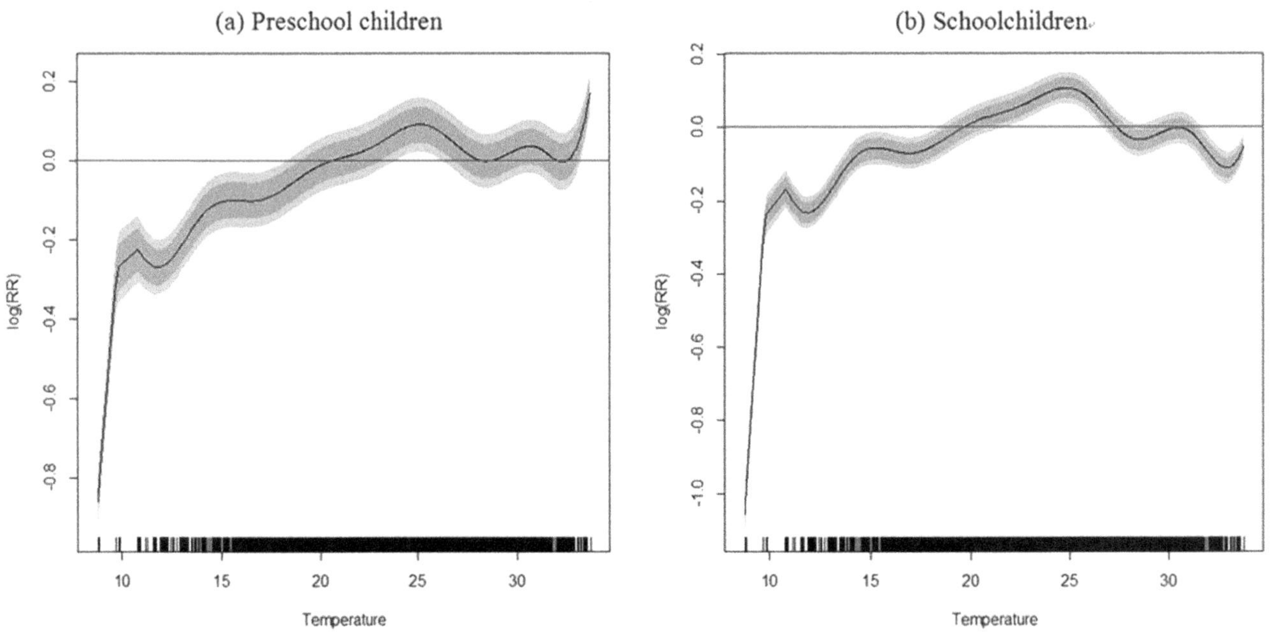

Figure 4. Temperature smoother for (a) preschool children's and (b) schoolchildren's conjunctivitis clinic visits. Dark grey and light grey colors represent 80% and 95% credible intervals, respectively.

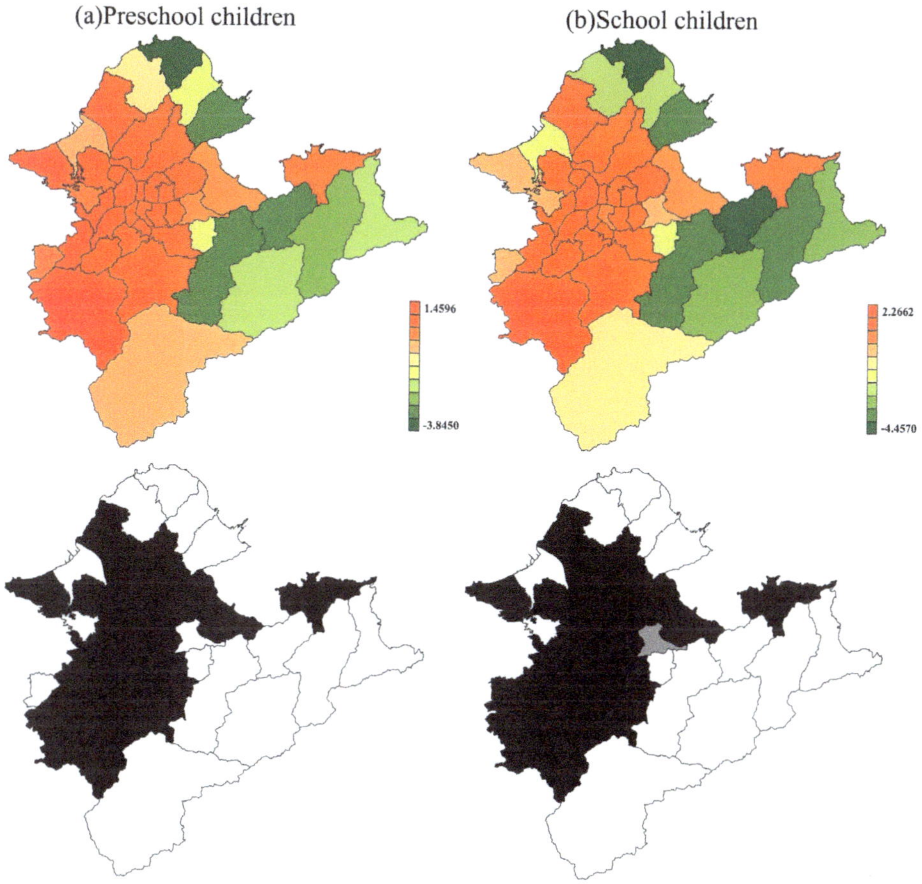

Figure 5. Maps of spatial effects (upper) with corresponding significance (lower) for (a) preschool children's and (b) schoolchildren's conjunctivitis clinic visits in Taipei, Taiwan, 2002–2007, presented by RR. In upper plots, the red color signifies higher RR, and the green color signifies lower RR. In lower plots, black and white areas demonstrate districts where the RR is statistically greater than 1 and smaller than 1, respectively. Grey areas demonstrate no significant difference.

popular oceanic recreational areas for swimmers and tourists, the numbers of well-equipped hospitals and clinics are much less numerous than in the Danshui District. In addition, the lack of eye departments in coastal area might propel residents to consult the medical center in Danshui district. Convenient transportation is another advantage in that eye clinics in the Danshui District are more accessible than nearby areas. As a result, medical services located in the Danshui District are most often the first choice for the tourists and local residents. Another important factor contributing to the increase in conjunctivitis clinic visits in this district relates to its geographical location. The Danshui District is located near an outlet where the Danshui River flows into the Taiwan Strait and therefore, sits at the opening of the Taipei Basin. Because of this location, wind speeds are generally higher in the Danshui District [42]. Studies have shown that dust and wind are the major irritating factors that often trigger eye diseases, such as conjunctivitis [12,43,44]. The distinct features of the spatial function in the STAR model not only control for spatial autocorrelation, but also facilitate the analysis of the geographical heterogeneity in conjunctivitis clinic visit. In addition, short-term and long-term temporal pattern modeling could be performed as in other diseases and health outcomes [26–28]. After consideration of the general spatial and temporal patterns of conjunctivitis clinic visit rates and their associations with covariates, ambient pollutants may better differentiate the health impact from ADS exposure on the subsequent development of conjunctivitis.

This study has three main limitations: First, the study period of this research is restricted to only 6 years because of inconsistent disease coding without the use of ICD-9 before 2002 plus a funding shortage after 2007. Second, some potential allergies to conjunctivitis, such as pollen grain and fungal spores, do not have district-level measurements, so this study is unable to include them as confounding predictors. Third, the STAR model has a complicated estimating algorithm in that, sometimes, unknown parameters cannot converge. This is especially when considering pre-ADS periods for 7 days prior to ADS periods or longer post-ADS periods up to 14 days.

Conclusions

This study demonstrates significantly elevated risks in children's clinic visits due to conjunctivitis in both preschool children and schoolchildren during ADS periods in Taipei, Taiwan. This acute impact produced an increased percentage of RR for clinic visits due to conjunctivitis in schoolchildren during the ADS period, and lasted during the 1 week post-ADS period. In addition, new evidence about the spatial disparities for the adverse effects of ADS events on children's eye health in northern Taiwan was also discovered. Children in all ages are suggested to reduce their overall outdoor exposure time during the ADS period and the post-ADS period, especially for schoolchildren who live in high risk districts. The results and findings of this study should be of particular concern to policy makers or media outlets that are responsible for issuing ADS warnings in advance.

Acknowledgments

We appreciate the Bureau of National Health Insurance for providing the clinic visit database. We also thank Dr. Shyh-Dye Lee for his constructive comments for the result interpretation, as well as Mary Trottier and Dr. Robert Woods for editing the English writing of the article.

Author Contributions

Conceived and designed the experiments: HLY LCC. Performed the experiments: LCC YJL CHY. Analyzed the data: LCC YJL. Contributed reagents/materials/analysis tools: LCC CHY HLY. Wrote the paper: HLY LCC.

References

1. Tam WWS, Wong TW, Wong AHS, Hui DSC (2011) Effect of dust storm events on daily emergency admissions for respiratory diseases. Respirology: no-no.
2. Lee EC, Leem J, Hong YC, Kim H, Kim HC (2008) Effects of Asian Dust Storm Events on Daily Admissions for Asthma and Stroke in Seven Metropolitans of Korea. Epidemiology 19: S145 110.1097/1001.ede.0000339954.000035 5923.cc.
3. Chiu HF, Tiao MM, Ho SC, Kuo HW, Wu TN, et al. (2008) Effects of Asian dust storm events on hospital admissions for chronic obstructive pulmonary disease in Taipei, Taiwan. Inhalation toxicology 20: 777–781.
4. Cheng MF, Ho SC, Chiu HF, Wu TN, Chen PS, et al. (2008) Consequences of exposure to Asian dust storm events on daily pneumonia hospital admissions in Taipei, Taiwan. Journal of toxicology and environmental health Part A 71: 1295–1299.
5. Chan CC, Chuang KJ, Chen WJ, Chang WT, Lee CT, et al. (2008) Increasing cardiopulmonary emergency visits by long-range transported Asian dust storms in Taiwan. Environmental Research 106: 393–400.
6. Yang CY, Tsai SS, Chang CC, Ho SC (2005) Effects of Asian dust storm events on daily admissions for asthma in Taipei, Taiwan. Inhalation toxicology 17: 817–821.
7. Chen YS, Sheen PC, Chen ER, Liu YK, Wu TN, et al. (2004) Effects of Asian dust storm events on daily mortality in Taipei, Taiwan. Environmental research 95: 151–155.
8. Lee HN, Tanaka T, Chiba M, Igarashi Y (2003) Long Range Transport of Asian Dust from Dust Storms and its Impact on Japan. Water, Air, & Soil Pollution: Focus 3: 231–243.
9. Tuominen IS, Konttinen YT, Vesaluoma MH, Moilanen JA, Helinto M, et al. (2003) Corneal innervation and morphology in primary Sjogren's syndrome. Investigative ophthalmology & visual science 44: 2545–2549.
10. Novaes P, do Nascimento Saldiva PH, Kara-Jose N, Macchione M, Matsuda M, et al. (2007) Ambient levels of air pollution induce goblet-cell hyperplasia in human conjunctival epithelium. Environmental health perspectives 115: 1753–1756.
11. Cakmak S, Dales RE, Burnett RT, Judek S, Coates F, et al. (2002) Effect of airborne allergens on emergency visits by children for conjunctivitis and rhinitis. The Lancet 359: 947–948.
12. Bourcier T, Viboud C, Cohen J-C, Thomas F, Bury T, et al. (2003) Effects of air pollution and climatic conditions on the frequency of ophthalmological emergency examinations. British Journal of Ophthalmology 87: 809–811.
13. Ezzati M, Saleh H, Kammen DM (2000) The Contributions of Emissions and Spatial Microenvironments to Exposure to Indoor Air Pollution from Biomass Combustion in Kenya. Environmental health perspectives 108: 833–839.
14. Ma C-J, Kasahara M, Höller R, Kamiya T (2001) Characteristics of single particles sampled in Japan during the Asian dust-storm period. Atmospheric Environment 35: 2707–2714.
15. Yang C-Y (2006) Effects of Asian Dust Storm Events on Daily Clinical Visits for Conjunctivitis in Taipei, Taiwan. Journal of Toxicology and Environmental Health, Part A 69: 1673–1680.
16. Schwartz J (2004) Air pollution and children's health. Pediatrics 113: 1037–1043.
17. Dockery DW, Ware JH, Ferris BG Jr, Speizer FE, Cook NR, et al. (1982) Change in pulmonary function in children associated with air pollution episodes. Journal of the Air Pollution Control Association 32: 937–942.
18. Dassen W, Brunekreef B, Hoek G, Hofschreuder P, Staatsen B, et al. (1986) Decline in children's pulmonary function during an air pollution episode. Journal of the Air Pollution Control Association 36: 1223–1227.
19. van der Zee S, Hoek G, Boezen HM, Schouten JP, van Wijnen JH, et al. (1999) Acute effects of urban air pollution on respiratory health of children with and without chronic respiratory symptoms. Occupational and environmental medicine 56: 802–812.
20. Boezen HM, van der Zee SC, Postma DS, Vonk JM, Gerritsen J, et al. (1999) Effects of ambient air pollution on upper and lower respiratory symptoms and peak expiratory flow in children. Lancet 353: 874–878.
21. Pope CA 3rd (1989) Respiratory disease associated with community air pollution and a steel mill, Utah Valley. American Journal of Public Health 79: 623–628.
22. Jedrychowski W, Flak E, Mroz E (1999) The adverse effect of low levels of ambient air pollutants on lung function growth in preadolescent children. Environmental health perspectives 107: 669–674.
23. Horak F Jr, Studnicka M, Gartner C, Spengler JD, Tauber E, et al. (2002) Particulate matter and lung function growth in children: a 3-yr follow-up study in Austrian schoolchildren. The European respiratory journal: official journal of the European Society for Clinical Respiratory Physiology 19: 838–845.
24. McConnell R, Berhane K, Gilliland F, London SJ, Vora H, et al. (1999) Air pollution and bronchitic symptoms in Southern California children with asthma. Environmental health perspectives 107: 757–760.
25. Middleton N, Yiallouros P, Kleanthous S, Kolokotroni O, Schwartz J, et al. (2008) A 10-year time-series analysis of respiratory and cardiovascular morbidity in Nicosia, Cyprus: the effect of short-term changes in air pollution and dust storms. Environmental health: a global access science source 7: 39.
26. Chien L-C, Yang C-H, Yu H-L (2012) Estimated Effects of Asian Dust Storms on Spatiotemporal Distributions of Clinic Visits for Respiratory Diseases in Taipei Children (Taiwan). Environmental health perspectives 7: e41317.
27. Yu H-L, Chien L-C, Yang C-H (2012) Asian Dust Storm Elevates Children's Respiratory Health Risks: A Spatiotemporal Analysis of Children's Clinic Visits across Taipei (Taiwan). PloS one 7: e41317.
28. Yu H-L, Yang C-H, Chien L-C (2013) Spatial vulnerability under extreme events: A case of Asian dust storm's effects on children's respiratory health. Environment international 54: 35–44.
29. TWEPA (2011) Dust storm identification. in Asian dust storm monitoring network. Taipei.
30. Lang S, Brezger A (2004) Bayesian P-Splines. Journal of Computational and Graphical Statistics 13: 183–212.
31. Brezger A, Lang S (2008) Simultaneous probability statements for Bayesian P-splines. Statistical Modelling 8: 141–168.
32. Kindermann R, Snell JL, American Mathematical Society (1980) Markov random fields and their applications. Providence, R.I.: American Mathematical Society. ix, 142 p. p.
33. Belitz C, Lang S (2008) Simultaneous selection of variables and smoothing parameters in structured additive regression models. Computational Statistics & Data Analysis 53: 61–81.
34. Fahrmeir L, Lang S (2001) Bayesian Inference for Generalized Additive Mixed Models Based on Markov Random Field Priors. Journal of the Royal Statistical Society Series C (Applied Statistics) 50: 201–220.
35. Akaike H (1974) A new look at the statistical model identification. Automatic Control, IEEE Transactions on 19: 716–723.
36. Fromont A, Binquet C, Sauleau EA, Fournel I, Bellisario A, et al. (2010) Geographic variations of multiple sclerosis in France. Brain: a journal of neurology 133: 1889–1899.
37. Belitz C, Brezger A, Kneib T, Lang S (2012) BayesX - Software for Bayesian inference in structured additive regression models. Version 2.1.
38. Chen PS, Tsai FT, Lin CK, Yang CY, Chan CC, et al. (2010) Ambient Influenza and Avian Influenza Virus during Dust Storm Days and Background Days. Environmental Health Perspectives 118: 1211–1216.
39. Yang CY, Cheng MH, Chen CC (2009) Effects of Asian dust storm events on hospital admissions for congestive heart failure in Taipei, Taiwan. Journal of toxicology and environmental health Part A 72: 324–328.
40. Kuo H-W, Shen H-Y (2010) Indoor and outdoor PM2.5 and PM10 concentrations in the air during a dust storm. Building and Environment 45: 610–614.
41. TWDOH (2012) Regulations Governing the Medical Services Covered under National Health Insurance. In: Department of Health EY, editor. Taipei, Taiwan.
42. NCU (2005) Taiwan Wind Query System. Chungli, Taiwan: National Central University.
43. Liu Z (2009) Acute Conjunctivitis. Essentials of Chinese Medicine: 443–445.
44. Stoss M, Michels C, Peter E, Beutke R, Gorter RW (2000) Prospective cohort trial of Euphrasia single-dose eye drops in conjunctivitis. The Journal of Alternative and Complementary Medicine 6: 499–508.

6

Analysis of Fundus Shape in Highly Myopic Eyes by Using Curvature Maps Constructed from Optical Coherence Tomography

Masahiro Miyake, Kenji Yamashiro*, Yumiko Akagi-Kurashige, Akio Oishi, Akitaka Tsujikawa, Masanori Hangai, Nagahisa Yoshimura

Department of Ophthalmology and Visual Sciences, Kyoto University Graduate School of Medicine, Kyoto, Japan

Abstract

Purpose: To evaluate fundus shape in highly myopic eyes using color maps created through optical coherence tomography (OCT) image analysis.

Methods: We retrospectively evaluated 182 highly myopic eyes from 113 patients. After obtaining 12 lines of 9-mm radial OCT scans with the fovea at the center, the Bruch's membrane line was plotted and its curvature was measured at 1-µm intervals in each image, which was reflected as a color topography map. For the quantitative analysis of the eye shape, mean absolute curvature and variance of curvature were calculated.

Results: The color maps allowed staphyloma visualization as a ring of green color at the edge and as that of orange-red color at the bottom. Analyses of mean and variance of curvature revealed that eyes with myopic choroidal neovascularization tended to have relatively flat posterior poles with smooth surfaces, while eyes with chorioretinal atrophy exhibited a steep, curved shape with an undulated surface ($P<0.001$). Furthermore, eyes with staphylomas and those without clearly differed in terms of mean curvature and the variance of curvature: 98.4% of eyes with staphylomas had mean curvature $\geq 7.8\times10^{-5}$ [1/µm] and variance of curvature $\geq 0.26\times10^{-8}$ [1/µm].

Conclusions: We established a novel method to analyze posterior pole shape by using OCT images to construct curvature maps. Our quantitative analysis revealed that fundus shape is associated with myopic complications. These values were also effective in distinguishing eyes with staphylomas from those without. This tool for the quantitative evaluation of eye shape should facilitate future research of myopic complications.

Editor: Bang V. Bui, University of Melbourne, Australia

Funding: This study was supported in part by grants-in-aid for scientific research (Nos. 21249084 and 200791294) from the Japan Society for the Promotion of Science, Tokyo, Japan, and the Japan National Society for the Prevention of Blindness, Tokyo, Japan. The funders had no role in study design, data collection and analysis, decision to publish, or preparation of the manuscript. Financial Disclosures: Nagahisa Yoshimura: Canon (Financial support), Topcon (Financial support); Masanori Hangai: Canon (Financial support), Topcon (Financial support).

Competing Interests: The authors have read the journal's policy and have the following conflicts: Nagahisa Yoshimura: Canon (Financial support), Topcon (Financial support); Masanori Hangai: Canon (Financial support), Topcon (Financial support).

* Email: yamashro@kuhp.kyoto-u.ac.jp

Introduction

Myopia is one of the most common visual disorders worldwide, representing a major public health concern among East Asian populations. [1–4] Myopic eyes with very long axial lengths (≥ 26.0 mm, ≥26.5 mm, or ≥28.0 mm) or a high degree of myopic refractive error (≤−5D, ≤−6D, or ≤−8D) are classified as highly myopic. [5–11] High myopia is typically associated with excessive elongation of the globe and, in middle-aged individuals, often leads to pathological changes such as posterior staphyloma. [12,13] Moriyama et al. analyzed the shapes of eyes with pathologic myopia using three-dimensional magnetic resonance imaging (MRI). The results demonstrated a clear association between eye shape and the likelihood of optic neuropathy. [14] However, eyeball shape as classified by MRI was not associated with myopic complications at the posterior pole such as myopic choroidal neovascularization (mCNV), chorioretinal atrophy (CRA), or myopic tractional maculopathy. Owing to the resolutional limitations of MRI, this technique cannot be used for detailed morphological investigations of the posterior pole, where most major myopic complications develop.

Today, optical coherence tomography (OCT) is emerging as a popular modality by which we can obtain precise cross-sectional images of retina and fundus, though its scan width is limited. While MRI is a very useful device with which to macroscopically evaluate eyeball shape, [14–16] OCT is more suitable for microscopic evaluation owing to its high resolution. The rapid scanning speed utilized for spectral-domain OCT can minimize the effects of ocular movement, allowing for a more precise analysis of retinal structure. [17] To date, several studies have examined staphylomas using OCT. [18,19] Notably, the height of a posterior staphyloma affects the development of mCNV. Previous reports investigated this phenomenon using several narrow 6-mm scans, which collectively captured only a small portion of the entire staphyloma. [18] In the current study, we evaluated twelve 9-mm radial OCT scans in each highly myopic eye studied. This information was used to create a curvature map for the nearly entirety of Bruch's membrane; the staphyloma edge and degree of staphyloma were clearly visualized with the aid of this map. Subsequent analyses revealed associations between posterior pole shape and myopic complications.

Materials and Methods

We examined 192 eyes respectively, having axial length ≥ 26 mm from 120 consecutive patients who underwent the analysis below during the period from April 2010 to March 2012. All procedures in this study adhered to the tenets of the Declaration of Helsinki. The ethics committee (Ethics Committee of Kyoto University Graduate School and Faculty of Medicine, Japan) approved the study protocol. All of the patients were fully informed about the purpose and procedures of this study, and written consent was obtained from each. Patient records/information was anonymized and de-identified prior to analysis.

Data collection

Of the 192 eyes, 10 eyes from 7 patients were excluded either because the OCT images and/or color fundus photographs were of poor quality or because they had a history of ocular surgery other than cataract surgery. A total of 182 highly myopic eyes from 113 patients were analyzed. Each subject underwent a complete ophthalmic examination, including axial length measurement using an IOL master (Carl Zeiss Meditec, Dublin, CA), indirect ophthalmoscopy and slit-lamp biomicroscopy, and optical coherence tomography (RS-3000, Nidek, Tokyo, Japan). Fluorescein angiography was performed if mCNV was suspected.

Mapping fundus curvature

In this analysis, we used Burch's membrane lines as representative lines of the fundus shape instead of the retina or RPE lines, which allowed us to overcome the drawbacks of previous method using retinal topography [20,21]; retinal or RPE topography can be easily biased by complications such as CNV, schisis, and MHRD.

We built new software to calculate the eye curvatures from their OCT images and construct a color curvature map. This software presents a measure of retinal shape with distribution of local curvature. By calculating the local curvature, it was possible to detect small unevenness of the retina. After obtaining 12 lines of a 9-mm radial OCT scan at center of the fovea, Bruch's membrane line was plotted (Figure 1A). The size of each OCT image was adjusted to correct for the difference in pixel resolution in the transverse and longitudinal directions. A case in which a curvature of the Bruch's membrane was used as shape analysis is described below using the OCT image shown in Figure 1. The curvature of the Bruch's membrane line as an analysis target was calculated. The curvature κ can be obtained by calculating, at respective points at the Bruch's membrane line:

$$\kappa = \frac{\frac{d^2z}{dx^2}}{\left(1+\left(\frac{dz}{dx}\right)^2\right)^{\frac{3}{2}}} \quad (1)$$

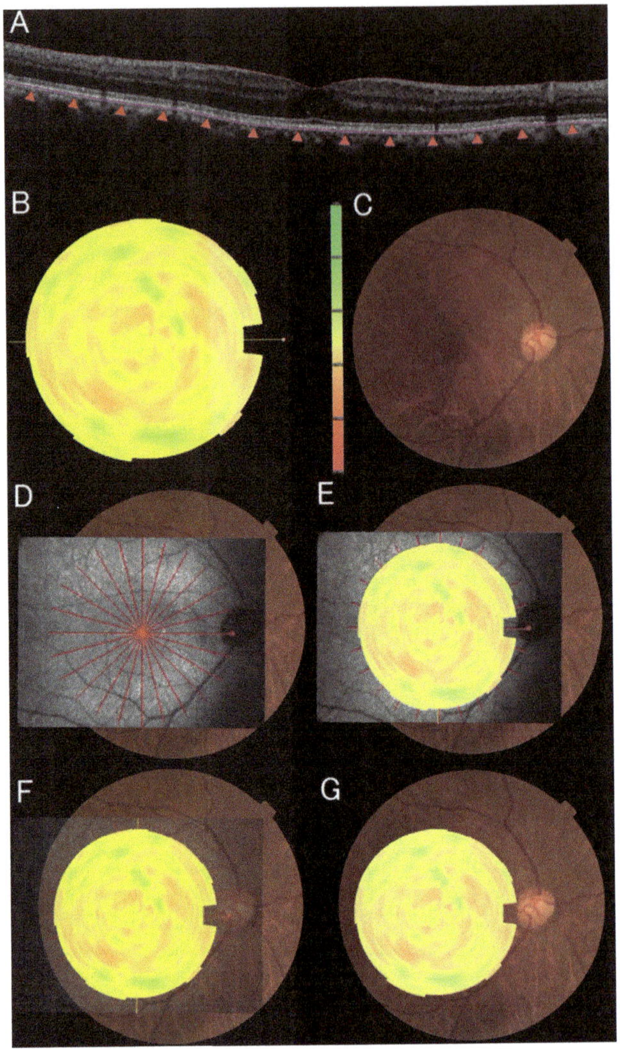

Figure 1. Construction of the curvature map for a normal eye. A, Bruch's membrane was plotted in each of 12 radial OCT scans with the fovea at the center. Local curvature was measured from 3 sequential points (sampled at 500-µm intervals). The sine of curvature was defined as positive when the membrane was convex upward. **B,** The value of curvature was mapped using yellow (RGB(255, 255, 0)) to represent zero curvature (flat), green (gradient from RGB(255, 255, 0) to RGB(0, 192, 32) according to curvature [1/µm]) for positive curvature (convex-upward), and red (gradient from RGB(255, 255, 0) to RGB(255, 0, 0) according to curvature [1/µm]) for negative curvature (convex-downward). **C,** Color fundus photograph on which the topographic maps will be overlaid. **D,** Scanning Laser Ophthalmoscope (SLO) images are overlaid on the fundus photographs. **E,** Topographic maps are overlaid on the SLO images. **F and G,** SLO image transparency was increased for an accurate superimposition.

The differentials in equation (1) were calculated by central difference. These equations are represented by:

$$\frac{dz}{dx} = \frac{f(x+h)-f(x-h)}{2h} \quad (2)$$

$$\frac{d^2z}{dx^2} = \frac{f(x+h)-2f(x)+f(x-h)}{h^2} \quad (3)$$

where f(x) is the Bruch's membrane line, and h is the spacing between two adjacent A-scans (500-µm apart). The curvature κ was measured using 3 sequential A-scans. Therefore, it represents local shape in the range of 1,000-µm (Local curvature). The values of the local curvature were calculated using all A-scans except in regions within 500-µm from right and left boundaries of an image. The unit of curvature κ was inverse micrometer. Positive, negative, or zero value of the curvature κ represents upward concave, downward convex, or flat respectively. In this study, the curvature was calculated with three points on the Bruch's membrane line. Because distance from the first point to the third point was 1000-µm, this localized curvature was allowed to be zero.

The degree of curvature was measured for the radial OCT scans with the fovea at the center. The distribution of the local curvature was presented as a color map overlaid on a c-scan retinal image: yellow (RGB(255, 255, 0)) for the local curvature value of 0.0 (1/infinity) [1/µm], green (RGB(0, 192, 32)) for the local curvature value of +0.0005 (1/2000) [1/µm], and red (RGB(255, 0, 0)) for the local curvature value of −0.0005 (1/2000) [1/µm]. The color of curvature map was limited to 1/2000 [1/µm]. The curvature map set a color to show a gradient from green to yellow as a local curvature value changes from 0.0005 to 0.0, and a gradient from red to yellow as a local curvature value changes from −0.0005 to 0.0. Examples of correspondence between fundus shape, curvature, and color were presented in Figure 2. Generated color map was then superimposed on a fundus photo, being intermediated by a Scanning Laser Ophthalmoscope (SLO) image (Figure 1B–1F). Figure 1G depicts a normal eye. Considering the spherical shape of a normal eye, the curvature of its posterior pole should be negative. However, its curvature is very low so that the map shows an overall yellow appearance.

A

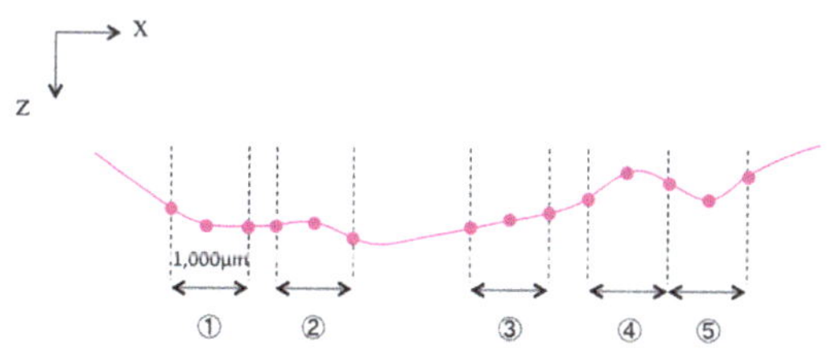

B

	Shape	Sign	Curvature	Color
①		negative	small	
②		positive	small	
③		zero	zero	
④		positive	large	
⑤		negative	large	

Figure 2. Image of correspondence between fundus shape, curvature, and color. A, An imaginary Bruch's membrane line to exemplify the correspondence. The curvature of one point was measured using 3 sequential A-scans (500-µm apart) so that it represented local shape in the range of 1,000-µm (Local curvature). Five points are exemplified in this figure. **B,** Corresponding curvature [1/µm] and color image for each 5 point. Positive, negative, or zero value of the curvature κ represents upward concave, downward convex, or flat, respectively. The color of curvature map showed a gradient from green (RGB(0, 192, 32)) to yellow (RGB(255, 255, 0)) as a local curvature value changes from 0.0005 to 0.0, and a gradient from red (RGB(255, 0, 0)) to yellow (RGB(255, 255, 0)) as a local curvature value changes from −0.0005 to 0.0.

Segmentation Method

A smoothing filter (Median filter) was applied to OCT images to remove noise components. Layer boundary extraction could be implemented by edge detection filter (Sobel filter) and the layer structure-emphasized filter (Hessian filter).

As for the inner limiting membrane, a peak of the layer structure emphasizing filter was searched for in the depth direction of fundus from the vitreum side, and a first peak position equal to or larger than a threshold was detected as an initial value of the inner limiting membrane and nerve fiber layer boundary. From that initial value, a gradient feature was searched for toward the vitreum side, and a gradient peak position was detected as the inner limiting membrane.

Likewise, as for the nerve fiber layer boundary, a gradient feature was searched for from that initial value in the depth direction of the fundus, and a gradient peak position was detected as the nerve fiber layer boundary.

As for the Bruch's membrane line, a peak of the layer structure emphasizing filter is searched for further in the depth direction of the fundus, and the last peak position equal to or larger than the threshold is detected as an initial value of the Bruch's membrane line. A gradient feature was searched for from that initial value in the depth direction of the fundus, and a gradient peak position was detected as the Bruch's membrane line.

By applying Snakes [22] using the detected boundary as the initial position, the boundary shape became smooth.

Data analysis

We evaluated the curvature maps for eyes with foveal retinal detachments (RDs), retinoschisis, mCNV, and severe CRA. In addition, differences in the curvature maps were compared between eyes with staphyloma and eyes without staphyloma. The presence of retinoschisis, RD, CRA, and staphyloma was determined using color fundus photographs and OCT images. FA images were used to identify mCNV. The images of each eye were examined by 2 retina specialists (K.Y and A.T), and any discrepancies were settled by a third specialist (N.Y). Cases showing patchy CRA >3 disc diameters in area were diagnosed as having severe CRA. The eyes with both retinoschisis and RD were classified as RD. Multiple comparisons of numerical values such as patient age and axial length were performed with analysis of variance (ANOVA) and Tukey–Kramer's tests. Single comparisons were performed using an unpaired *t*-test. The male:female ratio and other 2×2 or 2×3 tables were compared using Fisher's exact test and Tukey's test for post-hoc analysis. A p-value of ≤5% was considered statistically significant.

Results

Among these 113 patients, 37 were men and 76 were women, with a mean age of 61.9±14.1 years. The mean axial length was 28.68±1.74 mm. RD with or without retinoschisis was seen in 13 eyes (7.1%), retinoschisis without RD in 34 eyes (18.7%), mCNV in 33 eyes (18.1%), and severe CRA in 20 eyes (11.0%). The highly myopic patients with retinoschisis, RD, and severe CRA were significantly older than the highly myopic patients without these 3 complications ($P = 1.6 \times 10^{-4}$, 0.0017, 0.0012, respectively). There were more women than men with mCNV, retinoschisis, and CRA (Table 1). Axial length was significantly longer in eyes with retinoschisis, RD, and CRA as compared to eyes without

Table 1. Characteristics of the included eyes according to complications.

Variable		No complications	mCNV	Retinoschisis	RD	CRA	P-value†
n		88	33	34	13	20	
Age (years ± SD)		56.2±13.9	60.3±16.1	67.9±11.9	71.0±8.56	68.9±6.51	1.16×10^{-6}
p-value*	No complications	-	0.54	<0.001	0.002	0.001	
	mCNV	-	-	0.13	0.10	0.14	
	Retinoschisis	-	-	-	0.95	1.00	
	RD	-	-	-	-	0.99	
Sex (male:female)		44:44	5:28	6:28	4:9	3:17	2.03×10^{-4}
p-value*	No complications	-	0.002	0.004	0.60	0.02	
	mCNV	-	-	1.00	0.82	1.00	
	Retinoschisis	-	-	-	0.90	1.00	
	RD	-	-	-	-	0.86	
Axial length (mm ± SD)		28.02±1.49	28.35±1.20	29.46±1.54	29.31±1.38	30.96±1.11	5.47×10^{-11}
p-value*	No complications	-	0.82	<0.001	0.04	<0.001	
	mCNV	-	-	0.03	0.31	<0.001	
	Retinoschisis	-	-	-	1.00	0.05	
	RD	-	-	-	-	0.11	

*Tukey-Kramer's multiple comparison.
†Analysis of variance.
CNV: choroidal neovascularization, RD: retinal detachment, CRA: chorioretinal atrophy.

complications, while the axial length of eyes with mCNV was not significantly different from eyes without these 4 complications.

Constructing fundus curvature maps

Fundus curvature maps were successfully obtained and superimposed on color fundus photographs in all 182 cases. In 4 eyes with staphylomas, the entire staphyloma edge could be visualized clearly using this method (Figure 3A and 3B). Because the staphyloma edge must have an inflection point, the edge curvature theoretically ranges from zero to plus, which would be represented on the curvature map as yellow to green shading along the staphyloma edge. The area inside the staphyloma is depicted as red to orange, which represents a relatively high degree of concave curvature. This image can be contrasted with that of a representative normal eye, which yielded a topographical map that was yellow in overall appearance (Figure 1).

In this analysis, however, manual correction was needed in all cases more or less. While we required re-plot of less than 10 points per slice in eyes without staphyloma, re-plot of more than or equal to 10 points per slice was needed in most eyes with staphyloma to obtain correct curvature of Bruch's membrane. When image inversion towards the edges of the OCT scan existed, we could not construct curvature map at the corresponding area. In the studied eyes, however, mean coverage area was 86.4±10.2%, which corresponds to 87.3%–98.3% coverage of diameter.

Some of the participants underwent several OCT examinations within 3 months. In these eyes, the color map did not show notable change within 3 months, suggesting our method has acceptable repeatability.

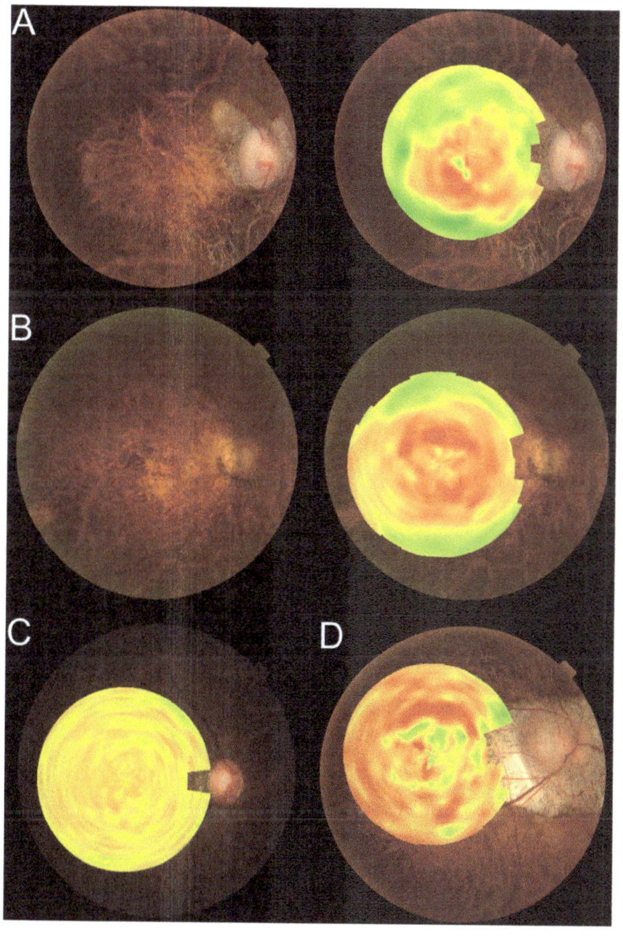

Figure 3. Representative color maps of highly myopic eyes. A, Right eye from a 58-year-old woman with axial length of 29.01 mm. The staphyloma edge is depicted in green-yellow. **B,** Right eye of a 72-year-old woman with axial length of 28.37 mm. Upper and lower edges of the staphyloma can be visualized clearly. **C,** Right eye of a 38-year-old woman, with axial length of 26.38 mm. The yellow-dominant color map represents a relatively flat fundus. **D,** Right eye from a 65-year-old woman with axial length of 34.64 mm. The mosaic color pattern indicates an undulated fundus.

Quantitative evaluation of the curvature maps

When we evaluated the color maps for 182 eyes, we found roughly 3 patterns of curvature maps: a yellow dominant curvature map (Figure 3C), a map with an orange-red color at the center (Figure 3A and 3B), and one with a mosaic pattern of red and green (Figure 3D). The comparison between eyes with yellow-dominant curvature maps and eyes that yielded maps with an orange-red color at the center suggested that the degree of staphyloma could be represented by the mean curvature value. In addition, the mosaic patterns of red and green suggested that the smoothness of the staphyloma surface could be represented by the variance in curvature. Hence, we calculated the mean absolute curvature and variance of curvature for each eye as an index for fundus shape. This approach allowed for a quantitative evaluation of the characteristics of fundus shape. With mean curvature values assigned to the horizontal axis and the variance values assigned to the vertical axis, a scatter plot was used to illustrate the consecutive distribution of all eyes evaluated (Figure 4A).

Characteristics of fundus curvature in eyes with myopic complications

Scatter plots showed that each myopic complication evaluated had a specific profile, as represented by mean curvature and variance. Eyes with mCNV exhibited low-to-moderate levels of curvature and minimal variance (Figure 4B). In contrast, eyes with severe CRA exhibited higher levels of both curvature and variance (Figure 4C). When we drew a splitting line at 1.5×10^{-4} for mean curvature and 1×10^{-8} for the variance of curvature, most eyes with mCNV were distributed throughout the left-lower area, while most eyes with CRA were distributed throughout the right-upper area. Eyes with RD and retinoschisis were similar in exhibiting moderate levels of both curvature and variance (Figure 4D).

The quantitative evaluation of mean curvature and variance of curvature revealed additional differences in fundus shape that distinguished each of the complications studied from the others. Mean curvature was significantly larger in eyes with complications than in eyes without any of the complications studied (Table 2). When the values of eyes with RD and eyes with retinoschisis were combined for further analysis, mean curvature values were significantly smaller in eyes with mCNV as compared to eyes with RD or retinoschisis, and significantly smaller in eyes with RD or retinoschisis as compared to eyes with CRA. Similar to the mean curvature results, variance of curvature was significantly larger in eyes with retinoschisis, RD, and CRA than in eyes without complications (Table 3). However, there was no significant difference in the variance of curvature between eyes with mCNV and eyes without complications. Among the eyes with complications, the variance of curvature also showed significant trends: smaller in eyes with mCNV, intermediate in eyes with RD or retinoschisis, and larger in eyes with CRA.

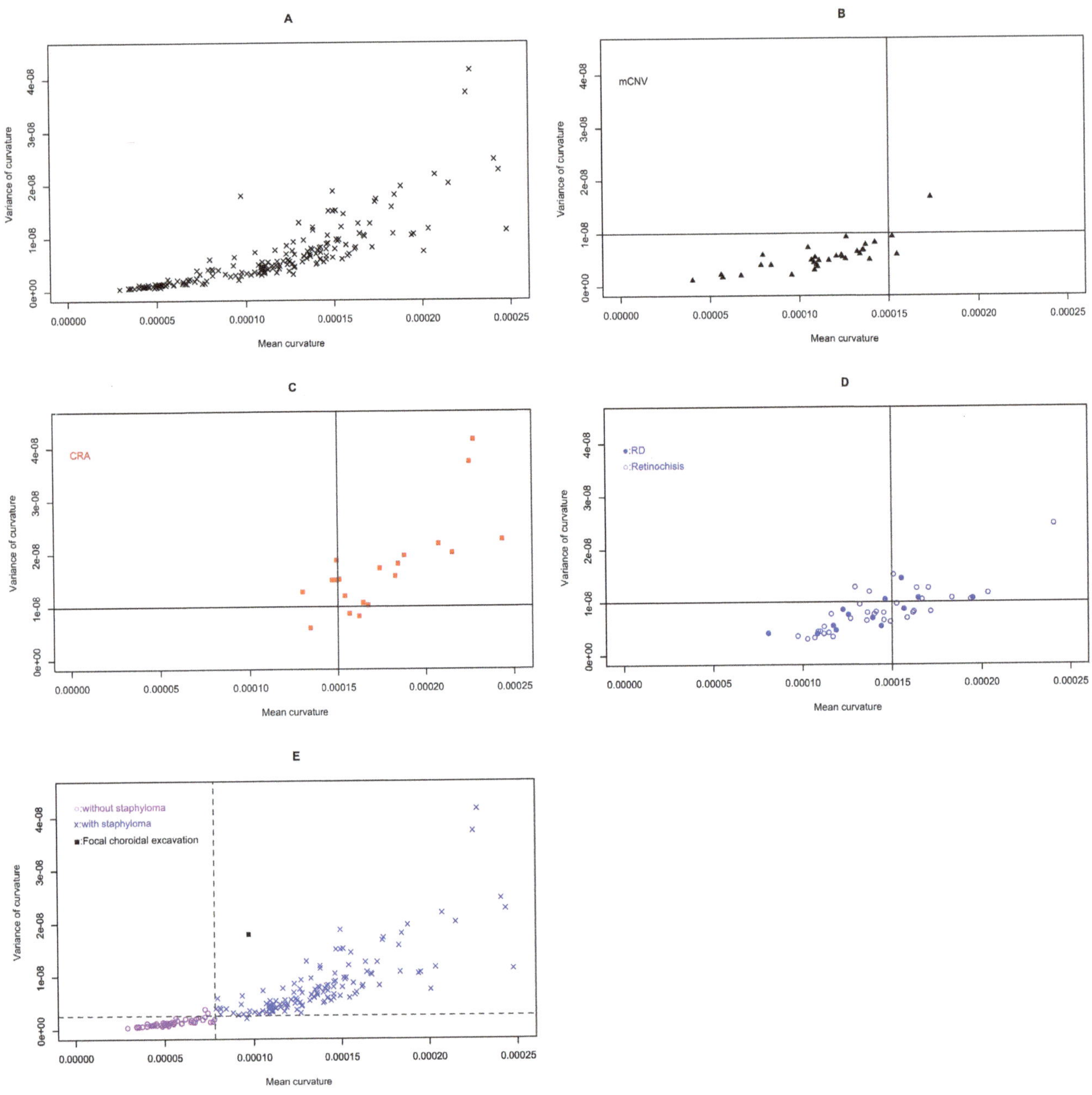

Figure 4. Scatter plot assigning mean curvature to the horizontal axis and variance of curvature to the vertical axis. A, All 182 highly myopic eyes are plotted. **B,** 33 eyes with myopic choroidal neovascularization (mCNV) are highlighted. Most values localize to the lower segment of the splitting line at 0.00015 for mean curvature and 1×10^{-8} for variance of curvature. **C,** 17 eyes with severe chorioretinal atrophy (CRA) are highlighted. Most of these values localize to the higher segment of the splitting line. **D,** 33 eyes with retinoschisis (open circles) and 11 eyes with foveal retinal detachments (filled circles) are plotted. **E,** Eyes with and without staphylomas. The groups are easily separated into 2 groups by broken lines that indicate 0.000078 in mean curvature and 0.26×10^{-8} in curvature variance. One eye without a staphyloma had focal choroidal excavation (square).

Characteristics of fundus curvature in eyes with staphylomas

Of the 182 eyes evaluated, 129 eyes were judged to have staphylomas, while 52 eyes were not. One eye without staphyloma had focal choroidal excavation, which was visualized clearly as a red spot on the color map. When the eye with focal choroidal excavation was excluded from the analysis, the highly myopic patients with staphylomas were found to be older than those without. There also more women than men with staphylomas (Table 4). Furthermore, eyes with staphylomas had significantly greater axial length, mean curvature, and variance of curvature. Figure 4E shows the distribution of eyes with staphylomas vs. those without in the scatter plot of mean curvature and variance of curvature. When we drew a watershed line at 7.8×10^{-5} for mean curvature and 0.26×10^{-8} for variance of curvature, 98.4% of eyes with staphyloma were distributed in areas of the plot corresponding to greater curvature and greater

Table 2. Mean absolute curvature of eyes with each complication.

Complication	No complications	mCNV	Retinoschisis	RD	CRA
value (x10^5: mean ± SD)	8.61±4.27	11.27±3.01	14.39±3.17	13.64±2.89	17.54±3.28
No complications	-	0.005	<0.001	<0.001	<0.001
mCNV	-	-	0.006	0.29	<0.001
Retinoschisis	-	-	-	0.97	0.02
RD	-	-	-	-	0.03

P-values* are shown.
*Tukey-Kramer's multiple comparison.
CNV: choroidal neovascularization, RD: retinal detachment, CRA: chorioretinal atrophy.

variance, while 96.2% of eyes without staphylomas aggregated to the zones of low curvature and low variance.

Discussion

In the current study, we successfully visualized the shape of the posterior pole by using a novel method to analyze the curvature of 12 lines of 9-mm radial OCT scans. The color map of curvature effectively localized the staphyloma itself as well as the surrounding border. Furthermore, mean curvature and variance of curvature calculations were used to quantitatively evaluate fundus shape, which revealed associations between myopic complications and fundus shape. Our findings suggest that mean curvature and variance of curvature values could be used to define staphylomas and quantitatively evaluate staphylomas.

At present, the process of mCNV development has not been fully elucidated. Lacquer cracks and CRA often lead to mCNV in highly myopic eyes. [23] Curtin and Karlin showed that axial length was associated with the development of lacquer cracks and CRA in high myopia. [24] They also showed that the development of mCNV was not dependent on increases in axial length. Our study also showed that axial length did not differ significantly between highly myopic eyes with mCNV and highly myopic eyes without myopic complications.

The analysis of posterior fundus shape could provide valuable insights for mCNV development. Our findings suggest that mCNV develops in eyes with moderate curvature without undulation. Considering that mCNV was observed in eyes with staphyloma as well as in eyes without staphyloma, the presence of a staphyloma itself was not able to predict the development of mCNV in this study. Previous reports on the relationship between staphyloma and the development of mCNV were inconsistent. Although 2 reports graded staphyloma using B-scan ultrasonographic images, one study reported that the prevalence of mCNV was not associated with staphyloma grade, [13] while another reported that mCNV development was inversely correlated with staphyloma severity. [25] In contrast to these reports using B-scan ultrasonographic images, a study using OCT images reported a direct correlation between mCNV development and staphyloma severity. [18] Quantitative evaluations of the entire posterior pole should elucidate the relationship between eye shape and mCNV development.

In contrast to eyes with mCNV, eyes with severe CRA tended to have severe staphylomas with undulated surfaces. Considering that patchy and diffuse CRA are reported to predispose the patient to the development of mCNV [23,26] while CRA also develops in the area proximal to regressed mCNV, [27,28] it might be expected that eyes with mCNV and eyes with CRA would exhibit similar shape. The observed differences in mean curvature and variance of curvature could be explained by the fact that severe CRA can develop after the inactivation of mCNV, causing concave deformation in the posterior pole [29]. The imaging strategy outlined in this study could be used to capture such temporal changes in fundus shape. The evaluation of time-course changes in fundus shape and the association with mCNV and CRA development might elucidate a causal relationship between mCNV and CRA. Such analysis might also identify factors that can be used to predict progression from mCNV to CRA, or vice versa.

The present study could not detect significant differences in fundus shape between eyes with retinoschisis and eyes with RD. The number of eyes with retinoschisis or RD may not have been sufficient for statistical evaluation. Since RD in highly myopic eyes are reported to originate from retinoschisis [30] while retinoschisis does not always lead to RD, the ability to predict RD development from retinoschisis could prevent severe visual loss in highly myopic

Table 3. Mean variance of curvature for eyes with each complication.

Complication	No complications	mCNV	Retinoschisis	RD	CRA
value (x10^9: mean ± SD)	3.37±3.08	5.53±2.87	8.42±4.29	7.87±3.15	17.40±8.88
No complications	-	0.10	<0.001	0.004	<0.001
mCNV	-	-	0.047	0.45	<0.001
Retinoschisis	-	-	-	0.99	<0.001
RD	-	-	-	-	<0.001

P-values* are shown.
*Tukey-Kramer's multiple comparison.
CNV: choroidal neovascularization, RD: retinal detachment, CRA: chorioretinal atrophy.

Table 4. Characteristics of the included eyes according to the presence of staphylomas.

Variable	without staphyloma	with staphyloma	P-value*
n	52	129	
Age (years ± SD)	49.4±12.5	65.7±12.1	<0.01
Sex (male:female)	29:23	33:96	<0.01†
Axial length (mm ± SD)	27.34±1.08	29.24±1.66	<0.01
Mean absolute curvature (x10^5: mean ± SD)	5.36±1.24	13.71±3.50	<0.01
Variance of curvature (x10^9: mean ± SD)	1.35±0.65	8.26±6.03	<0.01

*unpaired *t*-test.
†Fisher's exact test.

eyes. Currently, factors such as age, refractive error, axial length, staphyloma, CRA, and vitreoretinal interface quality are hypothesized to play a role in progression from retinoschisis to RD, [31,32] but the mechanisms involved have not been thoroughly elucidated. Further quantitative study of fundus shape might elucidate mechanisms of the progression form retinoschisis to RD.

Our methodology also allows for the quantification of staphyloma severity. Using the technology described here, staphylomas could be graded objectively on the basis of mean curvature and variance of curvature. Furthermore, our method might be able to distinguish eyes with staphyloma and eyes without staphyloma by the numerical values of mean curvature and variance of curvature. We may be able to define staphyloma by cut-off value of such parameters as well as high myopia by spherical equivalents of ≤-5D, ≤-6D, or ≤-8D, or axial length of $\geq$26.0 mm, $\geq$26.5 mm, or $\geq$28.0 mm. Similarly, mean curvature and variance of curvature could objectively define staphyloma, and further study should verify the value of mean curvature as $>7.8\times10^{-5}$ and the mean variance of curvature as $>0.26\times10^{-8}$ used in this study. Currently, staphylomas are usually graded in a subjective manner based on slit-lamp biomicroscopy. [12] Our method with wider OCT could be used to elaborate a standardized system for objective staphyloma classification.

This study has certain limitations. One is a segmentation problem. The auto-segmentation used for this research is accurate when studying the normal eye but not as well when studying highly myopic eyes, because the OCT images obtained in the latter case are often of poor quality. Manual segmentation support was therefore used in such cases presented here. The second issue involves scan width. The 9-mm scan width employed for this study is actually wider than that used in previous studies. However, it was not sufficiently wide to include the entire staphyloma border in all cases. We could detect the entire staphyloma edge only in 4 eyes out of 129 eyes with staphyloma. Third, this study utilized a cross-sectional study design using case series, which precluded causational analysis. Future studies should measure changes in curvature and variance over time. Associations between myopic complications and posterior fundus curvature should be further examined in high myopic patients without subjective complaint or myopic but not highly myopic eyes. Fourth, in a strict sense, the lines we plotted may not simply be attributed to Bruch's membrane line. Although fourth hyperreflective line in OCT is generally recognized as retinal pigment epithelium and the line we plotted as Bruch's membrane, [33,34] Spaide and Curcio discussed that the origin of the fourth hyperreflective line in OCT remained to be determined. [35] Lastly, the current study is evaluating the curvature of OCT images, not the true curvature of the eyeball. As being reported by Kuo et al., [36] the OCT images were more flattened than MRI images. Indeed, as shown in the Supplemental Note, Bruch's membrane line in OCT becomes considerably steeper after correction. However, since we evaluated the local curvature by every 1,000-µm distance rather than by eye shape as a whole, the curvature map did not notably change after correction (Details are shown in Supplemental Note). For the clinical setting, evaluating OCT images is more practical than evaluating true eye shape, from the viewpoint of accessibility. Considering the minor effect of correction to the local curvature evaluation, it would be more helpful for ophthalmologist to use the OCT image without correction.

Despite these limitations, this novel quantitative approach allowed us to correlate fundus shape and myopic complications. Furthermore, we demonstrated how these maps could be used to evaluate fundus shape. The ability to evaluate staphylomas quantitatively will facilitate investigations into the associations between myopic complications and staphylomas.

Acknowledgments

I am very grateful to Yoshihiko Iwase for his valuable cooperation in developing software.

Author Contributions

Conceived and designed the experiments: MM KY. Performed the experiments: MM. Analyzed the data: MM. Contributed reagents/materials/analysis tools: KY YAK AO AT MH NY. Wrote the paper: MM KY.

References

1. Kempen JH, Mitchell P, Lee KE, Tielsch JM, Broman AT, et al. (2004) The prevalence of refractive errors among adults in the United States, Western Europe, and Australia. Arch Ophthalmol 122: 495–505.
2. Saw SM (2003) A synopsis of the prevalence rates and environmental risk factors for myopia. Clin Exp Optom 86: 289–294.
3. Sawada A, Tomidokoro A, Araie M, Iwase A, Yamamoto T (2008) Refractive errors in an elderly Japanese population: the Tajimi study. Ophthalmology 115: 363–370 e363.
4. Wong TY, Foster PJ, Johnson GJ, Seah SK (2002) Education, socioeconomic status, and ocular dimensions in Chinese adults: the Tanjong Pagar Survey. Br J Ophthalmol 86: 963–968.
5. Jacobi FK, Zrenner E, Broghammer M, Pusch CM (2005) A genetic perspective on myopia. Cellular and molecular life sciences: CMLS 62: 800–808.
6. Chang L, Pan CW, Ohno-Matsui K, Lin X, Cheung GC, et al. (2013) Myopia-related fundus changes in Singapore adults with high myopia. Am J Ophthalmol 155: 991–999 e991.

7. Pan CW, Zheng YF, Anuar AR, Chew M, Gazzard G, et al. (2013) Prevalence of refractive errors in a multiethnic Asian population: the Singapore epidemiology of eye disease study. Invest Ophthalmol Vis Sci 54: 2590–2598.
8. Ohno-Matsui K, Akiba M, Modegi T, Tomita M, Ishibashi T, et al. (2012) Association between shape of sclera and myopic retinochoroidal lesions in patients with pathologic myopia. Invest Ophthalmol Vis Sci 53: 6046–6061.
9. Miyake M, Yamashiro K, Akagi-Kurashige Y, Kumagai K, Nakata I, et al. (2013) Vascular Endothelial Growth Factor Gene and the Response to Anti-Vascular Endothelial Growth Factor Treatment for Choroidal Neovascularization in High Myopia. Ophthalmology.
10. Khor CC, Miyake M, Chen LJ, Shi Y, Barathi VA, et al. (2013) Genome-wide association study identifies ZFHX1B as a susceptibility locus for severe myopia. Hum Mol Genet 22: 5288–5294.
11. Miyake M, Yamashiro K, Nakanishi H, Nakata I, Akagi-Kurashige Y, et al. (2013) Evaluation of pigment epithelium-derived factor and complement factor I polymorphisms as a cause of choroidal neovascularization in highly myopic eyes. Invest Ophthalmol Vis Sci 54: 4208–4212.
12. Curtin BJ (1977) The posterior staphyloma of pathologic myopia. Trans Am Ophthalmol Soc 75: 67–86.
13. Hsiang HW, Ohno-Matsui K, Shimada N, Hayashi K, Moriyama M, et al. (2008) Clinical characteristics of posterior staphyloma in eyes with pathologic myopia. Am J Ophthalmol 146: 102–110.
14. Moriyama M, Ohno-Matsui K, Hayashi K, Shimada N, Yoshida T, et al. (2011) Topographic analyses of shape of eyes with pathologic myopia by high-resolution three-dimensional magnetic resonance imaging. Ophthalmology 118: 1626–1637.
15. Cheng HM, Singh OS, Kwong KK, Xiong J, Woods BT, et al. (1992) Shape of the myopic eye as seen with high-resolution magnetic resonance imaging. Optom Vis Sci 69: 698–701.
16. Atchison DA, Pritchard N, Schmid KL, Scott DH, Jones CE, et al. (2005) Shape of the retinal surface in emmetropia and myopia. Invest Ophthalmol Vis Sci 46: 2698–2707.
17. van Velthoven ME, Faber DJ, Verbraak FD, van Leeuwen TG, de Smet MD (2007) Recent developments in optical coherence tomography for imaging the retina. Prog Retin Eye Res 26: 57–77.
18. Ikuno Y, Jo Y, Hamasaki T, Tano Y (2010) Ocular risk factors for choroidal neovascularization in pathologic myopia. Invest Ophthalmol Vis Sci 51: 3721–3725.
19. Chae JB, Moon BG, Yang SJ, Lee JY, Yoon YH, et al. (2011) Macular gradient measurement in myopic posterior staphyloma using optical coherence tomography. Korean journal of ophthalmology: KJO 25: 243–247.
20. Szkulmowski M, Wojtkowski M, Sikorski B, Bajraszewski T, Srinivasan VJ, et al. (2007) Analysis of posterior retinal layers in spectral optical coherence tomography images of the normal retina and retinal pathologies. J Biomed Opt 12: 041207.
21. Kaluzny JJ, Wojtkowski M, Sikorski BL, Szkulmowski M, Szkulmowska A, et al. (2009) Analysis of the outer retina reconstructed by high-resolution, three-dimensional spectral domain optical coherence tomography. Ophthalmic Surg Lasers Imaging 40: 102–108.
22. Kass M, Witkin A, Terzopoulos D (1988) Snakes: Active contour models. Int J Comput Vision 1: 321–331.
23. Hayashi K, Ohno-Matsui K, Shimada N, Moriyama M, Kojima A, et al. (2010) Long-term pattern of progression of myopic maculopathy: a natural history study. Ophthalmology 117: 1595–1611, 1611 e1591–1594.
24. Curtin BJ, Karlin DB (1971) Axial length measurements and fundus changes of the myopic eye. Am J Ophthalmol 71: 42–53.
25. Steidl SM, Pruett RC (1997) Macular complications associated with posterior staphyloma. Am J Ophthalmol 123: 181–187.
26. Ohno-Matsui K, Yoshida T, Futagami S, Yasuzumi K, Shimada N, et al. (2003) Patchy atrophy and lacquer cracks predispose to the development of choroidal neovascularisation in pathological myopia. Br J Ophthalmol 87: 570–573.
27. Yoshida T, Ohno-Matsui K, Yasuzumi K, Kojima A, Shimada N, et al. (2003) Myopic choroidal neovascularization: a 10-year follow-up. Ophthalmology 110: 1297–1305.
28. Kojima A, Ohno-Matsui K, Teramukai S, Yoshida T, Ishihara Y, et al. (2004) Factors associated with the development of chorioretinal atrophy around choroidal neovascularization in pathologic myopia. Graefe's archive for clinical and experimental ophthalmology = Albrecht von Graefes Archiv fur klinische und experimentelle Ophthalmologie 242: 114–119.
29. Teramura T (1993) [The shape of posterior staphyloma in high myopia]. Nippon Ganka Gakkai Zasshi 97: 873–880.
30. Shimada N, Ohno-Matsui K, Yoshida T, Sugamoto Y, Tokoro T, et al. (2008) Progression from macular retinoschisis to retinal detachment in highly myopic eyes is associated with outer lamellar hole formation. Br J Ophthalmol 92: 762–764.
31. Morita H, Ideta H, Ito K, Yonemoto J, Sasaki K, et al. (1991) Causative factors of retinal detachment in macular holes. Retina 11: 281–284.
32. Wu PC, Chen YJ, Chen YH, Chen CH, Shin SJ, et al. (2009) Factors associated with foveoschisis and foveal detachment without macular hole in high myopia. Eye 23: 356–361.
33. Farsiu S, Chiu SJ, O'Connell RV, Folgar FA, Yuan E, et al. (2013) Quantitative Classification of Eyes with and without Intermediate Age-related Macular Degeneration Using Optical Coherence Tomography. Ophthalmology.
34. Chiu SJ, Izatt JA, O'Connell RV, Winter KP, Toth CA, et al. (2012) Validated automatic segmentation of AMD pathology including drusen and geographic atrophy in SD-OCT images. Invest Ophthalmol Vis Sci 53: 53–61.
35. Spaide RF, Curcio CA (2011) Anatomical correlates to the bands seen in the outer retina by optical coherence tomography: literature review and model. Retina 31: 1609–1619.
36. Kuo AN, McNabb RP, Chiu SJ, El-Dairi MA, Farsiu S, et al. (2013) Correction of ocular shape in retinal optical coherence tomography and effect on current clinical measures. Am J Ophthalmol 156: 304–311.

7

Regulation of Nitric Oxide Production by δ-Opioid Receptors during Glaucomatous Injury

Shahid Husain*, Yasir Abdul, Sudha Singh, Anis Ahmad, Mahvash Husain

Hewitt Laboratory of the Ola B. Williams Glaucoma Center, Department of Ophthalmology, Storm Eye Institute, Medical University of South Carolina, Charleston, South Carolina, United States of America

Abstract

To determine the roles of nitric oxide in glaucomatous injury and its regulation by δ-opioid-receptor activation, animals were treated with: 1) a selective inducible nitric oxide synthase (iNOS) inhibitor (aminoguanidine; AG; 25 mg/kg, i.p.); 2) δ-opioid-receptor agonist (SNC-121; 1 mg/kg, i.p.); or 3) with both drugs simultaneously for 7 days, once daily. The loss in retinal ganglion cell (RGC) numbers and their function in glaucomatous eyes were significantly improved in the presence of AG or SNC-121; however, we did not see any significant additive or synergistic effects when animals were treated with both drugs simultaneously. The levels of nitrate-nitrite were significantly increased in the glaucomatous retina when compared with normal retina (normal retina 86±9 vs. glaucomatous retina 174±10 mM/mg protein), which was reduced significantly when animals were treated either with SNC-121 (121±7 mM/mg protein; $P<0.05$) or AG (128±10 mM/mg protein; $P<0.05$). Additionally, SNC-121-mediated reduction in nitrate-nitrite levels was not only blocked by naltrindole (a δ-opioid-receptor antagonist), but naltrindole treatment potentiated the nitrate-nitrite production in glaucomatous retina (235±4 mM/mg protein; $P<0.001$). As expected, naltrindole treatment also fully-blocked SNC-121-mediated retina neuroprotection. The nitrotyrosine level in the glaucomatous retina was also increased, which was significantly reduced in the SNC-121-treated animals. Additionally, the expression level of iNOS was clearly increased over the control levels in the glaucomatous retina and optic nerves, which was also reduced by SNC-121 treatment. In conclusion, our data support the notion that nitric oxide plays a detrimental role during glaucomatous injury and inhibition of nitric oxide production provided RGC neuroprotection. Furthermore, δ-opioid receptor activation regulates the production of nitric oxide via inhibiting the activity of iNOS in the retina and optic nerve.

Editor: Steven Barnes, Dalhousie University, Canada

Funding: Supported in part by National Institutes of Health/National Eye Institute grant EY019081 (SH), and an unrestricted grant to MUSC-SEI from Research to Prevent Blindness, New York, New York. This work was conducted in a facility constructed with support from the National Institutes of Health, Grant Number C06 RR015455 from the Extramural Research Facilities Program of the National Center for Research Resources. The funders had no role in study design, data collection and analysis, decision to publish, or preparation of the manuscript.

Competing Interests: The authors have declared that no competing interests exist.

* Email: Husain@musc.edu

Introduction

Glaucoma is a slowly progressing optic neuropathy that causes loss of retinal ganglion cells (RGCs), optic disc changes, and visual-field loss [1,2]. Currently, intraocular pressure (IOP) lowering strategies are the only effective way to control the disease progression. However, reduction in IOP is not always successful and many patients continue to experience the progressive loss of vision [3,4]. The mechanisms that lead to the RGC death during disease progression are unclear. However, accumulating literature suggests that multiple mechanisms are involved in RGC death in glaucoma including inflammation [5–8], apoptosis [9–11], neurotrophic factor deprivation [12,13], and nitric oxide production [14–16]. During the progression of glaucoma, glial cells, mainly astrocytes within the optic nerve head (ONH) [17], also play key roles in the initiation of lesions in glaucomatous optic neuropathy [18]. While astrocytes play a vital role in maintaining a normal physiological state in RGCs, they become activated in response to glaucomatous injury and produce neurotoxic substances like proinflammatory cytokines [7,8] and nitric oxide which ultimately leads to axonal and RGC loss [14,15,19].

Nitric oxide is an important signaling molecule, which regulates various physiological processes in numerous tissues. In the eye it regulates IOP [20,21], and small quantities could be beneficial to maintain metabolites and blood circulation [22]. However, sustained levels of nitric oxide production may result in direct tissue toxicity and contribute to neuronal degeneration [23]. Nitric oxide is produced by nitric oxide synthase (NOS); three isoforms of NOS have been cloned: constitutive (NOS-1 or nNOS), endothelial (NOS-3 or eNOS), and inducible (iNOS or NOS-2). Inducible NOS has been implicated in several neurodegenerative human diseases including Parkinson and stroke [24]. However, conflicting data have been reported for the role of nitric oxide and nitric oxide synthase in glaucoma-induced retina degeneration and RGC loss [14–16,25,26].

To clarify the role of nitric oxide in glaucoma pathology we have used a chronic ocular-hypertensive rat glaucoma model [27] and determined if δ-opioid-receptor activation regulates nitric oxide production. Additionally, we determined if δ-opioid-receptor-mediated retina neuroprotection is partly via nitric-oxide-dependent pathways. The data we provide herein support the idea that nitric oxide, mainly produced by iNOS, played a detrimental role during glaucomatous injury, and its inhibition either by its selective inhibitor, aminoguanidine (AG), or by δ-opioid-receptor agonist (SNC-121), provided retina neuroprotection against glaucomatous injury.

Materials and Methods

Animals

Adult female Brown Norway rats (3–5 months of age; 150–200 grams; Harlan Laboratories, Inc., Indianapolis, IN, and Charles River laboratory, San Diego, CA) were used in this study. Female rats were chosen because they are calm and easy to handle when measuring IOP in conscious rats. Rats were kept under a cycle of 12-hours light and 12-hours dark for all the studies. Animal handling was performed in accordance with the ARVO Statement for the Use of Animals in Ophthalmic and Vision Research; and the study protocol was approved by the Animal Care and Use Committee at the Medical University of South Carolina.

Drug Preparation

Delta (δ)-opioid-receptor agonist, SNC-121 (Santa Cruz Biotechnology, Dallas, TX), was dissolved in normal saline (0.9%). SNC-121 (1 mg/kg) was injected intraperitoneally (i.p.) into Brown Norway rats 30 minutes after glaucomatous injury, and treatment was continued for 7 days, once daily. Inducible nitric oxide synthase (iNOS or NOS-2) inhibitor, 25 mg/kg aminoguanidine hydrochloride (AG; Sigma-Aldrich, St. Louis, MO) was also intraperitoneally (i.p.) injected 30 minutes after glaucoma surgery. The AG treatment was continued for 7 days, once daily. In a separate group, animals were treated with both AG and SNC-121 simultaneously for 7 days, once daily. In this group, animals were first treated with AG (25 mg/kg, i.p.) 30 minutes after glaucomatous injury, followed by SNC-121 (1 mg/kg, i.p.) treatment at an interval of 15 minutes. A group of animals was also treated with a selective δ-opioid-receptor antagonist, naltrindole (3 mg/kg; i.p.), 30 minutes after glaucomatous injury, followed by SNC-121 treatment for 7 days, once daily. Drug administration (150–200 μL) was performed daily at the same time between 9 am-11 am. The control group was handled

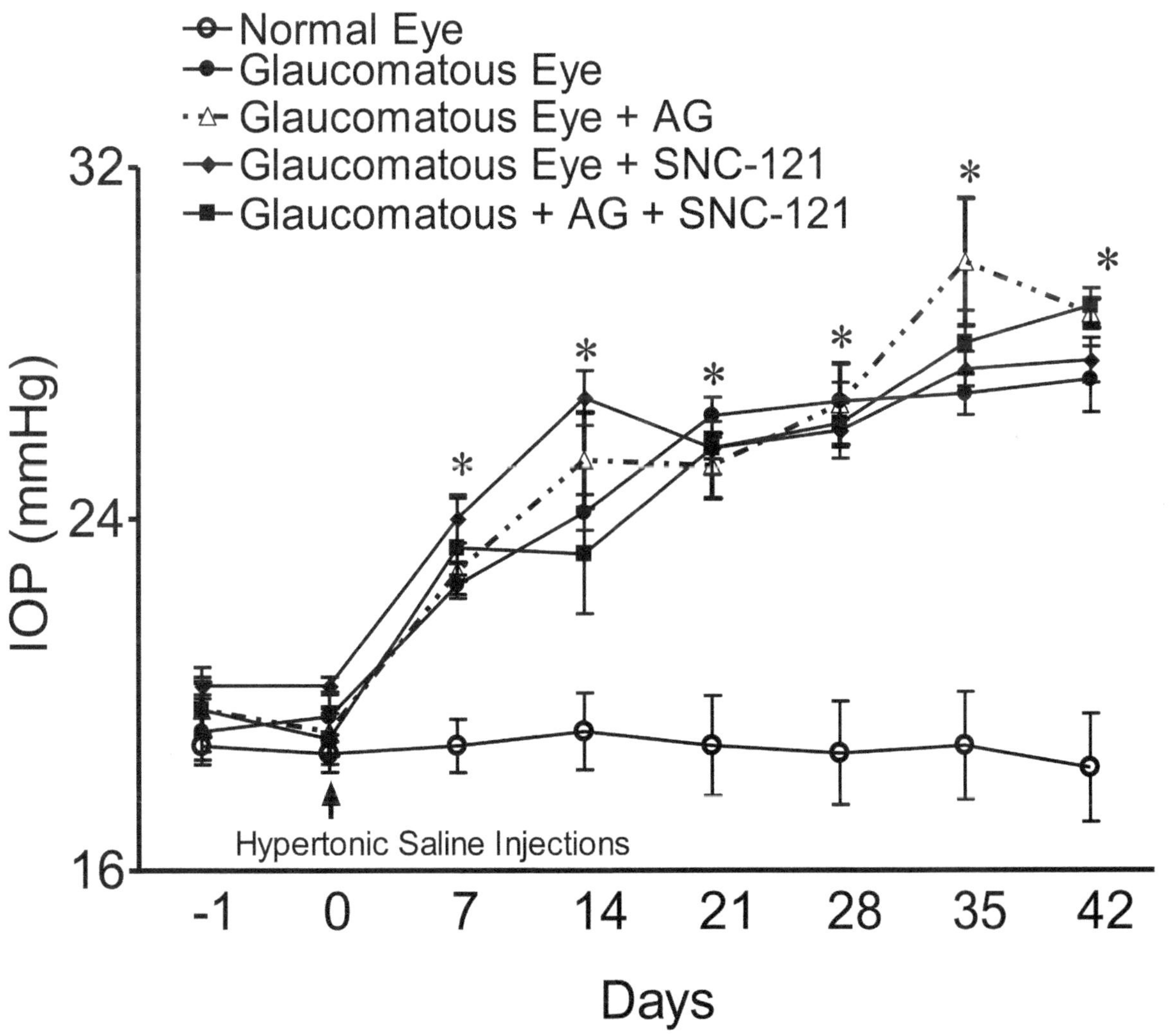

Figure 1. Intraocular pressure (IOP) measurements in normal and glaucomatous eyes. IOP of normal eyes and eyes from a chronic glaucoma model with and without AG (25 mg/kg; i.p.) and SNC-121 (1 mg/kg) treatment for 7 days (once daily) was measured as described in the Methods. IOP was elevated in one eye of Brown Norway rats by injecting approximately 50 μL of 2.0 M hypertonic saline, while the contralateral eye served as the control. Rats were maintained for up to 6 weeks post-surgery. Data are mean ± SE. *$P<0.05$; n = 6–8 for each group.

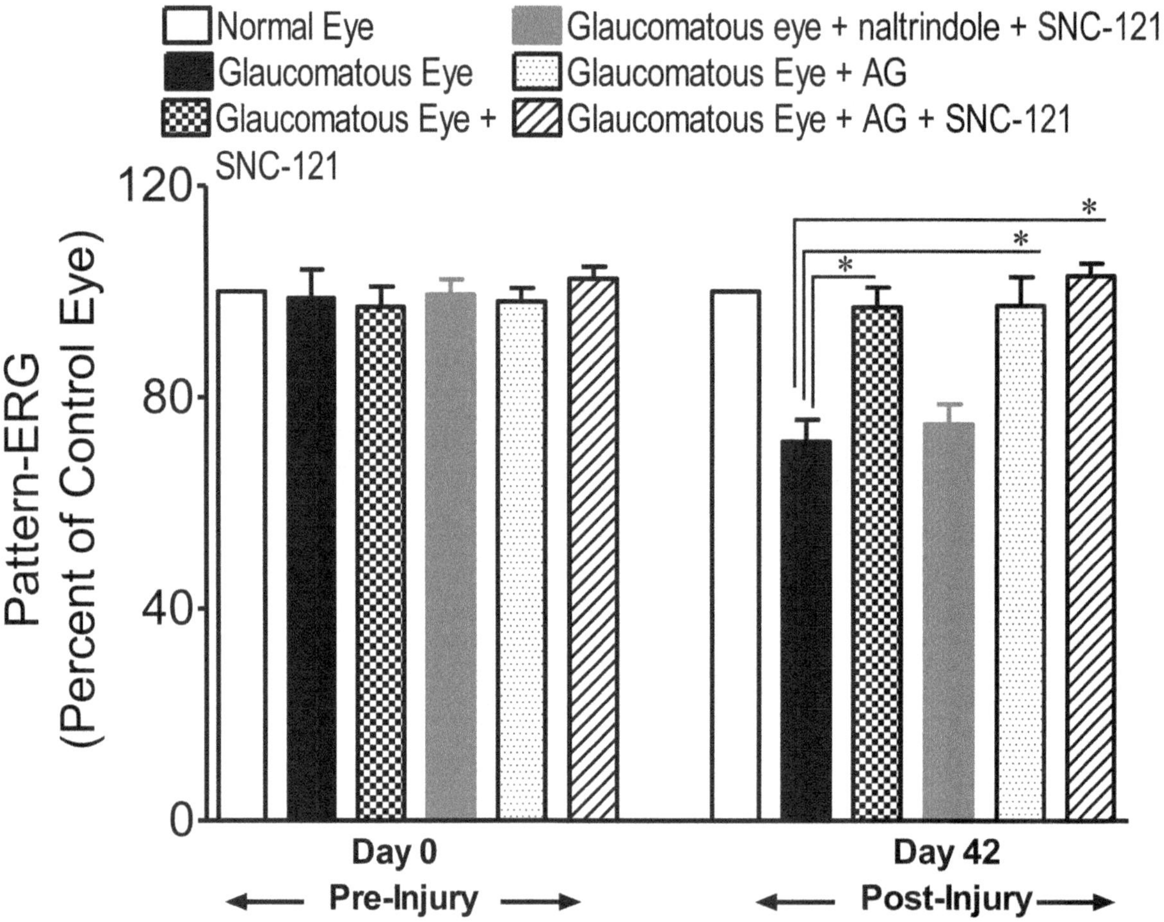

Figure 2. Pattern ERG recordings in normal and glaucomatous eyes. Changes observed in Pattern ERGs of untreated, AG or SNC-121-treated glaucomatous rat eyes are shown as a percentage of the contralateral control eye. In these experiments, Brown Norway rats were treated with AG (25 mg/kg, i.p.) or SNC-121 (1 mg/kg, i.p.), individually or together simultaneously, 30 minutes after hypertonic saline injections. Animals were treated with naltrindole 30 minutes after glaucomatous injury followed by SNC-121 treatment. The drug treatment was continued once daily for 7 days in all groups. Data are mean ± SE; *$P<0.05$; n = 7–8.

in a similar fashion except that normal saline was injected without SNC-121 or AG.

Development of Glaucoma Model by Hypertonic Saline Injection

Brown Norway rats (150–200 gm body weight) were housed under a standard 12:12 (light:dark) cycle. A stable baseline IOP was documented prior to hypertonic saline injection. Rats were anesthetized with ketamine (75 mg/kg) and xylazine (8 mg/kg) and body temperature was maintained at 37°C with a heating pad. Topical proparacaine (0.5%) was applied to the cornea. IOP was elevated using 50 µL of 2 M hypertonic saline into the circumferential limbal vein near the cornea as described earlier [7,27]. After surgery, an antibacterial ointment (neomycin) was applied at the injection site of each animal to prevent infections. As inclusion criteria following hypertonic saline injection, only animals with an elevated IOP that was at least 25% over baseline were included in the study.

Pattern Electroretinogram (Pattern-ERG) Recordings

Rats were anesthetized with ketamine (75 mg/kg) and xylazine (8 mg/kg) and body temperature was maintained at 37°C with a heating pad. Pattern-ERG recordings (without dark adaptation) were conducted in both eyes (sequentially) 3 days prior to IOP elevation by hypertonic saline injection, and then weekly post-surgery as described earlier [7,27]. For the Pattern-ERG amplitudes, measurements were made between a peak and adjacent trough of the waveform as described earlier [27]. Pattern-ERG amplitudes were obtained for each eye by collecting 300 sweeps at an interval of 1 second. The final pattern-ERG amplitude was an average of 300 sweeps for each eye.

Retinal Ganglion Cell (RGC) Counting

RGCs were visualized and counted by retrograde-labeling using fluorogold as described earlier [7,27]. Briefly, animals were anesthetized with ketamine (75 mg/kg, i.p.) and xylazine (8 mg/kg, i.p.), and 5% Fluorogold (Fluorochrome, LLC; Denver, CO) was injected into the superior colliculus in animals immobilized in a stereotaxic apparatus. Seven days after injection, animals were euthanized and their eyes were enucleated and fixed in 4% paraformaldehyde for 24 hours at 4°C. After rinsing with PBS, each retina was detached from the eyecup and prepared as a flatmount by mounting with the vitreous side-up. RGCs were counted and averaged per 8 microscopic fields of identical size (150 μm^2; 20x magnification) per retina by using Image J software (NIH, Bethesda, MD). The automated RGC numbers generated

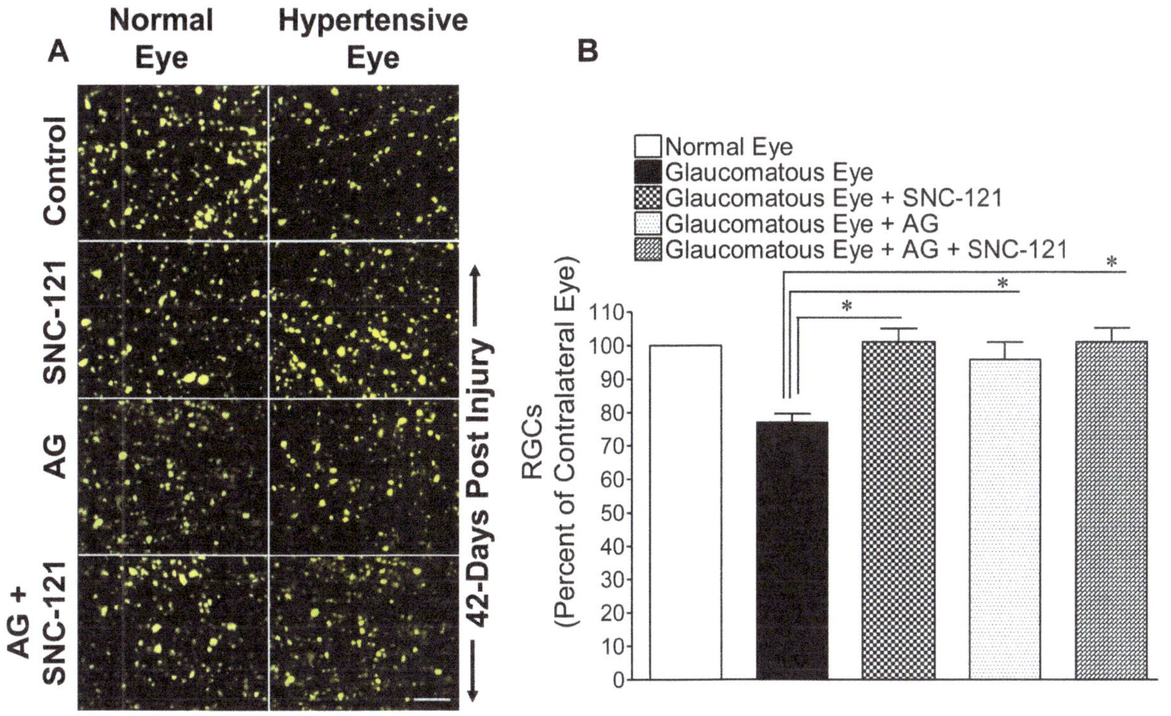

Figure 3. Retina flat mounts of normal and glaucomatous eyes. Fluorescence micrographs of flatmounted retinas depicting Fluorogold-labeled retina ganglion cells (RGCs) in normal and glaucomatous eyes in the absence or presence of drugs (**A**). Briefly, 3 μL of a 5% solution of Fluorogold was injected into the superior colliculus of anesthetized animals. Seven days post injection, animals were euthanized and retinas were prepared as flatmounts, vitreous-side facing up. Fluorescent RGCs were visualized under Zeiss microscopy. Bar = 20 μm. Total RGC tallies in glaucomatous eyes in the absence or presence of drugs. RGCs were counted in 8 microscopic fields of identical size (150 μm^2 area) for each retina, using Image J software (**B**). **P*<0.05; n = 6 for each group.

by Image J software were comparable when RGCs were counted manually by two operators in a masked fashion.

Immunohistochemistry

Optic nerves and eyes of normal and glaucomatous animals were collected at the 7th and 42nd day post glaucomatous injury, as described earlier [7,27]. Optic nerves and eyes were fixed in paraformaldehyde (4%) overnight at 4°C, then cryoprotected in a 30% sucrose solution overnight at 4°C. Optic nerves and eyes were washed with cold PBS and embedded in OCT compound embedding medium over dry ice. Cryosections of optic nerve and retina were cut in a cryostat at −20°C and tissues were incubated with primary antibody (anti iNOS at 1:100 dilution; BD BioSciences, San Jose, CA) followed by incubation with FITC-conjugated secondary antibody (1:400 dilutions; Jackson Immuno Research Laboratories, Inc., West Grove, PA). Negative control slides were incubated with 0.5% BSA instead of primary antibodies. Tissue sections were viewed under a fluorescent microscope and digitized images were captured by a digital camera (Zeiss).

Western Blotting

An equivalent amount of retina lysate (15 μg/lane) was loaded onto 10% SDS-PAGE. Proteins were separated and transferred to nitrocellulose membrane. The membranes were blocked with 5% nonfat dry milk, and then incubated with appropriate primary antibody (anti-Nitrotyrosine at a 1:1000 dilution; anti-iNOS at a 1:1000 dilution; or anti-β-actin at a 1:3000 dilution) for 12 hours at 4°C. After washing, membranes were incubated with appropriate secondary antibodies (HRP-conjugated at 1:3000 dilution). The membranes were treated with enhanced chemiluminescent reagent to detect the signals using a Biorad Versadoc imaging system (Biorad, Hercules, CA).

Measurements of Nitrate Nitrite in Retina Extracts

Nitrate-nitrite was estimated by using "Cayman's Assay Kit" (Cayman, Item number-780001, Ann Arbor, MI). This method involves a two-step process. Briefly, the retinas were homogenized and centrifuged at 10,000 *g* for 10 minutes. The supernatant was collected to measure nitrates-nitrites. The reaction was started by adding 80 μL of retina samples, 10 μL of enzyme cofactor, and 10 μL nitrate reductase in a 96-well plate. After 1 hour, 50 μL Greiss reagents were added and allowed to incubate for 30 minutes. The changes in absorbance were measured at 550 nm. The amount of nitrate-nitrite was expressed as mM of nitrate-nitrite per milligram protein.

Statistical Analysis

The data are expressed as mean ± SEM. The comparisons were made using Student *t* test for paired samples or ANOVA with Bonferroni post test for multiple comparisons (Graph Pad Software, Inc., San Diego, CA). A *P* value of <0.05 is considered significant.

Results

Intraocular pressure (IOP) was raised by injecting 2 M hypertonic saline into limbal veins and IOP was measured up to 42 days at an interval of 7 days, as described earlier [7]. A significant elevation in IOP was seen as early as 7 days post

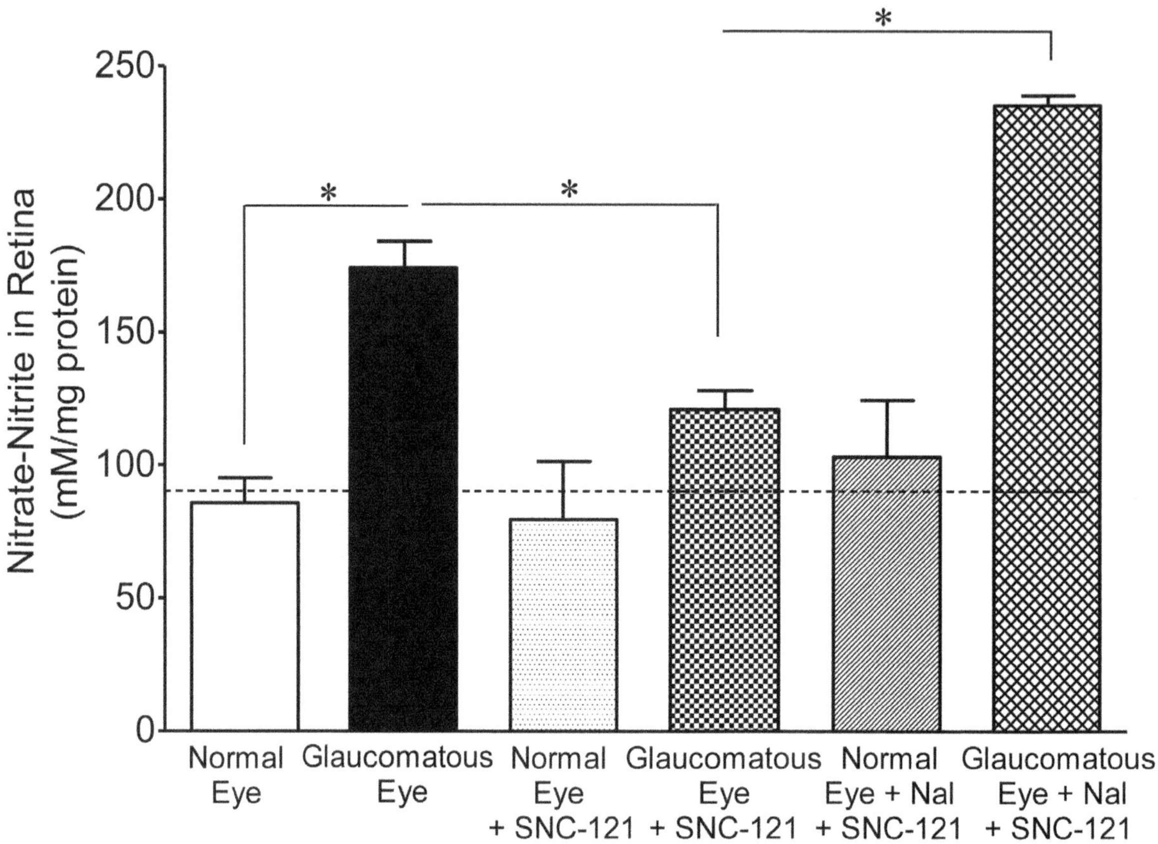

Figure 4. Measurements of nitrate-nitrite in normal and glaucomatous eyes in the presence of SNC-121. Animals were treated with SNC-121 (1 mg/kg, i.p.) 30 minutes after glaucomatous injury, and continued once daily for 7 days. A separate group of animals was pretreated with naltrindole (Nal; 3 mg/kg, i.p.) followed by SNC-121 (1 mg/kg, i.p.) treatment 30 minutes after glaucomatous injury, and continued for 7 days, once daily. The absorbance was read at 550 nm and absorbance was plotted against the nitrate standards. The amount of nitrate-nitrite is expressed as millimolar nitrates-nitrites per milligram protein. Data are expressed as mean ± SEM, (*$P<0.05$; n =4–7).

surgery and was maintained up to 42 days following IOP elevation. Similar to our previous studies, we did not see any significant changes in IOP of normal and glaucomatous eyes when animals were treated with a selective δ-opioid-receptor agonist, SNC-121 (1 mg/Kg, i.p.), for 7 days [7] (**Figure 1**). To determine the effects of aminoguanidine (AG) alone or in combination with SNC-121 on IOP, animals were either treated with AG (25 mg/kg, i.p.) alone for 7 days, once daily, or with AG (25 mg/kg, i.p.) and SNC-121 (1 mg/Kg, i.p.) simultaneously for 7 days, once daily. As shown in **Figure 1**, elevated IOP in glaucomatous animals was not changed significantly when animals were treated either with AG or AG plus SNC-121 simultaneously. The functional response of retinal ganglion cells (RGCs) in normal and glaucomatous eyes was measured by pattern-electroretinogram (Pattern-ERG) at 42nd day, post glaucomatous injury. To determine if δ-opioid-receptor-mediated retina neuroprotection was partly mediated via nitric oxide-dependent pathways, animals were treated with a selective iNOS inhibitor (AG; 25 mg/kg, i.p.), a selective δ-opioid-receptor agonist (SNC-121; 1 mg/kg, i.p.) individually or with both drugs simultaneously for 7 days, once daily. As shown in **Figure 2**, the Pattern-ERG amplitudes were reduced by 35% in glaucomatous animals (control eyes 100±00% vs. glaucomatous eyes 65±6%; $P<0.05$). Treatment of animals with AG for 7 days provided retina neuroprotection against glaucomatous injury (glaucomatous eyes, 65±6% vs. glaucomatous eyes + AG, 93±6%; $P<0.05$). Similar to our previous findings [7], SNC-121 treatment also provided a significant amount of retina neuroprotection; however, we did not see any significant additive or synergistic effects when animals were treated with both drugs (e.g., AG and SNC-121) simultaneously (glaucomatous eyes, 65±6% vs. glaucomatous eyes + AG + SNC-121, 110±8%; $P<0.05$). As expected, SNC-121-mediated retina neuroprotection was fully-blocked by pretreatment with δ-opioid-receptor antagonist, naltrindole (**Fig. 2**).

To confirm that declines in Pattern-ERG amplitudes were due to the loss of RGCs, they were visualized by retrograde-labeling with bilateral injections of fluorogold into the superior colliculus (**Fig. 3A**). The loss of RGCs in the glaucomatous eyes was reduced when animals were treated either with AG (25 mg/kg; i.p.) or SNC-121 (1 mg/kg; i.p.) for 7 days; however, we did not see any further decline in the rate of RGC loss when animals were treated with both drugs simultaneously. Quantification of RGCs in normal eyes, glaucomatous eyes, AG-treated glaucomatous eyes, SNC-121-treated glaucomatous eyes, or both drug-treated glaucomatous eyes are shown in **Figure 3B**. The mean number (± SE) of fluorogold-positive RGCs were: normal eyes, 2150±99 RGCs/mm^2; glaucomatous eyes, 1666±105 RGCs/mm^2 (23% less than normal eyes; $P<0.05$); AG-treated glaucomatous eyes, 2012±108.1 RGCs/mm^2 (21% greater than the glaucomatous eyes; $P<0.05$), SNC-121-treated glaucomatous eyes, 2223±75 RGCs/mm^2 (33% greater than the glaucomatous eyes; $P<0.05$),

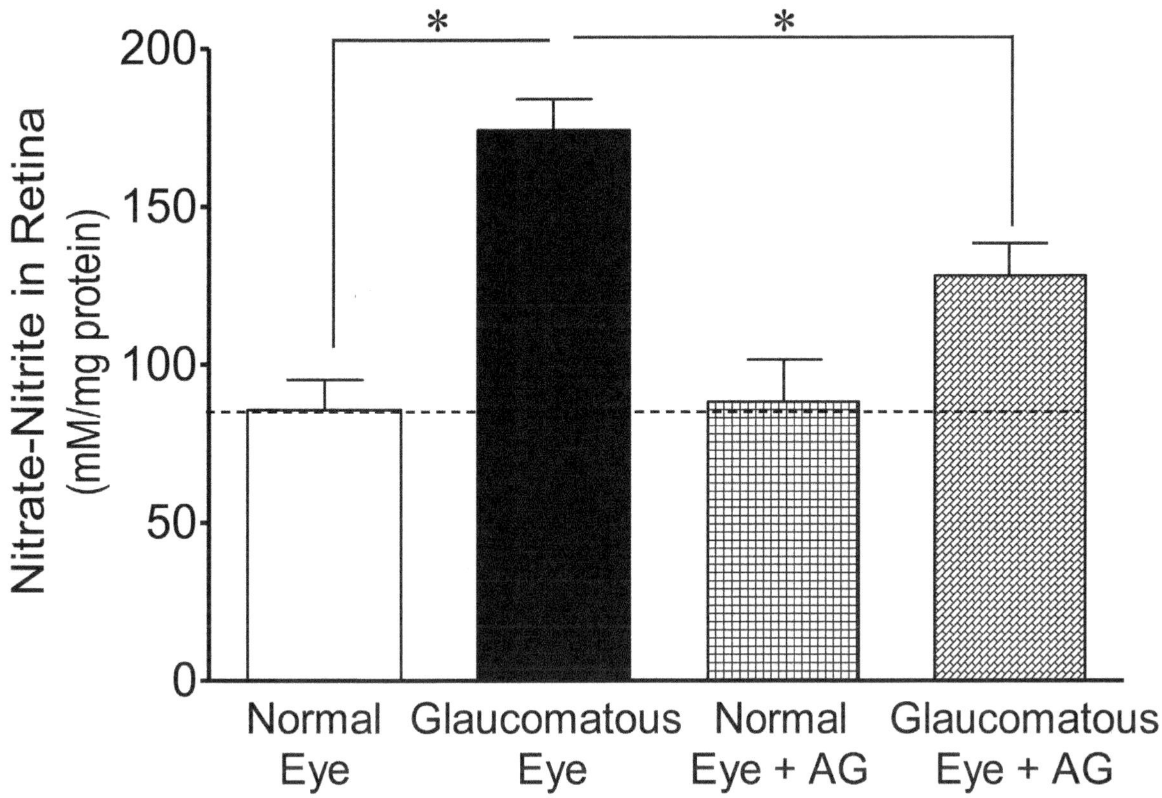

Figure 5. Measurements of nitrate-nitrite in normal and glaucomatous eyes in the presence of AG. Animals were treated with AG (25 mg/kg, i.p.) 30 minutes after glaucomatous injury and continued for 7 days, once daily. The absorbance was measured at 550 nm and absorbance was plotted against the nitrate standards. The amount of nitrate-nitrite is expressed as millimolar nitrates-nitrites per milligram protein. Data are expressed as mean ± SEM, (*$P<0.05$; n = 4–6).

and AG + SNC-121-treated glaucomatous eyes, 2181±94.59 RGCs/mm^2 (31% greater than the glaucomatous eyes; $P<0.05$).

To dissect out the molecular mechanisms, we measured the nitrate and nitrite levels, which are the end products of nitric oxide metabolism. We believe that nitric oxide is produced in an early stage of glaucoma; so we collected whole retina extracts to measure nitrates and nitrites at the 7th day, post glaucomatous injury. The levels of nitrate-nitrite were significantly increased in the retina sample of glaucomatous eyes when compared with normal eyes (normal eyes, 86±9 vs. glaucomatous eyes, 174±10 mM/mg protein; $P<0.001$; **Figs. 4–5**). The levels of nitrate-nitrite were significantly reduced in glaucomatous eyes when animals were treated either with SNC-121 (121±7 mM/mg protein; $P<0.05$; **Fig. 4**) or AG (128±10 mM/mg protein; $P<0.05$; **Fig. 5**) for 7 days, once a day. To confirm that SNC-121-mediated reduction in nitrate-nitrite levels was via activation of δ-opioid receptors, animals were treated with a selective δ-opioid-receptor antagonist, naltrindole. As shown in **Figure 4**, SNC-121-mediated reduction in nitrate-nitrite levels was not only blocked, but naltrindole treatment potentiated the nitrate-nitrite production in glaucomatous eyes (235±4 mM/mg protein; $P<0.001$; **Fig. 4**). Surprisingly, naltrindole increased the basal levels of nitrate-nitrite in normal eyes, although this change was not statistically significant. Nitric oxide is a versatile free-radical that mediates numerous biological functions. Although nitric oxide can modify numerous signaling pathways, the reaction of nitric oxide with cysteine residues in proteins, a process known as nitrosylation, is emerging as one of the most important mechanisms. This post-translational modification, *S*-nitrosylation, is a physiologically-important event that affects a wide variety of proteins involved in a number of cellular processes. As shown in **Figure 6**, an increase in the nitrotyrosine level in the retina sample of glaucomatous eyes was seen when compared with the normal eye on the 7th day, post injury. Interestingly, the nitrotyrosine levels were reduced in SNC-121-treated animals (**Fig. 6**).

To further confirm that elevation in nitric oxide production during glaucomatous injury is due to iNOS up-regulation and/or activation, we measured the iNOS levels in optic nerve at 7 and 42 days, post injury. As shown in **Figures 7–8**, the expression levels of iNOS were clearly increased over control levels in glaucomatous optic nerves, which was fully-attenuated in SNC-121-treated glaucomatous optic nerve. However, the iNOS expression pattern was not changed by SNC-121 treatment in normal optic nerves. Additionally, expression of iNOS was increased in the retina on day 7th and 42nd, post glaucomatous injury; which was significantly reduced by SNC-121 treatment (**Fig. 9**).

Discussion

We determined that activation of δ-opioid receptors by exogenous ligand (SNC-121) blocked nitric oxide production and subsequently rescued retinal ganglion cells (RGCs) from glaucomatous injury. Nitric oxide at physiological concentrations controls vascular inflammation and vascular injury by inhibiting the proinflammatory gene expression, but excessive production of nitric oxide can cause tissue toxicity and cell death [24]. Although the pathological role of nitric oxide in several neurodegenerative human diseases is somewhat clear, the pathological role of nitric

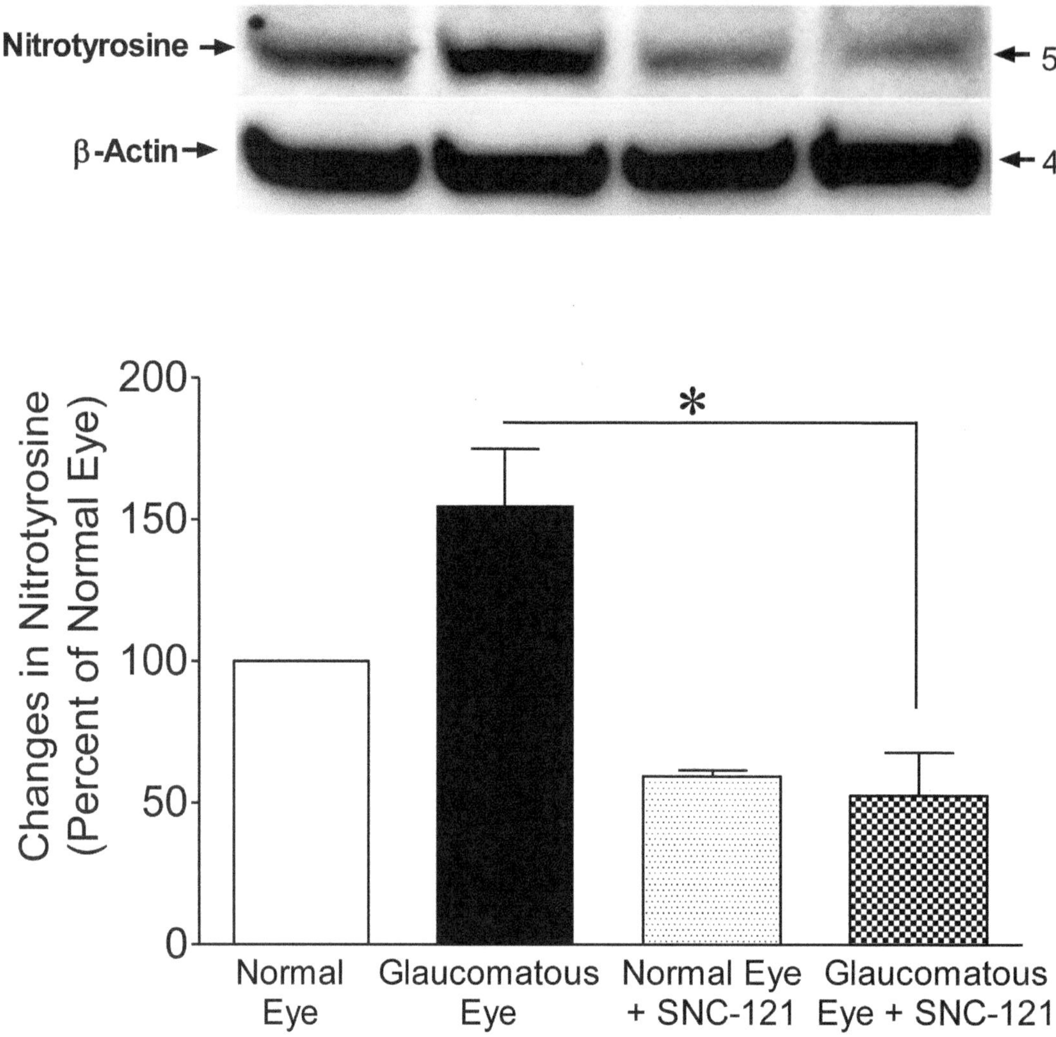

Figure 6. Measurement of protein nitrosylation in retina by Western blotting using nitrotyrosine antibodies in response to glaucomatous injury. Animals were treated with SNC-121 (1 mg/kg, i.p.) 30 minutes after glaucomatous injury and continued for 7 days, once daily. Retina extracts were collected at the 7th day, post injury, and analyzed using anti-nitrotyrosine antibodies and appropriate secondary antibodies (HRP-conjugated; dilution 1:3000). The signal was captured using enhanced chemiluminescent reagent and the Biorad Versadoc imaging system. Data shown are representative of four independent experiments. Data are expressed as mean ± SEM. *$P<0.05$; n = 4.

oxide in glaucoma remains in question. For example: an increase in the inducible nitric oxide synthase (iNOS) has been reported in astrocytes and the optic nerve head of primary open-angle glaucoma (POAG) patients [14,16,28]. Furthermore, aminoguanidine (AG), a selective iNOS inhibitor, treatment provides RGC neuroprotection in an extraocular vein cauterization glaucoma model [15]. There was a 36% loss in RGCs in this cautery glaucoma model which was reduced to 9.6% by 60 mg/kg AG treatment. In non-glaucoma models, nitric oxide is produced mainly by iNOS that has been implicated in ischemia-induced retinal degeneration [29,30]. The iNOS inhibition resulted in the RGC neuroprotection against ischemia [31] and axotomy [32]. In contrast, studies also have shown that iNOS levels are not changed in POAG patients [26] and iNOS does not play a detrimental role in glaucomatous injury in chronically-elevated IOP glaucoma model (i.e., a model of aqueous humor outflow obstruction). Moreover, iNOS expression was not correlated with the severity of optic nerve damage [26]. Additional studies have shown that iNOS does not play a detrimental role in optic neuropathy in the DBA/2J glaucoma model [25]. In view of these conflicting results obtained from different laboratories using different experimental glaucoma models, we decided to further test the potential involvement of nitric oxide and inducible NOS (iNOS) in glaucomatous injury. Additionally, we determined if δ-opioid-receptor activation regulates the nitric oxide production.

Although, contradictory reports have been presented in the literature for RGC and optic nerve neuroprotection by iNOS inhibitor (e.g., AG), but all the studies were agreed that AG treatment does not change IOP in normal and glaucomatous animals [15,26]. Our data is in agreement with previous reports showing that AG treatment had no significant effect on IOP (**Fig. 1**). Additionally, our data presented herein clearly demonstrated that blocking nitric oxide either directly by AG or indirectly via activating δ-opioid-receptors by SNC-121, provided RGC neuroprotection. The functional outcome (Pattern-ERG) of the retina is also changed in the δ-opioid-receptor agonist-treated animals, suggesting that SNC-121 possibly crosses the blood retinal barrier. The most striking findings were that iNOS

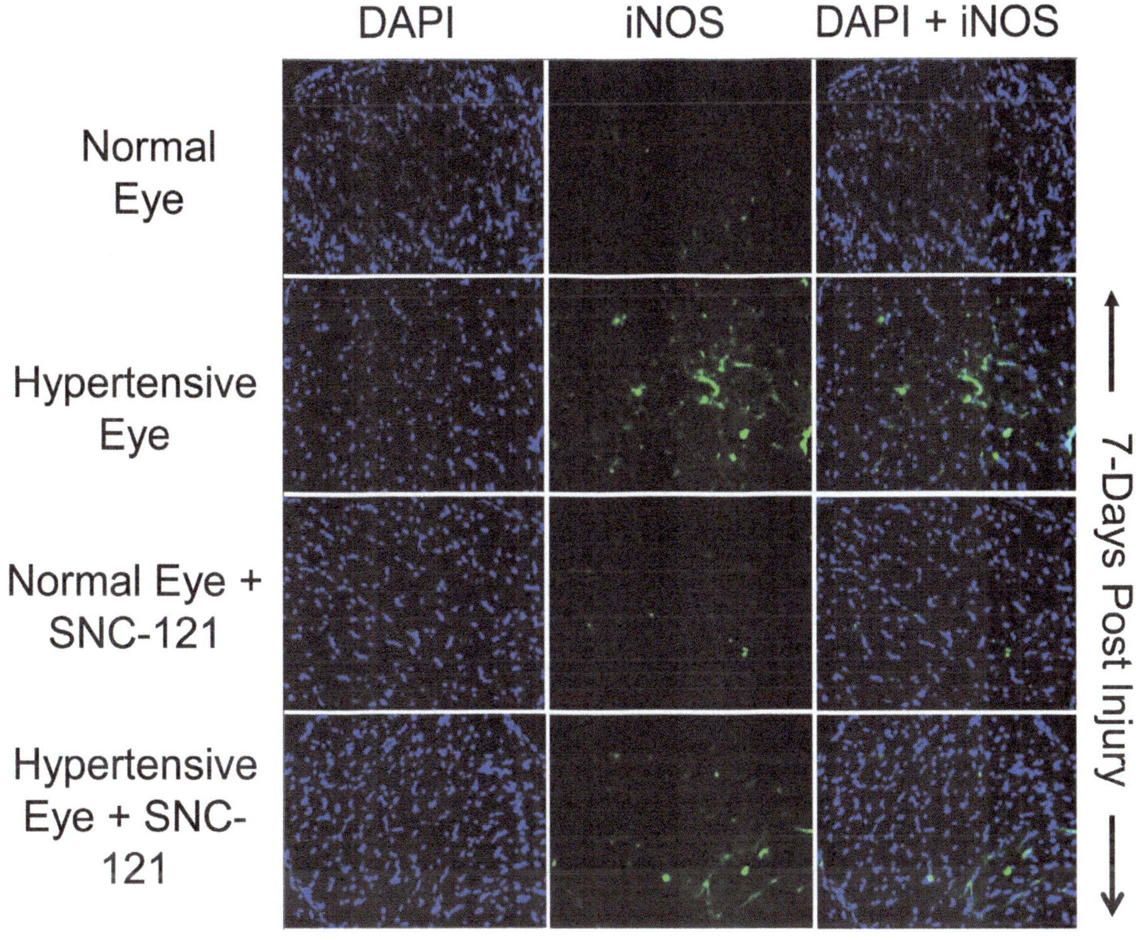

Figure 7. Changes in iNOS expression in glaucomatous optic nerve at 7 days, post injury. The optic nerve (non-myelinated; 2 mm post globe) of Brown Norway rats was removed 7-days post glaucomatous injury. Contralateral optic nerve was used as the normal control. Cryosections were immunostained by anti-iNOS antibodies as indicated horizontally. Ocular treatments are indicated vertically. Green color indicates staining for iNOS and blue nuclei for DAPI. There was no positive staining when primary antibodies were omitted (data not shown). Data shown here are representations of at least four independent experiments. A total of 10 animals were used in this experiment. Comparable staining for iNOS was seen in at least 4 animals in each treatment group.

production was not only elevated in the retina, but also increased in the optic nerve in response to glaucomatous injury, which was attenuated in the presence of SNC-121. Additionally, we have shown that changes in iNOS expression are occurring at an early stage of glaucoma progression (day 7), while other studies [15,26] have measured such changes in iNOS expression at 6–9 months, post glaucomatous injury. Our results confirmed that the enhanced levels of nitric oxide seen in glaucomatous eyes were due to up-regulation of iNOS not only in the retina, but also in the optic nerve, which may be playing a crucial role in orchestrating RGC death in a paracrine fashion during the pathogenesis of glaucoma.

Our findings are consistent with Shareef and Neufeld [15,16] who reported that treatment of glaucomatous rats with AG provide retina neuroprotection. However, our results do not agree with Pang and colleagues [26] while both studies have used a similar glaucoma rat model. However, there were numerous procedural differences in the two studies (e.g., Pang [26] and current study) and the discrepancies seen in these studies could be related to such variation in the protocols. For example: 1) normal and glaucomatous animals were kept under constant dim light that resulted in a higher baseline IOP (28 mmHg) versus dark-light cycle with baseline IOP (18–21 mmHg) in our studies; 2) pretreatment of animals with AG for 7 days prior to glaucomatous injury versus treatment of animals 30 minutes post glaucomatous injury in our studies; 3) duration of AG treatment in drinking water for 42 days versus AG treatment (intraperitoneally) for 7 days in our studies, 4) dosage differences of AG; and 5) the lack of RGC function measurement versus Pattern-ERG measurements in our studies. At this time, we cannot explain why genetic ablation of iNOS is not neuroprotective in the DBA/2J model. We believe, this area of research is still not fully-developed and more work is needed to understand a broader role of nitric oxide in general, and iNOS in particular for glaucoma pathology. Overall, our IHC data in retina and optic nerve, Western blotting data, and functional data (Pattern-ERG) support a neurodegenerative role of iNOS during glaucomatous injury.

Recently, we have shown that activation of δ-opioid receptors by a selective agonist (SNC-121) provides retina neuroprotection against glaucomatous injury via attenuation of p38 MAP kinase activity and TNF-α production [7]. Studies have shown that δ- and κ-opioid-receptor-activation provides brain neuroprotection via nitric oxide regulation [33,34]. The role of nitric oxide in δ-opioid-mediated retinal neuroprotection against glaucomatous

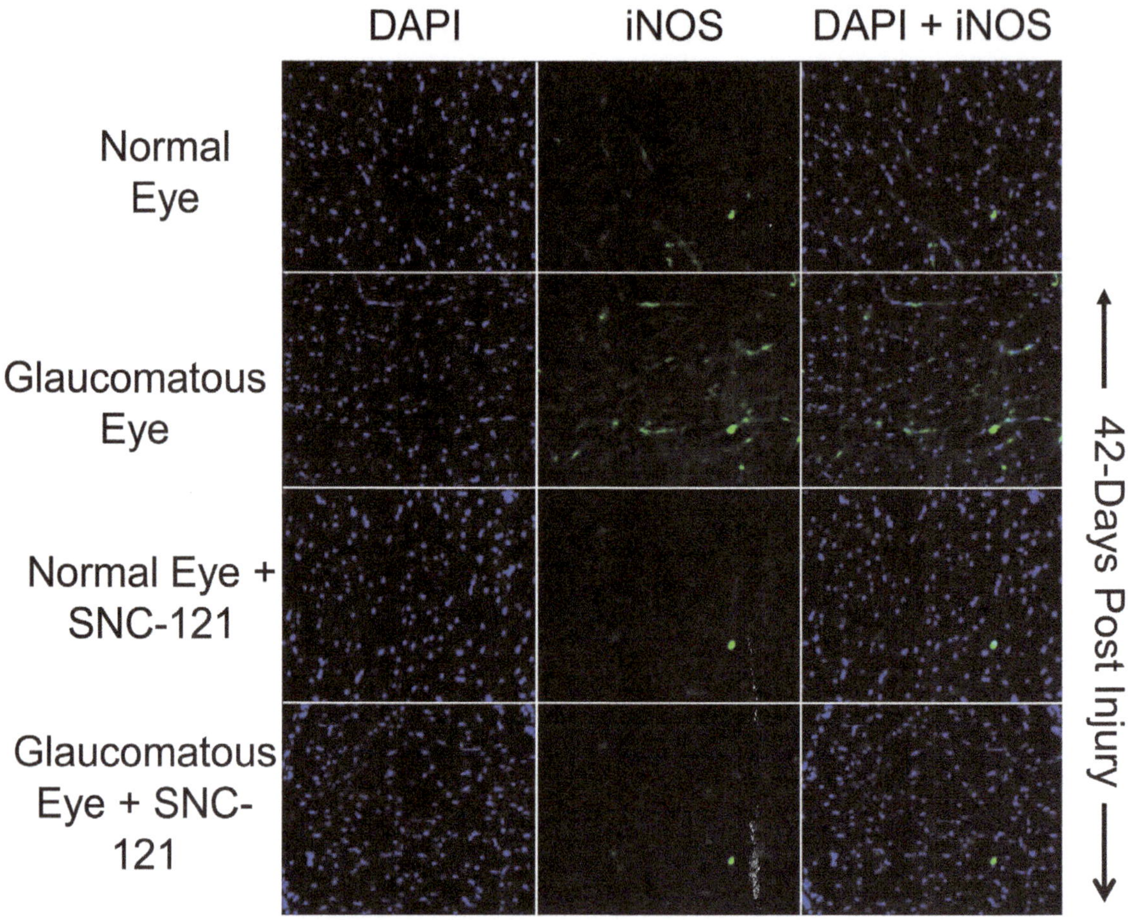

Figure 8. Changes in iNOS expression in glaucomatous optic nerve at 42 days, post injury. The optic nerve (non-myelinated; 2 mm post globe) of Brown Norway rats was removed 42-days post glaucomatous injury. Contralateral optic nerve was used as the normal control. Cryosections were immunostained by anti-iNOS antibodies as indicated horizontally. Ocular treatments are indicated vertically. Data shown in this Figure are a representation of at least four independent experiments. A total of 10 animals were used in this experiment. Comparable staining for iNOS was seen in at least 4 animals in each treatment group.

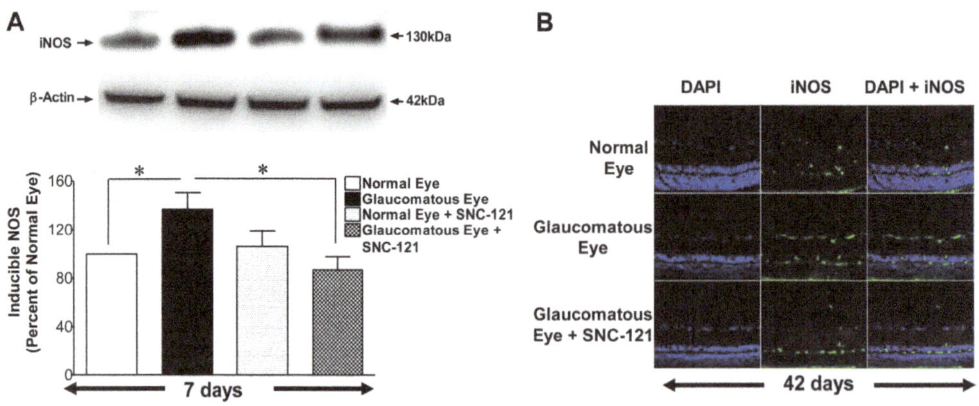

Figure 9. Changes in iNOS expression in glaucomatous retina at 7 and 42 days, post injury. (A) Brown Norway rats were treated with SNC-121 (1 mg/kg, i.p.) 30 minutes after glaucomatous injury and continued for 7 days, once daily. Retina extracts were collected at the 7th day, post injury, and analyzed using anti-iNOS antibodies and appropriate secondary antibodies (HRP-conjugated; dilution 1:3000). The signal was captured using enhanced chemiluminescent reagent and the Biorad Versadoc imaging system. Data are expressed as mean ± SEM. *$P<0.05$; n = 4. (B) The eyes of Brown Norway rats were removed 42-days post glaucomatous injury. Cryosections of retina were immunostained by anti-iNOS antibodies as indicated horizontally. Ocular treatments are indicated vertically. Data shown in this Figure are a representation of at least four independent experiments.

injury has not been defined. To determine the roles of iNOS in δ-opioid-receptor-mediated retina neuroprotection, we have treated animals with AG and SNC-121 after glaucomatous injury. We did not see any additional beneficial effects on RGC neuroprotection when animals were simultaneously-treated with AG and SNC-121, suggesting that SNC-121 treatment fully blocked the activity of iNOS. To further confirm the roles of δ-opioid-receptor-activation in iNOS regulation during glaucomatous injury, we measured the production of nitrates and nitrites in the presence or absence of SNC-121. It is very difficult to measure appreciable levels of nitric oxide due to its short life; however nitrites are the stable reservoir that can reduced to bioactive nitric oxide and other nitrogen reactive species during hypoxic conditions [35]. Both AG and SNC-121 treatment reduced the amount of nitrates-nitrites significantly in the glaucomatous eyes. As expected, SNC-121-mediated reduction in nitrates-nitrites was reversed by the δ-opioid-receptor antagonist, naltrindole. These data suggested that SNC-121-mediated reduction in nitrates-nitrites was due to δ-opioid-receptor-activation. It is important to emphasize that naltrindole treatment potentiated the levels of nitrate-nitrite production in both normal and glaucomatous retinas, suggesting that an endogenous tone of δ-opioid-receptor-activation is required to control endogenous levels of nitric oxide.

Nitrotyrosine is identified as an indicator or marker of cell damage, inflammation, and nitric oxide production. In general, oxidative stress increases the production of superoxide (O_2^-) and nitric oxide forming $ONOO^-$ (peroxynitrite). Under pathophysiological conditions, iNOS synthesizes excessive quantities of nitric oxide, which combines chemically with superoxide to form the highly reactive and destructive peroxynitrite [36]. Peroxynitrite causes the nitrosylation of cellular proteins, lipids, and DNA, which triggers apoptosis and ultimately cell death [37]. It is difficult to determine the production of peroxynitrite, usually nitrotyrosination of proteins is a detectable marker for peroxynitrite$^-$. Our data demonstrate that nitrotyrosination was increased in response to glaucomatous injury and δ-opioid-receptor-activation significantly reduced the nitrotyrosination in glaucomatous eyes.

In summary, the findings of the present study support the notion that nitric oxide plays a detrimental role during glaucomatous injury and inhibition of nitric oxide provides RGC neuroprotection. Furthermore, the activation of δ-opioid receptors regulates the iNOS activity/expression that will lead to the attenuation of nitric oxide production and rescue RGCs from glaucomatous injury.

Acknowledgments

The authors thankfully acknowledge Dr. Luanna Bartholomew (MUSC-SEI) for critical review of the manuscript.

Author Contributions

Conceived and designed the experiments: SH. Performed the experiments: SH YA SS AA MH. Analyzed the data: SH. Contributed reagents/materials/analysis tools: SH. Contributed to the writing of the manuscript: SH.

References

1. Quigley HA (1999) Neuronal death in glaucoma. Prog Retin Eye Res 18: 39–57.
2. Gupta N, Weinreb RN (1997) New definitions of glaucoma. Curr Opin Ophthalmol 8: 38–41.
3. Kass MA, Heuer DK, Higginbotham EJ, Johnson CA, Keltner JL, et al. (2002) The Ocular Hypertension Treatment Study: a randomized trial determines that topical ocular hypotensive medication delays or prevents the onset of primary open-angle glaucoma. Arch Ophthalmol 120: 701–713; discussion 829–730.
4. Lichter PR, Musch DC, Gillespie BW, Guire KE, Janz NK, et al. (2001) Interim clinical outcomes in the Collaborative Initial Glaucoma Treatment Study comparing initial treatment randomized to medications or surgery. Ophthalmology 108: 1943–1953.
5. Nakazawa T, Nakazawa C, Matsubara A, Noda K, Hisatomi T, et al. (2006) Tumor necrosis factor-alpha mediates oligodendrocyte death and delayed retinal ganglion cell loss in a mouse model of glaucoma. J Neurosci 26: 12633–12641.
6. Zhou H, Li XM, Meinkoth J, Pittman RN (2000) Akt regulates cell survival and apoptosis at a postmitochondrial level. J Cell Biol 151: 483–494.
7. Abdul Y, Akhter N, Husain S (2013) Delta-opioid agonist SNC-121 protects retinal ganglion cell function in a chronic ocular hypertensive rat model. Invest Ophthalmol Vis Sci 54: 1816–1828.
8. Tezel G, Li LY, Patil RV, Wax MB (2001) TNF-alpha and TNF-alpha receptor-1 in the retina of normal and glaucomatous eyes. Invest Ophthalmol Vis Sci 42: 1787–1794.
9. Fuchs C, Forster V, Balse E, Sahel JA, Picaud S, et al. (2005) Retinal-cell-conditioned medium prevents TNF-alpha-induced apoptosis of purified ganglion cells. Invest Ophthalmol Vis Sci 46: 2983–2991.
10. McKinnon SJ, Lehman DM, Tahzib NG, Ransom NL, Reitsamer HA, et al. (2002) Baculoviral IAP repeat-containing-4 protects optic nerve axons in a rat glaucoma model. Mol Ther 5: 780–787.
11. Reichstein D, Ren L, Filippopoulos T, Mittag T, Danias J (2007) Apoptotic retinal ganglion cell death in the DBA/2 mouse model of glaucoma. Exp Eye Res 84: 13–21.
12. Quigley HA, McKinnon SJ, Zack DJ, Pease ME, Kerrigan-Baumrind LA, et al. (2000) Retrograde axonal transport of BDNF in retinal ganglion cells is blocked by acute IOP elevation in rats. Invest Ophthalmol Vis Sci 41: 3460–3466.
13. Pease ME, McKinnon SJ, Quigley HA, Kerrigan-Baumrind LA, Zack DJ (2000) Obstructed axonal transport of BDNF and its receptor TrkB in experimental glaucoma. Invest Ophthalmol Vis Sci 41: 764–774.
14. Neufeld AH, Hernandez MR, Gonzalez M (1997) Nitric oxide synthase in the human glaucomatous optic nerve head. Arch Ophthalmol 115: 497–503.
15. Neufeld AH, Sawada A, Becker B (1999) Inhibition of nitric-oxide synthase 2 by aminoguanidine provides neuroprotection of retinal ganglion cells in a rat model of chronic glaucoma. Proc Natl Acad Sci U S A 96: 9944–9948.
16. Shareef S, Sawada A, Neufeld AH (1999) Isoforms of nitric oxide synthase in the optic nerves of rat eyes with chronic moderately elevated intraocular pressure. Invest Ophthalmol Vis Sci 40: 2884–2891.
17. Anderson DR (1969) Ultrastructure of human and monkey lamina cribrosa and optic nerve head. Arch Ophthalmol 82: 800–814.
18. Varela HJ, Hernandez MR (1997) Astrocyte responses in human optic nerve head with primary open-angle glaucoma. J Glaucoma 6: 303–313.
19. Neufeld AH, Shareef S, Pena J (2000) Cellular localization of neuronal nitric oxide synthase (NOS-1) in the human and rat retina. J Comp Neurol 416: 269–275.
20. Dortch-Carnes J, Russell K (2007) Morphine-stimulated nitric oxide release in rabbit aqueous humor. Exp Eye Res 84: 185–190.
21. Dortch-Carnes J, Russell KR (2006) Morphine-induced reduction of intraocular pressure and pupil diameter: role of nitric oxide. Pharmacology 77: 17–24.
22. Sugiyama T, Oku H, Ikari S, Ikeda T (2000) Effect of nitric oxide synthase inhibitor on optic nerve head circulation in conscious rabbits. Invest Ophthalmol Vis Sci 41: 1149–1152.
23. Dawson VL, Dawson TM, Bartley DA, Uhl GR, Snyder SH (1993) Mechanisms of nitric oxide-mediated neurotoxicity in primary brain cultures. J Neurosci 13: 2651–2661.
24. Dawson VL, Dawson TM (1998) Nitric oxide in neurodegeneration. Prog Brain Res 118: 215–229.
25. Libby RT, Howell GR, Pang IH, Savinova OV, Mehalow AK, et al. (2007) Inducible nitric oxide synthase, Nos2, does not mediate optic neuropathy and retinopathy in the DBA/2J glaucoma model. BMC Neurosci 8: 108.
26. Pang IH, Johnson EC, Jia L, Cepurna WO, Shepard AR, et al. (2005) Evaluation of inducible nitric oxide synthase in glaucomatous optic neuropathy and pressure-induced optic nerve damage. Invest Ophthalmol Vis Sci 46: 1313–1321.
27. Husain S, Abdul Y, Crosson CE (2012) Preservation of retina ganglion cell function by morphine in a chronic ocular-hypertensive rat model. Invest Ophthalmol Vis Sci 53: 4289–4298.
28. Liu B, Neufeld AH (2000) Expression of nitric oxide synthase-2 (NOS-2) in reactive astrocytes of the human glaucomatous optic nerve head. Glia 30: 178–186.
29. Sennlaub F, Courtois Y, Goureau O (2002) Inducible nitric oxide synthase mediates retinal apoptosis in ischemic proliferative retinopathy. J Neurosci 22: 3987–3993.
30. Neufeld AH, Kawai S, Das S, Vora S, Gachie E, et al. (2002) Loss of retinal ganglion cells following retinal ischemia: the role of inducible nitric oxide synthase. Exp Eye Res 75: 521–528.
31. Geyer O, Almog J, Lupu-Meiri M, Lazar M, Oron Y (1995) Nitric oxide synthase inhibitors protect rat retina against ischemic injury. FEBS Lett 374: 399–402.

32. Koeberle PD, Ball AK (1999) Nitric oxide synthase inhibition delays axonal degeneration and promotes the survival of axotomized retinal ganglion cells. Exp Neurol 158: 366–381.
33. Yang Y, Xia X, Zhang Y, Wang Q, Li L, et al. (2009) delta-Opioid receptor activation attenuates oxidative injury in the ischemic rat brain. BMC Biol 7: 55.
34. Goyagi T, Toung TJ, Kirsch JR, Traystman RJ, Koehler RC, et al. (2003) Neuroprotective kappa-opioid receptor agonist BRL 52537 attenuates ischemia-evoked nitric oxide production in vivo in rats. Stroke 34: 1533–1538.
35. Lundberg JO, Weitzberg E, Gladwin MT (2008) The nitrate-nitrite-nitric oxide pathway in physiology and therapeutics. Nat Rev Drug Discov 7: 156–167.
36. Beckman JS, Koppenol WH (1996) Nitric oxide, superoxide, and peroxynitrite: the good, the bad, and ugly. Am J Physiol 271: C1424–1437.
37. Muijsers RB, Folkerts G, Henricks PA, Sadeghi-Hashjin G, Nijkamp FP (1997) Peroxynitrite: a two-faced metabolite of nitric oxide. Life Sci 60: 1833–1845.

8

Whole Exome Analysis Identifies Frequent *CNGA1* Mutations in Japanese Population with Autosomal Recessive Retinitis Pigmentosa

Satoshi Katagiri[1,2], Masakazu Akahori[1], Yuri Sergeev[3], Kazutoshi Yoshitake[4], Kazuho Ikeo[4], Masaaki Furuno[5], Takaaki Hayashi[2], Mineo Kondo[6], Shinji Ueno[7], Kazushige Tsunoda[8], Kei Shinoda[9], Kazuki Kuniyoshi[10], Yohinori Tsurusaki[11], Naomichi Matsumoto[11], Hiroshi Tsuneoka[2], Takeshi Iwata[1]*

1 Division of Molecular and Cellular Biology, National Institute of Sensory Organs, National Hospital Organization Tokyo Medical Center, Tokyo, Japan, **2** Department of Ophthalmology, The Jikei University School of Medicine, Tokyo, Japan, **3** National Eye Institute, National Institutes of Health, Bethesda, MD, United States of America, **4** Laboratory of DNA Data Analysis, National Institute of Genetics, Shizuoka, Japan, **5** RIKEN Center for Life Science Technologies, Division of Genomic Technologies, Life Science Accelerator Technology Group, Transcriptome Technology Team, Yokohama, Japan, **6** Department of Ophthalmology, Mie University Graduate School of Medicine, Tsu, Japan, **7** Department of Ophthalmology, Nagoya University Graduate School of Medicine, Nagoya, Japan, **8** Laboratory of Visual Physiology, National Institute of Sensory Organs, Tokyo, Japan, **9** Department of Ophthalmology, Teikyo University School of Medicine, Tokyo, Japan, **10** Department of Ophthalmology, Kinki University Faculty of Medicine, Osaka, Japan, **11** Department of Human Genetics, Yokohama City University, Yokohama, Japan

Abstract

Objective: The purpose of this study was to investigate frequent disease-causing gene mutations in autosomal recessive retinitis pigmentosa (arRP) in the Japanese population.

Methods: In total, 99 Japanese patients with non-syndromic and unrelated arRP or sporadic RP (spRP) were recruited in this study and ophthalmic examinations were conducted for the diagnosis of RP. Among these patients, whole exome sequencing analysis of 30 RP patients and direct sequencing screening of all *CNGA1* exons of the other 69 RP patients were performed.

Results: Whole exome sequencing of 30 arRP/spRP patients identified disease-causing gene mutations of *CNGA1* (four patients), *EYS* (three patients) and *SAG* (one patient) in eight patients and potential disease-causing gene variants of *USH2A* (two patients), *EYS* (one patient), *TULP1* (one patient) and *C2orf71* (one patient) in five patients. Screening of an additional 69 arRP/spRP patients for the *CNGA1* gene mutation revealed one patient with a homozygous mutation.

Conclusions: This is the first identification of *CNGA1* mutations in arRP Japanese patients. The frequency of *CNGA1* gene mutation was 5.1% (5/99 patients). *CNGA1* mutations are one of the most frequent arRP-causing mutations in Japanese patients.

Editor: Namik Kaya, King Faisal Specialist Hospital and Research center, Saudi Arabia

Funding: This study was supported by the grants to T.I. from the Ministry of Health, Labor, and Welfare of Japan (13803661); to M.A. and T.H. from the Ministry of Education, Culture, Sports, Science, and Technology of Japan (Grant-in-Aid for Scientific Research C, 25462744 and 25462738); to T.H. from the Vehicle Racing Commemorative Foundation; and to M.F. from the Research Grant for RIKEN Omics Science Center MEXT. The funders had no role in study design, data collection and analysis, decision to publish, or preparation of the manuscript.

Competing Interests: The authors have declared that no competing interests exist.

* Email: iwatatakeshi@kankakuki.go.jp

Introduction

Retinitis pigmentosa (RP; OMIM #268000) is a heterogeneous group of inherited disorders characterized by visual field loss, night blindness, abnormal color vision and fundus degeneration. The prevalence of RP is approximately 1 per 4,000 persons and more than 1 million individuals are affected worldwide [1]. The inheritance of RP shows various patterns including autosomal recessive (arRP), autosomal dominant, X-linked, sporadic (spRP), mitochondrial [2] and digenic [3] inheritance. Among the various patterns of RP inheritance, arRP is the most frequent inheritance pattern and accounts for approximately 50% to 60% of all RP patients [1]. To date, 42 arRP-causing genes and three loci have been reported in the Retinal Information Network (RetNet; https://sph.uth.edu/retnet/). Among these arRP-causing genes, mutations in Usher syndrome 2A (*USH2A*) are the most frequent and account for approximately 17% cases including cases with additional hearing loss [1]. In non-syndromic arRP, the most frequent arRP genes are eyes shut homolog (*EYS*), *USH2A* and ATP-binding cassette sub-family A member 4 (*ABCA4*), which

Table 1. Autosomal recessive retinitis pigmentosa (arRP)-causing mutations and potential arRP-causing variants found by exome sequencing.

Family ID	Gene Name	GenBank ID	Exon	Nucleotide Change	Amino Acid Change	State	Frequency*	SNP ID	Reference	Pathogenicity
RP#002	*CNGA1*	NM_000087	5	c.191delG	p.G64VfsX29	Homo	2		HGVB	Disease-causing
RP#004	*EYS*	NM_001142800	33	c.6714delT	p.P2238PfsX16	Hetero	0		Collin et al. 2008	Disease-causing
	EYS	NM_001142800	35	c.C7002A	p.C2334X	Hetero	0		This study	
RP#014	*EYS*	NM_001142800	4	c.A141T	p.E47D	Hetero	0		This study	Potential disease-causing
	EYS	NM_001142800	26	c.4957dupA	p.S1653KfsX2	Hetero	2		Iwanami et al. 2012	
RP#016	*TULP1*	NM_003322	1	c.G3A	p.M1I	Hetero	0		This study	Potential disease-causing
	TULP1	NM_003322	13	c.C1246T	p.R416C	Hetero	0	rs200769197	dbSNP	
RP#017	*EYS*	NM_001142800	26	c.4022delC	p.S1341FfsX11	Hetero	0		This study	Disease-causing
	EYS	NM_001142800	26	c.4957dupA	p.S1653KfsX2	Hetero	2		Iwanami et al. 2012	
RP#019	*CNGA1*	NM_000087	6	c.265delC	p.L89FfsX4	Hetero	2		Chen et al. 2013	Disease-causing
	CNGA1	NM_000087	11	c.1429delG	p.V477YfsX17	Hetero	0		This study	
RP#021	*CNGA1*	NM_000087	5	c.191delG	p.G64VfsX29	Homo	2		HGVB	Disease-causing
RP#023	*USH2A*	NM_206933	49	c.C9676T	p.R3226X	Hetero	0		This study	Potential disease-causing
	USH2A	NM_206933	55	c.T10859C	p.I3620T	Hetero	0		HGVB	
RP#026	*EYS*	NM_001142800	26	c.4957dupA	p.S1653KfsX2	Homo	2		Iwanami et al. 2012	Disease-causing
RP#027	*SAG*	NM_000541	11	c.926delA	p.T309TfsX12	Homo	6		Fuchs et al. 1995	Disease-causing
RP#028	*USH2A*	NM_206933	41	c.T7880C	p.I2627T	Hetero	0		This study	Potential disease-causing
	USH2A	NM_206933	55	c.C10931T	p.T3644M	Homo	1	rs185823130	dbSNP	
	USH2A	NM_206933	70	c.T15178C	p.S5060P	Hetero	0		This study	
RP#029	*CNGA1*	NM_000087	6	c.265delC	p.L89FfsX4	Homo	2		Chen et al. 2013	Disease-causing
RP#030	*C2orf71*	NM_001029883	1	c.C85T	p.R29W	Hetero	4	rs201706430	dbSNP	Potential disease-causing
	C2orf71	NM_001029883	2	c.C3748T	p.R1250C	Hetero	0		This study	

HGVB = Human Genetic Variation Browser (http://www.genome.med.kyoto-u.ac.jp/SnpDB/about.html); dbSNP = (http://www.ncbi.nlm.nih.gov/SNP/); Frequency* show the number of mutations or variants found in 1150 alleles of 575 controls.

account for approximately 10%, 8% and 5% to 6% of cases, respectively [1,4–10].

Large scale screening of selective exons in 30 RP-causing genes was previously performed in 193 Japanese RP families [11]. Although it only targeted exons with known mutations, the study failed to identify high frequency RP genes [11]. Another study of the Japanese RP population focused on the RP genes *RHO* [12–14] and *EYS* [15,16], and found that *EYS* was a frequent arRP gene with a prevalence rate of 9% to 16% [15,16]. However, almost all reported *EYS* gene mutations in these studies have not been reported in Western populations suggesting that Japanese individuals have a different genetic background [15,16]. These results suggest that the genetic background of RP in the Japanese population is different from that in the Western population.

The recent technological development of exon capture with 99% coverage of all exons and its combination with next generation sequencing enables effective genetic studies for hereditary diseases [17–20] and the investigation of novel mutations in multiple candidate genes [21].

The purpose of this study was to find frequent arRP genes in the Japanese population. In this study, we performed whole exome analysis of 30 Japanese arRP/spRP patients with confirmation in an additional 69 arRP/spRP patients. We found frequent arRP-causing mutations in the cyclic nucleotide gated channel alpha 1 (*CNGA1*) gene.

Materials and Methods

Informed consent

The protocol of this study was approved by the Institutional Review Board at the six participating institutions (National Hospital Organization Tokyo Medical Center, Jikei University School of Medicine, Mie University School of Medicine, Nagoya University Graduate School of Medicine, Teikyo University

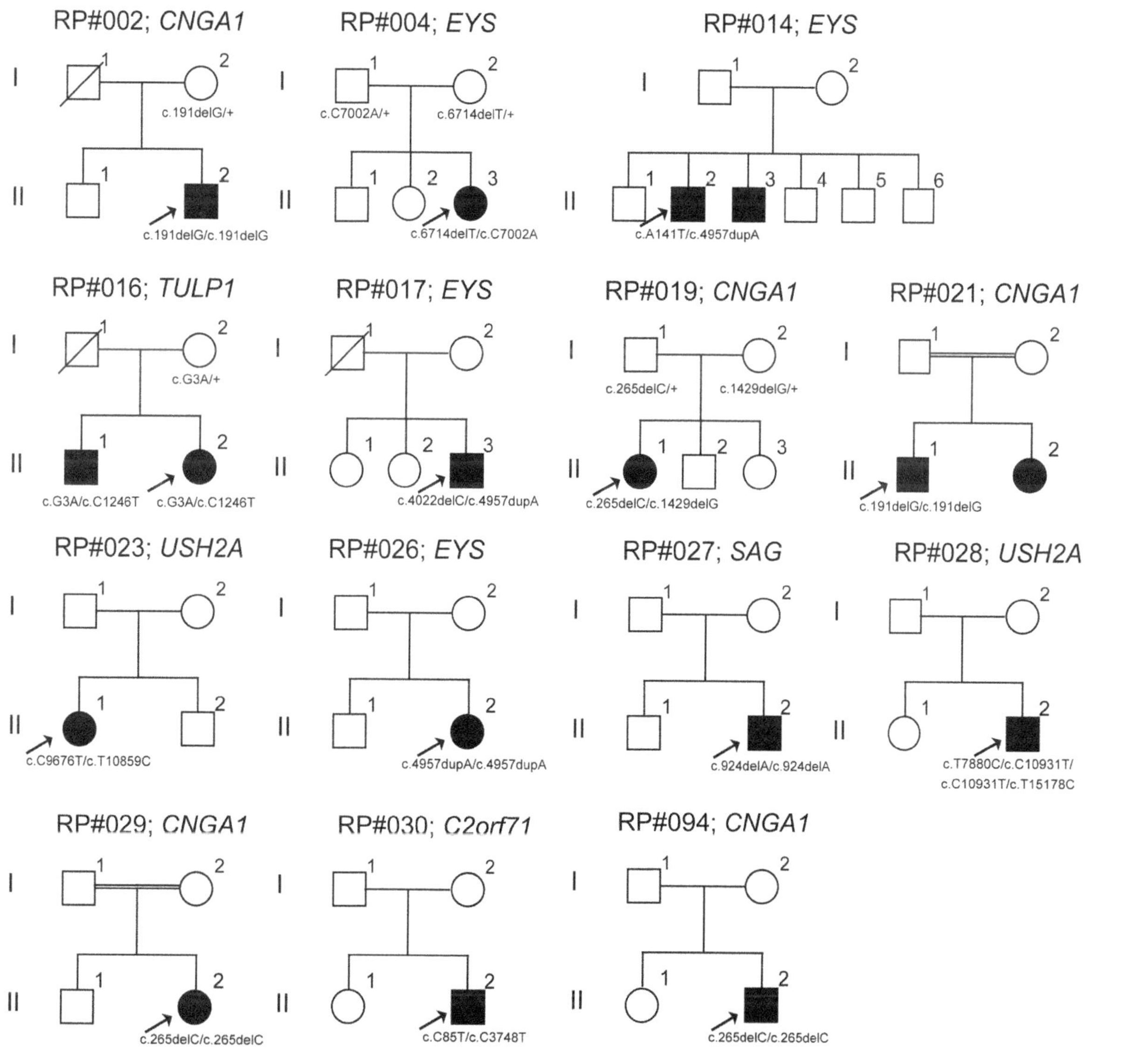

Figure 1. Pedigrees identified with arRP-causing mutations or potential arRP-causing variants. The solid squares (male) and circles (female) represent affected patients. The proband of each family is indicated by a black arrow. Unaffected family members are represented by white icons. The slash symbol indicates deceased individuals. The doubled line indicates consanguineous marriage. The generation number is shown on the left.

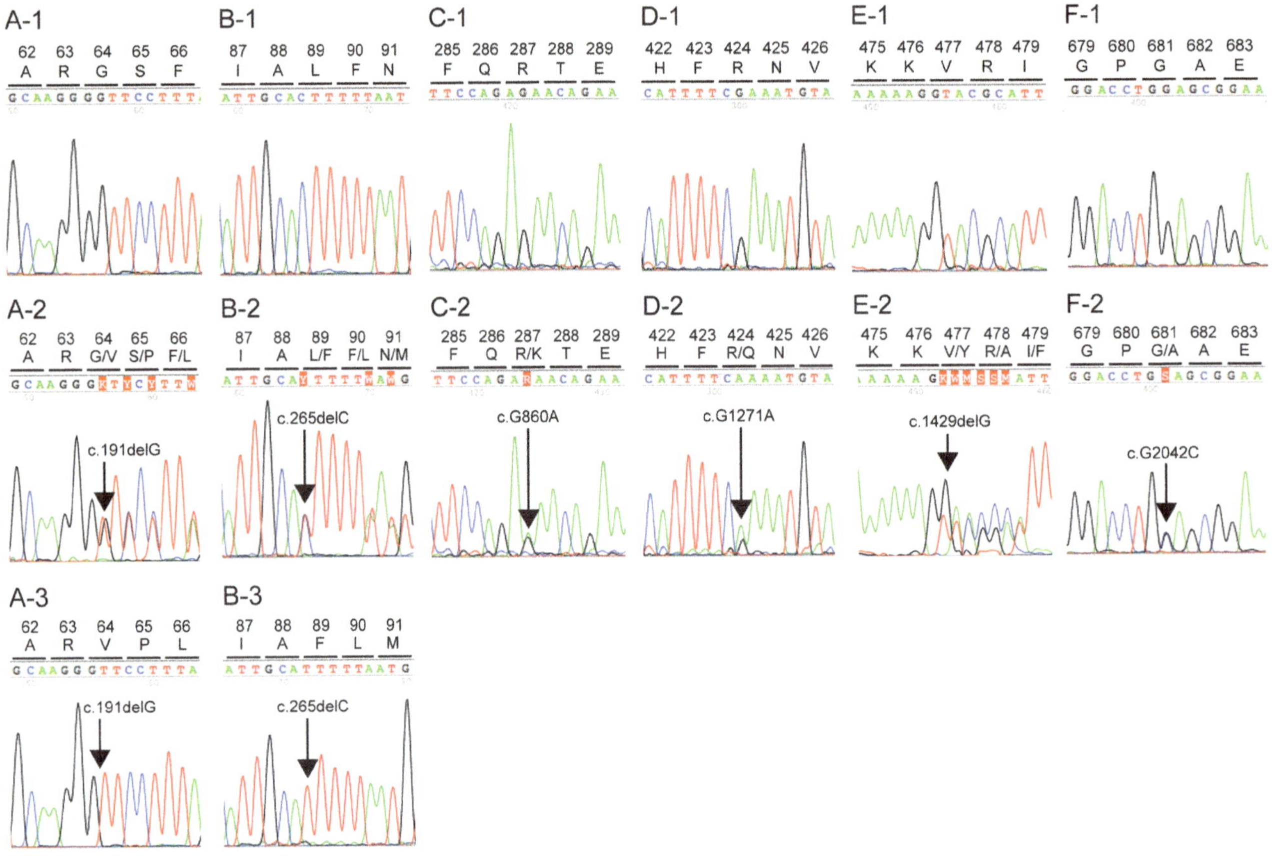

Figure 2. Sequence data of all six identified *CNGA1* mutations in this study. A-1 to F-1 show the normal sequence data for the *CNGA1* gene. A-2 to F-2 show the sequence data for heterozygous *CNGA1* mutations (c.191delG, c.265delC, c.G860A, c.G1271A, c.1429delG and c.G2042C, respectively). A-3 and B-3 show the sequence data for homozygous *CNGA1* mutations (c.191delG and c.265delC).

School of Medicine and Kinki University Faculty of Medicine). The protocol adhered to the tenets of the Declaration of Helsinki, and signed informed consent was obtained from all participants.

Clinical studies

In total, 99 unrelated arRP/spRP patients with no apparent syndrome were recruited from the National Hospital Organization Tokyo Medical Center, Jikei University School of Medicine, Mie University School of Medicine, Nagoya University Graduate School of Medicine, Teikyo University School of Medicine and Kinki University Faculty of Medicine. The patient history was taken and ophthalmic examinations were performed. Clinical diagnosis and evaluation for RP were based on the decimal best-corrected visual acuity (BCVA), slit-lamp examination, fundus examination, visual fields determined using kinetic perimetry (Goldmann perimeter [GP]; Haag Streit, Bern, Switzerland) and electroretinography (ERG) findings. Characteristic findings for diagnosis of RP include progressive visual field loss from peripheral, night blindness, abnormal color vision, fundus degeneration represented by bone spicule pigmentations and attenuation of retinal vessels, and the more or equally decreased rod responses compared with cone responses of ERG [1,22].

DNA preparation and exome sequencing analysis

We obtained venous blood samples from all participants and genomic DNA was extracted. Whole exome sequencing was performed for 30 arRP/spRP patients using a method previously described [23]. Briefly, construction of paired-end sequence libraries and exome capture were performed by using the Agilent Bravo automated liquid-handling platform with SureSelect XT Human All Exon kit V4+ UTRs kit (Agilent Technologies, Santa Clara, CA). Enriched libraries were sequenced by using an Illumina HiSeq2000 sequencer. Reads were mapped to the reference human genome (1000 genomes phase 2 reference, hs37d5) with Burrows–Wheeler Aligner software version 0.6.2 [24]. Duplicated reads were then removed by Picard Mark Duplicates module version 1.62, and mapped reads around insertion/deletion polymorphisms were realigned by using the Genome Analysis Toolkit (GATK) version 2.1–13 [25]. Base-quality scores were recalibrated by using GATK. To extract potentially RP-causing variants, we focused only on variants that could change the amino acid sequence, such as non-synonymous variants, splice acceptor and donor site variants, and insertion/deletion polymorphisms. The identified variants were filtered by a frequency of less than 1% in the 1000 Genomes project (http://www.1000genomes.org) and the Human Genetic Variation Browser (http://www.genome.med.kyoto-u.ac.jp/SnpDB/about.html). The remained variants were further screened within 212 genes registered as retinal disease-causing genes in the RetNet database updated on March 10, 2014. All remained variants of 30 arRP/spRP patients were summarized in Table S1 in File S1. Selection of disease-causing mutations was restricted to three genetic criteria: first, homozygosity or compound heterozygosity of known arRP-causing mutations; second, compound heterozygosity

Table 2. Identification of patients with *CNGA1* sequence mutations and variants in this study.

Family ID	Exon	Nucleotide Change	Amino Acid Change	State	Frequency*	Polyphen-2 (score)	SIFT (score)	SNP ID	Reference	Pathogenicity
RP#002	5	c.191delG	p.G64Vfs29X	Homo	2				HGVB	Disease-causing
RP#019	6	c.265delC	p.L89FfsX4	Hetero	2				Chen et al. 2013	Disease-causing
	11	c.1429delG	p.V477YfsX17	Hetero	0				This study	
RP#021	5	c.191delG	p.G64Vfs29X	Homo	2				HGVB	Disease-causing
RP#029	6	c.265delC	p.L89FfsX4	Homo	2				Chen et al. 2013	Disease-causing
RP#040	11	c.G1271A	p.R424Q	Hetero	7	Benign (0.266)	Damaging (0)	rs192912733	Jin et al. 2008	Not disease-causing
RP#063	11	c.G2042C	p.G681A	Hetero	1	Benign (0.001)	Tolerated (0.36)		HGVB	Not disease-causing
RP#087	11	c.G860A	p.R287K	Hetero	5	Benign (0.101)	Tolerated (0.32)		HGVB	Not disease-causing
RP#094	6	c.265delC	p.L89FfsX4	Homo	2				Chen et al. 2013	Disease-causing

Polyphen-2 (http://genetics.bwh.harvard.edu/pph2/); SIFT (http://sift.jcvi.org); HGVB = Human Genetic Variation Browser (http://www.genome.med.kyoto-u.ac.jp/SnpDB/about.html); Frequency* show the number of mutations or variants found in 1150 alleles of 575 controls.

of known and predicted arRP-causing mutations; and third, homozygosity or compound heterozygosity of predicted arRP-causing mutations. Mutations were defined as disease causing only if these criteria were fulfilled. Mutations causing exon truncation through frameshift, splicing and termination were considered to be more severe than missense mutations with unknown pathogenic relevance. In addition, to investigate the potential disease-causing variants, we added three genetic criteria: first, compound heterozygosity of known arRP-causing mutation and missense potential arRP-causing variant; second, compound heterozygosity of predicted arRP-causing mutation and potential arRP-causing variant; and third, homozygosity or compound heterozygosity of potential arRP-causing variants.

Direct sequencing of the *CNGA1* gene

The *CNGA1* mutations identified by whole exome sequencing were further confirmed by direct sequencing. An additional 69 arRP/spRP patients were analyzed by direct sequencing for all coding exons (4 to 11) of *CNGA1*. The targeted exons (4 to 11) of the *CNGA1* gene were amplified by PCR using the primer pairs given in Table S2 in File S1. The PCR products were purified using Agencourt APMure XP (Beckman Coulter, Brea, CA) and used as a template for sequencing. Both DNA strands were sequenced by an automated sequencer (3730*xl* DNA Analyzer; Life Technologies Corporation, Carlsbad, CA) using the BigDye Terminator kit V3.1 (Life Technologies Corporation).

Assessment of found mutations or variants in this study

Novel mutations and variants were defined as those not present in the literature, dbSNP database (http://www.ncbi.nlm.nih.gov/SNP/), Human Genetic Variation Browser, 1000 Genome project database or the Human Gene Mutation Database (http://www.hgmd.cf.ac.uk). In addition, the frequency of identified mutations or variants in this study was investigated using in-house exome sequencing data from 575 unaffected Japanese controls at Yokohama City University. Segregation was confirmed for both the arRP-causing mutations and potential arRP-causing variants by direct sequencing when parent samples were available.

Results

Whole exome sequencing analysis and identification of frequent arRP gene mutations

To identify frequent arRP-causing genes, we performed whole exome sequencing in non-syndromic 30 arRP/spRP patients. We focused on 212 retinal disease-causing genes registered in RetNet database updated on March 10, 2014. The average of mean depth for all 30 samples reached 71.11±7.68-fold and the average of coverage at 4- and 12-fold for all 30 samples reached 98.1% and 92.5% respectively. The analysis of arRP-causing mutations and potential arRP-causing variants was conducted according to the criteria described in Materials and Methods. Segregation of identified arRP-causing mutations and potential arRP-causing variants were conducted in five families: RP#002, RP#004, RP#011, RP#016 and RP#019. Although the results of segregation in RP#002, RP#004, RP#016 and RP#019 matched the inheritance pattern, two *USH2A* variants in RP#011 (Table S1 in File S1) did not match the inheritance pattern because the father of RP#011 carried two identical *USH2A* variants. Therefore, we concluded that the two *USH2A* variants in RP#011 were not arRP-causing. Consequently, the exome analysis identified eight arRP-causing mutations including three novel mutations and five known mutations in eight arRP/spRP patients [6,16,26,27] and identified potential arRP-causing

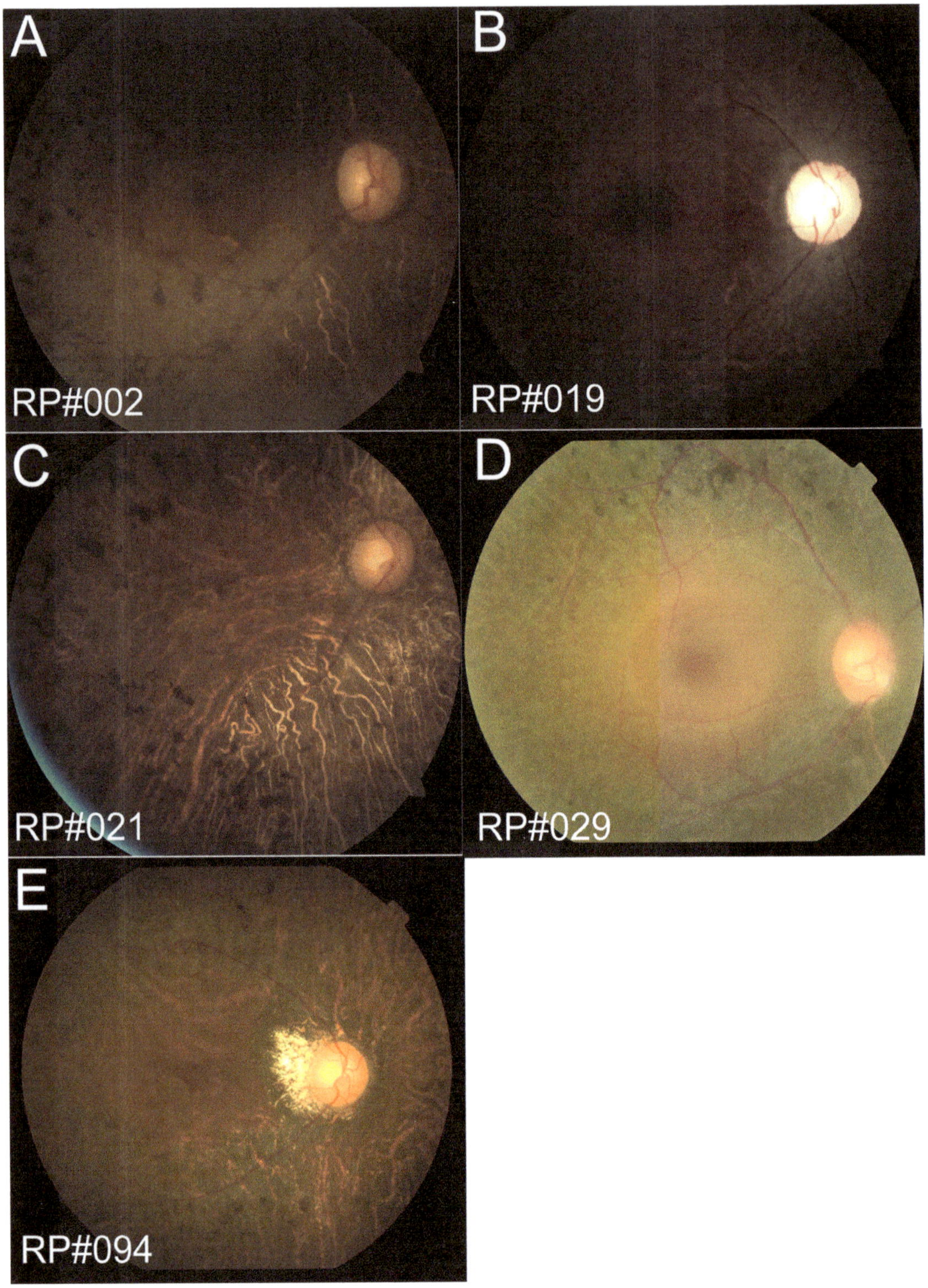

Figure 3. Fundus photographs of the patients with heterozygous or homozygous *CNGA1* mutations. Funduscopy indicates retinal degeneration with pigmentation and attenuation of retinal vessels in all patients. Macular edema does not existed in any patient, although retinal degeneration in the macular region is observed in RP#002, RP#021 and RP#094 (A, C and E).

variants including six novel variants and five known variants in five arRP/spRP patients (Table 1). The arRP-causing mutations were found in *CNGA1* (four patients), *EYS* (three patients) and S-antigen retina and pineal gland (*SAG*) (one patient). Potential arRP-casing variants were found in *USH2A* (two patients), *EYS* (one patient), tubby like protein 1 (*TULP1*) (one patient) and chromosome 2 open reading frame 71 (*C2orf71*) (one patient). Among these genes, the most frequent arRP-causing gene was

Table 3. Ophthalmic findings in five patients with retinitis pigmentosa with compound heterozygous or homozygous *CNGA1* mutations.

Patient	Diagnosed Age, Examined Age, Sex	Onset of night blindness	BCVA		ERG	Visual field	Mutations
			Right	Left			
RP#002	42, 51, M	Childhood	0.5	0.7	Non-recordable	Severely constricted	c.191delG/c.191delG
RP#019	26, 35, F	Childhood	1.0	1.0	Non-recordable	Ring scotoma	c.265delC/c.1429delG
RP#021	60, 65, M	Childhood	0.2	0.1	Non-recordable	Severely constricted	c.191delG/c.191delG
RP#029	25, 51, F	Childhood	1.0	1.0	Non-recordable	Severely constricted	c.265delC/c.265delC
RP#094	16, 46, M	Childhood	0.4	0.3	Non-recordable	Severely constricted	c.265delC/c.265delC

BCVA = decimal corrective visual acuity; ERG = electroretinography; M = male; F = female.

CNGA1. In particular, pedigree RP#002 with a homozygous c.191delG (p.G64VfsX29) mutation, RP#019 with compound heterozygous c.265delC (p.L89FfsX4) and c.1429delG (p.V477YfsX17) mutations, RP#021 with a homozygous c.191delG mutation and RP#029 with a homozygous c.265delC mutation were identified. Further direct sequencing confirmed that the parents in pedigree RP#019 had c.265delC or c.1429delG respectively. The *CNGA1* sequence was compared with the NCBI reference sequence for the *CNGA1* transcript (GenBank ID; NM_000087.3).

Screening of all *CNGA1* exons in 69 additional arRP/spRP Japanese patients

Direct sequencing of the coding region of the *CNGA1* gene in 69 arRP/spRP patients identified homozygous c.265delC mutation in pedigree RP#094 and three heterozygous variants c.G860A (p.R287K), c.G1271A (p.R424Q) and c.G2042C (p.G681A) in pedigrees RP#040, RP#063 and RP#087 respectively. All pedigrees identified to have arRP-causing mutations or potential arRP-causing variants are shown in Figure 1.

Identified *CNGA1* mutations and variants

Among the three arRP-causing mutations and three variants found in this study, two (c.265delC and c.G1271A) were previously reported as arRP-causing or potential arRP-causing [11,26] and four were not reported as arRP-causing or potential arRP-causing (c.191delG, c.265delC, c.G860A and c.G2042C). The polyphen-2 program predicted that all three missense variants in p.R287K (c.G860A), p.R424Q (c.G1271A) and p.G681A (c.G2042C) were benign. In contrast, the SIFT program predicted that p.R424Q (c.G1271A) potentially could cause severe damage to the protein, whereas p.G681A (c.G2042C) and p.R287K (c.G860A) potentially could cause mild damage. All identified mutations and variants in *CNGA1* gene are summarized in Table 2 and sequence data are given in Figure 2.

Haplotype analysis

The haplotypes of *CNGA1* and the surrounding sequences were determined for four arRP patients, RP#002, RP#019, RP#021 and RP#029. Single-nucleotide polymorphisms (SNPs) with a frequency higher than 5% (1000 Genomes project database) were determined within 1 kb upstream and downstream of *CNGA1* (chromosome 4, positions 47,937,994–48,014,961) as shown in Table S3 in File S1. The haplotype analysis determined an identical haplotype for four alleles in patients RP#002 and RP#021 suggesting a common ancestor for the c.191delG mutation. Moreover, identical haplotypes for one allele in patient RP#019 and for both alleles in patient RP#029 were detected suggesting a common ancestor for the c.265delC mutation.

Clinical features of *CNGA1* mutations

To characterize the clinical features of patients with *CNGA1* mutations, we additionally investigated the clinical data of five patients with compound heterozygous or homozygous *CNGA1* mutations (Table 3). All five patients reported that they noticed night blindness from childhood. Funduscopy showed retinal degeneration with pigmentation and attenuation of retinal vessels in all patients (Fig. 3). Macular edema was not observed in any patients, although retinal degeneration in macular regions was detected in RP#002, RP#021 and RP#094 (Fig. 3A, 3C and 3E). The BCVA of RP#019 and RP#029 remained at 1.0, whereas that of RP#002, RP#021 and RP#094 was reduced. ERG showed no recordable pattern in four patients and could not be conducted in one patient. The GP of RP#022 showed ring scotoma with a preserved peripheral visual field, whereas that of another four patients was severely constricted.

Discussion

Mutations in the *CNGA1* gene were identified for the first time in a Japanese population with a high frequency of 5.1% for homozygous or compound heterozygous mutations. The exome analysis of arRP/spRP patients revealed that 43.3% carried arRP-causing mutations or potential arRP-causing variants in *CNGA1* (13.3%), *EYS* (13.3%), *USH2A* (6.7%), *C2orf71* (3.3%), *SAG* (3.3%) and *TULP1* (3.3%). Although the prevalence of other five gene mutations was consistent with that in previous studies [1,4–8,28–30], the prevalence of *CNGA1* was clearly higher than in population of European descent [31,32]. We screened for mutation in all the coding exons of *CNGA1* in an additional 69 arRP/spRP Japanese patients to further investigate the prevalence of *CNGA1* mutations in the Japanese population. We identified an arRP-causing homozygous *CNGA1* mutation in one patient. Consequently, three *CNGA1* frameshift mutations (c.191delG, c.265delC and c.1429delG) were identified as arRP-causing mutations in five patients (Table 2).

Rod cyclic nucleotide-gated ion channels contain CNGA1 and CNGB1 protein at a ratio of 3 CNGA1:1 CNGB1 [33]. Each molecule of CNGA1 protein has at least three functional domains as described in the UniProtKB (acc. # P29973, http://www.uniprot.org, Cross-References, ProteinModelPortal); these domains function as a cation-transporter domain (residues 202–396, the Pfam ion_trans motif, http://pfam.sanger.ac.uk), cGMP-binding domain (residues 404–596, SWISSMODEL structure based on the PDB file: 4hbn_A, http://www.rcsb.org/pdb/home/home.do) and carboxy-terminal leucine zipper (CLZ) domain (residues 623–690, experimental structure based on the PDB file:3swf). The p.G64VfsX29 (c.191delG) and p.L89FfsX4 (c.265delC) protein had no transmembrane lesions, and most of the protein structure including all three functional domains was abolished. In contrast, the p.V477YfsX17 (c.1429delG) mutant protein had the correct structure up to 5th transmembrane domain helix, but lacked the 6th transmembrane domain helix, the cGMP-binding site, and the coiled-coil CLZ domain. The cGMP-binding site is important for the function of CNGA1 as a cation channel. Loss of the cGMP-binding site is likely to influence the final stage of the photo transduction pathway [31]. In addition, the absence of the coiled-coil CLZ domain completely disrupts the 3:1 stoichiometry in CNG channels [33]. Although the p.V477YfsX17 (c.1429delG) mutant may retain part of its structure, the protein function is predicted to be completely lost.

We additionally identified the heterozygous *CNGA1* missense variants c.G860A (p.R287K), c.G1271A (p.R424Q) and c.G2042C (p.G681A) (Table 2). Heterozygous c.G1271A variant has been previously reported [11]. Based on the mild score given by the polyphen-2 program and the severe score given by the SIFT program, we also predicted that this variant is potentially disease causing. In contrast, the two novel missense variants c.G860A and c.G2042C were predicted to cause mild damage by both the polyphen-2 and SIFT programs suggesting that it is non-pathogenic. Overall, all three missense *CNGA1* variants (c.G860A, c.G1271A and c.G2042C) were found in only one allele of *CNGA1*. We conclude that these three *CNGA1* variants were not disease causing in nature, at least from the phenotypic observation.

The clinical course of the five patients with compound heterozygous or homozygous *CNGA1* mutations included night blindness from childhood, visual field loss in middle age, non-recordable ERG and characteristic retinal degeneration pattern of RP, which were consistent with previously reported phenotypes of *CNGA1* mutations [32,34]. Retinal degeneration in the macular region and severely decreased BCVA occurred in 3/5 patients suggesting that the advanced stage of *CNGA1* mutations included degeneration of the entire retina with both rod and cone photoreceptors. Although the genotype-phenotype correlation for *CNGA1* mutations was not clear in this study, all five patients with *CNGA1* mutations showed typical phenotypes of RP.

Previous reports have shown a strong association of *CNGA1* with arRP [11,26,31,32,34,35]. Dryja et al. estimated the prevalence of *CNGA1* mutations in arRP patients to be between 1.7 and 2.3% (3 or 4 of 173 patients) [31]. The prevalence of *CNGA1* mutations in a Spanish arRP population was 2.1% (1 of 46 patients) [32], whereas that in a Chinese population with hereditary retinal dystrophy was 4.0% (1 of 25 patients) [26]. The average prevalence of *CNGA1* mutations in arRP/spRP patients was 7.6% (1 of 13 patients) [26]. These findings suggest that the prevalence of *CNGA1* mutations is higher in Asian population than in populations of European descent. The prevalence of *CNGA1* mutations in Chinese populations requires further study because only one Chinese patient has been reported to have a homozygous mutation in this gene [26]. Jin et al. investigated *CNGA1* exons 6, 8 and partial 11 in 193 Japanese RP families and found a single heterozygous *CNGA1* variant (c.1271G>A) [11]. In our study, all coding exons of *CNGA1* were screened and the estimate prevalence of *CNGA1* mutations reached at 5.1% (5 of 99 patients) including four homozygous and one compound heterozygous patients. Our findings suggest that the prevalence of *CNGA1* mutations is higher in Asian populations than in European populations. Moreover, c.191delG mutation has only been reported in Human Genetic Variation Browser (the database of genetic variations in Japanese population, http://www.genome.med.kyoto-u.ac.jp/SnpDB/), c.265delC mutation only reported in Chinese population [26] and c.1429delG mutation identified as novel. The *CNGA1* mutations found in this study only overlapped with mutations identified in studies of Asian individuals indicating that the founder is specific to Asian populations. Lastly, the haplotypes for the *CNGA1* mutations found in this study were individually unique (Table S3 in File S1). Further investigation of haplotypes is required to clarify the origin of these *CNGA1* mutations.

Supporting Information

File S1 Supporting Tables. Table S1, All rare variants of 30 arRP/spRP paients of this study, focusing on 212 retinal disease-causing genes registered in the Retinal Information Network (https://sph.uth.edu/retnet/). Table S2, *CNGA1* primers and PCR conditions. Table S3, Haplotype analysis of four retinitis pigmentosa patients with *CNGA1* mutations.

Acknowledgments

We thank the patients and their families for participation in this study. The authors wish to acknowledge RIKEN GeNAS for the sequencing of the exome-enriched libraries using the Illumina HiSeq2000.

Author Contributions

Conceived and designed the experiments: TI SK. Performed the experiments: SK MA YS KY KI MF TH MK SU KT KS KK YT NM. Analyzed the data: SK MA TI. Contributed reagents/materials/analysis tools: HT. Wrote the paper: SK TI.

References

1. Hartong DT, Berson EL, Dryja TP (2006) Retinitis pigmentosa. Lancet 368: 1795–1809.
2. Mansergh FC, Millington-Ward S, Kennan A, Kiang AS, Humphries M, et al. (1999) Retinitis pigmentosa and progressive sensorineural hearing loss caused by a C12258A mutation in the mitochondrial MTTS2 gene. Am J Hum Genet 64: 971–985.
3. Kajiwara K, Berson EL, Dryja TP (1994) Digenic retinitis pigmentosa due to mutations at the unlinked peripherin/*RDS* and *ROM1* loci. Science 264: 1604–1608.
4. Rivolta C, Sweklo EA, Berson EL, Dryja TP (2000) Missense mutation in the *USH2A* gene: association with recessive retinitis pigmentosa without hearing loss. Am J Hum Genet 66: 1975–1978.
5. Abd El-Aziz MM, Barragan I, O'Driscoll CA, Goodstadt L, Prigmore E, et al. (2008) *EYS*, encoding an ortholog of Drosophila spacemaker, is mutated in autosomal recessive retinitis pigmentosa. Nat Genet 40: 1285–1287.
6. Collin RW, Littink KW, Klevering BJ, van den Born LI, Koenekoop RK, et al. (2008) Identification of a 2 Mb human ortholog of Drosophila eyes shut/spacemaker that is mutated in patients with retinitis pigmentosa. Am J Hum Genet 83: 594–603.
7. Abd El-Aziz MM, O'Driscoll CA, Kaye RS, Barragan I, El-Ashry MF, et al. (2010) Identification of novel mutations in the ortholog of Drosophila eyes shut gene (*EYS*) causing autosomal recessive retinitis pigmentosa. Invest Ophthalmol Vis Sci 51: 4266–4272.
8. Audo I, Sahel JA, Mohand-Said S, Lancelot ME, Antonio A, et al. (2010) *EYS* is a major gene for rod-cone dystrophies in France. Hum Mutat 31: E1406–1435.
9. Bandah-Rozenfeld D, Littink KW, Ben-Yosef T, Strom TM, Chowers I, et al. (2010) Novel null mutations in the *EYS* gene are a frequent cause of autosomal recessive retinitis pigmentosa in the Israeli population. Invest Ophthalmol Vis Sci 51: 4387–4394.
10. Klevering BJ, Yzer S, Rohrschneider K, Zonneveld M, Allikmets R, et al. (2004) Microarray-based mutation analysis of the *ABCA4* (*ABCR*) gene in autosomal recessive cone-rod dystrophy and retinitis pigmentosa. Eur J Hum Genet 12: 1024–1032.
11. Jin ZB, Mandai M, Yokota T, Higuchi K, Ohmori K, et al. (2008) Identifying pathogenic genetic background of simplex or multiplex retinitis pigmentosa patients: a large scale mutation screening study. J Med Genet 45: 465–472.
12. Fujiki K, Hotta Y, Hayakawa M, Sakuma H, Shiono T, et al. (1992) Point mutations of rhodopsin gene found in Japanese families with autosomal dominant retinitis pigmentosa (ADRP). Jpn J Hum Genet 37: 125–132.
13. Saga M, Mashima Y, Akeo K, Oguchi Y, Kudoh J, et al. (1994) Autosomal dominant retinitis pigmentosa. A mutation in codon 181 (Glu->Lys) of the rhodopsin gene in a Japanese family. Ophthalmic Genet 15: 61–67.
14. Fujiki K, Hotta Y, Murakami A, Yoshii M, Hayakawa M, et al. (1995) Missense mutation of rhodopsin gene codon 15 found in Japanese autosomal dominant retinitis pigmentosa. Jpn J Hum Genet 40: 271–277.
15. Hosono K, Ishigami C, Takahashi M, Park DH, Hirami Y, et al. (2012) Two novel mutations in the *EYS* gene are possible major causes of autosomal recessive retinitis pigmentosa in the Japanese population. PLoS One 7: e31036.
16. Iwanami M, Oshikawa M, Nishida T, Nakadomari S, Kato S (2012) High prevalence of mutations in the *EYS* gene in Japanese patients with autosomal recessive retinitis pigmentosa. Invest Ophthalmol Vis Sci 53: 1033–1040.
17. Shendure J, Ji H (2008) Next-generation DNA sequencing. Nat Biotechnol 26: 1135–1145.
18. Mardis ER (2008) The impact of next-generation sequencing technology on genetics. Trends Genet 24: 133–141.
19. Mardis ER (2008) Next-generation DNA sequencing methods. Annu Rev Genomics Hum Genet 9: 387–402.
20. Ansorge WJ (2009) Next-generation DNA sequencing techniques. N Biotechnol 25: 195–203.
21. Shanks ME, Downes SM, Copley RR, Lise S, Broxholme J, et al. (2013) Next-generation sequencing (NGS) as a diagnostic tool for retinal degeneration reveals a much higher detection rate in early-onset disease. Eur J Hum Genet 21: 274–280.
22. Berson EL (1993) Retinitis pigmentosa. The Friedenwald Lecture. Invest Ophthalmol Vis Sci 34: 1659–1676.
23. Katagiri S, Yoshitake K, Akahori M, Hayashi T, Furuno M, et al. (2013) Whole-exome sequencing identifies a novel *ALMS1* mutation (p.Q2051X) in two Japanese brothers with Alström syndrome. Molecular Vision 19: 2393–2406.
24. Li H, Durbin R (2009) Fast and accurate short read alignment with Burrows-Wheeler transform. Bioinformatics 25: 1754–1760.
25. McKenna A, Hanna M, Banks E, Sivachenko A, Cibulskis K, et al. (2010) The Genome Analysis Toolkit: a MapReduce framework for analyzing next-generation DNA sequencing data. Genome Res 20: 1297–1303.
26. Chen X, Zhao K, Sheng X, Li Y, Gao X, et al. (2013) Targeted sequencing of 179 genes associated with hereditary retinal dystrophies and 10 candidate genes identifies novel and known mutations in patients with various retinal diseases. Invest Ophthalmol Vis Sci 54: 2186–2197.
27. Fuchs S, Nakazawa M, Maw M, Tamai M, Oguchi Y, et al. (1995) A homozygous 1-base pair deletion in the arrestin gene is a frequent cause of Oguchi disease in Japanese. Nat Genet 10: 360–362.
28. Hagstrom SA, North MA, Nishina PL, Berson EL, Dryja TP (1998) Recessive mutations in the gene encoding the tubby-like protein TULP1 in patients with retinitis pigmentosa. Nat Genet 18: 174–176.
29. Nakazawa M, Wada Y, Tamai M (1998) Arrestin gene mutations in autosomal recessive retinitis pigmentosa. Arch Ophthalmol 116: 498–501.
30. Collin RW, Safieh C, Littink KW, Shalev SA, Garzozi HJ, et al. (2010) Mutations in *C2ORF71* cause autosomal-recessive retinitis pigmentosa. Am J Hum Genet 86: 783–788.
31. Dryja TP, Finn JT, Peng YW, McGee TL, Berson EL, et al. (1995) Mutations in the gene encoding the alpha subunit of the rod cGMP-gated channel in autosomal recessive retinitis pigmentosa. Proc Natl Acad Sci U S A 92: 10177–10181.
32. Paloma E, Martinez-Mir A, Garcia-Sandoval B, Ayuso C, Vilageliu L, et al. (2002) Novel homozygous mutation in the alpha subunit of the rod cGMP gated channel (*CNGA1*) in two Spanish sibs affected with autosomal recessive retinitis pigmentosa. J Med Genet 39: E66.
33. Shuart NG, Haitin Y, Camp SS, Black KD, Zagotta WN (2011) Molecular mechanism for 3:1 subunit stoichiometry of rod cyclic nucleotide-gated ion channels. Nat Commun 2: 457.
34. Zhang Q, Zulfiqar F, Riazuddin SA, Xiao X, Ahmad Z, et al. (2004) Autosomal recessive retinitis pigmentosa in a Pakistani family mapped to CNGA1 with identification of a novel mutation. Mol Vis 10: 884–889.
35. Gonzalez-del Pozo M, Borrego S, Barragan I, Pieras JI, Santoyo J, et al. (2011) Mutation screening of multiple genes in Spanish patients with autosomal recessive retinitis pigmentosa by targeted resequencing. PLoS One 6: e27894.

9

Arginase 2 Deficiency Prevents Oxidative Stress and Limits Hyperoxia-Induced Retinal Vascular Degeneration

Jutamas Suwanpradid[1,2], Modesto Rojas[1,2,3], M. Ali Behzadian[1], R. William Caldwell[2,3], Ruth B. Caldwell[1,2,4]*

1 Vascular Biology Center, Georgia Regents University, Augusta, Georgia, United States of America, **2** Culver Vision Discovery Institute, Georgia Regents University, Augusta, Georgia, United States of America, **3** Department of Pharmacology and Toxicology, Department of Cellular Biology & Anatomy, Georgia Regents University, Augusta, Georgia, United States of America, **4** Charlie Norwood VA Medical Center, Augusta, Georgia, United States of America

Abstract

Background: Hyperoxia exposure of premature infants causes obliteration of the immature retinal microvessels, leading to a condition of proliferative vitreoretinal neovascularization termed retinopathy of prematurity (ROP). Previous work has demonstrated that the hyperoxia-induced vascular injury is mediated by dysfunction of endothelial nitric oxide synthase resulting in peroxynitrite formation. This study was undertaken to determine the involvement of the ureahydrolase enzyme arginase in this pathology.

Methods and Findings: Studies were performed using hyperoxia-treated bovine retinal endothelial cells (BRE) and mice with oxygen-induced retinopathy (OIR) as experimental models of ROP. Treatment with the specific arginase inhibitor 2(S)-amino-6-boronohexanoic acid (ABH) prevented hyperoxia-induced apoptosis of BRE cells and reduced vaso-obliteration in the OIR model. Furthermore, deletion of the arginase 2 gene protected against hyperoxia-induced vaso-obliteration, enhanced physiological vascular repair, and reduced retinal neovascularization in the OIR model. Additional deletion of one copy of arginase 1 did not improve the vascular pathology. Analyses of peroxynitrite by quantitation of its biomarker nitrotyrosine, superoxide by dihydroethidium imaging and NO formation by diaminofluoroscein imaging showed that the protective actions of arginase 2 deletion were associated with blockade of superoxide and peroxynitrite formation and normalization of NOS activity.

Conclusions: Our data demonstrate the involvement of arginase activity and arginase 2 expression in hyperoxia-induced vascular injury. Arginase 2 deletion prevents hyperoxia-induced retinal vascular injury by preventing NOS uncoupling resulting in decreased reactive oxygen species formation and increased nitric oxide bioavailability.

Editor: Jing Chen, Children's Hospital Boston, United States of America

Funding: The work was supported in part by grants from National Institutes of Health (NIH grant R01-EY11766), the Department of Veterans Affairs, Veterans Health Administration, Office of Research and Development, Biomedical Laboratory Research and Development (BX001233), and the Culver Vision Discovery Institute at Georgia Regents University. The contents do not represent the views of the Department of Veterans Affairs or the United States Government. The funders had no role in study design, data collection and analysis, decision to publish, or preparation of the manuscript.

Competing Interests: The authors have declared that no competing interests exist.

* Email: rcaldwel@gru.edu

Introduction

Retinopathy of prematurity (ROP) is a major cause of vision loss in premature infants. In the United States, the Centers of Disease Control reports that almost 500,000 babies, one out of every eight, are born prematurely, each year. [1] Many of them develop ROP. The incidence of ROP is inversely proportional to birth weight and ~50% of infants born weighing less than 1700 g develop ROP. [2] Clinical observations in human infants and studies in animal models indicate that exposure of the immature retinal blood vessels to relative hyperoxia damages the immature retinal capillaries and impairs vascular development. [3] The resulting vascular insufficiency results in a condition of relative hypoxia as development of the retina continues. This up-regulates growth factors, such as vascular endothelial growth factor (VEGF), leading to pathological angiogenesis. [4,5]

The mechanisms underlying the vascular injury during ROP are not fully understood. However, disruption of amino acid metabolism may be involved. Preterm infants have been shown to have a deficit in L-arginine, which is nutritionally essential for neonatal development. [6] L-arginine is the substrate of both nitric oxide synthase (NOS) and arginase. NOS catalyzes L-arginine to produce NO and L-citrulline, whereas arginase uses L-arginine to produce urea and ornithine. Hepatic urea production is crucial for ammonia detoxification and L-arginine deficiency in preterm infants can cause severe hypoargininemia, which results in hyperammonemia and organ dysfunction. [6] Studies using a mouse model of oxygen-induced retinopathy (OIR) showed that treatment of neonatal mice with supplemental arginine and glutamine prepared as a dipeptide reduced retinal neovascularization and reduced vascular hyperpermeablity following hyperpoxia exposure. [7] Therefore, alterations in L-arginine metabolism may play a role in the microvascular injury.

The products of L-arginine metabolism by NOS and arginase have been strongly implicated in a variety of angiogenic responses. NO can promote angiogenesis and also regulates vascular tone and remodeling. [8–12] Ornithine is processed to form L-proline and polyamines, important for collagen synthesis and cell growth, respectively. Thus, products of both enzymes are needed for proper vascular growth and remodeling. However, dysfunction of both enzymes has been implicated in vascular and retinal injury. Our previous studies have shown that hyperoxia induced death of cultured retinal endothelial cells and vaso-obliteration in the immature retina is associated with NOS mediated increases in peroxynitrite formation. [13,14] Our studies in models of diabetes and oxidative stress-induced vascular disease have shown that elevated arginase can lead to vascular dysfunction and injury by reducing the availability of L-arginine to NOS, causing it to become uncoupled and to form superoxide which reacts with NO to form peroxynitrite. [15,16] Our studies in the OIR model also have shown involvement of the mitochondrial arginase isoform, arginase 2, in hyperoxia-induced death of retinal neuronal cells. [17,18] Thus, the overall aim of the present study was to determine whether the arginase pathway is also involved in hyperoxia-induced retinal vascular injury. Here we present data to show involvement of arginase activity and arginase 2 expression in hyperoxia-induced injury of the retinal microvasculature.

Results

Hyperoxia-Induced Endothelial Cell Apoptosis

We first determined the involvement of arginase activity in hyperoxia-induced endothelial cell death by using a highly selective competitive inhibitor of arginase 2(S)-amino-6-boronohexanoic acid (ABH, 100 μM). [19,20] BREC treated with or without ABH, were maintained under normoxia (21% O_2) or hyperoxia (40% O_2) for 48 hours and stained with propidium iodide. The effect of hyperoxia on apoptosis was evaluated by flow cytometry. This analysis showed that hyperoxia treatment caused a significant increase in numbers of apoptotic cells with hypodiploid nuclei as compared with cells maintained in normoxia (Figure 1A, 1B). Inhibition of arginase activity markedly attenuated hyperoxia-induced apoptosis (Figure 1A, 1B). Next, we quantified the accumulation of nitrite (NO_2^-), a product of nitric oxide, in media collected from BREC exposed to normoxia or hyperoxia with and without ABH as described above. Nitrite accumulation was decreased in BREC treated with hyperoxia (Figure 1C). The hyperoxia-induced decrease in nitrite was prevented with ABH treatment (100 μM). This study suggests that inhibition of arginase prevented hyperoxia-induced endothelial cell injury and preserved nitric oxide bioavailability.

Hyperoxia-Induced Vaso-Obliteration

In order to evaluate the potential role of arginase activity in hyperoxia-induced retinal vascular injury *in vivo*, we performed experiments in the OIR mouse model. For this, mice were treated with ABH (15 mg/kg/day, ip) beginning on P7 and maintained in 70% oxygen for various times. The isolectin B4-labeled retinas of mice treated with vehicle (saline) and maintained in hyperoxia from P7–12, showed extensive capillary obliteration with a maximal loss at P9 (Figure 1D, 1E). This vessel loss was significantly attenuated in mice treated with ABH, implying a role for arginase in the vascular injury. In order to examine the role of arginase gene expression in this process, we performed similar experiments using mice lacking both copies of the arginase 2 gene alone (A1+/+A2−/−) or in combination with deletion of 1 copy of arginase 1 (A1+/−A2−/−). Deletion of both copies of arginase 1 is lethal by P10 due to hyperammonemia. These data show that the hyperoxia-induced vaso-obliteration was significantly reduced in the A1+/+A2−/− mice as compared with the wild type mice (Figure 2A, 2B). The area of vaso-obliteration in the A1+/−A2−/− mice was not significantly different from that in the mice lacking A2 alone (Figure 2B), suggesting that arginase 1 is not involved in the hyperoxia-induced vaso-obliteration. Time course analysis showed that the protective effect of arginase 2 deletion was evident within 1 day after the onset of hyperoxia and persisted throughout the hyperoxia treatment (Figure 2C). In order to confirm that the retinas of arginase knockout mice develop normally, we also compared retinal morphology in tissue sections prepared from retinas of adult WT, A2−/− and A1+/−A2−/−. As shown in Figure 2D retinal structure qualitatively normal in both lines of mutant mice.

Vitreo-Retinal Neovascularization during Relative Hypoxia

In order to assess involvement of arginase expression in pathological angiogenesis that occurs during the hypoxia phase of OIR, we maintained mice in 70% oxygen from P7 to P12, returned them to normal atmosphere for 5 days and labeled their retinas with isolectin B4 to detect the blood vessels. On P17 extensive vitreo-retinal neovascularization was evident in the wild type mice (Figure 3A). We quantified this pathological angiogenesis by measuring the area occupied by neovascular tufts relative to the total retinal surface area. This analysis revealed that the area of neovascularization in the A1+/+A2−/− retina was significantly reduced as compared to the wild type retina (Figure 3B). Furthermore, in the double mutant mice lacking one copy of arginase 1 as well as both copies of arginase 2, the neovascular tuft formation showed a pattern closer to that in the wild type mice (Figure 3B).

Intra-Retinal Neovascularization during Relative Hypoxia

We next examined the involvement of arginase expression in physiological retinal angiogenesis/vascular repair during the hypoxia phase of OIR. For this, we measured the capillary-free area relative to the total retinal surface area in the P17 retinas. This analysis showed that vascular repair was significantly enhanced in the A1+/+A2−/− mice as compared with the wild type mice (Figure 3A, 3C). Moreover, the capillary dropout area was slightly increased in the double knockout A1+/−A2−/− as compared with the A1+/+A2−/−mice, suggesting that arginase 1 is not involved in the vascular damage.

Arginase Expression during Relative Hypoxia

Figure 4 shows the expression of arginase 2 in the retinas of hyperoxia treated mice and their room air (RA) controls. As we have reported previously, immunolocalization analysis showed robust immunoreactivity for arginase 2 in horizontal cells of hyperoxia-treated wild type mice (Figure 4A). [17,18] Sections prepared from arginase 2 deficient mice were negative, demonstrating specificity of the immunolabeling for arginase 2. Western blot analysis of retinal extracts prepared from wild type mice exposed to hyperoxia for 48 hours showed no change in total levels of arginase 2 as compared with the normoxia controls (Figure 4B). Similarly, western blots prepared after 6, 12, or 24 hours of hyperoxia also showed no change in total levels of arginase 2 as compared with the normoxia controls (data not shown).

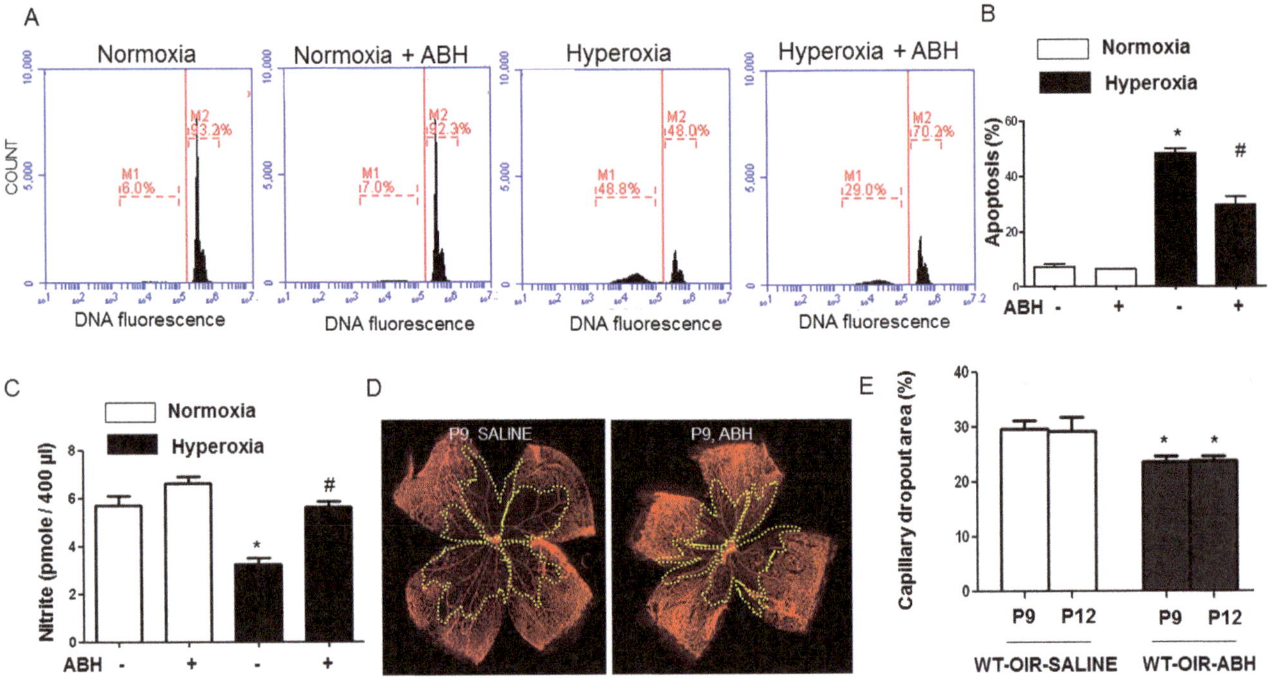

Figure 1. Inhibiting arginase inhibits hyperoxia-induced cell death and preserves nitrite accumulation *in vitro* and vaso-obliteration *in vivo*. For *in vitro* studies, BRECs were treated with hyperoxia (40% O_2, 5% CO_2) or normoxia (21% O_2, 5% CO_2) with and without ABH (100 µM) for 48 hours. Groups of cells were stained with propidium iodide and the percentage of apoptotic nuclei (hypodiploid, M1) and normal nuclei (diploid, M2) were quantified by flow cytometry (A, B). n = 4–5, * P≤0.05 vs normoxia and hyperoxia treated with ABH, # P≤0.05 vs hyperoxic and normoxic treatment. NO release was detected using chemiluminescence to measure nitrite levels in conditioned media from the treated cells (C. n = 6–9. * P≤ 0.05 vs normoxia with or without ABH, # P≤0.05 vs hyperoxia without ABH. For *in vivo* analyses, wild type mice were treated with daily i.p. injections of vehicle (saline) or ABH (15 mg/kg) from P7 to P9 or P12. Retinal vessels were visualized by lectin labeling (D) and the area of capillary dropout (yellow) was quantified in fluorescence micrographs using ImageJ (E). n = 7–9, *P≤0.05 vs saline.

Formation of Peroxynitrite, Superoxide and Nitric Oxide during Hyperoxia

Previous studies have linked arginase activity to vascular dysfunction and injury by a mechanism involving uncoupling of NOS leading to formation of superoxide which reacts rapidly with NO to produce peroxynitrite. [21] Our previous studies have shown that hyperoxia-induced degeneration of retinal microvascular endothelial cells is associated with increased NOS-dependent peroxynitrite formation. [13,14] To examine the involvement of arginase 2 in this process, we assayed nitrotyrosine levels in wild type and arginase 2-deficient mice following hyperoxia exposure. While peroxynitrite is short-lived at physiological pH, nitrotysine is a stable end product of the peroxynitrite reaction with tyrosine residues in proteins. Thus, nitrotyrosine serves as a biomarker for peroxynitrite. [22–24] Our analysis demonstrated a two fold increase in levels of nitrated proteins in retinas of hyperoxia treated wild type mice as compared with the normoxia controls (Figure 5A, 5B). By contrast, nitrotyrosine levels remained low in the hyperoxia-treated arginase 2 deficient mice, suggesting involvement of arginase 2 expression in the hyperoxia-induced increase in peroxynitrite formation.

To examine the involvement of NOS uncoupling in this process, we used DHE imaging to determine the effects of the hyperoxia treatment on NOS-dependent formation of superoxide in flash frozen retina sections pre-treated with and without the NOS inhibitor L-NAME. This analysis showed a 2 fold increase in DHE fluorescence intensity in the retinas of the hyperoxia-treated wild type mice compared with the normoxia controls (Figure 5C, 5D). Since DHE can be oxidized by other ROS beside superoxide, [25] Control experiments were performed using SOD which catalyzes superoxide to hydrogen peroxide. The SOD treatment markedly blunted the DHE fluorescence, indicating involvement of superoxide in the reaction. The hyperoxia-induced increase in DHE fluorescence was also markedly reduced by pre-treatment of the retina sections with the NOS inhibitor L-NAME, This implies that NOS activity is an important contributor to superoxide production. Moreover, the hyperoxia-induced increase in DHE staining was suppressed in the arginase 2 deficient mice. Taken together, these data suggest that arginase 2 has an important role in hyperoxia-induced superoxide formation by a mechanism involving NOS uncoupling.

We further examined the role of arginase 2 expression in hyperoxia-induced NOS dysfunction by analyzing NO formation using DAF-FM imaging of retina sections from wild type and arginase 2-deficient mice pre-treated with and without L-NAME. The NO signal was markedly reduced in sections from hyperoxia-treated wild type mice as compared with the other groups (Figure 5E, 5F). By contrast the NO signal was preserved in the retinas of the hyperoxia-treated arginase 2-deficient mice. L-NAME treatment abrogated the DAF-FM signal in both wild type and arginase 2 deficient retinas, demonstrating specificity of the reaction for NO. These data indicate that arginase 2 deletion preserves normal NOS function and NO formation in the OIR mouse model.

Discussion

Hyperoxia-induced obliteration of newly formed blood vessels in the immature retina has been well established as a primary

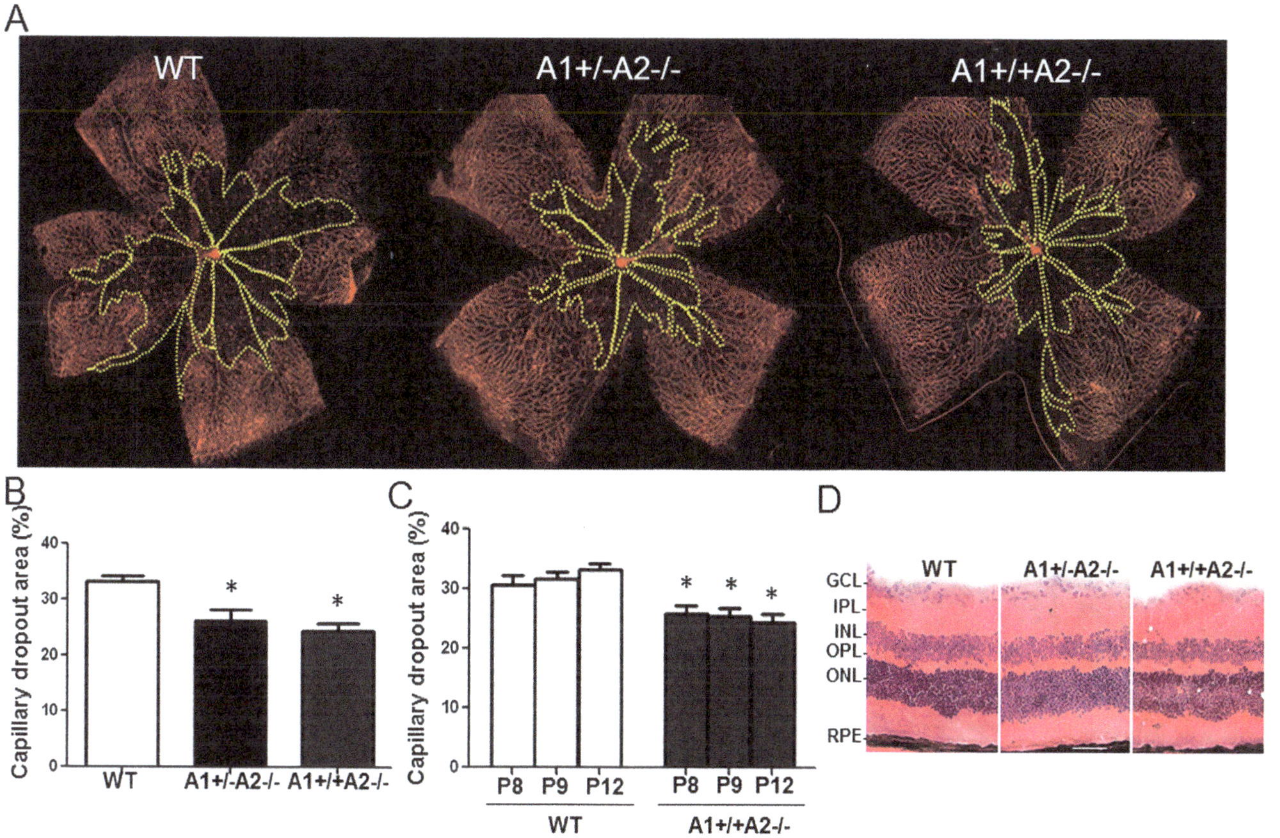

Figure 2. Arginase 2 deletion limits hyperoxia-induced retinal vaso-obliteration. Wild type (WT), arginase 2-deficient mice (A1+/+A2−/−) and arginase-deficient mice lacking one copy of arginase 1 (A1+/−A2−/−) were placed in 70% oxygen on P7 and prepared for analysis on P8, P9 or P12. Retinal vessels were visualized by lectin labeling (A) and the area of capillary dropout (yellow) was quantified in fluorescence micrographs using ImageJ (B, C). n = 5–9, *P≤0.05 vs WT. Images of hematoxylin and eosin stained cryostat sections from adult mice show comparable retinal morphology in WT, A2−/− and A1+/−A2−/− retinas (D, GCL: ganglion cell layer, IPL: inner plexiform layer, INL: inner nuclear layer, OPL: outer plexiform layer, ONL: outer nuclear layer, RPE: retinal pigment epithelium, scale bar = 50 μm).

mediator of retinopathy of prematurity. [3] Our previous studies *in vivo* and *in vitro* have shown involvement of NOS mediated increases in peroxynitrite formation in hyperoxia-induced vaso-obliteration and endothelial cell death. [14,26] Now we demonstrate involvement of the arginase enzyme in this pathology. Studies in retinal endothelial cells showed that treatment with the specific arginase inhibitor ABH blocked hyperoxia-induced apoptosis and preserved NO availability. *In vivo* experiments using the mouse OIR model showed that inhibition of arginase activity or deletion of the arginase 2 gene significantly reduced hyperoxia-induced vaso-obliteration. Deletion of arginase 2 also limited pathological vitreoretinal neovascularization while enhancing vascular repair during the relative hypoxia phase of OIR. Interestingly, deletion of one copy of the arginase 1 gene in combination with both copies of arginase 2 was less effective in reducing vitreoretinal neovascularization. This suggests that arginase 2 is the predominant isoform involved in the vascular injury. Immunoblot analyses of the peroxynitrite biomarker nitrotyrosine showed that deletion of the arginase 2 gene also limited peroxynitrite formation. Our studies further indicated that arginase 2 expression is involved in hyperoxia-induced superoxide formation by a mechanism requiring activity of NOS. Moreover, NO formation by NOS was suppressed in retinas of hyperoxia-treated mice and the hyperoxia-induced suppression of NO formation was prevented in arginase 2 deficient mice. Taken together, these data indicate that hyperoxia induced vascular injury is mediated by arginase 2-induced uncoupling of NOS.

Interestingly, pathological neovascularization was slightly increased in mice lacking 1 copy of arginase as well as both copies of arginase 2 as compared with the mice lacking both copies of arginase 2 alone. Therefore, we performed additional studies to determine the impact of arginase 1 deletion on vascular regrowth into the area of vaso-obliteration following hyperoxia treatment. The data show that deletion of 1 copy of arginase impairs vascular repair during the hypoxic phase of the OIR model (manuscript in preparation). The mechanisms controlling expression and function of arginase 1 and 2 in the retina are as yet unknown. However, studies using human lung endothelial cells have shown that HIF-2 regulates arginase 2 expression and activity during hyperoxia treatment. [27] In addition, ROS-induced upregulation and activation of endothelial arginase 1 is regulated by AP1 mediated activation of the Rho A/ROCK system leading to p38 MAPK activation. [28,29] In models of artherosclerosis, liver X receptors (LXRs) were found to regulate macrophage arginase 1 [30] while arginase 2 in endothelial cells is regulated by epigenetic mechanisms involving activity of histone deacetylase 2. [31] In the immune system, arginase 1 in macrophage can be regulated by PTEN pathway [32].

This study is the first we know of to show that inhibiting the arginase enzyme or deleting the arginase 2 gene limits hyperoxia-

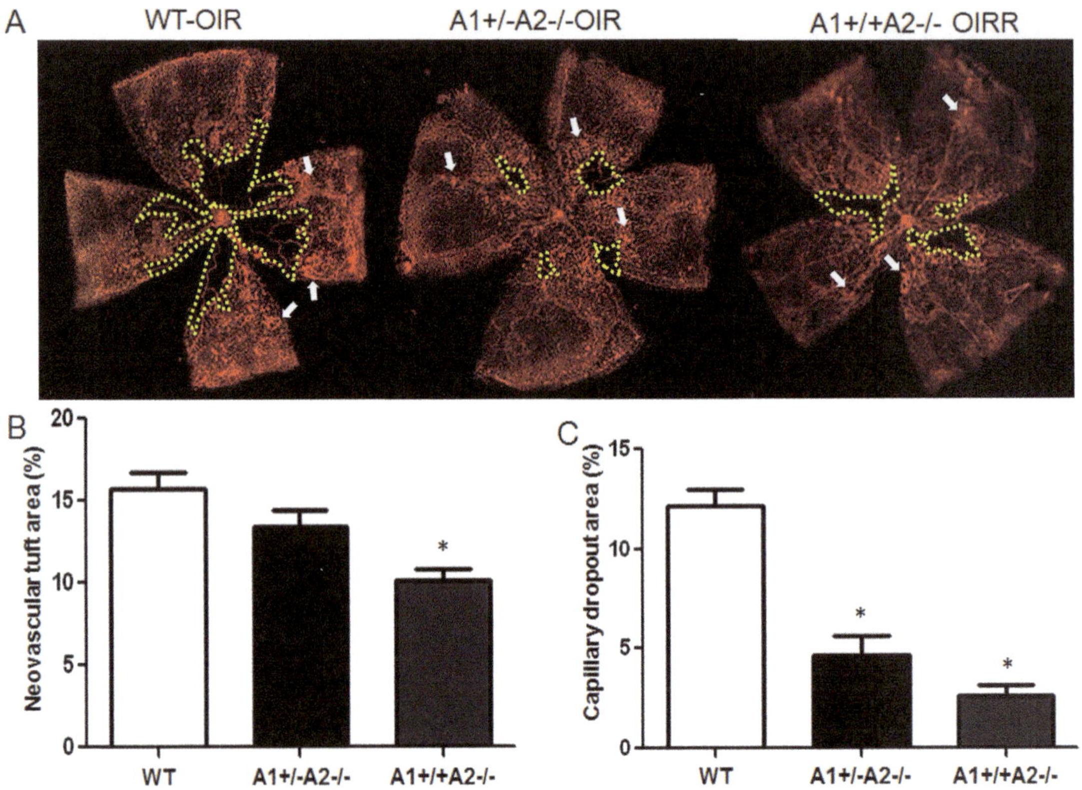

Figure 3. Arginase 2 deletion limits pathological vitreo-retina neovascularization while enhancing intra-retinal neovascularization. Wild type (WT), arginase 2-deficient mice (A1+/+A2−/−) and arginase 2-deficient mice lacking one copy of arginase 1 (A1+/−A2−/−) were maintained in 70% oxygen from P7 to P12, returned to normoxia for 5 days and prepared for analysis on P17. Retinal vessels were visualized by lectin labeling (A) and areas of vitreoretinal neovascular tufts (arrows) and capillary dropout (yellow) were quantified in fluorescence micrographs using ImageJ (B,C). n = 11–13, *P≤0.05 vs WT and A1+/−A2−/− in B and WT in C.

induced injury of the immature retinal vessels. Interestingly, a previous study reported that higher levels of arginase 2 mRNA and an apparent decrease in iNOS activity were associated with decreases in neuronal cell injury during the hypoxia phase of OIR in mice that lack the TNFα gene, implying a neuroprotective role for arginase 2 in OIR. [33] However, our previous studies have shown that deletion of arginase 2 prevents hyperoxia-induced death of retinal neurons during both hyperoxia and relative hypoxia phases of OIR. [17,18] The neuronal cell death was found to be mediated by a process involving hyperoxia-induced increases in polyamine oxidation.[18] Studies are now in progress to examine the involvement of alterations in polyamine metabolism in the retinal vascular injury during OIR. Further study is required to reconcile this discrepancy between the effects of arginase 2 deletion in limiting neuronal and vascular injury as shown in our current and previous studies and the association between upregulation of arginase 2 and decreased neuronal injury as shown in the TNF-α deficient mice.

Our data showing decreases in superoxide and peroxynitrite along with increases in NO formation in the arginase 2 deficient retina strongly indicate involvement of arginase 2 mediated uncoupling of NOS in the hyperoxia-induced vascular injury during OIR. One limitation of our results is that we were unable to detect any change in the total amount of arginase 2 protein in the OIR retinas. The lack of an effect of OIR on arginase 2 protein expression can be explained by the fact that arginase 2 is localized mainly in mitochondria and expression levels are low in most cell types. As shown in Figure 4, arginase 2 is strongly expressed in horizontal cells which are few in number and restricted a single layer at the outer border of the inner nuclear layer. The arginase 2 signal appears high in the horizontal cells of the OIR retina as compared with the room air controls. However, our previous work has shown that horizontal cells undergo degeneration in the OIR retina as indicated by TUNEL labeling within calbindin-positive horizontal cells and decreases in number of calbindin-positive cells. By contrast the horizontal cell death is limited in the arginase 2 knockout mice. [18] Thus, the hyperoxia-induced increase in arginase 2 expression may be offset by decreases in the number of arginase 2-positive cells. It is possible that arginase 2 activation is involved in hyperoxia-induced horizontal cell death. The role of retinal horizontal cells in the control of retinal vascular survival and function is not yet known. However, the horizontal cells are distributed in a network across the entire retina and their processes are in contact with the photoreceptors, bipolar cells and amacrine cells as well as with the outermost layer of retinal vessels. [34,35] They are known to modulate signaling between photoreceptors and bipolar cells. [36] An important function of horizontal cells is sending inhibition signals to enhance spatial contrast of image. [36] Therefore, it is likely that loss of horizontal cells leads to poor vision outcome in ROP patient. Our previous work has shown that arginase 2 deletion reduces OIR-induced impairment of visual function as shown by electroretinography. [17] Thus the horizontal cells are ideally positioned to regulate microvascular function in relation to neuronal activity. The specific functions of these neurovascular interactions are as yet unknown. Further study

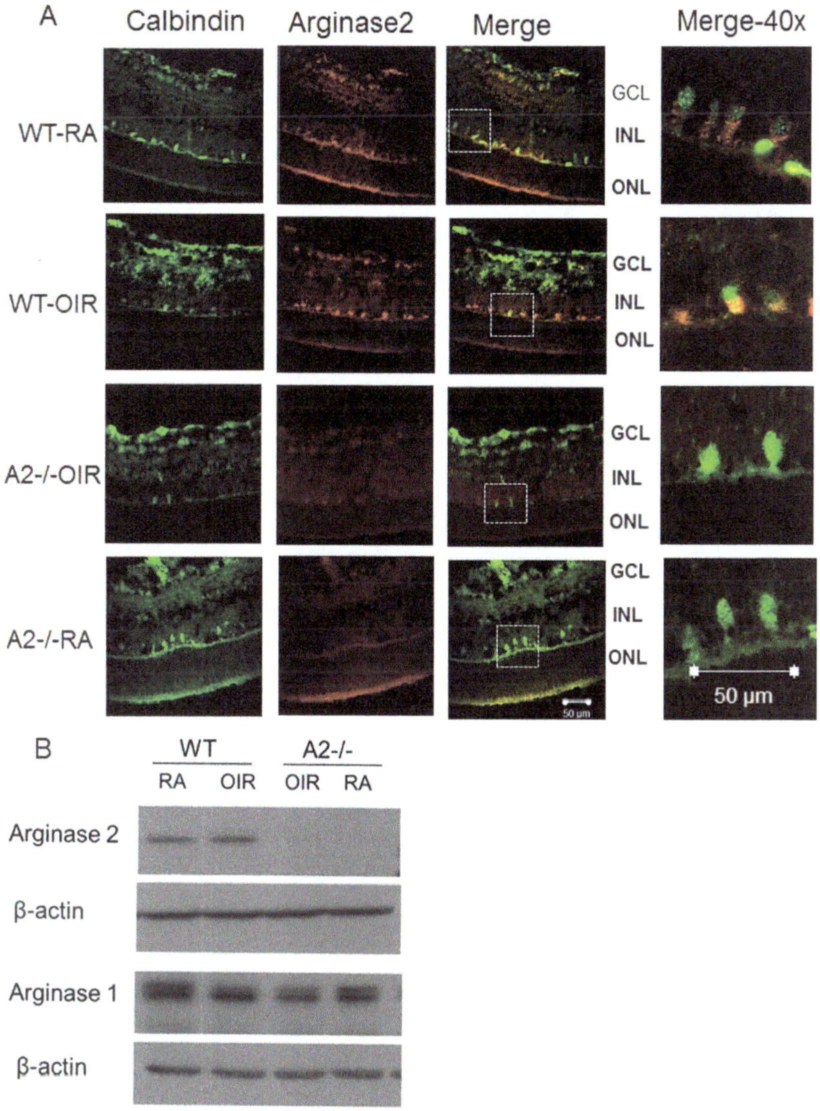

Figure 4. Hyperoxia treatment and Arginase 2 expression in OIR retina. Wild type mice (WT) and mice wild type for arginase 1 and deficient in arginase 2 (A2−/−) were placed in 70% oxygen (OIR) or room air (RA) on P7 and prepared for analysis on after 24 (A) or 48 hr (B). Immunofluorescence imaging (A) of arginase 2 and calbindin in retinal cryosections shows that arginase 2 (red) is highly expressed in horizontal cells (green). Scale bar = 50 µm, n = 3. Western blot analysis (B) showing arginase 1 and 2 levels following normoxia and hyperoxia treatment, n = 5.

is needed to elucidate the role of the horizontal cell alterations in the vascular and neuronal injury during ischemic retinopathy.

Due to the limited resolution of confocal microscope imaging and the small volume of vascular tissue in the 10 µm frozen sections used for our immunolocalization studies, we were unable to clearly localize arginase 2 within the retinal vascular cells. Our previous analyses have demonstrated arginase 2 expression in retinal vessels isolated from mice as well as in cultured BRECs. [37] More studies will be needed to determine the specific effects of hyperoxia exposure on arginase 2 expression and activity in vascular endothelial cells.

Our finding that deletion of arginase 2 in mice prevents hyperoxia-induced obliteration of the retinal vasculature while preventing NOS-dependent ROS formation and preserving NO availability is consistent with previous studies showing involvement of excessive arginase 1 in hyperoxia-induced vascular injury in the developing lung [38] and excessive arginase 2 in vascular dyfunction associated with atherosclerosis and aging. [39,40], [41] Moreover, in other retinal disease models, including acute inflammation and diabetes, excessive arginase 1 has been shown to dysregulate endothelial function through interfering with NOS function. [8,42,43] These differences suggest that differences in vascular maturity, target tissue and/or specific disease-associated triggers determine the arginase isoform involved in vascular injury.

Further work is needed to define the specific mechanisms by which arginase 2 deletion limits ROS formation, preserves NOS function and protects the retinal vessels during hyperoxia treatment. Several studies have shown that arginase 2 up-regulation in endothelial cells causes vascular dysfunction and injury via NOS uncoupling. [39,40,44] It is possible that hyperoxia-induced activation of arginase 2 triggers NOS uncoupling by depleting L-arginine, oxidizing tetrahydrobiopterin (BH4) and/or increasing endogenous methylarginine, all of which can lead to reduction in NO availability and buildup of ROS. [45] A

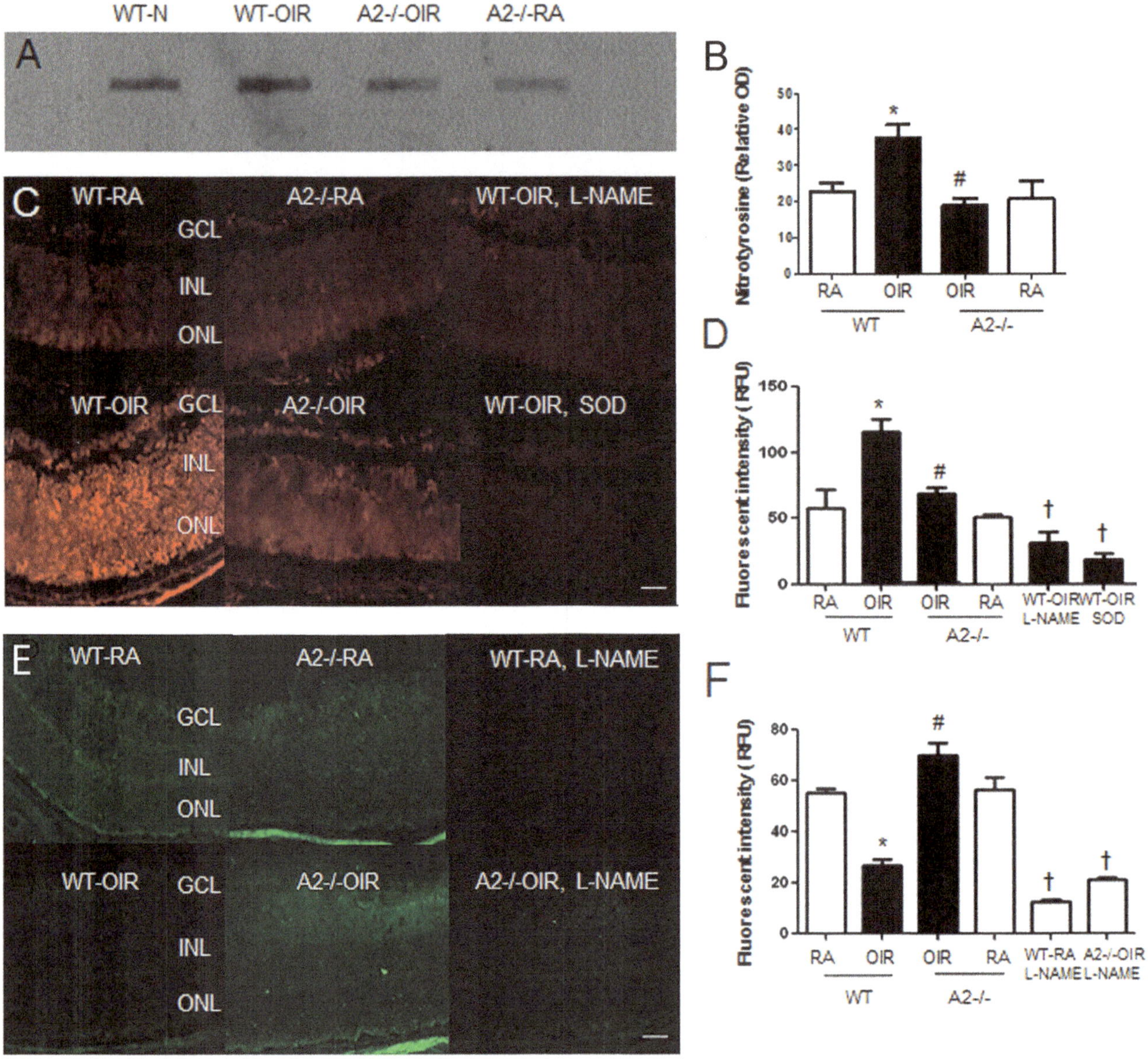

Figure 5. Arginase 2 deletion prevents hyperoxia-induced increases in retinal nitrotyrosine (A) and superoxide (C) levels and preserves NO formation (E). Wild type (WT) and mice wild type for arginase 1 and deficient in arginase 2 (A2−/−) were placed in 70% oxygen (OIR) or room air (RA) on P7 and prepared for analysis on P8. Nitrotyrosine levels in retina samples were detected by slot blot (A) and quantified using ImageJ software (B). n = 6, *P≤0.05 vs WT-RA, # P≤0.05 vs WT-OIR. DHE imaging of superoxide formation was performed using flash frozen retinal sections (C). Results were quantified using Metamorph Imaging System (D). n = 3–5, scale bar = 50 μm, *P≤0.05 WT-OIR vs all groups; # = P≤0.05 vs WT-OIR. † P<0.05 vs WT-OIR. NO formation in situ was determined by DAF-2-DA fluorescence imaging (E). Results were quantified using Metamorph Imaging System (F). n = 3, scale bar = 50 μm, * P≤0.05 vs WT-RA, # P≤0.05 vs WT OIR, † P<0.05 vs WT-RA, A2-/-OIR, A2-/-RA.

previous study using the OIR mouse model indicated that eNOS over-expression reduced BH4 leading to vascular injury during hyperoxia. [46] Arginase 2 activation can also increase oxidative stress in multiple cell types by increasing polyamine oxidation due to activation of the ornithine/polyamine pathway. Our previous studies have shown that arginase 2 deletion limits hyperoxia-induced increases in oxidative stress and reduces injury and death of the retinal neurons by a mechanism involving suppression of hyperoxia-induced activation of polyamine oxidase. [17,18,37] Arginase 2 deletion also limits microglial activation in our OIR model (manuscript in preparation). Studies are in progress to better understand the relationship between the neuronal and vascular cell injury and the role of the arginase pathway in this pathology.

Conclusions

In summary, clinical studies have shown low levels of L-arginine and L-glutamine in infants with ROP, [6] and treatment with an arginyl-glutamine dipeptide supplement was found to lessen vascular damage in the OIR mouse model. [7] Reduction in L-arginine appears to involve up-regulation of arginase activity. Excessive arginase activity is not only involved in L-arginine deficiency, but it is apparently associated with enhanced polyamine production along with polyamine oxidation which is toxic to cells. Our studies suggest that limiting arginase activity, particularly arginase 2, is a promising means of treating oxidative stress-related retinopathy.

Materials and Methods

Cell Culture Analysis and Nitric Oxide Measurement

Primary cultures of BREC were prepared as described previously. [47] Cells from *passages 5–8* were used in all experiments. Cells were maintained in M199 supplemented with 10% FBS, 10% CS-C complete medium, 2 mM glutamine, 100 U/ml penicillin, and 100 μg/ml streptomycin at 37°C in a humidified CO_2 incubator. For analysis of hyperoxia effects on apoptosis, BREC were grown to 70% confluence and switched to serum-free medium. The next day they were placed in a hyperoxic (40% O_2, 5% CO_2) or normoxic (21% O_2, 5% CO_2) environment for 48 h as described by us previous. [14] Cells were treated with or without ABH (100 μM). To quantify apoptosis, cells were trypsinized, washed with phosphate buffer saline (PBS) and resuspended in propidium iodide (PI) solution (0.1% triton, 0.1% sodium citrate, and 50 mg/L PI, Sigma-Aldrich, St. Louis, MO) for one hour. [48] A minimum of 30,000 cells/sample were analyzed on a flow cytometer (BD Accuri C6, San Jose, CA) using a 488-nm laser line for excitation and >600 nm for detecting the emission. The percentage of apoptotic (M1) and normal nuclei (M2) was obtained by analysis of the DNA histogram. For analysis of NO release, conditioned media (200 μl) was collected from cells treated as described for the apoptosis study was treated with ethanol (200 μl) to remove proteins and refluxed in sodium iodide/glacial acetic acid to convert NO_2^- to NO. NO was measured via NO-specific chemiluminescence after reaction with ozone using a Sievers NO analyzer (GE Analytical Instruments, Boulder, CO). [49] Net NO_2^- release from cells treated with ABH or vehicle under normoxic or hyperoxic condition was calculated after subtracting NO_2^- content in the base media.

Ethics Statement

All procedures with animals were carried out in strict accordance with the recommendations in the Guide for the Care and Use of Laboratory Animals of the National Institutes of Health. The protocol was approved by the Committee on the Ethics of Animal Experiments of Georgia Regents University Animal Care and Use Committee (Animal Welfare Assurance no. A3307-01). Euthanasia was performed by thoracotomy under avertin (2, 2, 2 tribromoethanol, Sigma) anesthesia, and all efforts were made to minimize suffering.

Treatment of Animals

Experiments were performed with C57BL/6J wild-type mice and mice deficient in arginase 1 or/and arginase 2 (A1+/−A2−/−, A1+/−A2+/+, A1+/+A2−/−). These lines were developed by Drs. S. D. Cederbaum [50] and W. E. O'Brien [51] and were provided by Dr. Cederbaum with the permission of Dr. O'Brien. Some mice were treated with the arginase inhibitor 2(S)-amino- 6-boronohexanoic acid (ABH, kindly provided by Dr. Dan Berkowitz). Room temperature was maintained at 20°C, and illumination was provided by standard fluorescent lighting on a 12-hour light–dark cycle.

Oxygen-induced retinopathy was induced in newborn mice according to the protocol of Smith, et al. with some adjustment. [52] On postnatal day 7 (P7), mice were placed along with their dams into 70% oxygen for up to 5 days, after which they were transferred back to room air. The 70% oxygen concentration was used because the mutant mice do not tolerate 75% oxygen treatment. The animals were sacrificed at various times. Following deep anesthesia with Avertin (250 mg/kg, ip), mice were euthanized by thoracotomy and the eyeballs were taken out and fixed in 4% paraformaldehyde (PFA) overnight. Retina flat-mounts were dissected and labeled with biotinylated *Griffonia simplicifolia* isolectin B4 (Vector Laboratories). Retinas were viewed with fluorescence microscopy (Axiophot, Zeiss, Chester, VA) and the images captured in digital format (Spot System; Diagnostic Instruments, Sterling Heights, MI). Central capillary dropout Image-J software [52].

Histology and Morphology of Retina Cross Sections

Retinal morphology was studied on retinal cryostat sections from WT, A2-/-, and A1+/−A2−/− OIR adult mice. Sections (10 μm) containing the optic nerve were collected 20 um apart from one another, and stained with hematoxylin and eosin (H&E, Fisher Scientific).

Immunofluorescence

Eyes were removed, fixed in 4% paraformaldehyde, washed in PBS and retinas were isolated and cryoprotected. Cryostat sections (10 um) were permeabilized in 1% Triton (20 min) and blocked in 10% normal goat serum containing 1% BSA (1 h). Sections were then incubated overnight in primary antibodies (4°C): (rabbit polyclonal anti-arginase 2, 1:250, Santa Cruz Biotechnology, Dallas, TX; mouse monoclonal anti-calbindin, 1:200, Sigma-Aldrich, St. Louis, MO) followed by reaction with fluorescein or Texas red conjugated secondary antibodies (Life Technologies, Grand Island, NY), washed in PBS and mounted with Vectashield (Vector Laboratories, Burlingame, CA).

Western Blotting

Retinas were homogenized in a modified RIPA buffer [20 mmol/L Tris-HCl (pH 7.4), 2.5 mmol/L ethylenediamine tetraacetic acid, 50 mmol/L NaF, 10 mmol/L Na4P2O7, 1% TritonX-100, 0.1% sodium dodecyl sulfate, 1% sodium deoxycholate, 1 mmol/L phenylmethyl sulfonyl fluoride] and 10 μg protein samples were separated by 10% sodium dodecyl sulfate polyacrylamide gel electrophoresis, transferred to nitrocellulose membrane, and reacted with antibodies (chicken polyclonal anti-arginase 1, 1:20,000, kindly provided by Dr. Sidney Morris; rabbit polyclonal anti Arginase 2 antibody (1:250, Santa Cruz Biotechnology, Dallas, TX) followed by horseradish peroxidase-linked secondary antibody and enhanced chemiluminescence (Amersham Pharmacia, San Francisco, CA). Membranes were stripped and reprobed for β-actin to demonstrate equal loading.

Nitrotyrosine Slot Blot

Relative amounts of proteins nitrated on tyrosine were measured by use of slot-blot techniques. Assay lysate was transferred onto nitrocellulose membrane using a slot-blot microfiltration unit (Bio-Rad Laboratories, Hercules, CA). Nitrotyrosine was detected by use of a mouse monoclonal anti-nitrotyrosine antibody (Cayman Chemical, Ann Harper, MI) followed by followed by horseradish peroxidase-conjugated secondary antibody (1:2000, GE Healthcare Bio-Sciences, Pittsburgh, PA). Immunoreactive proteins were detected using the enhanced chemiluminescence (ECL) system (GE Healthcare Bio-Sciences, Pittsburgh, PA). Relative levels of nitrotyrosine immunoreactivity were determined by Image J software.

Dihydroethidium Fluorescence Imaging of Superoxide

Superoxide production was evaluated in retinal frozen sections by the dihydroethidium (DHE) method, as described previously. [43] Briefly, frozen sections were preincubated in NADPH (100 μM) with or without PEG-SOD (400 U/mL) or NOS inhibitor L-NG-nitroarginine methyl ester (L-NAME, 100 μmol, 1 mM) for 20 minutes, followed by reaction with DHE (2 μM) for 20 minutes at 37°C. DHE images from serial sections treated with or without inhibitors were obtained using a fluorescence microscope (AxioVision; Carl Zeiss, Thornwood, NY). DHE was excited at 470 nm with an emission spectrum of 610 nm. The images were analyzed for reaction intensity using computer assisted morphometry (Metamorph Image System; Molecular Devices, Downingtown, PA).

Diaminofluorescein Diacetate Imaging of Nitric Oxide

NO production was evaluated in retinal frozen sections using 4,5-diaminofluorescein diacetate (DAF-2 DA, EMD Millipore, Billerica, MA). [43] Briefly, frozen sections were pre-incubated with HEPES or NOS inhibitor L-NG-nitroarginine methyl ester (L-NAME; 100 μmol (1 mM) for 20 minutes, followed by reaction with DAF-2 DA for 20 minutes at 37°C. Slices were then washed 3 times for total of 15 min with fresh HEPES. NO images from serial sections treated with or without inhibitors were obtained using a fluorescence microscope (AxioVision). DAF was excited at 488 nm with an emission spectrum at 515 nm. The images were analyzed for reaction intensity (Metamorph Image System).

Statistical Analysis

All data were summarized as means ±SEM. Statistical methods to were used to compare treatment groups and determine significance of observed differences in all experiments. In each case the data were reviewed to see how well they fit the assumptions of the tests. In most cases the comparisons were between multiple groups and the overall differences were analyzed by ANOVA followed by Tukey multiple comparison to evaluate group differences. P values <0.05 were taken as significant.

Acknowledgments

This research was completed in partial fulfillment of requirements for J. Suwanpradid's PhD degree. The authors thank Tahira Lemtalsi for technical assistance, Dr. Julia Brittain for advice on flow cytometry, Dr. Yunchao Su and Dr. Dmitry Kondrikov for providing a hyperoxia chamber, Dr. Dan Berkowitz for providing ABH and Dr. Sidney Morris for providing the arginase 1 antibody.

Author Contributions

Conceived and designed the experiments: JS MR RWC RBC. Performed the experiments: JS MR MAB. Analyzed the data: JS MR RBC MAB. Contributed reagents/materials/analysis tools: RBC RWC MAB. Wrote the paper: JS MR. Edited and revised the manuscript: MAB RWC RBC.

References

1. Premature Babies. U.S. National Library of Medicine (2013).
2. Fulton AB, Hansen RM, Moskowitz A, Akula JD (2009) The neurovascular retina in retinopathy of prematurity. Prog Retin Eye Res 28: 452–482.
3. Ashton N, Ward B, Serpell G (1954) Effect of oxygen on developing retinal vessels with particular reference to the problem of retrolental fibroplasia. Br J Ophthalmol 38: 397–432.
4. Smith LE (2008) Through the eyes of a child: understanding retinopathy through ROP the Friedenwald lecture. Invest Ophthalmol Vis Sci 49: 5177–5182.
5. Smith LE, Wesolowski E, McLellan A, Kostyk SK, D'Amato R, et al. (1994) Oxygen-induced retinopathy in the mouse. Invest Ophthalmol Vis Sci 35: 101–111.
6. Wu G, Jaeger LA, Bazer FW, Rhoads JM (2004) Arginine deficiency in preterm infants: biochemical mechanisms and nutritional implications. J Nutr Biochem 15: 442–451.
7. Neu J, Afzal A, Pan H, Gallego E, Li N, et al. (2006) The dipeptide Arg-Gln inhibits retinal neovascularization in the mouse model of oxygen-induced retinopathy. Invest Ophthalmol Vis Sci 47: 3151–3155.
8. Zhang W, Baban B, Rojas M, Tofigh S, Virmani SK, et al. (2009) Arginase activity mediates retinal inflammation in endotoxin-induced uveitis. Am J Pathol 175: 891–902.
9. Jenkinson CP, Grody WW, Cederbaum SD (1996) Comparative properties of arginases. Comp Biochem Physiol B Biochem Mol Biol 114: 107–132.
10. Kielczewski JL, Jarajapu YP, McFarland EL, Cai J, Afzal A, et al. (2009) Insulin-like growth factor binding protein-3 mediates vascular repair by enhancing nitric oxide generation. Circ Res 105: 897–905.
11. Hardy P, Dumont I, Bhattacharya M, Hou X, Lachapelle P, et al. (2000) Oxidants, nitric oxide and prostanoids in the developing ocular vasculature: a basis for ischemic retinopathy. Cardiovasc Res 47: 489–509.
12. Sessa WC (2009) Molecular control of blood flow and angiogenesis: role of nitric oxide. J Thromb Haemost 7 Suppl 1: 35–37.
13. Brooks SE, Gu X, Samuel S, Marcus DM, Bartoli M, et al. (2001) Reduced severity of oxygen-induced retinopathy in eNOS-deficient mice. Invest Ophthalmol Vis Sci 42: 222–228.
14. Gu X, El-Remessy AB, Brooks SE, Al-Shabrawey M, Tsai NT, et al. (2003) Hyperoxia induces retinal vascular endothelial cell apoptosis through formation of peroxynitrite. Am J Physiol Cell Physiol 285: C546–554.
15. Romero MJ, Platt DH, Tawfik HE, Labazi M, El-Remessy AB, et al. (2008) Diabetes-induced coronary vascular dysfunction involves increased arginase activity. Circ Res 102: 95–102.
16. Romero MJ, Iddings JA, Platt DH, Ali MI, Cederbaum SD, et al. (2012) Diabetes-induced vascular dysfunction involves arginase I. Am J Physiol Heart Circ Physiol 302: H159–166.
17. Narayanan SP, Suwanpradid J, Saul A, Xu Z, Still A, et al. (2011) Arginase 2 deletion reduces neuro-glial injury and improves retinal function in a model of retinopathy of prematurity. PLoS One 6: e22460.
18. Narayanan SP, Xu Z, Putluri N, Sreekumar A, Lemtalsi T, et al. (2014) Arginase 2 deficiency reduces hyperoxia-mediated retinal neurodegeneration through the regulation of polyamine metabolism. Cell Death Dis 5: e1075.
19. Morris SM Jr. (2009) Recent advances in arginine metabolism: roles and regulation of the arginases. Br J Pharmacol 157: 922–930.
20. Christianson DW (2005) Arginase: structure, mechanism, and physiological role in male and female sexual arousal. Acc Chem Res 38: 191–201.
21. Durante W, Liao L, Reyna SV, Peyton KJ, Schafer AI (2001) Transforming growth factor-beta(1) stimulates L-arginine transport and metabolism in vascular smooth muscle cells: role in polyamine and collagen synthesis. Circulation 103: 1121–1127.
22. Xia Y, Dawson VL, Dawson TM, Snyder SH, Zweier JL (1996) Nitric oxide synthase generates superoxide and nitric oxide in arginine-depleted cells leading to peroxynitrite-mediated cellular injury. Proc Natl Acad Sci U S A 93: 6770–6774.
23. Beckman JS, Koppenol WH (1996) Nitric oxide, superoxide, and peroxynitrite: the good, the bad, and ugly. Am J Physiol 271: C1424–1437.
24. Gow AJ, Duran D, Malcolm S, Ischiropoulos H (1996) Effects of peroxynitrite-induced protein modifications on tyrosine phosphorylation and degradation. FEBS Lett 385: 63–66.
25. Zhao H, Joseph J, Fales HM, Sokoloski EA, Levine RL, et al. (2005) Detection and characterization of the product of hydroethidine and intracellular superoxide by HPLC and limitations of fluorescence. Proc Natl Acad Sci U S A 102: 5727–5732.
26. Brooks SE, Gu X, Kaufmann PM, Marcus DM, Caldwell RB (1998) Modulation of VEGF production by pH and glucose in retinal Muller cells. Curr Eye Res 17: 875–882.
27. Krotova K, Patel JM, Block ER, Zharikov S (2010) Hypoxic upregulation of arginase II in human lung endothelial cells. Am J Physiol Cell Physiol 299: C1541–1548.
28. Shatanawi A, Romero MJ, Iddings JA, Chandra S, Umapathy NS, et al. (2011) Angiotensin II-induced vascular endothelial dysfunction through RhoA/Rho kinase/p38 mitogen-activated protein kinase/arginase pathway. Am J Physiol Cell Physiol 300: C1181–1192.
29. Chandra S, Romero MJ, Shatanawi A, Alkilany AM, Caldwell RB, et al. (2012) Oxidative species increase arginase activity in endothelial cells through the RhoA/Rho kinase pathway. Br J Pharmacol 165: 506–519.
30. Pourcet B, Feig JE, Vengrenyuk Y, Hobbs AJ, Kepka-Lenhart D, et al. (2011) LXRalpha regulates macrophage arginase 1 through PU.1 and interferon regulatory factor 8. Circ Res 109: 492–501.
31. Pandey D, Sikka G, Bergman Y, Kim JH, Ryoo S, et al. (2014) Transcriptional regulation of endothelial arginase 2 by histone deacetylase 2. Arterioscler Thromb Vasc Biol 34: 1556–1566.
32. Sahin E, Haubenwallner S, Kuttke M, Kollmann I, Halfmann A, et al. (2014) Macrophage PTEN Regulates Expression and Secretion of Arginase I Modulating Innate and Adaptive Immune Responses. J Immunol.

33. Stevenson L, Matesanz N, Colhoun L, Edgar K, Devine A, et al. (2010) Reduced nitro-oxidative stress and neural cell death suggests a protective role for microglial cells in TNFalpha-/- mice in ischemic retinopathy. Invest Ophthalmol Vis Sci 51: 3291–3299.
34. Knabe W, Ochs M (1999) Horizontal cells invest retinal capillaries in the tree shrew Tupaia belangeri. Cell Tissue Res 298: 33–43.
35. Mojumder DK (2008) Capillary-contacting horizontal cells in the rodent retina. J Anat Soc India 57: 34–36.
36. Poche RA, Reese BE (2009) Retinal horizontal cells: challenging paradigms of neural development and cancer biology. Development 136: 2141–2151.
37. Narayanan SP, Rojas M, Suwanpradid J, Toque HA, Caldwell RW, et al. (2013) Arginase in Retinopathy. Prog Retin Eye Res.
38. Ali NK, Jafri A, Sopi RB, Prakash YS, Martin RJ, et al. (2012) Role of arginase in impairing relaxation of lung parenchyma of hyperoxia-exposed neonatal rats. Neonatology 101: 106–115.
39. Ryoo S, Lemmon CA, Soucy KG, Gupta G, White AR, et al. (2006) Oxidized low-density lipoprotein-dependent endothelial arginase II activation contributes to impaired nitric oxide signaling. Circ Res 99: 951–960.
40. Ryoo S, Gupta G, Benjo A, Lim HK, Camara A, et al. (2008) Endothelial arginase II: a novel target for the treatment of atherosclerosis. Circ Res 102: 923–932.
41. Shin WS, Berkowitz DE, Ryoo SW (2012) Increased arginase II activity contributes to endothelial dysfunction through endothelial nitric oxide synthase uncoupling in aged mice. Exp Mol Med 44: 594–602.
42. Elms SC, Toque HA, Rojas M, Xu Z, Caldwell RW, et al. (2013) The role of arginase I in diabetes-induced retinal vascular dysfunction in mouse and rat models of diabetes. Diabetologia 56: 654–662.
43. Patel C, Rojas M, Narayanan SP, Zhang W, Xu Z, et al. (2013) Arginase as a mediator of diabetic retinopathy. Front Immunol 4: 173.
44. Que LG, Kantrow SP, Jenkinson CP, Piantadosi CA, Huang YC (1998) Induction of arginase isoforms in the lung during hyperoxia. Am J Physiol 275: L96–102.
45. Forstermann U, Sessa WC (2012) Nitric oxide synthases: regulation and function. Eur Heart J 33: 829–837, 837a–837d.
46. Edgar K, Gardiner TA, van Haperen R, de Crom R, McDonald DM (2012) eNOS overexpression exacerbates vascular closure in the obliterative phase of OIR and increases angiogenic drive in the subsequent proliferative stage. Invest Ophthalmol Vis Sci 53: 6833–6850.
47. Feng Y, Venema VJ, Venema RC, Tsai N, Behzadian MA, et al. (1999) VEGF-induced permeability increase is mediated by caveolae. Invest Ophthalmol Vis Sci 40: 157–167.
48. Riccardi C, Nicoletti I (2006) Analysis of apoptosis by propidium iodide staining and flow cytometry. Nat Protoc 1: 1458–1461.
49. Jagnandan D, Sessa WC, Fulton D (2005) Intracellular location regulates calcium-calmodulin-dependent activation of organelle-restricted eNOS. Am J Physiol Cell Physiol 289: C1024–1033.
50. Deignan JL, Livesay JC, Yoo PK, Goodman SI, O'Brien WE, et al. (2006) Ornithine deficiency in the arginase double knockout mouse. Mol Genet Metab 89: 87–96.
51. Shi O, Morris SM Jr., Zoghbi H, Porter CW, O'Brien WE (2001) Generation of a mouse model for arginase II deficiency by targeted disruption of the arginase II gene. Mol Cell Biol 21: 811–813.
52. Connor KM, Krah NM, Dennison RJ, Aderman CM, Chen J, et al. (2009) Quantification of oxygen-induced retinopathy in the mouse: a model of vessel loss, vessel regrowth and pathological angiogenesis. Nat Protoc 4: 1565–1573.

Rhegmatogenous Retinal Detachment Surgery in Elderly People over 70 Years Old: Visual Acuity, Quality of Life, and Cost-Utility Values

Yingyan Ma[1]❡, Xiaohua Ying[2]❡, Haidong Zou[1,3]*, Xiaocheng Xu[2], Haiyun Liu[1], Lin Bai[1], Xun Xu[1], Xi Zhang[1]

1 Department of Ophthalmology, Shanghai First People's Hospital, Shanghai Jiao Tong University, Shanghai, China, **2** School of Public Health, Fudan University, Shanghai, China, **3** Shanghai Eye Disease Prevention & Treatment Center, Shanghai, China

Abstract

Background and Purpose: To evaluate the influence of rhegmatogenous retinal detachment (RRD) surgery on elderly patients in terms of visual acuity, vision-related quality of life and its cost-effectiveness.

Methods: Elderly patients over 70 years old, who were diagnosed and underwent RRD surgery at Shanghai First People's Hospital, Shanghai Jiao Tong University, China, from January 1, 2009, through January 1, 2013. The participants received scleral buckling surgery and vitreous surgery with or without scleral buckling under retrobulbar anesthesia. We followed the patients for 1 year and collected best-corrected visual acuity (BCVA), vision-related quality of life, and direct medical costs data. Utility values elicited by time-trade-off were analyzed to determine the quality of life. Quality-adjusted life years (QALYs) gained in life expectancy were calculated and discounted at 3% annually. Costs per QALY gained were reported using the bootstrap method. Further analyses were made for two age groups, age 70–79 and age over 80 years. Sensitivity analyses were performed to test stability of the results.

Results: 98 patients were included in the study. The BCVA significantly improved by 0.53±0.44 (Logarithm of the Minimum Angle of Resolution (logMAR)) at the 1-year postoperative time point ($p<0.001$). Utility values increased from 0.77 to 0.84 ($p<0.001$), and an average of 0.4 QALYs were gained in the life expectancy. Costs per QALY gained from the RRD surgery were 33,186 Chinese Yuan (CNY) (5,276 US dollars (USD))/QALY; 24,535 CNY (3,901 USD)/QALY for the age group of 70–79 years and 71,240 CNY (11,326 USD)/QALY for the age group over 80 years.

Conclusions: RRD surgery improved the visual acuity and quality of life in the elderly patients over 70 years old. According to the World Health Organization's recommendation, at a threshold of willingness to pay of 115,062 CNY (18,293 USD)/QALY, RRD surgery is cost effective in the elderly patients.

Editor: Haotian Lin, Sun Yat-sen University, China

Funding: This study was funded by a key grant from the Shanghai Health Bureau (20114007), a grant from the Shanghai Leading Talent Reserve Programme (40311), and a grand from National Population and Family Planning Commission: Researches on modern hospital management system-costs calculation in hospital (SJYF2014XD010B). ZHD received the funding. The funders had no role in study design, data collection and analysis, decision to publish, or preparation of the manuscript.

Competing Interests: The authors have declared that no competing interests exist.

* Email: zouhaidong@hotmail.com

❡ These authors contributed equally to this work.

Introduction

Rhegmatogenous retinal detachment (RRD) is the most common type of retinal detachment, and it severely threatens visual acuity and vision-related quality of life [1–3]. Proper and timely treatments, such as scleral buckling surgery and vitreous surgery, can largely restore visual acuity and permit a certain degree of improvement in vision-related quality of life [4], [5]. However, in most developing countries with limited medical resources, the treatment for retinal detachment has been a low priority [6]. Despite the effectiveness of RRD surgery, the costs are not small. Brown and associates reported the costs for vitreoretinal surgery to be between 7,109 US dollars (USD) and 9,607 USD in patients with severe proliferative vitreoretinopathy [7]. Two recent studies performed in America calculated the costs for the two types of surgery varying from 4,048 USD to 7,940 USD [8], [9]. In our previous study, an average cost of 11,384 Chinese Yuan (CNY) (1,810 USD, 1 USD = 6.29 CNY, 2012.12.31) was determined for RRD surgery in Shanghai [10]. Although comparatively lower than the cost reported in America, it is still a large burden for most families in China.

The annual incidence of RRD ranged from 6.3 to 17.9 per 100,000 population globally [11]. Age is one risk factor for RRD [11–13]. In elderly people who are 70 to 79 years old, the incidences vary from 15.21 to 50 per 100,000 worldwide [11]. In a recent study conducted in the Netherlands, the annual incidence of RRD was reported to be 21.43 per 100,000 for people aged 85–89 years old [14]. However, age was also a negative predictor for optimal visual outcomes after RRD surgery. As demonstrated in many previous studies, patients of older age have inferior functional results, namely best-corrected visual acuity, than younger patients [15–19]. Therefore, in clinical practice, it is not unusual that many elderly people give up on the surgery considering the expensive medical costs, the uncertain visual outcomes, and the relatively short remaining life years. These elderly people will definitely experience severe visual impairment, and as a result, losses of quality of life. As shown in a survey of a community population aged over 60 years in Shanghai, retinal detachment was the fifth leading cause of blindness [20].

Cost-utility analysis is one method of economic evaluation that incorporates the utility value in the form of quality-adjusted life years (QALYs) with costs to calculate how much money should be spent on each QALY gained for certain medical interventions [21], [22]. One advantage of cost-utility analysis is that it allows comparison among different disciplines by a common unit of measure (costs/QALY). Therefore, policymakers can identify relative priorities when determining resource allocation among medical interventions [21], [22]. In Brown's study, the costs/QALY were between 40,252 USD/QALY and 62,383 USD/QALY for vitreous surgery in patients complicated with severe proliferative vitreoretinopathy [7]. In the recent American study, the costs/QALY varied from 1,377 USD/QALY to 2,243 USD/QALY for scleral buckling and vitreous surgery [9]. In Shanghai, the costs/QALY were 13,794 CNY (2,193 USD)/QALY for normal RRD patients throughout their life expectancies [10]. However, the cost-effectiveness of RRD surgery for elderly patients has not been evaluated in the existing literatures.

As we enter an aging society, along with the popularity of cataract surgery and high rates of myopia, we anticipate a greater number of elderly patients suffering from RRD [11]. Therefore, it is worthwhile to explore how much the elderly people could benefit from RRD surgery and whether performing RRD surgery is cost-effective in this population. This study presented the outcomes of RRD surgery in terms of visual acuity and vision-related quality of life and calculated its cost-effectiveness in an elderly population.

Methods

Ethics

All participants gave their written informed consent. The study was conducted according to the tenets of the Declaration of Helsinki and was approved by the Institutional Review Board at Shanghai First People's Hospital, Shanghai Jiao Tong University.

Participants and investigations

Between January 1, 2009, and January 1, 2013, study participants included elderly patients over the age of 70 years who were newly diagnosed with RRD (in at least one eye) and subsequently underwent surgery in the Shanghai First People's Hospital, Shanghai Jiao Tong University. Patients were excluded if they had other severe eye diseases, physical disability or mental disorders.

Participants were interviewed before and one year after surgery. Data were collected for age, gender, educational level, systemic diseases, duration of time from RRD symptoms to RRD surgery (or, if no symptoms, time since diagnosis), range of detachment in quadrants, macular-on or macular-off, RRD surgery type, surgical procedures, best-corrected visual acuity (BCVA), costs, utility value, and complications of surgery. BCVA was also collected at the 3-month postoperative time point. Surgical procedures were classified as scleral buckling surgery and vitreous surgery with or without scleral buckling. A skilled interviewer (HDZ), who did not take part in any of the examinations or follow-up with the participants, administered the questionnaire and provided assistance when required.

Utility values and costs

Utility values were obtained by using the time trade-off (TTO) method at pre-operative and 1-year post-operative time points. Participants were asked how many additional years they expected to live and how many of these theoretical remaining years they would be willing to give up in return for guaranteed, permanently perfect vision. The utility value was then calculated by subtracting the quotient of these numbers (years given up/years to live) from 1.0 [23]. For example, if a 70-year-old RRD patient with a self-perceived life expectancy of 10 additional years would like to trade 2 years to get rid of his or her visual impairment caused by RRD, the utility value related to his or her RRD would be $(1.0-2/10)=0.8$.

Costs were calculated from the patient perspective, and all of these costs were inflated to 2012 values by utilizing the consumer price index for health care [24]. Self-designed investigation forms were distributed to record the medical costs associated with RRD surgery for the first diagnosed eye, including costs of pharmaceuticals, examinations, treatment, anesthesia, surgery, hospitalization, and transportation fees. Downstream costs induced by surgery were also collected during the 1-year follow up, such as the costs for the removal of silicone oil and treatment for complications including cataract surgery, treatment of corneal edema, and intraocular hypertension. If the second eye also received RRD surgery during the 1-year study period, costs incurred by this surgery were also recorded. The costs collected in this research were associated with the Chinese medical insurance unified prices; hence, they were representative of the medical costs charged by other hospitals in Shanghai and in other cities in China. Only direct costs were included. Indirect costs, such as loss of productivity and leisure time, were not incorporated into this investigation.

Model design

According to our previous research [25], we assumed that the utility value in RRD patients increased steadily in the first year and then remained stable. Hypothetical patients designed as no-treatment controls were expected to obtain the same pre-operative utility values as the participants. Additionally, it was assumed that their utility values remained constant and that no medical costs related to RRD treatment had ever been incurred in our hypothetical patients.

Because the benefits of RRD surgery are life-long, we carried out a cost-utility analysis over the remaining life expectancy for RRD surgery. Lacking evidence of utility change over the remaining lifetime of RRD patients, and in accord with other economic evaluations within ophthalmology [7], [26], [27], we assumed that the vision-related quality of life would remain constant over the life expectancy. The age and gender-specific life expectancy table from the Health Profile China was used to calculate life expectancy QALYs gained [28]. In the control group, hypothetical patients who did not receive surgery would also

Table 1. Characteristics and surgical data for 98 elderly RRD patients.

	Total	70s	80s	P value*
No. of patients	98	57	41	
Average age [Mean (SD)]	78.49(4.36)	75.33(2.48)	82.88(1.90)	<0.001
Male [No. (%)]	54(55.1)	35(61.40)	19(46.34)	0.139
Education time >10 years [No. (%)]	50(51.02)	32(56.14)	18(43.90)	0.232
Duration of symptoms [Weeks, Median (Range)]	5[1–27]	6[1–23]	4[1–27]	0.550
More than 2 quadrants detached [No. (%)]	78(79.60)	46(80.70)	32(78.05)	0.748
Macular-off [No. (%)]	68(69.39)	40(70.18)	28(68.29)	0.842
Types of surgery				0.191
Scleral buckling surgery [No. (%)]	31(31.63)	21(36.84)	10(24.39)	
Vitreous surgery [No. (%)]	67(68.37)	36(63.16)	31(75.61)	
Bilateral surgery rate [No. (%)]	13(13.27)	9(15.79)	4(9.76)	0.385
Complication rate [No. (%)]	66(67.35)	35(61.40)	31(75.61)	0.139

*A comparison was made between age groups of patients in their 70s and 80s. An independent sample t-test was used for continual data of normal distribution, a Mann Whitney U test for non-normal distribution data, and the Pearson chi-square test for the categorical data. A value of $P<0.05$ was regarded as statistically significant.
RRD, rhegmatogenous retinal detachment; SD, standard deviation.

remain at their preoperative health status throughout their life expectancies with no medical expenditures related to RRD. The QALYs were discounted at 3% annually in the baseline analysis. Because all medical costs were paid over a 1-year period, they were not discounted. The incremental cost-effectiveness ratio (ICER) was then calculated to evaluate the life-span cost-utility result of RRD surgery, compared with the no-treatment option.

Moreover, we performed subgroup analyses by dividing the participants into two age groups: 70–79-year-olds and over 80-year-olds. Costs, QALYs gained, and the ICER were calculated for each age group to explore the cost-effectiveness of RRD surgery in different age intervals. Additional analyses for scleral buckling surgery and vitreous surgery were also calculated.

Threshold ratio of willingness to pay

In China, there is no official guiding document or consensus on the threshold ratio of willingness to pay (WTP); hence, we adopted the standard posed by the World Health Organization (WHO). As recommended by the WHO, if the ICER is less than three times the gross domestic product (GDP) per capita, it can be regarded as cost-effective, and if the ICER is less than the GDP per capita, the intervention can be regarded as highly cost-effective [29]. This approach has already been utilized in several economic evaluations in China [30], [31]. With a 2012 GDP per capita in China of 38,354 CNY, we used 115,062 CNY (18,293 USD)/QALY as the threshold ratio of willingness to pay to determine whether the RRD surgery was cost-effective in the elderly population.

Statistical analysis

Costs and QALYs are usually highly skewed, and the uncertainty of the ICER is difficult to present using traditional statistical methods; therefore, we performed a bootstrapping with 1,000 replications to calculate mean costs, mean QALYs, the ICERs and the uncertainty of those results [32–34]. The percentile method (2.5 and 97.5 percentiles from the bootstrapped sample) was used to estimate 95% confidence intervals (CIs) for the incremental costs and QALYs [21], [33]. Furthermore, cost-effectiveness acceptability curves (CEACs) were drawn, representing the probability of RRD surgery being more cost-effective than no treatment for different thresholds of willingness to pay per QALY [35], [36]. The Mann-Whitney U test was used to compare the differences of costs, utility values, QALYs, and duration time of RRD between the two age groups for the non-normal distribution of the variables. An independent sample t-test was used for continual data of normal distribution, and the Pearson chi-square test was used for the categorical data. The paired sample t-test was used for testing differences between BCVA

Table 2. Outcomes of visual acuity for RRD surgery in an elderly population (n = 98).

	Total	70s	80s	P value*
BCVA before surgery [LogMAR, Mean (SD)]	1.06(0.50)	1.05(0.50)	1.09(0.52)	0.682
BCVA 3 months after surgery [LogMAR, Mean (SD)]	0.74(0.35)	0.71(0.34)	0.78(0.36)	0.334
Difference of BCVA during the 3 months [LogMAR, Mean (SD)]	0.32(0.35)	0.34(0.36)	0.31(0.34)	0.709
BCVA 1 year after surgery [LogMAR, Mean (SD)]	0.54(0.26)	0.53(0.25)	0.55(0.29)	0.650
Difference of BCVA during the 1 year [LogMAR, Mean (SD)]	0.53(0.44)	0.52(0.40)	0.54(0.49)	0.845

*A comparison was made between age groups of patients who were in their 70s and 80s using independent samples t-tests. A value of $P<0.05$ was regarded as statistically significant.
RRD, rhegmatogenous retinal detachment; BCVA, best-corrected visual acuity; LogMAR, Logarithm of the Minimum Angle of Resolution; SD, standard deviation.

Table 3. Results of the baseline cost-utility analysis for RRD surgery in an elderly population (bootstrap, n = 1000).

	Total	70s	80s	P value*
Utility value before surgery [Mean (SD)]	0.77(0.12)	0.76(0.13)	0.79(0.11)	0.131
Utility value 1-year after surgery [Mean (SD)]	0.84(0.08)	0.84(0.07)	0.84(0.09)	0.352
Difference of utility values during the 1 year [Mean (SD)]	0.07(0.07)	0.08(0.08)	0.05(0.06)	0.096
QALYs gained in life-expectancy [Mean (95% CI)]	0.40(0.31–0.50)	0.55(0.41–0.72)	0.18(0.12–0.24)	
Mean Costs [CNY(USD)]	12,992(2,066)	13,319(2,117)	12,484(1,985)	
Costs 95% CI [CNY(USD)]	11,984(1,905) –14,088(2,239)	11,818(1,879)– 14,800(2,353)	11,131(1,769)– 13,910(2,211)	
Mean ICER [CNY(USD)/QALY]	33,186(5,276)	24,536(3,901)	71,240(11,326)	

*Comparisons were made between age groups of patients in their 70s and 80s using a Mann Whitney U test. A value of P<0.05 was regarded as statistically significant. RRD, rhegmatogenous retinal detachment; CNY, Chinese Yuan; USD, US dollar; SD, standard deviation; QALY, quality-adjusted life year; CI, confidence interval; ICER, incremental cost-effectiveness ratio.

before and after surgery, and the Wilcoxon signed rank test was used for differences between utility values.

A value of $P<0.05$ was regarded as statistically significant. All bootstrap analyses were performed using Microsoft Excel 2007 software, and other analyses were calculated by SPSS 16.0.

Sensitivity analyses

We conducted sensitivity analyses to test the robustness of the results. First, we tested the impact of varying the discount rate from the 3% assumed in the baseline scenario to between 0% and 5% for lifespan analyses, as recommended [21]. Second, we floated the costs and QALYs to 10% individually and simultaneously. Subsequently, we calculated the upper limits for the extent of the increasing costs, or the decreasing QALYs, to overturn the final determination. Finally, we performed an additional analysis by excluding patients who had undergone bilateral RRD surgery, which might have had a potential influence on the results [7].

Results

A total of 98 patients fulfilled study inclusion criteria, with 57 patients aged 71 to 79 years old and 41 patients aged 81 to 87 years old. Basic socio-demographic and clinical data for the patients appear in Table 1. There was no significant difference between the two age groups in terms of basic characteristics, including type of surgery. During the 1-year follow up, no severe systemic diseases occurred in any participant.

The best-corrected visual acuity significantly improved at the 3-month post-operative time point compared with the preoperative time (paired sample t-test, $p<0.001$ for overall participants,

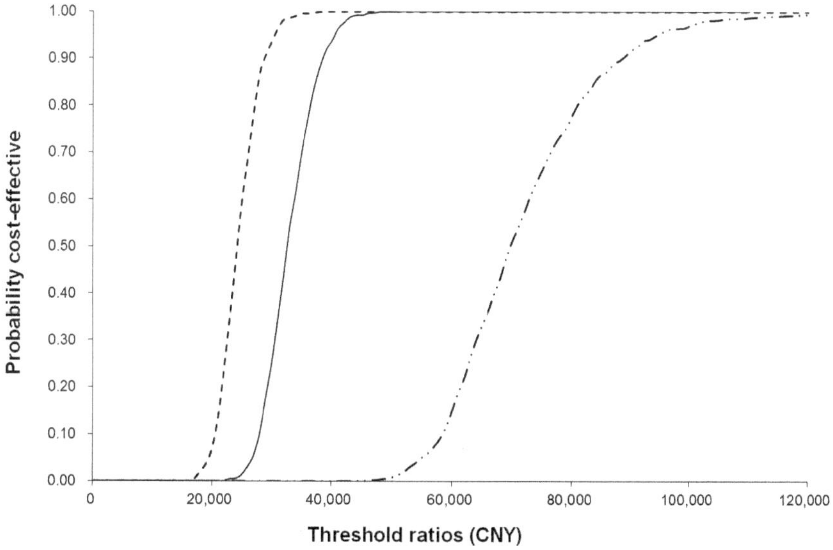

Figure 1. CEACs of life expectancy analysis for RRD surgery in the 70–79-year-olds, the above-80-year-olds, and all the elderly patients. The upper most dashed line represents the CEAC for RRD surgery in the 70–79-year-olds. The solid line represents the CEAC for RRD surgery in all of the elderly people. The dot-dashed line represents the CEAC for RRD surgery in the above-80-year-olds. RRD, Rhegmatogenous retinal detachment; CNY, Chinese yuan; QALY, quality-adjusted life year; CEAC, Cost-effectiveness acceptability curve.

Table 4. Threshold ratios of WTP (CNY (USD)/QALY) for RRD surgery to be cost-effective at probabilities of 50%, 70% and 90% compared with no treatment option.

	WTP [CNY(USD)/QALY]		
Probability of being cost-effective	**All (n = 98)**	**70s (n = 57)**	**80s (n = 41)**
50%	33,000(5,246)	24,000(3,816)	70,000(11,129)
70%	35,000(5,564)	26,000(4,134)	76,000(12,083)
90%	39,000(6,200)	29,000(4,610)	88,000(13,991)

WTP, willingness to pay; CNY, Chinese Yuan; USD, US dollar; QALY, quality-adjusted life year.

patients in their 70s, and patients in their 80s). At the 1-year postoperative time point, BCVA also improved significantly (paired sample t-test, $p<0.001$ for overall participants, patients in their 70s, and patients in their 80s) (Table 2). The utility values significantly increased 1 year after the surgery (Wilcoxon signed rank test, $p<0.001$ for the whole group, patients in their 70s, and patients in their 80s). The results of the baseline cost-utility analysis for the two age groups are shown in Table 3.

Over their remaining life expectancies, participants could achieve an average of 0.4 QALYs by having the retinal detachment surgery. For patients in their 70s, the QALYs gained were more than three times greater than for those of the patients in their 80s. According to the threshold willingness to pay, which was 115,062 CNY (18,293 USD)/QALY in 2012, the retinal detachment surgery is cost-effective for all elderly patients. The ICER for patients in their 80s is approximately three times higher than that of those in their 70s, though it is still a cost-effective intervention.

With a WTP of 115,062 CNY (18,293 USD) per QALY, there is a 100%, 100%, and 99.2% chance of RRD surgery being cost-effective for all of the elderly, patients in their 70s, and patients in their 80s, respectively. The CEAC (Figure 1) of the over-age-80 group is lower than that of the 70–79-year-old group, which indicates that RRD surgery is more cost-effective for those in their 70s than in their 80s. In the absence of an officially recognized threshold WTP, we further listed the threshold ratios of WTP for the surgery with cost-effective chances of 50%, 70%, and 90% (Table 4).

The results of additional analyses for the two major types of surgery were presented in table 5. The vitreous surgery was a little more expensive than the scleral buckling surgery, however obtained more QALYs for the elderly patients as well; hence, the costs per QALYs for vitreous surgery were less expensive than for scleral buckling surgery in the elderly population.

Table 6 presents the results of the sensitivity analyses. In general, the sensitivity analyses do not influence the decisions based on the results of the baseline analysis. Altering the discount rate from 3% in the baseline scenario to 0% decreases the ICERs; however, using a 5% discount rate increases the ICERs. Raising the costs by 10% and reducing the QALYs gained by 10% mildly increases the ICERs. With changes in both the costs and the QALYs, the ICERs still did not exceed the threshold of 115,062 CNY (18,293 USD)/QALY. To overturn the cost-effectiveness of the RRD surgery, the costs have to be 2.5 times more than the existing costs and the QALYs gained should be decreased by 75% from the baseline. Excluding bilateral RRD patients enhances the ICERs and makes RRD surgery less cost-effective for all of the elderly patients and in each age group.

Discussion

This article is the first to evaluate the visual outcomes and health economic value of RRD surgery in the elderly population. RRD surgery improved the visual acuity and quality of life for the elderly patients and was cost-effective in consideration of their life expectancies, with ICERs ranging from 30,142 CNY (4,792 USD)/QALY to 40,607 CNY (6,456 USD)/QALY. For patients above 80 years of age, although the ICER was about three times higher than that for patients aged 70–79 years, the RRD surgery remained a cost-effective intervention.

Compared with other studies, the patients in this study are relatively older, as most studies included patients with an average age of approximately 60 years old [37–39]. Additionally, the duration of symptoms until surgery is longer, although it is similar to those reported in developing countries [40], [41]. In China, 60–70% of RRD patients reside in remote areas or small villages and lack knowledge about RRD [42]; thus, the elderly patients received treatment after a longer time period from their diagnoses, which resulted in relatively poorer preoperative visual acuity and higher rates of macular-off compared with participants in other studies.

Table 5. Results of cost-utility analysis for the two surgery types in an elderly RRD population (bootstrap, n = 1000).

	Scleral buckling surgery (n = 31)	Vitreous surgery (n = 67)
Mean Costs [CNY(USD)]	12,804(2,036)	13,027(2,071)
Costs 95% CI [CNY(USD)]	10,813(1,719)−14,737(2,343)	11,698(1,859)−14,343(2,281)
QALYs gained in life-expectancy [Mean (95% CI)]	0.36(0.24–0.50)	0.41(0.29–0.56)
Mean ICER [CNY(USD)/QALY]	36,513(5,805)	32,287(5,133)

RRD, rhegmatogenous retinal detachment; CNY, Chinese Yuan; USD, US dollar; QALY, quality-adjusted life year; ICER, incremental cost-effectiveness ratio.

Table 6. A summary of ICERs (CNY (USD)/QALY) in sensitivity analyses for RRD surgery in an elderly population (n = 98).

	All	70s	80s
0% discount	30,142(4,792)	22,072(3,509)	69,756(10,091)
5% discount	35,092(5,579)	25,933(4,123)	73,961(11,758)
Cost+10%	36,111(5,740)	26,849(4,269)	78,790(12,526)
QALYs−10%	37,049(5,891)	27,160(4,318)	80,863(12,856)
Costs+10% and QALYs−10%	40,607(6,456)	29,743(4,729)	89,210(14,183)
Costs limit	+250%	+365%	+68%
QALYS limit	−75%	−81%	−42%
Excluding bilateral RRD patients	38,243(6,080)	25,825(4,106)	72,250(11,486)

ICER, incremental cost-effectiveness ratio; CNY, Chinese Yuan; USD, US dollar; RRD, rhegmatogenous retinal detachment; QALY, quality-adjusted life year.

However, the surgery brought significant improvement to the visual acuity of these patients. The BCVA of the elderly patients increased continuously from 3 months to 1 year postoperatively in the study. The average improvement in BCVA was 0.53±0.44 at the 1-year postoperative time point for all of the participants. Although age was reported to be a negative predictor of visual acuity outcomes after RRD surgery in many publications [15–19], the increase in BCVA in our study was no less than that reported in other studies that also included younger patients whose average age was approximately 60 years old [25], [37], [38], [43]. Similarly, in the SPR study, no relationship was observed between age and inferior visual outcomes [44]. Due to the inconsistency of the baseline status of RRD between the different study groups, the results in our study cannot be directly compared with other studies and we are therefore not be able to conclude whether age is a negative predictor for visual outcome. In any case, the significant improvement in BCVA indicates that RRD surgery is beneficial for patients over 80 years old as well as patients 70–79 years old.

In recent years, increasing emphasis has been put on evaluating the vision-related quality of life in ocular diseases. To reflect how the retinal detachment surgery influences the patients' quality of life, we investigated preference-based utility values before and 1 year after the surgery among the elderly patients. Utility analysis, unlike some other quality of life measurements, enables comparisons of quality of life across different health statuses in medicine and further analyses of cost-utility results for resource allocations [45]. The patients reported statistically significant increases in utility values postoperatively, rising from an average of 0.77 to

Table 7. Comparisons of surgical outcomes between the normal RRD patients and the elderly patients [4], [10].

	Normal population	Elderly population	P value*
No. of Patients	117	98	
Age [Mean (SD)]	54.28(10.30)	78.49(4.36)	<0.001
Type of surgery			<0.001
Scleral buckling surgery [No. (%)]	68(58.12)	31(31.63)	
Vitreous surgery [No. (%)]	49(41.89)	67(68.37)	
Preoperative BCVA	1.06(0.63)	1.06(0.50)	0.832
BCVA after 3 months	0.68(0.40)	0.74(0.35)	0.227
BCVA after 1 year	0.51(0.32)	0.54(0.26)	0.456
Difference of BCVA in 3 months	0.38(0.40)	0.32(0.35)	0.314
Difference of BCVA in 1 year	0.55(0.48)	0.53(0.44)	0.773
Utility value before surgery	0.77(0.12)	0.77(0.12)	0.806
Utility value after 1 year	0.83(0.10)	0.84(0.08)	0.610
Difference of utility value in 1 year	0.06(0.09)	0.07(0.07)	0.427
Costs [Bootstrap 1000 times; Mean (95% CI); CNY]	11,384(10,338–12,563)	12,992(11,984–14,088)	
QALYs gained in life time [Bootstrap 1000 times; Mean (95% CI)]	0.88(0.64–1.13)	0.40(0.31–0.50)	
ICERs [Bootstrap 1000 times; Mean; CNY/QALY]	13,794	33,186	

*An independent sample t-test was used for continual data of normal distribution, a Mann Whitney U test for non-normal distribution data, and the Pearson chi-square test for the categorical data. A value of $P<0.05$ was regarded as statistically significant.
RRD, rhegmatogenous retinal detachment; SD, standard deviation; BCVA, best -corrected visual acuity; CI, confidence interval; CNY, Chinese Yuan; QALY, quality-adjusted life year.

0.84. The patients above 80 years old seem to benefit less than those in the 70 to 79 years old group do, as demonstrated by the 1-year postoperative utility value; however, the ambiguous p value (0.096) makes it difficult to determine whether this difference is meaningful. Moreover, the change in utility values in the elderly population is similar to what we investigated in a younger population with an average age of 54 years old ($P = 0.427$) [4]. A summary of comparisons with our previous study is presented in Table 7.

When the benefit of lifetime was considered, the QALYs gained in patients aged 70–79 years old were approximately three times greater than in patients over 80 years old. Compared with our previous study [10], the QALYs gained in the elderly population were relatively small: 0.40 QALYs for the elderly compared to 0.88 QALYs for an average group of patients (Table 7). This is likely because older people have theoretically fewer remaining life years than younger people do. Consequently, the ICER, which combined the costs and QALYs gained, was higher in the elderly population compared to an average group of patients. The ICER in patients over 80 years old was three times higher than that in patients in their 70s. Despite the lower cost-effectiveness of RRD surgery in the elderly patients, the treatment was still below the threshold of willingness to pay of China, even for patients over 80 years old.

In the subgroup analyses for the two types of surgery, the vitreous surgery was less expensive for each QALYs gained than scleral buckling surgery in the elderly population, however, the discrepancy was not large. Unlike what we observed in the normal patients [10], the elderly people seemed to benefit less from scleral buckling surgery, probably because that the elderly patients usually have more complicated and diverse conditions than the normal patients do, which enables the comparable costs for the two types surgery. This might also be the reason that the proportion of vitreous surgery was higher in the elderly population than in the normal patients (Table 7), since surgeons' preference of choosing the vitreous surgery for complicated situation.

Elderly patients do not always accept surgery for RRD. On the one hand, the costs of RRD surgery are still relatively high for most people in our country, despite the fact that the National Health Insurance policy might cover some of the expenses [46]. On the other hand, elderly people might have fewer demands for vision-related quality of life because daily life activities are reduced and their life expectancy is relatively short. Additionally, lacking knowledge about health, they might be anxious about the disadvantages of the surgery, such as discomfort, complications, or risk of death. As a result, quite a few elderly people ultimately choose not to undertake the surgical option, which is the reason for the relatively small sample size in this population. It is difficult to persuade such patients to have surgery, yet it is considered unethical for an ophthalmologist to allow these patients to return home without treatment. Our study provides evidence that RRD surgery can improve visual acuity and the quality of life, and it is a cost-effective intervention in people over 70 years old. Therefore, ophthalmologists should persuade such elderly RRD patients to have surgery. In the interim, this health economic evaluation of RRD surgery may also provide a valuable tool for governmental agencies in formulating the National Health Insurance policy.

There are some limitations of this study. First, the study lacks real patient controls; however, not offering treatment for RRD patients violates the tenets of the Declaration of Helsinki, preventing approval by an ethical committee. Secondly, the study period was not long enough to truly reflect the long-term cost-utility of RRD surgery. The results of the long-term analysis were based on the assumption that no more costs associated with RRD surgery would be incurred and that patients would retain their utility value of the 1-year postoperative time point throughout their remaining life years. In the real world, outpatient service fees and transportation fees should be included as well, even if the costs are trivial compared with the surgery expenditures during the first year. Additionally, the utility value would deteriorate both in the treatment group and in the control group over the course of the life expectancy; however, some of the declining factors might counteract each other, making their influence unclear. Third, the study population was relatively small, and all the participants were from one teaching hospital. The results might be more presentative for large cities with similar economic conditions as Shanghai than for small towns in China. In future work, studies with more participants from different regions and longer follow-up times are desirable to facilitate cost-utility analyses that are more comprehensive. Finally, we did not include indirect costs, and this exclusion would probably underestimate the economic value of the surgery, as people in the control group had severe visual impairment, which might influence their living independency and incur expenses for nursing.

To conclude, the RRD surgery greatly improves visual acuity and the quality of life in elderly people in China. Compared to other studies that include younger populations, the visual acuity and vision-related quality of life outcomes were similar. Considering the shorter life expectancy, the elderly patients obtain fewer QALYs from RRD surgery, and thus, a higher cost per QALY was found. However, it is still cost-effective for elderly people to have RRD surgery, even for patients over 80 years old.

Author Contributions

Conceived and designed the experiments: HDZ XZ XX. Performed the experiments: HYL LB. Analyzed the data: YYM XHY XCX. Contributed reagents/materials/analysis tools: XHY XCX. Contributed to the writing of the manuscript: YYM. Final approval of the version to be published: HDZ. Help to interpret data: HYL LB. Modified the manuscript: XX XZ HDZ.

References

1. Ross WH, Stockl FA (2000) Visual recovery after retinal detachment. Curr Opin Ophthalmol 11: 191–194.
2. Zou H, Zhang X, Xu X, Liu H (2008) Quality of life in subjects with rhegmatogenous retinal detachment. Ophthal Epidemiol 15: 215–217.
3. Okamoto F, Okamoto Y, Hiraoka T, Oshika T (2008) Vision-related quality of life and visual function after retinal detachment surgery. Am J Ophthalmol 1461: 85–90.
4. Zou H, Zhang X, Xu X, Liu H, Bai L, et al. (2011) Utility value and retinal detachment surgery. Ophthalmology 118: 601.
5. Sodhi A, Leung LS, Do DV, Gower EW, Schein OD, et al. (2008) Recent trends in the management of rhegmatogenous retinal detachment. Surv Ophthalmol 53: 50–67.
6. Yorston D, Jalali S (2002) Retinal detachment in developing countries. Eye 16: 353–358.
7. Brown GC, Brown MM, Sharma S, Busbee B, Landy J (2002) A cost-utility analysis of interventions for severe proliferative vitreoretinopathy. Am - J Ophthalmol 133: 365–372.
8. Seider MI, Naseri A, Stewart JM (2013) Cost comparison of scleral buckle versus vitrectomy for rhegmatogenous retinal detachment repair. Am J Ophthalmol 156: 661–666.
9. Chang JS, Smiddy WE (2014) Cost-effectiveness of retinal detachment repair. Ophthalmology 121: 946–951.
10. Ma Y, Ying X, Zou H, Xu X, Liu H, et al. (2014) Cost-utility Analysis of Rhegmatogenous Retinal Detachment Surgery in Shanghai, China. Ophthalmic Epidemiol, doi:10.3109/09286586.2014.884601.
11. Mitry D, Charteris DG, Fleck BW, Campbell H, Singh J (2010) The epidemiology of rhegmatogenous retinal detachment: geographical variation and clinical associations. Br J Ophthalmol 94: 678–684.

12. Park SJ, Choi NK, Park KH, Woo SJ (2013) Five year nationwide incidence of rhegmatogenous retinal detachment requiring surgery in Korea. PloS one. Available at http://www.plosone.org/article/info%3Adoi%2F10.1371%2Fjournal.pone.0080174#pone-0080174-g001. Accessed May 1,2014.
13. Mitry D, Charteris DG, Yorston D, Siddiqui MA, Campbell H, et al. (2010) The epidemiology and socioeconomic associations of retinal detachment in Scotland: a two-year prospective population-based study. Invest Ophthalmol Vis Sci 51: 4963–4968.
14. Van de Put MA, Hooymans JM, Los LI, Dutch Rhegmatogenous Retinal Detachment Study Group (2013) The incidence of rhegmatogenous retinal detachment in The Netherlands. Ophthalmology 120: 616–622.
15. Ross WH (2002) Visual recovery after macula-off retinal detachment. Eye (Lond) 16: 440–446.
16. Ahmadieh H, Entezari M, Soheilian M, Azarmina M, Dehghan MH, et al. (2000) Factors influencing anatomic and visual results in primary scleral buckling. Eur J Ophthalmol 10: 153–159.
17. Mowatt L, Shun Shin GA, Arora S, Price N (2005) Macula off retinal detachments. How long can they wait before it is too late? Eur J Ophthalmol 15: 109–117.
18. Pastor JC, Fernández I, Rodríguez de la Rúa E, Coco R, Sanabria Ruiz Colmenares MR, et al. (2008) Surgical outcomes for primary rhegmatogenous retinal detachments in phakic and pseudophakic patients: the Retina 1 Project–report 2. Br J Ophthalmol 92: 378–382.
19. Liu F, Meyer CH, Mennel S, Hoerle S, Kroll P (2006) Visual recovery after scleral buckling surgery in macula-off rhegmatogenous retinal detachment. Ophthalmologica 220: 174–180.
20. Huang XB, Zou HD, Wang N, Wang WW, Fu J, et al. (2009) A prevalence survey of blindness and visual impairment in adults aged equal or more than 60 years in Beixinjing blocks of Shanghai, China. Zhonghua Yan Ke Za Zhi 45: 786–792.
21. Drummond MF (2005) Methods for the economic evaluation of Health Care Programmes. United States: Oxford university press. 7–269p.
22. Muennig P (2008) Cost-effectiveness analyses in health: a practical approach. United States: John Wiley & Sons. 1–18p.
23. Sharma S, Brown GC, Brown MM, Hollands H, Robins R, et al. (2002) Validity of the time trade-off and standard gamble methods of utility assessment in retinal patients. Br J Ophthalmol 86: 493–496.
24. National Bureau of Statistics of China (2014) Statistical Communique of the People's Republic of China. Available at: http://www.stats.gov.cn/tjsj/tjgb/ndtjgb/. Accessed May 1, 2014.
25. Zou H, Zhang X, Xu X, Liu H, Bai L, et al. (2011) Vision-Related Quality of Life and Self-Rated Satisfaction Outcomes of Rhegmatogenous Retinal Detachment Surgery: 3-Year Prospective Study. PLoS one. Available at: http://www.plosone.org/article/info%3Adoi%2F10.1371%2Fjournal.pone.0028597. Accessed December 5, 2013.
26. Sach TH, Foss AJ, Gregson RM, Zaman A, Osborn F, et al. (2010) Second-eye cataract surgery in elderly women: a cost-utility analysis conducted alongside a randomized controlled trial. Eye (Lond) 24: 276–283.
27. Sharma S, Hollands H, Brown GC, Brown MM, Shah GK, et al. (2001) The cost-effectiveness of early vitrectomy for the treatment of vitreous hemorrhage in diabetic retinopathy. Curr Opin Ophthalmol 12: 230–234.
28. World Health Rankings. Health profile China. Available at http://www.worldlifeexpectancy.com/country-health-profile/china. Accessed Dec 3, 2013.
29. Commission on Macroeconomics, HealthWorld Health Organization (2001) Macroeconomics and Health: Investing in Health for Economic Development-Report of the Commission on Macroeconomics and HealthWorld Health Organization, Geneva, Switzerland.
30. Yuan Y, lloeje U, Li H, Hay J, Yao GB (2008) Economic implications of entecavir treatment in suppressing viral replication in chronic hepatitis B (CHB) patients in China from a perspective of the Chinese Social Security program. Value Health 11(Suppl): 11–22.
31. Yang L, Christensen T, Sun F, Chang J (2012) Cost-effectiveness of switching patients with type 2 diabetes from insulin glargine to insulin detemir in Chinese setting: a health economic model based on the PREDICTIVE study. Value Health 15(Suppl): 56–59.
32. Briggs AH, Gray AM (1999) Handling uncertainty when performing economic evaluation of healthcare interventions. Health Technol Assess 3: 1–134.
33. Polsky D, Glick HA, Willke R (1997) Confidence intervals for cost-effectiveness ratios: a comparison of four methods. Health Econ 6: 243–252.
34. Barber JA, Thompson SG (2000) Analysis of cost data in randomized trials: an application of the nonparametric bootstrap. Stat Med 19: 3219–3236.
35. van Hout BA, Al MJ, Gordon GS, Rutten FF (1994) Costs, effects and C/E-ratios alongside a clinical trial. Health Econ 3: 309–319.
36. Fenwick E, Claxton K, Sculpher M (2001) Representing uncertainty: the role of cost-effectiveness acceptability curves. Health Econ 10: 779–787.
37. Heimann H, Zou X, Jandeck C, Kellner U, Bechrakis NE, et al. (2006) Primary vitrectomy for rhegmatogenous retinal detachment: an analysis of 512 cases. Graefes Arch Clin Exp Ophthalmol 244: 69–78.
38. Salicone A, Smiddy WE, Venkatraman A, Feuer W (2006) Visual recovery after scleral buckling procedure for retinal detachment. Ophthalmology 113: 1734–1742.
39. Schneider EW, Geraets RL, Johnson MW (2012) Pars plana vitrectomy without adjuvant procedures for repair of primary rhegmatogenous retinal detachment. Retina 32: 213–219.
40. Ahmadieh H, Moradian S, Faghihi H, Parvaresh MM, Ghanbari H, et al (2005) Anatomic and visual outcomes of scleral buckling versus primary vitrectomy in pseudophakic and aphakic retinal detachment: six-month follow-up results of a single operation–report no. 1. Ophthalmology 112: 1421–1429.
41. Azad RV, Chanana B, Sharma YR, Vohra R (2007) Primary vitrectomy versus conventional retinal detachment surgery in phakic rhegmatogenous retinal detachment. Acta Ophthalmol Scand 85: 540–545.
42. Li X, Beijing Rhegmatogenous Retinal Detachment Study Group (2003) Incidence and epidemiological characteristics of rhegmatogenous retinal detachment in Beijing, China. Ophthalmology 110: 2413–2417.
43. Heimann H, Bartz Schmidt KU, Bornfeld N, Weiss C, Hilgers RD, et al. (2007) Scleral Buckling versus Primary Vitrectomy in Rhegmatogenous Retinal Detachment Study Group. Scleral buckling versus primary vitrectomy in rhegmatogenous retinal detachment: a prospective randomized multicenter clinical study. Ophthalmology 114: 2142–2154.
44. Heussen N, Feltgen N, Walter P, Hoerauf H, Hilgers RD, et al (2011) Scleral buckling versus primary vitrectomy in rhegmatogenous retinal detachment study (SPR Study): predictive factors for functional outcome. Study report no. 6. Graefes Arch Clin Exp Ophthalmol 249: 1129–1136.
45. Brown MM, Brown GC, Sharma S, Busbee B (2003) Quality of life associated with visual loss: a time tradeoff utility analysis comparison with medical health states. Ophthalmology 110: 1076–1081.
46. Shanghai Health Insurance. Information of urban basic health insurance programs in Shanghai. Available at http://www.shyb.gov.cn/ybzc/zcfg/03/201111/t20111101_1134638.shtml. Accessed Dec 3, 2013.

11

Angiogenic Potential of Vitreous from Proliferative Diabetic Retinopathy and Eales' Disease Patients

Ponnalagu Murugeswari[1¤a], Dhananjay Shukla[2¤b], Ramasamy Kim[2], Perumalsamy Namperumalsamy[2], Alan W. Stitt[3], Veerappan Muthukkaruppan[1*]

1 Department of Immunology and Cell Biology, Aravind Medical Research Foundation, Dr.G.Venkataswamy Eye Research Institute, Madurai, India, **2** Vitreous and Retina Service, Aravind Eye Care System, Madurai, India, **3** Centre for Experimental Medicine, Queens University, Belfast, United Kingdom

Abstract

Purpose: Proliferative Diabetic Retinopathy (PDR) and Eales' Disease (ED) have different aetiologies although they share certain common clinical symptoms including pre-retinal neovascularization. Since there is a need to understand if the shared end-stage angiogenic pathology of PDR and ED is driven by common stimulating factors, we have studied the cytokines contained in vitreous from both patient groups and analyzed the angiogenic potential of these samples *in vitro*.

Material and Methods: Vitreous samples from patients with PDR (n = 13) and ED (n = 5) were quantified for various cytokines using a cytokine biochip array and sandwich ELISA. An additional group of patients (n = 5) with macular hole (MH) was also studied for comparison. To determine the angiogenic potential of these vitreous samples, they were analyzed for their ability to induce tubulogenesis in human microvascular endothelial cells. Further, the effect of anti-VEGF (Ranibizumab) and anti-IL-6 antibodies were studied on vitreous-mediated vascular tube formation.

Results: Elevated levels of IL-6, IL-8, MCP-1 and VEGF were observed in vitreous of both PDR and ED when compared to MH. PDR and ED vitreous induced greater levels of endothelial cell tube formation compared to controls without vitreous ($P < 0.05$). When VEGF in vitreous was neutralized by clinically-relevant concentrations of Ranibizumab, tube length was reduced significantly in 5 of 6 PDR and 3 of 5 ED samples. Moreover, when treated with IL-6 neutralizing antibody, apparent reduction (71.4%) was observed in PDR vitreous samples.

Conclusions: We have demonstrated that vitreous specimens from PDR and ED patients share common elevations of pro-inflammatory and pro-angiogenic cytokines. This suggests that common cytokine profiles link these two conditions.

Editor: Rudolf Kirchmair, Medical University Innsbruck, Austria

Funding: Supported by grants from Department of Science and Technology (SR/SO/HS-04/2003), TIFAC-CORE in diabetic retinopathy, India, and Commonwealth Split-Site Scholarship programme. The funders had no role in study design, data collection and analysis, decision to publish, or preparation of the manuscript.

* Email: muthu@aravind.org

¤a Current address: Stem Cell Research Laboratory, Narayana Nethralaya Foundation, Bangalore, India
¤b Current address: Retina-Vitreous Service, Ratan Jyoti Nethralaya, Gwalior, India

Introduction

Proliferative Diabetic Retinopathy (PDR) and Eales' Disease (ED) are potentially blinding vitreoretinal diseases. ED is an idiopathic inflammatory venous occlusion that primarily affects the peripheral retina of healthy young men (20–30 years). Retinal changes in ED include periphlebitis, peripheral non-perfusion and neovascularization. In addition, visual loss is characteristically caused by bilateral recurrent vitreous hemorrhage [1], [2]. Although PDR and ED have different etiology, the symptoms and signs of these diseases run parallel to each other with some differences [3]. We have previously observed this commonality in the presence of inflammatory cytokines [interleukin-6 (IL-6), interleukin-8 (IL-8), monocyte chemoattractant protein-1 (MCP-1)] and vascular endothelial growth factor (VEGF) in vitreous [4].

Angiogenesis is a highly complex and coordinated process requiring multiple receptors and ligands in endothelial cells for which VEGF is a pivotal element in a variety of normal and pathological circumstances [5], [6]. VEGF is upregulated during retinal hypoxia and levels of this growth factor are raised in the vitreous of patients with PDR [7], [8] and VEGF-neutralizing antibodies are now being used for treatment of pathological ocular angiogenesis and macular oedema [9], [10], [11], [12].

Though the presence of pro-angiogenic and pro-inflammatory cytokines in the vitreous of PDR and ED patients has been demonstrated by several studies the functional potential of their vitreous has never been shown. Therefore, we have investigated the angiogenic potential of vitreous from these patients using the endothelial tube formation assay *in vitro*, and the effects of anti-VEGF and anti-IL6 neutralizing antibodies on this potential.

Materials and Methods

Ethics Statement

Patients were recruited in accordance with the Declaration of Helsinki and with the approval of the Institutional Review Board (IRB) of Aravind Eye Hospital. Written informed consent as per the procedure approved by IRB was obtained from the patients and maintained.

Study Subjects

Consecutive patients scheduled to undergo vitrectomy for proliferative ED, advanced PDR or Macular Hole (MH) were prospectively recruited in one of the three treatment groups. The clinical diagnosis of ED was made on the basis of peripheral venous sheathing in multiple quadrants in the fellow eye, or the operated eye, as observed intra-operatively. The patients with conditions which could secondarily cause venous sheathing, such as non-inflammatory retinal vein occlusions, diabetic or hypertensive retinopathy, sickle cell retinopathy, ocular inflammatory conditions like choroiditis, or pars planitis, or associated systemic infective/autoimmune/other inflammatory disease (as revealed by history, examination, or investigations), were excluded from the study. The indications for vitrectomy included best-corrected visual acuity less than 20/400 due to vitreous haemorrhage of at least 2 months duration with/without epiretinal membranes; rhegmatogenous/combined-mechanism retinal detachment; or a tractional retinal detachment involving the macula. Eventhough, haemorrhage is an important indication for vitrectomy; small samples of undiluted vitreous were obtained before isotonic infusion and aspiration. The samples which contained blood contamination were excluded from the study.

All the diabetic patients included in this study had type 2 diabetes mellitus. Like ED patients, they were also surgical inpatients, who presented with advanced PDR, as defined by the ETDRS study report number 12 [13]. The indications for vitrectomy were the same as mentioned above for ED patients.

Patients with idiopathic MH were chosen as control. MH is caused by vitreomacular traction, without any associated retinal ischaemia, vascular proliferation or inflammation, and is therefore least likely to be associated with local release of VEGF or other inflammatory cytokines. MH patients were evaluated to rule out a history or signs of ocular trauma or any other associated ocular pathology. The main preoperative investigation in MH was optical coherence tomography, to assess the morphology of MH for surgical feasibility and prognosis. MH patients had no systemic diabetes mellitus. Patients were recruited in accordance with the Declaration of Helsinki and with the approval of the Institutional Review Board of Aravind Eye Hospital. Informed consent was also obtained from the patients. All the cases had no history of a previous ocular surgery.

Thirteen PDR patients (11 males, 2 females), aged 54.2±7.8 years (mean ± SD) having diabetes for 13.0±9.7 years were included in the study. All 5 ED patients were males and 31±10 years old. Five MH patients (1 female, 4 males) aged 60.4±8.2 were included as controls. All the PDR and ED patients had retinal neovascularization and vitreous haemorrhage. As the etiology is different [14], the ED patients were males and relatively younger in age. Therefore, this difference in age and sex is admissible.

Sample Collection

At the beginning of vitrectomy, undiluted vitreous (200–700 µl) was aspirated via pars plana with a vitreous cutter, before opening the infusion port. These undiluted vitreous samples (13 PDR, 5 ED and 5 MH) were immediately frozen in aliquots in polypropylene tube at −80°C until assay.

Cytokine Assay

Vitreous samples (PDR, n = 8; ED, n = 2) were quantified for a range of cytokines (IL-2, IL-4, IL-6, IL-8, IL-10, IL-1α, IL-1β, IFN-γ, VEGF, TNF-α, MCP-1, EGF) using the Evidence

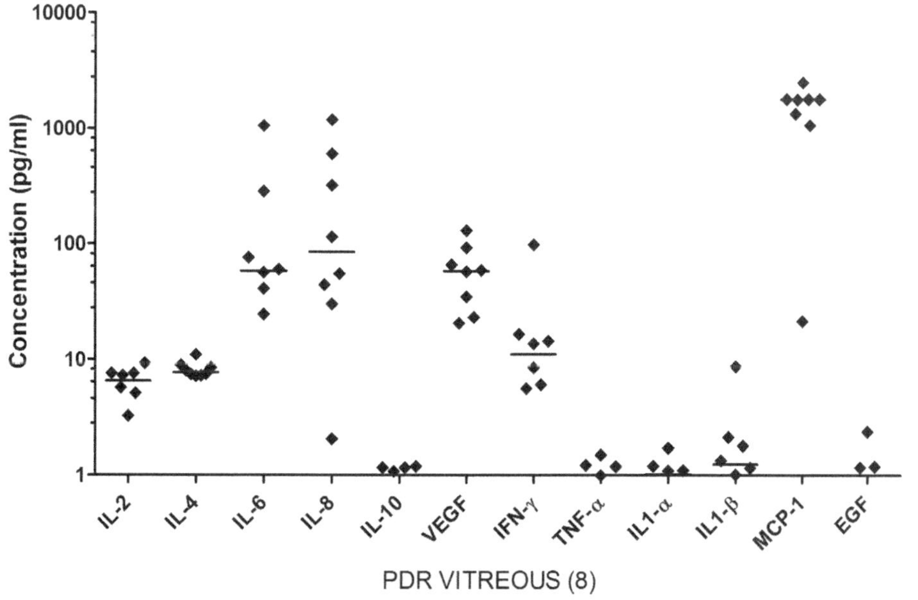

Figure 1. Scatter plot showing the distribution levels of 12 cytokines in vitreous from PDR (n = 8) patients, quantified using cytokine bio-chip array. Each sample represents the mean of duplicates. Solid line indicates the median. PDR-Proliferative diabetic retinopathy; ED- Eales' disease. IL - Interleukins, VEGF- Vascular endothelial growth factor, IFN-γ- Interferon gamma, TNF-α - Tumour necrosis factor alpha, MCP-1 - Monocyte chemoattractant protein-1, EGF - Epidermal growth factor.

Table 1. Levels of cytokines in PDR, ED and MH vitreous used for tubulogenesis assay.

Sample Code	IL6 (pg/ml)	IL8 (pg/ml)	VEGF (pg/ml)	IL-1β (pg/ml)	MCP1 (pg/ml)
*PDR-27	0	0	849.2	-	978.2
* PDR-29	0	0	0	0	0
* PDR-38	260.2	38.0	2401.4	0	2486.9
* PDR-40	225.1	89.4	682.7	0	2571.0
* PDR-45	0	228.3	5805.7	0	1863.6
† PDR-49	>530	30.1	130.2	0	1349.0
† PDR-53	0	2.1	20.6	2.1	21.6
† PDR-58	60.3	604.2	57.5	1.7	>900
† PDR-61	56.6	55.4	66.0	1.0	>900
† PDR-66	24.6	44.3	59.1	0.6	1071.0
* ED-09	0	290.2	105.7	23.8	2063.0
* ED-12	175.0	632.6	0	2.0	-
* ED-16	-	148.1	221.2	3.2	-
† ED-17	38.5	56.9	144.0	0.3	1017.9
† ED-19	158.9	961.0	204.9	2.6	>900
* MH-09	0	4.9	0	103.7	118.4
* MH-29	0	0	0	35.1	937.8
* MH-35	0	0	0	0	0
* MH-38	0	0	107.8	0	174.0
MH-44	-	-	-	-	-

The cytokine levels were analysed by cytokine bio-chip array for 5 PDR, 2 ED vitreous (indicated by †) and the remaining (PDR = 5, ED = 3, MH = 4) by sandwich ELISA (indicated by*). The values in the table represent the mean concentration duplicate of each sample. For the two ED (†) samples, cytokines not included in this table are: IL-2, 8.1 pg/ml; IL-4, 7.14 pg/ml; IFN- γ, 12.8 pg/ml and less than 1.6 pg/ml for IL-10, TNF-α, IL-1α. 0- Less than the detectable limit; - cytokine not analysed; > Higher than the maximum detectable limit. PDR - Proliferative diabetic retinopathy; ED - Eales' disease; MH - Macular Hole.

Investigator Cytokine Biochip Array (Randox, UK). For each sample, this assay was carried out in duplicate. It is a biochip with multiple cytokine antibodies coated on a solid substrate. After incubation with vitreous samples, cytokine specific enzyme-labelled secondary antibodies were added, and the cytokines were quantified by chemiluminescence using a charged coupled device (CCD) camera. The standard curves were constructed for each cytokine and the sample concentration was determined by the evidence investigator (Randox, UK). As a follow-up, IL-6, IL-8, MCP-1, and VEGF were also quantified by sandwich ELISA (BD Biosciences, R & D systems) according to the manufacturer's instructions for 5 PDR, 3 ED and 4 MH samples. The standard curve was prepared using recombinant human cytokines.

Tubulogenesis assay

Human dermal microvascular endothelial cells (HMECs) were purchased (PromoCell Gmbh, Heidelberg, Germany) and grown in T-25 Nunclon culture flasks (Nalge Nunc International,UK) with medium (PromoCell) supplemented with growth supplements (PromoCell) and Primocin (50 mg/ml) (Invitrogen,UK). The *in vitro* tubulogenesis assay was performed as previously described using confluent cells of passage four to six [15]. Briefly for each assay 2×10^4 HMECs in 5 µl were resuspended in 10 µl of vitreous and mixed with 15 µl of growth factor reduced matrigel (BD Biosciences,USA) (PDR, n = 6; ED, n = 5, MH n = 5). In place of vitreous 10 µl of medium was used in controls.

In another series of experiments, HMEC cultures were treated with ranibizumab (RZB) (0.125 mg/ml or 0.25 mg/ml; PDR, n = 6; ED, n = 5) (Genentech,Inc., South San Francisco) or anti-IL-6 (0.1 µg/ml; PDR,n = 7;ED,n = 2) neutralizing antibody (R & D systems, UK). IL-6 was chosen in preference to other cytokines and chemokines, since it is known to be elevated in vitreous and plays a role in the pathogenesis of ocular diseases [4], [16], [17]. Moreover, previous studies have demonstrated that IL-6 levels in aqueous and vitreous fluids from PDR patients significantly correlate with disease severity [17], [18], [19]. The above mixture of matrigel, HMEC, and RZB was prepared collectively for 3 assays (n = 3) and anti-IL-6 mixture for 2 assays for each sample. Thirty microliter aliquots from the mixture were spotted for each assay onto Nunclon 48-well culture plates. After matrigel polymerization at 37°C for 30 minutes, blobs were covered with endothelial cell supplement medium. Tube formation was observed after 48 hours, phase images were captured in five regions per well and tube length was quantified using NIS-Elements software (Nikon, UK). The mean tube length of all the five regions of triplicate/duplicate was obtained.

Statistical Analysis

The Man-Whitney U test was used to analyse the differences between the experimental and control groups. Values are expressed as mean ± SD. All analysis was done using statistical software Stata 11.0. The results were considered significant at $P<0.05$.

Results

Cytokine Profile

We have earlier demonstrated that significantly higher concentrations of IL-6, IL-8, MCP-1 and VEGF were observed in

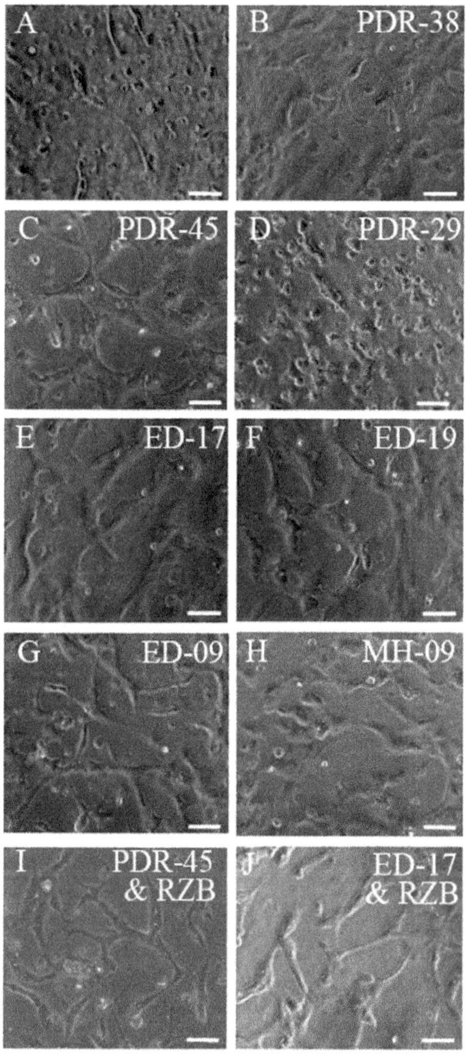

Figure 2. Representative phase images of tube formation induced by vitreous from PDR/ED/MH patients in human dermal microvascular endothelial cell (HMEC). 2×10^5 HMECs in triplicate were exposed to vitreous alone or with RZB (0.125 mg/ml). Tube formation was observed and images were captured after 48 hours incubation. Each panel shows a part of the representative well. The tube length was quantified by NIS-Elements software (Nikon). Scale bar = 100 µm. A. Control (without vitreous); B and C - PDR vitreous-induced tube formation, which had high levels of VEGF/IL-6/MCP-1; D-PDR vitreous with trace levels of cytokines showing a very few tube formation. E- G - ED vitreous-induced tube formation as in PDR. H - MH vitreous. I and J are images of vascular tubes in the presence of PDR/ED vitreous and anti-VEGF antibody, showing reduction in tube length compared to C and E respectively. Number in the images denotes the patient ID as in table 1. PDR - Proliferative diabetic retinopathy; ED-Eales' disease; MH- Macular Hole. RZB – Ranibizumab.

vitreous of PDR (n = 25) and ED (n = 10) than in that of MH patients (n = 25) [4]. The above study also showed strikingly similar cytokine profile in both PDR and ED vitreous and this finding is further confirmed by an extremely rapid cytokine biochip array (Figure 1, Table 1). Moreover, only trace levels of IL-10, TNF-α, IL1-α, IL1-β and EGF were observed in both groups.

Endothelial Tube Formation induced by patient vitreous

The tubulogenesis assay is an *in vivo* correlate of angiogenesis involving endothelial alignment, elongation and polygonal network [20]. Cytokine concentrations estimated by ELISA or Biochip for PDR, ED and MH vitreous, which have been used for tubulogenesis assay, are presented in Table 1. After 48 hours of culture the endothelial cells in the absence of vitreous formed a few short tubes and majority of them remained as individual cells (Fig. 2A). Mean tubular length was 122 µm in control (Fig. 3). In some of the vitreous samples, there were more prominent polygonal tubule network and these had correspondingly high concentrations of VEGF or IL-6 (Fig. 2B and C). On the other hand, vitreous with only trace amounts of cytokines produced minimal tubule formation similar to the control (endothelial cells without vitreous) (Fig. 2D and 3A). Among the 6 PDR vitreous samples tested, 5 showed a significant increase in tube formation (mean fold increase ranging from 0.3 to 0.5, $P<0.05$, Fig. 3A).

Interestingly a similar vascular response pattern was observed with ED vitreous containing either high (ED-17 and 19; Fig. 2E and F) or low levels of (ED-09, Fig. 2G) cytokines (Table 1). Among, the 5 vitreous samples from ED patients 4 showed significant increase in tube formation (mean fold increase ranging from 0.1 to 0.7) ($P<0.05$; Fig. 3B).

In MH patients though the retinal vascular reaction does not occur in vivo, we observed significant tube formation with vitreous from all these patients (Fig. 3C). The nature of the vascular assembly is shown in figure 2H for vitreous of MH-09 which contained substantial amount of MCP-1 and IL1-β and trace level of VEGF (Table-1). With limited number of samples studied, it was not possible to apply a test for correlation. However, the data indicate that tube formation in vitro is influenced by the levels of various pro-angiogenic factors present in the vitreous samples.

Effect of RZB on vitreous-induced Endothelial Tube Formation

HMECs were exposed to clinically-relevant concentrations of RZB in combination with the each of the vitreous samples from PDR and ED patients. Tube formation was observed and images were captured after 48 hours of incubation. Figures 2C and 2I show the nature of the vascular assembly in the presence or absence of RZB with PDR-45 vitreous. The tube length was reduced in all six cases with 0.125 mg/ml RZB and the mean fold decrease ranged from 0.2 to 0.7 though significantly in 5 cases (Fig. 4A). Interestingly, we have also observed the reduction in tube length when ED vitreous was treated with RZB (Fig. 2E and 2J). This anti-VEGF effect was observed in all five cases with a mean fold decrease ranging from 0.2 to 1.2, though showing a significant decrease in three cases (Fig. 4B).

Effect of IL-6 neutralizing antibody on vitreous-induced endothelial tube formation

Since IL-6 was observed at high levels in PDR as well as in ED vitreous, we carried out another set of experiments to test the effect of anti-IL6 neutralizing antibody (0.1 µg/ml) on tube formation. Among seven samples of PDR vitreous tested, tube length was reduced in 5 samples with a mean fold ranging from 0.06 to 0.3 (Fig. 5A, C and E). Even though a noticeable reduction was observed in tube length, there was no significant difference between the groups with anti-IL-6 treatment. Our study included only two ED samples for anti-IL-6 treatment due to its reduced availability of clinical samples and limited volume of vitreous; of the two an apparent reduction in tube length was observed in one sample (ED -17) (Fig. 5B, D and F).

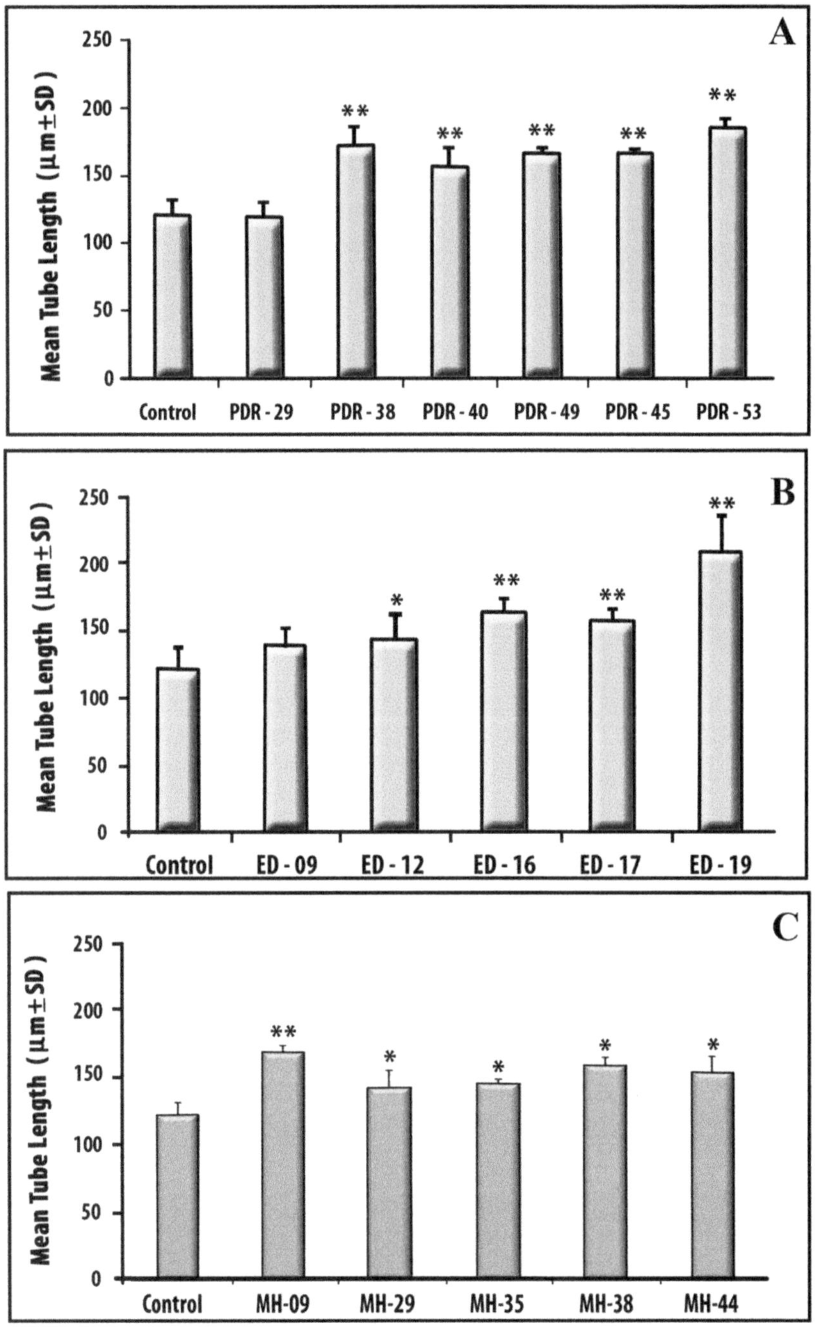

Figure 3. Angiogenic potential of vitreous in capillary tube formation. Experimental details are as in Fig. 2. (A) PDR vitreous, (B) ED vitreous, (C) MH vitreous. Bar graph shows the mean concentration of the triplicate of each sample. PDR-proliferative diabetic retinopathy; ED- Eales' disease; MH- Macular Hole. Number in X-axis denotes the patient number as in table 1. $^{**}P<0.001$; $^{*}P<0.05$.

Discussion

Angiogenic growth factors contribute to neovascularization that occurs in retinal diseases like DR and ED. In these vitreo-retinal diseases inflammatory processes are also considered to be critical, suggesting that a range of secreted factors in the vitreous cavity are associated with pathological processes [21], [22], [23]. The presence of inflammatory and angiogenic growth factors has been demonstrated in vitreous [4], [16], [24] from these patients. Though PDR & ED differ in their etiology the profile of proangiogenic factors in the vitreous is markedly similar. We have previously found no significant difference in the concentration of VEGF, IL-6, IL-8 and MCP-1 between these two diseases [4]. Moreover, the profile of twelve cytokines is also similar as shown by cytokine array (Fig. 1, Table 1) and this correlates with the other assays. This bio-chip approach is rapid and accurate taking <4 hours for analysis. It is known that some patients fail to respond to RZB therapy and in the future there may be a place for rapid vitreous analysis post-vitrectomy and establishing if certain growth factors or cytokines are absent or elevated. This would enable patient-specific tailoring the subsequent therapy.

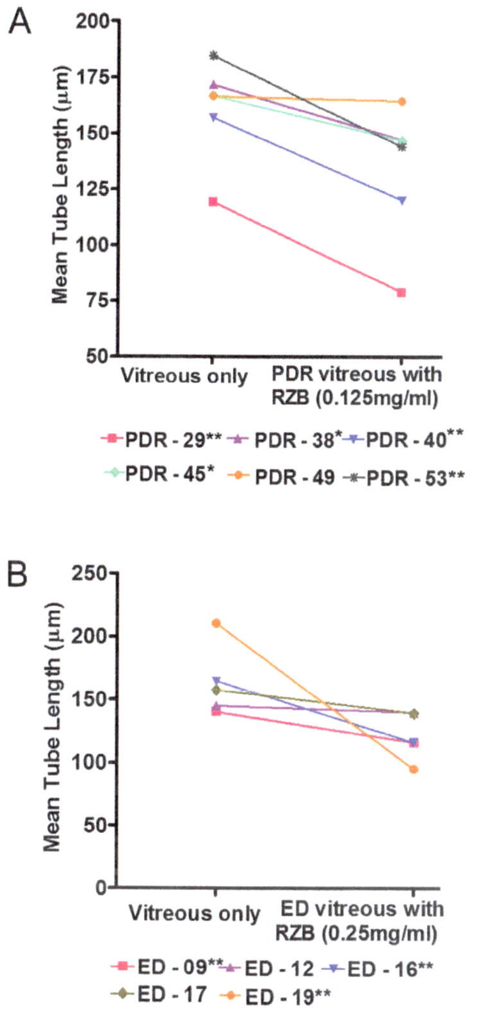

Figure 4. Effect of anti-VEGF antibody on vitreous-induced tube formation. HMECs were mixed with PDR vitreous in presence of RZB (in triplicate cultures). Tube formation was observed and images were captured after 48 hours incubation. (A) 0.125 mg/ml of RZB with PDR vitreous (B) 0.25 mg/ml of RZB with ED vitreous. The tube length was quantified by Nikon NIS-Elements software. Number in the legend denotes the patient ID as in table 1. PDR - Proliferative diabetic retinopathy; ED- Eales' disease; RZB-Ranibizumab. $^{**}P<0.001$;$^{*}P<0.05$.

Though there have been several reports on the presence of cytokines in vitreous of patients with vitreo-retinal diseases, to our knowledge, this is the first study to evaluate the angiogenic potential of vitreous from these patients. Using the *in vitro* tubulogenesis assay, we demonstrated the ability of PDR, ED, MH vitreous in inducing endothelial tube formation. In general, markedly increased number of vascular tubes and tubular network was observed with vitreous from the above patient groups than the control without vitreous. It is possible that the factors particularly VEGF, IL-6, IL-8 and MCP-1 might be responsible for vascular tube formation (Table 1, Fig. 3). Further, in addition to VEGF which is known to play a significant role in neovascularization in PDR [25], vitreous containing high levels of IL-6 and IL-8 or MCP-1 but with trace amount of VEGF also induced network of vascular tubes. (Table 1; Fig. 3; PDR-40, 49; ED-12, MH-09, 29). Therefore, in addition to VEGF, inflammatory cytokines are involved in inducing neovascularization.

There is substantial supporting evidence to indicate the interrelationship between the expression of inflammatory cytokines and vascular growth factors in different types of clinical conditions involving angiogenesis. The expression of IL-6, a multi-functional cytokine is elevated in tissues that undergo active angiogenesis, but it does not induce proliferation of endothelial cells. IL-6 has the ability to induce angiogenesis indirectly by the expression of VEGF [26] and possibly by increasing endothelial permeability [27].

Certain transcription factors like NF-Kappa B are known to activate synergistically transcription of cytokines such as IL-6 and chemokines IL-8 and MCP-1 [28], [29], [30]. Further, transcriptional activation of VEGF by IL-6 via STAT-3 pathway and transactivation of VEGF-R2 by IL-8 are associated with vascular permeability [31], [32]. Thus, IL-6, present in significant amount in vitreous of PDR and ED patients, may be able to function as indirect inducer of tube formation *in vitro*. Whether a similar IL-6 induced VEGF expression occurs in the endothelial cells in the tubulogenesis assay needs further studies.

RZB is a high affinity recombinant Fab which binds to the receptor–binding site of all biologically active forms of VEGF-A, thus preventing the activation of two related receptor tyrosine kinase, VEGFR-1 and VEGFR-2. Consequently, the endothelial cell proliferation, migration, permeability and vascular assembly are inhibited by RZB [33], [34], [35]. In this context our study was designed to evaluate the ability of RZB and anti-IL-6 antibodies to inhibit the angiogenic ability of PDR and ED vitreous. A marked reduction in vascular tube formation was observed when PDR vitreous was treated with RZB although this was not observed in all the samples. For example among the two PDR vitreous samples, though both contained low levels of VEGF, tube formation was significantly reduced by RZB in PDR-53 but not in PDR-49 and this difference may possibly be due to the presence of low levels of IL-6 and MCP-1 in the former but high levels of these cytokines in the latter. In general our results can be correlated with clinical studies wherein up to 38.6% of PDR patients did not respond to VEGF therapy [36].

In our context with IL-6 neutralizing antibody we observed tube length reduction in PDR; however, the reduction was not significant (Table-1, Fig. 5E). These samples contained high levels of MCP-1 and varying concentrations of other cytokines. In general, the present study suggests the involvement of inflammatory cytokines in addition to VEGF in inducing tube formation. Further studies are required to evaluate the inter-relationship between the expression of inflammatory cytokines and VEGF as well as their synergistic activity at the molecular level.

In conclusion, this is the first study to evaluate the angiogenic potential of vitreous from PDR and ED patients, demonstrating that VEGF present in ED vitreous is involved in inducing the vascular endothelial cell migration and assembly. Further, the importance of proinflammatory factors in addition to VEGF in retinal neovascularization is well-indicated. It is important to note that in patients, vitreous levels of growth factors and cytokines may not necessarily be due to the pathophysiology of the respective disease entity, but from intravitreal blood and associated cell sources such as thrombocytes. Nevertheless, in this study patient numbers are limited since the majority of vitreous samples we obtained needed to be excluded from the study due to blood contamination. Nevertheless, the study forms a basis for extending patient numbers and further investigating the cytokine profile in PDR and ED and how this influences key function endpoints such as pathological angiogenesis. Therefore, the current data is a useful platform for extending the investigation by using several functional endothelial cell migration, proliferation, and permeability assays [37], [38] to elucidate the importance of various factors (IL-8,MCP-1) and their

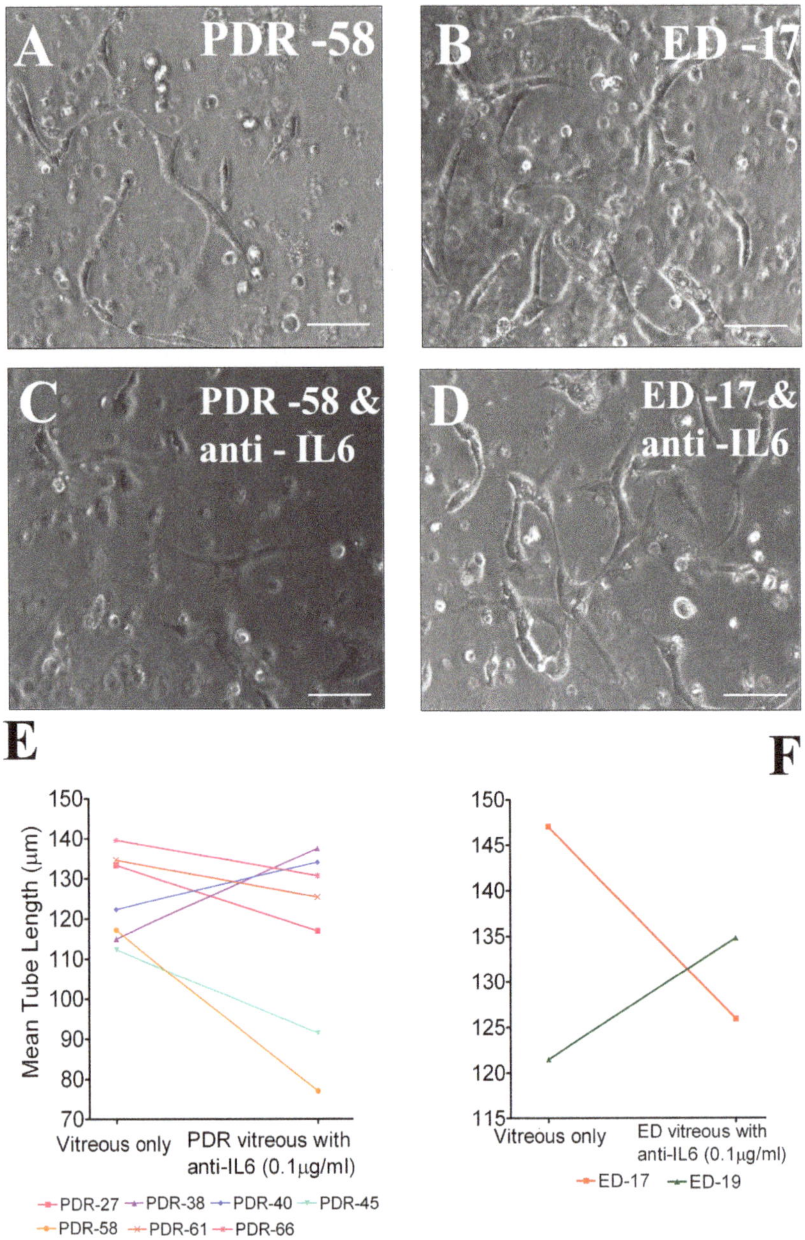

Figure 5. Effects of anti-IL-6 on vitreous-induced tube formation. HMECs were mixed with PDR or ED vitreous with or without anti-IL6 (0.1 μg/ml). Tube formation was observed and images were captured after 48 hours of incubation (in duplicate cultures). A and B are PDR or ED vitreous-induced tube formation. C and D are images of vascular tubes of corresponding vitreous with anti-IL6. E and F – shows the effect of anti-IL6 on vascular tube length for 6 PDR (E) and 2 ED (F) vitreous samples. The tube length was quantified by NIS-Elements software (Nikon). Number in the image denotes the patient ID as in table 1. PDR-Proliferative diabetic retinopathy; ED- Eales' disease. Scale bar = 100 μm.

interaction in neovascularization, by using the patients' vitreous and a combination of neutralizing antibodies.

Acknowledgments

We thank Dr. Carmel McVicar and Dr. Medina Reinhold for their technical support in tubulogenesis assay and Mr. B. Vijaya Kumar in statistical analysis.

Author Contributions

Conceived and designed the experiments: VRM AS PM. Performed the experiments: PM. Analyzed the data: PM AS VRM. Contributed reagents/materials/analysis tools: AS DS RK PN. Wrote the paper: PM VRM AS DS. Helped in getting the fund from TIFAC-CORE: PN.

References

1. Das T, Biswas J, Kumar A, Nagpal PN, Namperumalsamy P, et al. (1994) Eales' disease. Indian J Ophthalmol 42: 3–18.
2. Murthy KR, Abraham C, Baig SM,Badrinath SS (1977) Eales' disease. Proc All Ind Ophthalmol. pp. 323.

3. Atmaca LS, Batioglu F, Atmaca Sonmez P (2002) A long-term follow-up of Eales' disease. Ocul Immunol Inflamm 10: 213–221.
4. Murugeswari P, Shukla D, Rajendran A, Kim R, Namperumalsamy P, et al. (2008) Proinflammatory cytokines and angiogenic and anti-angiogenic factors in vitreous of patients with proliferative diabetic retinopathy and eales' disease. Retina 28: 817–824.
5. Ferrara N, Hillan KJ, Gerber HP, Novotny W (2004) Discovery and development of bevacizumab, an anti-VEGF antibody for treating cancer. Nat Rev Drug Discov 3: 391–400.
6. Ferrara N, Damico L, Shams N, Lowman H, Kim R (2006) Development of ranibizumab, an anti-vascular endothelial growth factor antigen binding fragment, as therapy for neovascular age-related macular degeneration. Retina 26: 859–870.
7. Aiello LP, Avery RL, Arrigg PG, Keyt BA, Jampel HD, et al. (1994) Vascular endothelial growth factor in ocular fluid of patients with diabetic retinopathy and other retinal disorders. N Engl J Med 331: 1480–1487.
8. Abu El-Asrar AM, Nawaz MI, Kangave D, Mairaj Siddiquei M, Geboes K (2013) Angiogenic and vasculogenic factors in the vitreous from patients with proliferative diabetic retinopathy. J Diabetes Res 2013: 539658.
9. Rosenfeld PJ, Brown DM, Heier JS, Boyer DS, Kaiser PK, et al. (2006) Ranibizumab for neovascular age-related macular degeneration. N Engl J Med 355: 1419–1431.
10. Boyer DS, Hopkins JJ, Sorof J, Ehrlich JS (2013) Anti-vascular endothelial growth factor therapy for diabetic macular edema. Ther Adv Endocrinol Metab 4: 151–169.
11. Koytak A, Altinisik M, Sogutlu Sari E, Artunay O, Umurhan Akkan JC, et al. (2013) Effect of a single intravitreal bevacizumab injection on different optical coherence tomographic patterns of diabetic macular oedema. Eye (Lond) 27: 716–721.
12. Osaadon P, Fagan XJ, Lifshitz T, Levy J (2014) A review of anti-VEGF agents for proliferative diabetic retinopathy. Eye (Lond) 28: 510–520.
13. ETDRS (1991) Fundus Photographic risk factors for progression of diabetic retinopathy. ETDRS Report Number 12. Ophthalmology. pp. 823–833.
14. Namperumalsamy P, Shukla D (2013) Eales' disease. In: Ryan SJ, editor-in-chief. Textbook of RETINA. St.Louis Elsevier. pp. 1479–1485.
15. Stitt AW, McGoldrick C, Rice-McCaldin A, McCance DR, Glenn JV, et al. (2005) Impaired retinal angiogenesis in diabetes: role of advanced glycation end products and galectin-3. Diabetes 54: 785–794.
16. Yoshimura T, Sonoda KH, Sugahara M, Mochizuki Y, Enaida H, et al. (2009) Comprehensive analysis of inflammatory immune mediators in vitreoretinal diseases. PLoS One 4: e8158.
17. Koskela UE, Kuusisto SM, Nissinen AE, Savolainen MJ, Liinamaa MJ (2013) High vitreous concentration of IL-6 and IL-8, but not of adhesion molecules in relation to plasma concentrations in proliferative diabetic retinopathy. Ophthalmic Res 49: 108–114.
18. Funatsu H, Yamashita H, Shimizu E, Kojima R, Hori S (2001) Relationship between vascular endothelial growth factor and interleukin-6 in diabetic retinopathy. Retina 21: 469–477.
19. Funatsu H, Yamashita H, Noma H, Mimura T, Nakamura S, et al. (2005) Aqueous humor levels of cytokines are related to vitreous levels and progression of diabetic retinopathy in diabetic patients. Graefes Arch Clin Exp Ophthalmol 243: 3–8.
20. Arnaoutova I, George J, Kleinman HK, Benton G (2009) The endothelial cell tube formation assay on basement membrane turns 20: state of the science and the art. Angiogenesis 12: 267–274.
21. Joussen AM, Poulaki V, Le ML, Koizumi K, Esser C, et al. (2004) A central role for inflammation in the pathogenesis of diabetic retinopathy. FASEB J 18: 1450–1452.
22. Adamis AP, Berman AJ (2008) Immunological mechanisms in the pathogenesis of diabetic retinopathy. Semin Immunopathol 30: 65–84.
23. Abcouwer SF (2013) Angiogenic Factors and Cytokines in Diabetic Retinopathy. J Clin Cell Immunol Suppl 1.
24. Bromberg-White JL, Glazer L, Downer R, Furge K, Boguslawski E, et al. (2013) Identification of VEGF-independent cytokines in proliferative diabetic retinopathy vitreous. Invest Ophthalmol Vis Sci 54: 6472–6480.
25. Tolentino MJ, Miller JW, Gragoudas ES, Chatzistefanou K, Ferrara N, et al. (1996) Vascular endothelial growth factor is sufficient to produce iris neovascularization and neovascular glaucoma in a nonhuman primate. Arch Ophthalmol 114: 964–970.
26. Cohen T, Nahari D, Cerem LW, Neufeld G, Levi BZ (1996) Interleukin 6 induces the expression of vascular endothelial growth factor. J Biol Chem 271: 736–741.
27. Maruo N, Morita I, Shirao M, Murota S (1992) IL-6 increases endothelial permeability in vitro. Endocrinology 131: 710–714.
28. Marumo T, Schini-Kerth VB, Busse R (1999) Vascular endothelial growth factor activates nuclear factor-kappaB and induces monocyte chemoattractant protein-1 in bovine retinal endothelial cells. Diabetes 48: 1131–1137.
29. Goebeler M, Gillitzer R, Kilian K, Utzel K, Brocker EB, et al. (2001) Multiple signaling pathways regulate NF-kappaB-dependent transcription of the monocyte chemoattractant protein-1 gene in primary endothelial cells. Blood 97: 46–55.
30. Grosjean J, Kiriakidis S, Reilly K, Feldmann M, Paleolog E (2006) Vascular endothelial growth factor signalling in endothelial cell survival: a role for NFkappaB. Biochem Biophys Res Commun 340: 984–994.
31. Wei LH, Kuo ML, Chen CA, Chou CH, Lai KB, et al. (2003) Interleukin-6 promotes cervical tumor growth by VEGF-dependent angiogenesis via a STAT3 pathway. Oncogene 22: 1517–1527.
32. Petreaca ML, Yao M, Liu Y, Defea K, Martins-Green M (2007) Transactivation of vascular endothelial growth factor receptor-2 by interleukin-8 (IL-8/CXCL8) is required for IL-8/CXCL8-induced endothelial permeability. Mol Biol Cell 18: 5014–5023.
33. Chen Y, Wiesmann C, Fuh G, Li B, Christinger HW, et al. (1999) Selection and analysis of an optimized anti-VEGF antibody: crystal structure of an affinity-matured Fab in complex with antigen. J Mol Biol 293: 865–881.
34. Olsson AK, Dimberg A, Kreuger J, Claesson-Welsh L (2006) VEGF receptor signalling - in control of vascular function. Nat Rev Mol Cell Biol 7: 359–371.
35. Schnichels S, Hagemann U, Januschowski K, Hofmann J, Bartz-Schmidt KU, et al. (2013) Comparative toxicity and proliferation testing of aflibercept, bevacizumab and ranibizumab on different ocular cells. Br J Ophthalmol 97: 917–923.
36. Arevalo JF, Wu L, Sanchez JG, Maia M, Saravia MJ, et al. (2009) Intravitreal bevacizumab (Avastin) for proliferative diabetic retinopathy: 6-months follow-up. Eye (Lond) 23: 117–123.
37. Reinhold HS, Buisman GH (1975) Repair of radiation damage to capillary endothelium. Br J Radiol 48: 727–731.
38. Williams MC, Wissig SL (1975) The permeability of muscle capillaries to horseradish peroxidase. J Cell Biol 66: 531–555.

12

Looking the Cow in the Eye: Deletion in the *NID1* Gene Is Associated with Recessive Inherited Cataract in Romagnola Cattle

Leonardo Murgiano[1], Vidhya Jagannathan[1], Valerio Calderoni[2], Monika Joechler[3], Arcangelo Gentile[3], Cord Drögemüller[1]*

1 Institute of Genetics, Vetsuisse Faculty, University of Bern, Bern, Switzerland, **2** Bovine practitioner, Fontanelice, Italy, **3** Department of Veterinary Medical Sciences, University of Bologna, Ozzano dell'Emilia, Italy

Abstract

Cataract is a known condition leading to opacification of the eye lens causing partial or total blindness. Mutations are known to cause autosomal dominant or recessive inherited forms of cataracts in humans, mice, rats, guinea pigs and dogs. The use of large-sized animal models instead of those using mice for the study of this condition has been discussed due to the small size of rodent lenses. Four juvenile-onset cases of bilateral incomplete immature nuclear cataract were recently observed in Romagnola cattle. Pedigree analysis suggested a monogenic autosomal recessive inheritance. In addition to the cataract, one of the cases displayed abnormal head movements. Genome-wide association and homozygosity mapping and subsequent whole genome sequencing of a single case identified two perfectly associated sequence variants in a critical interval of 7.2 Mb on cattle chromosome 28: a missense point mutation located in an uncharacterized locus and an 855 bp deletion across the exon 19/intron 19 border of the bovine nidogen 1 (*NID1*) gene (c.3579_3604+829del). RT-PCR showed that *NID1* is expressed in bovine lenses while the transcript of the second locus was absent. The *NID1* deletion leads to the skipping of exon 19 during transcription and is therefore predicted to cause a frameshift and premature stop codon (p.1164fs27X). The truncated protein lacks a C-terminal domain essential for binding with matrix assembly complexes. *Nidogen 1* deficient mice show neurological abnormalities and highly irregular crystal lens alterations. This study adds *NID1* to the list of candidate genes for inherited cataract in humans and is the first report of a naturally occurring mutation leading to non-syndromic catarct in cattle provides a potential large animal model for human cataract.

Editor: Andreas R. Janecke, Innsbruck Medical University, Austria

Funding: The authors have no support or funding to report.

Competing Interests: The authors have declared that no competing interests exist.

* Email: cord.droegemueller@vetsuisse.unibe.ch

Introduction

Cataract is a known condition affecting the internal integrity of the eye lens (crystalline) and leads to its opacification, interfering with normal sight. Vision can be compromised up to partial or total blindness, especially if both eyes are affected (bilateral cataract) [1–3]. The etiology of cataracts is heterogeneous like trauma, radiation, chronic disease, drugs or medications [4], [5]. A very important triggering factor of cataracts is aging; the majority of cataract cases manifest themselves in the later stages of life [6]. It is thought that nutrition could play a role in cataract development as well [7]. Nonetheless, a number of cases of cataracts are congenital or have an early onset [8], [9]. Approximately 1/3 of all congenital cataracts are caused by mostly autosomal dominant, rarely autosomal recessive or X-linked inherited mutations [9–12]. Almost 200 genes and a great number of loci identified as being causative of Mendelian and age-related cataract in humans are known [13]. The affected genes encode various proteins of importance for the crystalline structural stability [2], [12] most of them being crystallins, connexins and membrane junction proteins, but transcription factors like MAF are present as well [2], [13]. Many causative mutations change protein conformation and decrease their solubility and stability [12], [14] very likely leading to self-aggregation and precipitation [15].

In animals, most of the knowledge regarding cataractogenesis comes from genetic studies of hereditary cataracts in mice. Mutations causing inherited non-syndromic cataract have been identified in at least 18 mouse genes [16], and the use of animal models for the condition has been discussed for long time [17]. However, the need for a medium sized animal model has been pointed out due to the fact that rodents have small lenses which are hard to dissect and manipulate and need to be pooled for analysis. [18]. As an example, dogs showing breed specific forms of inherited cataract have been proposed as a complementary large animal model for molecular studies regarding cataract development, with the purpose of facilitating gene discovery and the development of therapies (OMIA-9615, [16]).

The occurrence of cataract in livestock probably is underestimated. This is somehow expected since, compared to other condition of greater severity, cataracts does not affect the health of the animal in such a way to hamper its production efficiency. One study has mapped a locus for an inherited cataract form in sheep to a region on chromosome 6 [19]. The authors stressed the necessity of developing a genetic test for cataract in sheep as predicting which animals will develop cataracts would make them suitable models for the development of the condition and to study possible therapies [19]. Indeed, the use of a sheep model for cataracts in which the potential therapeutic efficacy of a chemical has been tested has been reported [20]. Cataracts in cattle have been reported sporadically (OMIA-9913) and the mode of inheritance has been an object of debate [21], [22]. A recent case of congenital cataract in Ayrshire cattle with a high prevalence in a single herd was reported, but a genetic etiology has not been demonstrated [23], as well as in a population of Swiss calves [24]. One study has reported a dominant mutation in the *FNB1* gene as the cause of Marfan syndrome in cattle accompanied by cataract beside other defects [25].

Romagnola is a local variety of beef cattle bred in north central Italy of about twenty thousand animals. Due to a significant level of inbreeding, the Romagnola breed recently has experienced outbreaks of two recessive diseases, namely paunch calf syndrome and pseudomyotonia, for which gene tests for eradication were developed after successful identification of the causative gene mutations [26–27]. During the fall of 2013 cataracts in four inbred juvenile Romagnola cattle were observed, prompting an in depth study to identify the causative mutation.

Results and Discussion

A recessively inherited juvenile-onset form of cataract in cattle

In November 2013, four male Romagnola calves, varying in age from 3 to 4 months, were seen due to a visible clouding of both eyes causing obvious signs of impaired vision (**Figure 1**). The problem had been noticed by the owner some weeks prior to the request for consultation. According to the records of the owner the opacity was not present at birth. The clinical investigation carried out in dim light during the first on-farm visit showed a relatively less severe opacity of the lenses. Vision impairment was evident when the animal moved within the box, especially when forced to escape rapidly from the examiner. The body condition score of the animals was slightly reduced, whereas mental status was normal. According to the owner, all dams of the affected calves, as well as the other animals present at the farm, had no visible ocular problems. In addition, one of the affected animals also showed a slight head tilt towards the right side (**Video S1**). The cow-calf herd is made up of 60 Romagnola cows housed in a free stall barn with straw as bedding material, and are fed hay and barley-based concentrate (80% barley +20% mais). In the summer (May to November), the cows are allowed to graze in a hilly pasture and in a wood near the farm, which is also populated with wild animals. The hay and the concentrate are supplemented at the end of the grazing period when grass is reduced due to the dry season. The calving season is concentrated in winter and spring (November to May). Two sires are present in the herd and they are usually kept for a maximum of three years to avoid parental inbreeding. Cows and heifers are vaccinated annually against bovine viral diarrhea (BVD), rhinotracheitis (IBR), parainfluenza 3 (PI3), and bovine respiratory syncitial virus (BRSV) viruses using inactivated strains. At the time of our farm visit, the herd had not been treated against parasites for long time, and, in fact, gastrointestinal strongyles were detected using coprological investigation. During the first visit no elements suggestive of nutritional or potentially toxic environmental factors were detected. The suggested correlation of the cataracts to the proximity of mobile telephone masts [24] was excluded on the basis of the absence of such stations in the surrounding area.

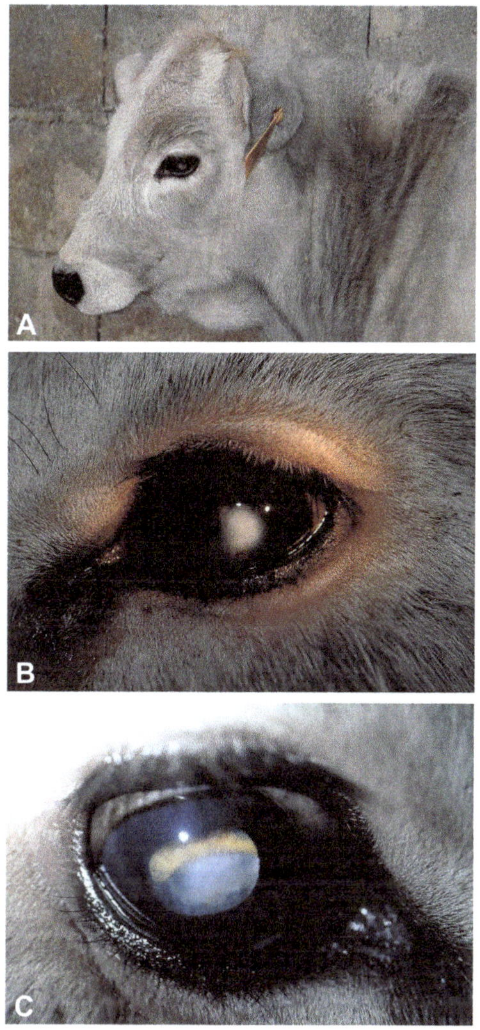

Figure 1. Cataract in Romagnola cattle. (**A**) Opacity of the left eye's noted from a distance. Case 3, born 27 July 2013, photo 4th November 2013. (**B**) Dioptric media opacity of the left eye. Case 2, born 16 th August 2013, photo 6 th November 2013. (**C**) Mild central nuclear opacity. Fundus only partially to view (yellow = tapetal retina; blue = papilla). Case 2, born 16 th August 2013, photo 6 th November 2013.

One calf was admitted to the teaching hospital of the Department of Veterinary Medical Sciences of the University of Bologna for in-depth clinical study. A thorough ophthalmologic examination was carried out in a darkened environment. The exam did not show any lid or and conjunctival problems, the menace was bilaterally positive, and the Shirmer tear tests as well as the intraocular pressure (IOP) values were normal. By direct focal light source stimulation, the direct and consensual pupillary reflexes were normal or slightly more accentuated. Direct ophthalomoscopy revealed a regular morphology and arrangement of the iris and net margins of the pupillary lumen. After mydriasis induction, examination of both lenses revealed mild central nuclear opacity irregularly extending towards the periphery. Partial fundus evaluation revealed a regular papilla and a normal tapetum. Hematological parameters and clinical biochemistry did not show notable alterations. The final diagnosis for this calf was bilateral incomplete immature nuclear cataract.

Analysis of the pedigree data revealed that all four affected animals were paternal half siblings of *Volturno* (**Figure 2**). Furthermore, their respective dams were also paternal half sibs belonging to another sire *Posimo* which had been culled some years before. We examined three other young calves with the same family relationship and approximately the same age as the affected animals and they did not show any visible ocular problems. Both bulls, *Volturno* and *Posimo*, had a common male ancestor (*Marte*) over 1 and 3 generations ago which was born in 1978. Although none of these three sires was still alive a visible cataract could probably be excluded as they were selected after a detailed clinical exam revealing no signs of genetic conditions before they were used as artificial insemination sires. Taken together, we assumed a monogenic recessive inheritance of the underlying mutation causing the cataract phenotype in that family of Romagnola cattle.

Mapping of the cataract mutation to a 7.2 Mb region on BTA 28

Hypothesizing a simple Mendelian recessive inheritance we initiated a positional cloning study to unravel the underlying genetics. Initially we genotyped 777,961 evenly spaced SNPs on the 4 affected calves, the sire and the 4 dams, and we merged these data along with a set of similar genotype data of 51 Romagnola cattle which had been generated in the course of a previous study [26]. After removing 236,126 non-informative markers, 549,341 SNPs were used for genome-wide association mapping (GWAS). The calculated genomic inflation factor (lambda) was 1.78 suggesting a fairly highly stratified population. We therefore decided to carry out the analysis using a mixed-model in order to take into account the population stratification; this showed significantly associated markers exceeding the threshold for genome-wide significance after a Bonferroni correction (raw P value $<7.7\times10^{-8}$). A best 14 markers were located in the same single contiguous genomic region (3.32–10.05 Mb) on bovine chromosome 28 (BTA 28) (**Figure 3A+B**; **Figure S1**; **Table S1**).

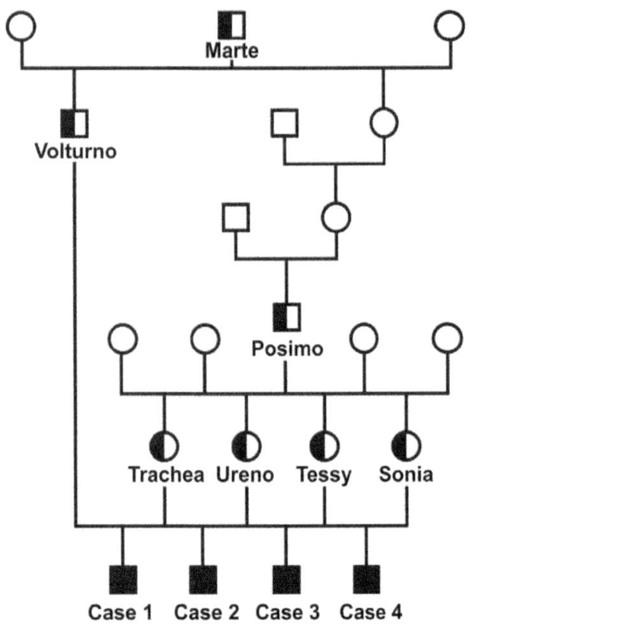

Figure 2. Family tree showing four Romagnola calves affected by cataract and their parents. Males are represented by squares, females by circles. Affected animals are shown with fully black symbols and genotyped carriers with a half-filled symbol. All unnamed animals with empty symbols were not available for genotyping. Note the inbreeding loop to the sire *Marte*.

In the light of the highly likely monogenic recessive inheritance (**Figure 2**) we assumed that the four affected animals were expected to be identical by descent (IBD) for the causative mutation and flanking chromosomal segments. Therefore, we searched for extended regions of homozygosity with simultaneous allele sharing and found five genome regions greater than 1 Mb that fulfilled these criteria whereas the largest homozygous segment corresponds to a 7.2 Mb interval from 2,870,897 to 10,073,583 on BTA 28 (**Figure 3C**; **Table S2**). Observing an almost matching overlap of the GWAS hit and the homozygous region on chromosome 28 we concluded that this single genome interval probably contains the causative mutation for the cataract phenotype. The mapped critical interval contains 42 annotated genes beside a number of uncharacterized loci. Consulting the database to understand their expected function revealed that the region contained no obvious candidates, except possibly tubulin folding cofactor E (*TBCE*) since tubulin folding is supposed to have a role in lens transparency [28].

A deletion in the *NID1* gene is associated with cataract in cattle

For mutation analysis we sequenced the entire genome of a single affected animal (case 2, **Figure 2**) in order to detect all the variants in the annotated genes and loci of the mapped 7.2 Mb interval on BTA 28. We collected 319,462,911 100 bp paired-end reads from a shotgun fragment library corresponding to roughly 13.5× coverage of the genome. The SNPs and short indel variants were called compared to the reference genome and 92,955 high quality variants across the whole exome including untranslated regions and 10 bp of flanking introns were detected, of which 27,597 were coding variants. Within the exome of the critical BTA 28 region we detected a total of 129 variants, of which 43 were located within coding sequences or within splice sites having a predicted effect on the amino acid sequence of the annotated genes (**Table S3**). Comparison of the DNA variants between the affected calf and 44 cow genomes of 15 different cattle breeds that had been sequenced in our laboratory in the course of other studies revealed that 42 of the coding variants occurred in the control genomes of animals from different breeds and could thus be excluded as causative variants. The single remaining variant was a missense mutation in the uncharacterized locus *ENSBTAG00000039845* (c.687G>C, p.Q229H). Furthermore, we used the Delly package [29] for looking for larger deletions in the sequenced case and in 41 control cow genomes with a genome-wide coverage of more than 10 fold. A total of 253 deletions were private structural variants occurring only in the genome of the affected Romagnola animal with cataract of which a single 855 bp deletion was detected in the critical region on BTA 28 (g.8733811_8734665del). Annotation showed that this deletion removes 26 nucleotides from the 3′-end of exon 19 (nts 3579 to 3604) and 829 nucleotides from the 5′-end of intron 19 (nts 3604+1 to +827) of of the bovine nidogen 1 (*NID1*) gene (c.3579_3604+829del; **Figure 4A+B**). We genotyped the two detected private coding variants in larger cohorts of Romagnola cattle. The *NID1* deletion was validated by PCR and subsequent agarose gel electrophoresis confirmed that all four affected animals were homozygous, while all five parents were heterozygous, which was confirmed by subsequent Sanger sequencing (**Figure 4C**). Later on, fragment size analyses were performed for *NID1* genotyping.

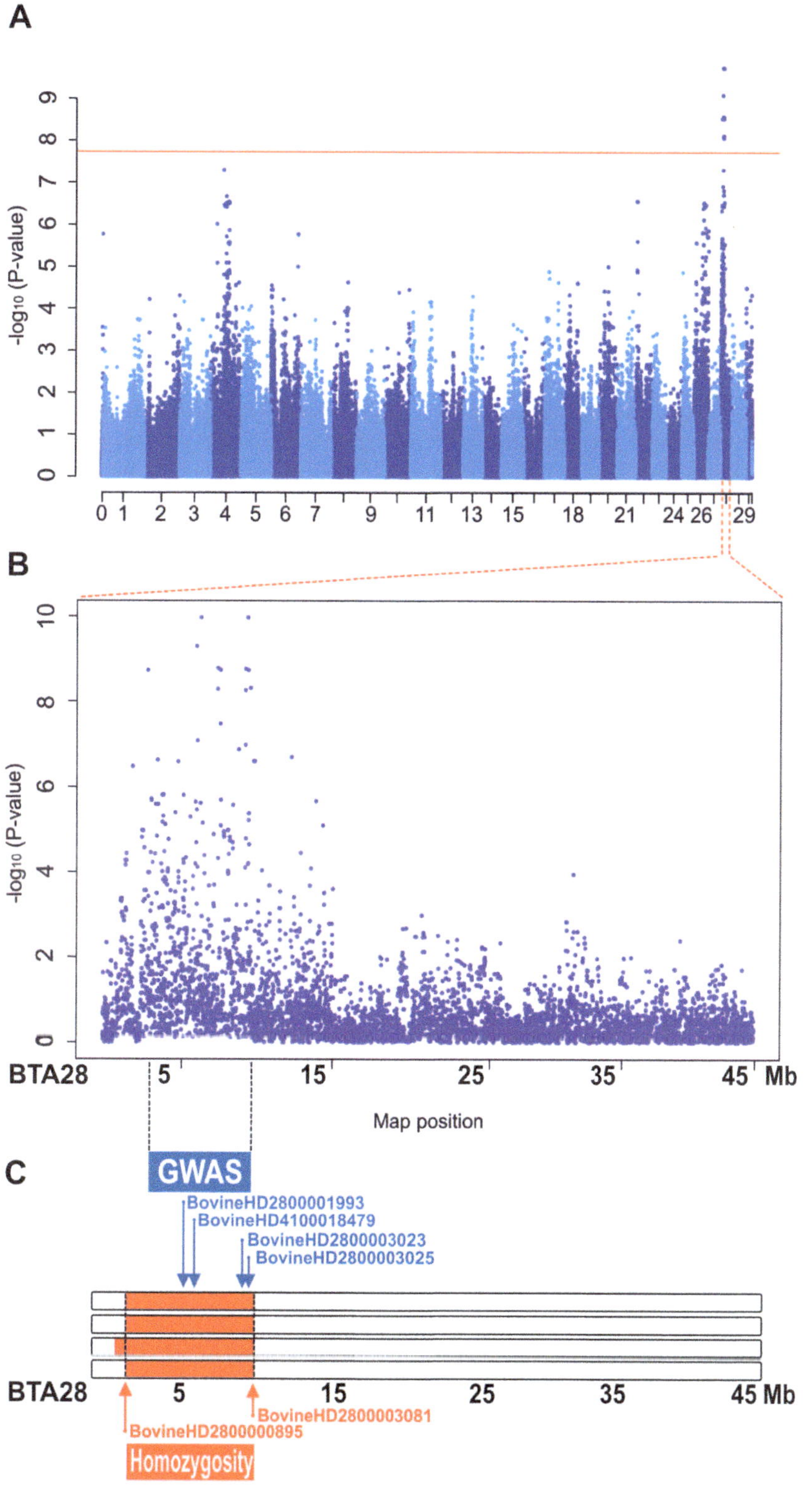

Figure 3. Mapping of the cataract mutation to BTA 28. (**A**) Results of the genome-wide association study (GWAS): Manhattan plot showing the negative log of the raw P values calculated with the mixed-model genotypic association test. Genome-wide significance thresholds are indicated ($P \leq 0.01$, solid red horizontal line at 7.7 10^{-8} $-\log_{10}$Pvalue). (**B**) Detailed view of Manhattan plot for chromosome 28. (**C**) (blue) the 4 most significantly associated BTA 28 SNPs from GWAS in combination with the identical by descent (IBD; red) segments of the four affected animals. The names of the SNPs lines are reported along with their positions on the map.

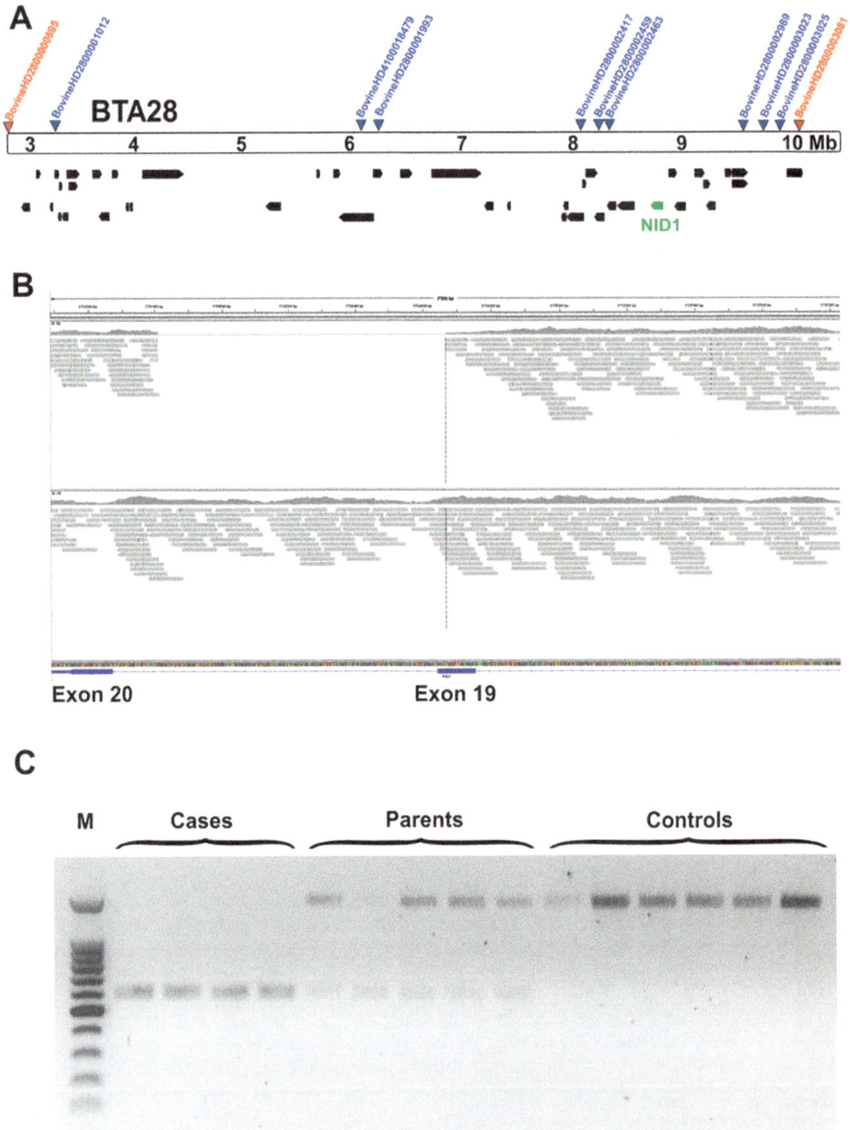

Figure 4. The *NID1* deletion. (**A**) Gene content of the fine-mapped critical interval Position of the two extreme homozygous marker (red) from homozygosity mapping and of the nine most significant markers from GWAS (blue) are indicated. Annotated genes in the region are shown in black, along with *NID1* (green). (**B**) Screenshot of the next generation sequence reads mapped against the reference sequence. Note the 855 bp deletion. (**C**) Detected genotypes of the *NID1* deletion. Note the shorter PCR product in affected animals, the longer in controls and the presence of both products in carriers.

PCR and Sanger sequencing was used for validation and genotyping of the *ENSBTAG00000039845* SNP. Both variants remained perfectly associated with the cataract phenotype in more than 500 animals (**Table 1**).

The *NID1* gene encodes a protein which is involved in matrix assembly and is expressed in various tissues and reportedly in lenses [30], [31]. A protein sequence based database search for the uncharacterized locus *ENSBTAG00000039845* revealed 70% sequence coverage and 57% sequence identity with the putative PRAME family member 24-like protein of *Bos taurus* (XP_606544.2). In addition, the result pointed out 63% sequence coverage and 98% identity with putative PRAME family member 25-like protein in *Bos mutus* (XP_005905668.1). PRAME family members are encoded by genes which are primarily involved in immunity and reproduction, and whose expression is restricted to the testis and a variety of cancers [32]. As an experimental control, we extracted RNA from skin and lenses of healthy cattle. RT-PCR revealed no evidence for expression of the *ENSBTAG00000039845* transcript neither in the skin nor in the lens, but interestingly, we observed *NID1* expression in both skin and lens (**Figure S2**). Thus we concluded that the *NID1* deletion is much more likely to cause cataract than the *ENSBTAG00000039845* variant. The *NID1* deletion consisting in the loss of hundreds of bases was potentially more disruptive compared to the exchange of a single less conserved amino acid in the uncharacterized locus which is not expressed in the lens.

None of the 1062 healthy Romagnola cattle genotyped for the *NID1* deletion had the homozygous mutant genotype, but 50 of them were determined to be carriers. All available ancestors of the 4 cases were shown to be carriers including the common founder

Table 1. Association of coding variants with the cataract phenotype in Romagnola cattle.

Genotype	Cases	Obligate carriers[a]	Romagnola population controls[b]
ENSBTAG00000039845: c.687G>C			
G/G			535
G/C		5	36
C/C	4		
NID1: c.3579_3604+829del			
wt/wt			1012
wt/del		5	45
del/del	4		

[a] Parents of affected offspring were classified as obligate carriers.
[b] A larger cohort was genotyped for the *NID* variant to evaluate the frequency of the defect allele within the breed.

sire *Marte* confirming the assumed recessive inheritance (**Figure 2**). In addition, a complete pedigree of all carriers with available records indicating that the mutation occurs restricted to a certain breeding line of Romagnola cattle was built (**Figure S3**). The mutation occurred at least two generations before the bull *Marte* thus confirming the initial suspicion that a recent mutation event in a common ancestor was responsible for the outbreak. The frequency of the deleterious *NID1* allele within this large sample of Romagnola cattle was 2.4%. This is quite low in comparison to recently determined frequencies for other recessive defects in Italian beef cattle [33], [34] and might explain the fact that until know no further affected animals have been observed.

The effect of the deletion on the *NID1* transcript was investigated with cDNA prepared from the skin tissue of an affected animal homozygous for the genomic deletion and a healthy control homozygous for the wild type allele. Sequencing of an RT-PCR product containing the exon 19- exon 20 junction showed that mRNA produced in the case, but not the control, lacked the entirety of exon 19 (**Figure 5**). This exon skipping results in a mutant transcript containing a frame-shift which predicts a truncation of 50 amino acids and contain 27 amino acids different from those found in the wild type protein (**Figure S4**). This predicts deletion of a portion of the G3 beta propeller domain which binds to laminin, and to the sixth EGF-like domain in the C-terminal part of the protein [35]. If not nonsense-mediated decay prevents transcription this would ultimately severely damage the role of *NID1* in the matrix assembly (**Figure 5**) [36].

Role of *NID1* during cataractogenesis

In mammals are two known multivalent basement membrane (BM) binding proteins of the nidogen family called NID1 and NID2 [37–40] Basement membranes are found between cell surfaces and the interstitium or between cells [41]. Pathological conditions can arise due to mutations which can disrupt the extracellular matrix and/or its linkages leading to the loss of matrix integrity, adhesion strength and/or receptor-mediated signaling, affecting nerves, muscles, skin, kidneys and various tissues [42]. Interactions of the NID1 and NID2 proteins with many other matrix components have been demonstrated *in vitro*, in particular with laminins and collagen IV having the role of a stabilizing bridge (**Figure 5**) [40], [43], [44]. Deletion of either *NID1* or *NID2* did not reveal alterations in the BM architecture [31], [45], [46] and it has been suggested that the two proteins may be partially redundant, each compensating for the contingent lack of the other [45], [47]; their tissue-specificity in development has been suggested [31], [48], [49]. Nonetheless, mice lacking both nidogens die shortly after birth from lung and heart anomalies, which are directly correlated to BM defects [50]. *Nid1* knockout mice showed differences in some of crystal lenses of 7-week-old *Nid1* null mice compared to wild type [31]. In detail, they described the border between elongating fiber cells and the posterior lens capsule as being highly irregular [31]. In the same study the authors reported that, in the brain and eye lenses, the intrinsic expression level of *Nid2* seems to be lower as compared to other tissues in wild-type mice. No obvious up-regulation of *Nid2* was detected in *Nid1 -/-* mice using western blot [31]. These authors suggested that both *Nid1* and *Nid2* can generally compensate for the non-functionality of the other. Nonetheless, the tissue-specific expression of a single variant can trigger a pathological condition if this variant, being the only one expressed in that tissue, is not functional (**Figure 5**). To verify if this is also the case in cattle, we investigated the presence of *NID1* and *NID2* transcript in normal bovine lenses compared to skin. RT-PCR indeed showed detectable level of *NID2* transcript in crystal lenses while in skin both *NID1* and *NID2* transcripts were expressed (**Figure S2**). We therefore concluded that the pathological condition is circumscribed to the eye (and possibly nervous tissue) because of tissue-specific expression of the *NID1* and *NID2* genes (**Figure 5**). One of the affected calves in our study showed an abnormal, albeit light, head movement (**Video S1**). Interestingly, head bobbing and seizure-like behavior have been reported in *Nid1* knockout mice, more severe if one *Nid2* allele was mutated as well [31], [51]. Furthermore, we found no evidence for the presence of other reported accompanied alterations affecting limb development [52]. This could suggest that, since the signs in our animals were less pronounced, it was possible that the deletion of larger portions of the protein could lead to a more severe condition, and, perhaps, this could also suggest that, in our calves, the altered *NID1* mRNA was translated into a shorter, but not completely defective, polypeptide. Gresham et al. have shown that different domains of NID1 activate distinct functions such as chemotaxis or phagocytosis [53]. Recently, a probably dominant acting *de novo* nonsense *NID1* mutation in a family with Dandy-Walker syndrome and occipital cephaloceles resulting in in the loss of the entire G2 and G3 regions of NID1 protein including all the EGF-like domains has been reported [54]. In our study the loss of the NID G3 domain is obviously not sufficient to create a pathological condition in heterozygous animals. Therefore, it is reasonable to assume that the milder phenotype observed in cattle

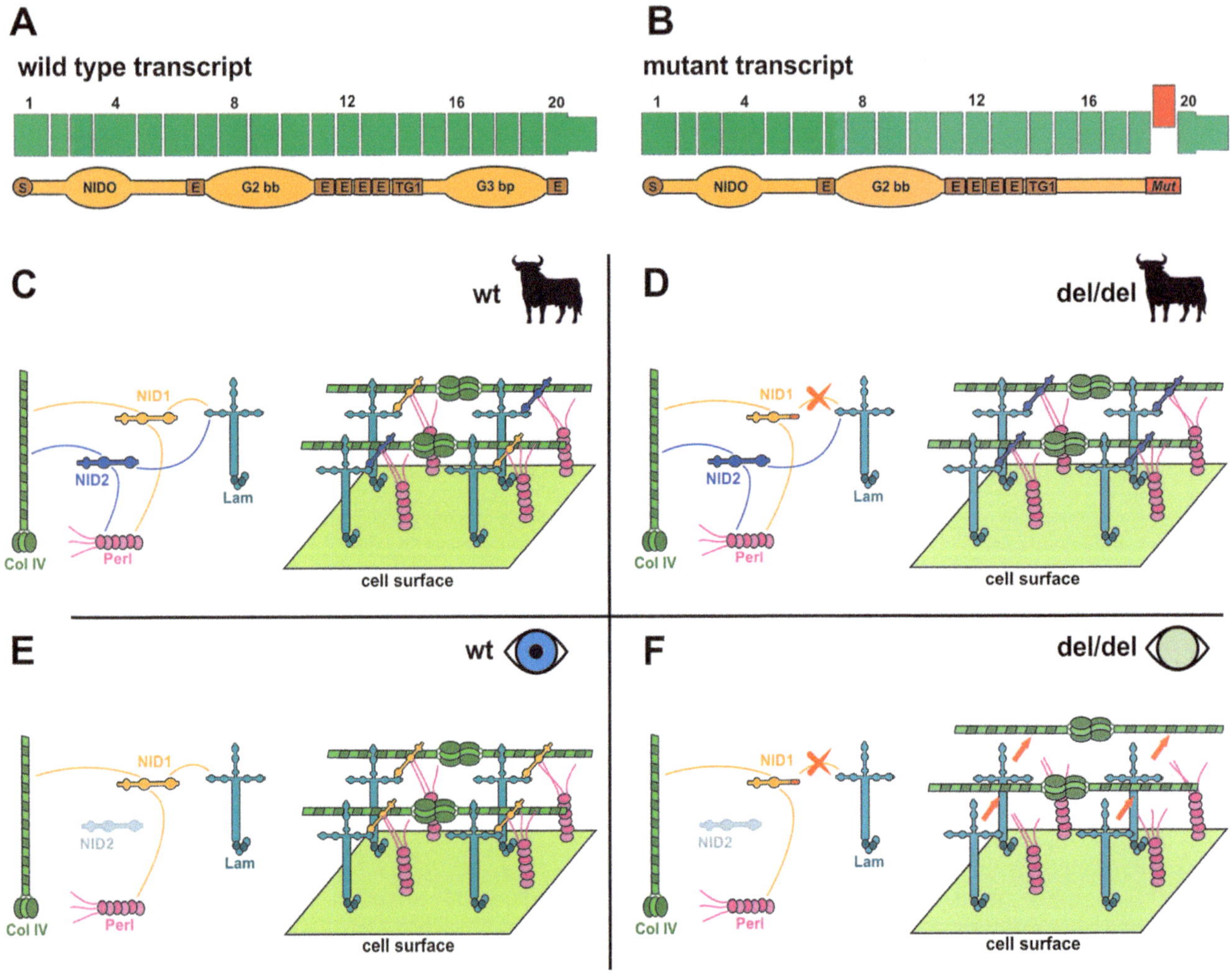

Figure 5. Tissue-specific inferred pathological mechanism. (**A**) Wild type transcript. The translated NID1 protein is shown. *S*: Signal peptide; *NIDO*: Nidogen domain; *E*: EGF-like domains *G2bb*: G2 beta-barrel domain; G3bp: G3 beta-propeller domain, binding laminin [36] (**B**) Mutated NID1. The skipped exon is represented in red. The C-terminal part of the protein is altered severely and part of the G3 domain is lost. (**C**) Matrix assembly in various body tisses of an animal (like muscle, heart, kidney, skin, [31]) with wild type NID; NID1 and NID2 are both expressed in detectable level; Both interact functionally with laminin and participate to the matrix assembly, probably compensating each for the lack of the other [41–45]. (**D**) Body tissues of an animal lacking a functional NID1: in all the tissue in which NID2 is expressed (all barring brain and lenses according to literature [31]) NID2 compensates for the lack of NID1 [45–47]. (**E**) Eye of an individual with functional NID1. NID2 is not expressed at detectable levels, but NID1 alone is enough in its role of bridge protein in the matrix assembly. (**F**) Eye of an individual lacking of functional NID1. NID1 cannot interact functionally with laminin, and this defect is not compensated in the lens tissue, leading to matrix instability and ultimately to a pathological condition. (**C-F**) Simplified version of basal membrane [38]. *NID1*: Nidogen 1. *NID2*: Nidogen 2. *Lam*: Laminins. *Col IV*: Collagen IV. *Perl*: Perlecan. Only interactions of the Nidogens with other elements are shown. Nidogens role is to bridge the interactions among the main matrix proteins [36].

could be due to the location of the mutation concerning only the terminal part of the protein. Overall, it appears that *NID* mutations can lead to very diverse phenotypes in mammals.

Because of the possible role played by *NID1* in eye lenses, Dong and colleagues actually suggested that *NID1* knockout mice could be used as a model system to further explore the role of the lens capsule in the cellular organization of the crystalline lens [31]. Still, the alterations reported are unclear, and there are authors reporting no alterations at all in crystal lenses [50]. In addition, the role of NID1 in signs other than those of a neurological nature is often overlooked [55], [56]. In his paper, May observed alterations in the inner limiting membrane in the posterior eye segment of *NID1 -/-* mice [57]. The author speculated that specific mechanical forces and eye size/proportion can play a role in the stress suffered by basement membranes, with NID1 being important to their stability [57]. Along the same lines, it could therefore be speculated that our cataract phenotype in cattle, caused by nonfunctional NID1, could be, at least in part, due to the anatomical differences in the bovine eye as compared to the murine eye. Following this line of thinking, it could then be asked whether mice would accurately model the eye membrane alteration of large mammals (humans included), at least the alterations involving basal membrane stability. Indeed, it has previously been reported that murine models, although being very important in the study of eye lens pathologies, are far from being related to their human counterparts with regard to genotype/phenotype correlation [58]. In our study, it can be verified that cataractic lenses in cattle with nonfunctional NID1 were detectable immediately and clearly macroscopically.

Conclusions

Our findings add the *NID1* gene to the list of candidates for nuclear cataract. In addition, the identification of a naturally occurring mutation for cataract in Romagnola cattle provides an interesting large animal model for human cataract. This study highlights the potential of the unique family structures of livestock populations in combination with state-of-the-art methods in order to determine causative mutations for a recessive defect in a short term. Furthermore, it was shown that, if reported and studied, a usually unreported condition, could possibly give to novel insights. To our knowledge, this is the first recorded causative mutation for recessive inherited cataract in cattle. It is the first time that *NID1* has been associated with crystal lens alteration in bigger mammals and a confirmation of the crucial involvement of *NID1* in crystal lens integrity as has previously been suggested in mice.

Material and Methods

Ethics Statement

All handling of the animals was conducted according to national and international guidelines for animal welfare. There is no permit number as this study was not based on an invasive animal experiment and used naturally occurring cases. This is a very special situation in veterinary medicine, as the data is from client-owned cattle which underwent veterinary exams; there was no "animal experiment" according to the legal definition in Italy. The samples used were taken a single cattle farm in Italy and the cattle owner agreed that the samples could be used in the study. Skin samples were taken from punches needed to clip the code ID numbers to the animal ears. Finally, the unaffected eye lenses came from routine necropsies on cattle with unrelated conditions which were carried out in the Department of Veterinary Medical Sciences of the University of Bologna.

Animals and SNP genotyping

Blood samples were collected from 4 affected calves and their parents from the same farm. Genotyping of these cases was performed using the BovineHD BeadChip (Illumina), including 777,961 evenly distributed SNPs and standard protocols as recommended by the manufacturer. In addition, stored DNA from 1057 healthy Romagnola cattle was also used, resulting in a total of 1066 samples from this breed.

Genome-wide association and homozygosity mapping

The GenAbel package in R studio was used for GWAS [59]. As a preliminary step in the analysis a first quality control to remove markers and individuals with call rates <90% from the analysis was carried out. Markers with minor allele frequency <5% were removed and also markers strongly deviating from the Hardy-Weinberg equilibrium ($p<10^{-6}$). This was followed by a mixed model association study. The threshold of $P\leq0.01$ for genome-wide significance was Bonferroni-adjusted to account for multiple testing ($0.01/549{,}341 = 1.82\times10^{-8}$). PLINK software [60] was used to search for extended intervals of homozygosity with shared alleles as described previously. Individuals and SNPs were selected using the commands –keep, and –extract while final files were generated through the –merge command. Homozygosity analysis was carried out on all cases using the commands –cow, –homozyg and –homozyg-group.

Whole genome re-sequencing and variant calling

We prepared a fragment library with a 300 bp insert size and collected one lane of Illumina HiSeq2500 paired-end reads (2×100 bp); the fastq files were created using Casava 1.8. We obtained a total of 356,094,795 paired-end reads which were then mapped to the cow reference genome UMD3.1/bosTau6 and aligned using Burrows-Wheeler Aligner (BWA) version 0.5.9-r16 [61] with default settings. The mapping showed 313,195,442 reads had unique mapping positions. The SAM file generated by BWA was then converted to BAM and the reads sorted by chromosome using samtools [62]. PCR duplicates were marked using Picard tools (http://sourceforge.net/projects/picard/). We used the Genome Analysis Tool Kit (GATK version 2.4.9, [63]) to perform local realignment and to produce a cleaned BAM file. The genome data has been made freely available under accession no. PRJEB5965 at the European Nucleotide Archive [64].

Variant calls were then made with the unified genotyper module of GATK. The variant data for each sample was obtained in variant call format (version 4.0) as raw calls for all samples and sites flagged using the variant filtration module of GATK. Variant filtration was performed, following best practice documentation of GATK version 4. The snpEFF software [65] together with the UMD3.1/bosTau Ensembl annotation was used to predict the functional effects of detected variants. The Delly package was used to detect structural variants in cleaned BAM files. Delly uses variation in pair-end reads distance and orientation to find deletions, duplications, inversions and translocations. Structural variation software that are based on coverage and orientation are unable to detect variations larger than the insert size, as read mapping software usually requires the library insert size as an argument for aligning within range. Hence, in order to avoid missing large inserts, deletions and false positives all detected variants in the candidate region were also manually inspected [29].

Sanger sequencing and genotyping

The associated variants were genotyped by re-sequencing of targeted PCR products using Sanger sequencing technology. PCR primers were designed using PRIMER3 [66]. PCR products were run on 0.8% agarose gel, 0.5 µg/ml ethidium bromide. PCR products were amplified using flanking primers (*NID1* (F) TCCAAGCGACAAAAGAGGTT, (R) TTTCCGCTCGATA-CAGTCAA; *ENSBTAG00000039845* (F) TGTGGCTCCTAA-ATGACCAA, (R) ACTTGGAGGATCCCAGGACT; *NID1* cDNA (F) TTTCCGCTCGATACAGTCAA, (R) CTTGAAGG-GCTGCAGCC with AmpliTaqGold360Mastermix (Life Technologies) and the products directly sequenced using the PCR primers on an ABI 3730 capillary sequencer (Life Technologies) after treatment with exonuclease I (N.E.B) and rAPid alkaline phosphatase (Roche). Sequence data were analyzed using Sequencher 5.1 (GeneCodes). We used an alternative fragment size analysis assay to genotype additional cattle for the *NID1* deletion using three primers: (F) CATCAGGGAAATCCTGC-TGT and ($R_{wild\ type}$) CAGGTGGGTTACCTTCAGGA, and (R_{mutant}) GTGACCTGGAAAAGGCAGAA. Products were visualized on an ABI 3730 capillary sequencer and analyzed with the GeneMapper 4.0 software (Life Technologies). Fragments with the deletion are 286 bp in length and fragments without the deletion are 176 bp in length.

RNA extraction and cDNA product amplification

The RNA was extracted from skin tissue and crystal lenses with the same procedure using RNeasy mini kit (Qiagen). First, the tissue was finely crushed in TRIZOL (Ambion) using mechanical means, chloroform was then added and the RNA separated through centrifugation. Additional passages were carried out as described by the manufacturer. Genomic DNA contamination was eliminated enzymatically using the Quantitect Reverse Transcription Kit (Qiagen). The same kit was used to synthetize cDNA, as described by the manufacturer. The cDNA fragments of target genes PCR products were amplified using the following primers: *NID1*: (F) CTTGAAGGGCTGCAGTATCC, (R) TTTCCGC-TCGATACAGTCAA; *NID2* (F) GACTCAGCTGTGACCTG-CAC, (R) AAGACCCGGTCAACATTCAG; *ENSBTAG00000 039845*: (F) TGTGGCTCCTAAATGACCAA, (R) ACTTG-GAGGATCCCAGGACT; *GADPH* (F) ACCCAGAAGACTG-TGGATGG, (R) CCAGCAGCTGAGGAACTCTT. The PCRs were carried out with AmpliTaqGold360Mastermix (Life Technologies). The PCR products were run on 2% agarose gel and 0.5 μg/ml ethidium bromide.

Supporting Information

Figure S1 QQ-plot. QQ- plots showing the observed versus expected -log p-values. The diagonal line in the QQ plots indicates the distribution of SNP markers under the null hypothesis, and the skewing of a marker toward the upper side suggests that it has a stronger association with the pathological condition than one would expected by mere chance. The deviation of observed values from the expected is clearly visible and indicates a consistent difference between cases and controls and reflects the GWAS result obtained.

Figure S2 Tissue specific gene expression. The picture shows the amplified fragment of cDNA extracted from skin (left) and crystal lenses (right) of healthy cattle. *GADPH*: Glyceraldehyde 3-phosphate dehydrogenase. The samples are from 1-year old calves slaughtered *NID1*: nidogen-1; *NID2*: Nidogen-2; *PRAME*: uncharacterized locus *ENSBTAG00000039845*; Mk: 100 bp ladder. Note that the PRAME like transcript is absent in both skin and crystal lens and that the *NID2* transcript is absent in the crystal lens albeit to skin.

Figure S3 Extended family tree. The family tree in Figure 2 expanded adding all the carriers detected within the population whose the ancestry was known and able to be reconstructed. Males are represented by squares, females by circles. Affected animals are shown with fully black symbols and genotyped carriers with a half-filled symbol. All animals with empty symbols were not available for genotyping. The purpose of this picture is to show the recessive inheritance of the mutation and to find a common ancestor. Note how most animals show having *Marte* as a common ancestor. *Marte* shares common ancestry with a number of carriers in *Emiro*, son of *Titano* and ancestor of another carrier.

Figure S4 NID protein sequences. Predicted amino acid sequence of the wild type and mutated NID1 protein. In green fragment of the protein present only in the wild type, in red the predicted change in the mutant.

Table S1 Top 14 significant SNPs.

Table S2 Region of homozygosity among the affected animals.

Table S3 List of all the variants in the BTA 28 candidate region. Non-synonymous variants are bolded.

Video S1 Neurological abnormalities in a single cataract case.

Acknowledgments

The authors wish to thank Michaela Drögemüller, Mandy Otto, and Irene Reber for their help, and Michèle Ackermann, Brigitta Colomb and Muriel Fragnière for their precious technical assistance. We would like to express our appreciation to the University of Bern for the use of the Next Generation Sequencing Platform in performing the whole genome re-sequencing experiment and the Vital-IT high-performance computing center of the Swiss Institute of Bioinformatics for performing computationally intensive tasks (http://www.vital-it.ch/).

Author Contributions

Conceived and designed the experiments: LM VJ AG CD. Performed the experiments: LM VJ VC MJ AG CD. Analyzed the data: LM VJ CD. Contributed reagents/materials/analysis tools: VC MJ AG CD. Wrote the paper: LM AG CD.

References

1. Koenigsberg R (1989) Churchill's Medical Dictionary. Churchill Livingstone Inc. 308 p.
2. Deng H, Yuan L (2014) Molecular genetics of congenital nuclear cataract. Eur J Med Genet 57: 113–122.
3. Yi J, Yun J, Li ZK, Xu CT, Pan BR (2011) Epidemiology and molecular genetics of congenital cataracts. Int J Ophthalmol 4: 422–432.
4. Mesa R, Bassnett S (2013) UV-B-induced DNA damage and repair in the mouse lens. Invest Ophthalmol Vis Sci 54: 6789–6797.
5. Sinha R, Kumar C, Titiyal JS (2009) Etiopathogenesis of cataract: Journal review. Indian J Ophthalmol 2009 57: 245–249.
6. Petrash JM (2013) Aging and age-related diseases of the ocular lens and vitreous body. Invest Ophthalmol Vis Sci 54: ORSF54-59.
7. Chew EY (2013) Nutrition effects on ocular diseases in the aging eye. Invest Ophthalmol Vis Sci 54: ORSF42–47.
8. Churchill A, GrawJ (2011) Clinical and experimental advances in congenital and paediatric cataracts. Philos Trans R Soc Lond B Biol Sci 366: 1234–1249.
9. Hejtmancik JF (2008) Congenital cataracts and their molecular genetics. Semin Cell Dev Biol 19: 134–149
10. He W, Li S (2000) Congenital cataracts: gene mapping. Hum Genet 106: 1–13.
11. Huang B, He W (2010) Molecular characteristics of inherited congenital cataracts. Eur J Med Genet 53: 347–357
12. Liang J (2004) Interactions and chaperone function of A-crystallin with T5PgC-crystallin mutant. Protein Sci 13: 2476–2482.
13. Shiels A, Bennett TM, Hejtmancik JF (2010) Cat-Map: putting cataract on the map. MolVis 16: 2007–2015.
14. Liu B, Song S, Hanson H, Liang J (2008) Protein-protein interactions involving congenital cataract T5P γC-crystallin mutant: a confocal fluorescence microscopy study. Exp Eye Res 87: 515–520.
15. Talla V, Narayanan C, Srinivasan N, Balasubramanian D (2006) Mutation causing self-aggregation in human γC-crystallin leading to congenital cataract. Invest Ophthalmol Vis Sci 47: 5212–5217.
16. Hunter LS, Sidjanin DJ, Johnson JL, Zangerl B, Galibert F, et al. (2006) Radiation hybrid mapping of cataract genes in the dog. Mol Vis 12: 588–596.
17. Gelatt KN, Das ND (1984) Animal models for inherited cataracts: a review. Curr Eye Res 3: 765–778.
18. Tripathi BJ, Tripathi RC, Borisuth NS, Dhaliwal R, Dhaliwal D (1991) Rodent models of congenital and hereditary cataract in man. Lens Eye Toxic Res 8: 373–413.
19. Wilson GR, Morton JD, Palmer DN, McEwan JC, Gately K, et al. (2012) The locus for an inherited cataract in sheep maps to ovine chromosome 6. Mol Vis 18: 1384–1394.
20. Morton JD, Lee HY, McDermott JD, Robertson LJ, Bickerstaffe R, et al. (2013) Macrocyclic calpain inhibitor slows the development of inherited cortical cataracts in a sheep model. Invest Ophthalmol Vis Sci 54: 389–395.
21. Detlefson JA, Yapp WW (1920) The inheritance of congenital cataract in cattle. Amer Nat 54: 277–280.
22. Gregory PW, Mead SW, Regan WM (1943) A congenital hereditary eye defect of cattle. J Hered 34: 125–128.
23. Krump L, O'Grady L, Lorenz I, Grimes T (2014) Congenital cataracts in an Ayrshire herd: a herd case report. Ir Vet J 67: 2.

24. Hässig M, Jud F, Naegeli H, Kuppe J, Spiess M (2009) Prevalence of nuclear cataract in Swiss veal calves and its possible association with mobile telephone antenna base stations. Schweiz Archiv Tierheilkd 151: 471–478.
25. Hirano T, Matsuhashi T, Kobayashi N, Watanabe T, Sugimoto Y (2012) Identification of an FBN1 mutation in bovine Marfan syndrome-like disease. Anim Genet 43: 11–17.
26. Testoni S, Bartolone E, Rossi M, Patrignani A, Bruggmann R, et al. (2012) KDM2B is implicated in bovine lethal multi-organic developmental dysplasia. PLoS One 7: e45634.
27. Murgiano L, Sacchetto R, Testoni S, Dorotea T, Mascarello F, et al. (2012) Pseudomyotonia in Romagnola cattle caused by novel ATP2A1 mutations. BMC Vet Res 8: 186.
28. Clark JI, Matsushima H, David LL, Clark JM (1999) Lens cytoskeleton and transparency: a model. Eye (Lond) 13: 417–424.
29. Rausch T, Zichner T, Schlattl A; Stütz AM, Benes V, et al. (2012) DELLY: structural variant discovery by integrated paired-end and split-read analysis Bioinformatics 28: i333–i339.
30. Salmivirta K, Talts JF, Olsson M, Sasaki T, Timpl R, et al. (2002) Binding of mouse nidogen-2 to basement membrane components and cells and its expression in embryonic and adult tissues suggest complementary functions of the two nidogens. Exp Cell Res 279: 188–201.
31. Dong L, Chen Y, Lewis M, Hsieh JC, Reing J, et al. (2002) Neurologic defects and selective disruption of basement membranes in mice lacking entactin-1/nidogen-1. Lab Invest 82: 1617–1630.
32. Chang TC, Yang Y, Yasue H, Bharti AK, Retzel EF (2011) The expansion of the PRAME gene family in Eutheria. PLoS One 6: e16867.
33. Murgiano L, Testoni S, Drögemüller C, Bolcato M, Gentile A (2013) Frequency of bovine congenital pseudomyotonia carriers in selected Italian Chianina sires. Vet J 195: 238–240.
34. Murgiano L, Drögemüller C, Sbarra F, Bolcato M, Gentile A (2014). Prevalence of paunch calf syndrome carriers in Italian Romagnola cattle. Vet J 200: 459–461.
35. Darbro BW, Mahajan VB, Gakhar L, Skeie JM, Campbell E, et al. (2013) Mutations in extracellular matrix genes NID1 and LAMC1 cause autosomal dominant Dandy-Walker malformation and occipital cephaloceles. Hum Mutat 34: 1075–1079.
36. Takagi J, Yang Y, Liu JH, Wang JH, Springer TA (2003) Complex between nidogen and laminin fragments reveals a paradigmatic beta-propeller interface. Nature 424: 969–974.
37. Carlin B, Jaffe R, Bender B, Chung AE (1981) Entactin, a novel basal lamina-associated sulfated glycoprotein. J Biol Chem 256: 5209–5214.
38. Timpl R, Dziadek M, Fujiwara S, Nowack H, Wick G (1983) Nidogen: a new, self-aggregating basement membrane protein. Eur J Biochem 137: 455–465.
39. Kimura N, Toyoshima T, Kojima T, Shimane M (1998) Entactin-2: a new member of basement membrane protein with high homology to entactin/nidogen. Exp Cell Res 241: 36–45.
40. Kohfeldt E, Sasaki T, Göhring W, Timpl R (1998) Nidogen-2: a new basement membrane protein with diverse binding properties. J Mol Biol 282: 99–109.
41. Yurchenco PD, Amenta PS, Patton BL (2004) Basement membrane assembly, stability and activities observed through a developmental lens. Matrix Biol 22: 521–538.
42. Yurchenco PD, Patton BL (2009) Developmental and pathogenic mechanisms of basement membrane assembly. Curr Pharm Des 15: 1277–1294.
43. Fox J, Mayer U, Nischt R, Aumailley M, Reinhardt D, et al. (1991) Recombinant nidogen consists of three globular domains and mediates binding of laminin to collagen type IV. EMBO J 10: 3137–3146.
44. Aumailley M, Battaglia C, Mayer U, Reinhardt D, Nischt R, et al. (1993) Nidogen mediates the formation of ternary complexes of basement membrane components. Kidney Int 43: 7–12.
45. Murshed M, Smyth N, Miosge M, Karolat J, Krieg T, et al. (2000) The absence of nidogen-1 does not affect murine basement membrane development. Mol Cell Biol 20: 7007–7012.
46. Schymeinsky J, Nedbal S, Miosge N, Pöschl E, Rao C, et al. (2002) Gene structure and functional analysis of the mouse nidogen-2 gene: nidogen-2 is not essential for basement membrane formation in mice. Mol Cell Biol 22: 6820–6830.
47. Miosge N, Sasaki T, Timpl R (2002) Evidence of nidogen-2 compensation for nidogen-1 deficiency in transgenic mice. Matrix Biol 21: 611–621.
48. Miosge N, Holzhausen S, Zelent C, Sprysch P, Herken R (2001) Nidogen-1 and nidogen-2 are found in basement membranes during human embryonic development. Histochem J 33: 523–530.
49. Neu R, Adams S, Munz B (2006) Differential expression of entactin-1/nidogen-1 andentactin-2/nidogen-2 in myogenic differentiation. Differentiation 74: 573–582.
50. Bader B, Smyth N, Nedbal S, Miosge N, Baranowsky A, et al. (2005) Compound genetic ablation of nidogen 1 and 2 causes basement membrane defects and perinatal lethality in mice. Mol Cell Biol 25: 6846–6856.
51. Vasudevan A, Ho MS, Weiergräber M, Nischt R, Schneider T (2010) Basement membrane protein nidogen-1 shapes hippocampal synaptic plasticity and excitability. Hippocampus 20: 608–620.
52. Böse K, Nischt R, Page A, Bader BL, Paulsson M, et al. (2006) Loss of nidogen-1 and -2 results in syndactyly and changes in limb development. J Biol Chem 281: 39620–39629.
53. Gresham HD, Graham IL, Griffin GL, Hsieh JC, Dong LJ, et al. (1996) Domain-specific interactions between entactin and neutrophil integrins: G2 domain ligation of integrin alpha3beta1 and E domain ligation of the leukocyte response integrin signal for different responses. J Biol Chem 271: 30587–30594.
54. Darbro BW, Mahajan VB, Gakhar L, Skeie JM, Campbell E, et al. (2013) Mutations in extracellular matrix genes NID1 and LAMC1 cause autosomal dominant Dandy-Walker malformation and occipital cephaloceles. Hum Mutat 34: 1075–1079.
55. Aszódi A, Legate KR, Nakchbandi I, Fässler R (2006) What mouse mutants teach us about extracellular matrix function. Annu Rev Cell Dev Biol 22: 591–621.
56. Breitkreutz D, Koxholt I, Thiemann K, Nischt R (2013) Skin Basement Membrane: The Foundation of Epidermal Integrity—BM Functions and Diverse Roles of Bridging Molecules Nidogen and Perlecan. BioMed Research Int DOI: 10.1155.
57. May CA (2012) Distribution of nidogen in the murine eye and ocular phenotype of the nidogen-1 knockout mouse. ISRN Ophthalmol doi:10.5402.
58. Marchitti SA, Bateman JB, Petrash JM, Vasiliou V (2008) Mouse Models of the Cornea and Lens: Understanding Ocular Disease. In: Tsonis PA, editor, animal models in eye research. Academic Press, Elsiever.
59. Aulchenko YS, Ripke S, Isaacs A, van Duijn CM (2007) GenABEL: an R library for genome-wide association analysis. Bioinformatics 23: 1294–1296.
60. Purcell S, Neale B, Todd-Brown K, Thomas L, Ferreira MAR, et al. (2007) PLINK: a toolset for whole-genome association and population-based linkage analysis. Am J Hum Genet 81: 559–575.
61. Li H, Durbin R (2009) Fast and accurate short read alignment with Burrows-Wheeler transform. Bioinformatics 25: 1754–1760.
62. Hompage Samtools (2014). Available: http://samtools.sourceforge.net. Accessed 2014 Feb 27.
63. McKenna A, Hanna M, Banks E, Sivachenko A, Cibulskis K, et al. (2010) The genome analysis toolkit: a MapReduce framework for analyzing next-generation DNA sequencing data. Genome Res 20: 1297–1303.
64. Homepage European Nucleotide Archive (2014). Available: http://www.ebi.ac.uk/ena/data/view/PRJEB5965. Accessed 2014 Jul 14.
65. Cingolani P, Platts A, Coon M, Nguyen T, Wang L, et al. (2012) A program for annotating and predicting the effects of single nucleotide polymorphisms, SnpEff: SNPs in the genome of Drosophila melanogaster strain w1118; iso-2; iso-3. Fly 6: 80–92.
66. Untergrasser A, Cutcutache I, Koressaar T, Ye J, Faircloth BC, et al. (2012) Primer3 - new capabilities and interfaces. Nucleic Acids Res 40: e115.

13

The Whole Macular Choroidal Thickness in Subjects with Primary Open Angle Glaucoma

Shunsuke Nakakura[1]*, Minami Yamamoto[1], Etsuko Terao[1], Toshihiko Nagasawa[1], Hitoshi Tabuchi[1], Yoshiaki Kiuchi[2]

1 Department of Ophthalmology, Saneikai Tsukazaki Hospital, Himeji, Japan, **2** Department of Ophthalmology and Visual Sciences, Graduate School of Biomedical Sciences, Hiroshima University, Hiroshima, Japan

Abstract

Purpose: We investigated the whole macular choroidal thickness in subjects with glaucoma in order to evaluate the effects of glaucoma and glaucoma visual field damage on the choroidal thickness.

Subjects and Methods: We examined 40 primary open angle glaucoma patients with only superior visual field defects and 48 normal controls. The macular choroidal thickness was measured using swept-source optical coherence tomography according to the three-dimensional raster scan protocol (6×6 mm). We used the choroidal thickness within a 1.0-mm circle measured on ETDRS grids as the central sector and then used a 6×6 rectangular grid to divide the area into six sectors.

Results: No significant differences were found in the choroidal thickness values between the glaucoma and normal subjects in any of the sectors after adjusting for the age and axial length (all P>0.4, ANCOVA). According to a stepwise analysis of the glaucoma subjects performed using the parameters of age, axial length, central corneal thickness and mean deviation (MD value) obtained by static perimetry, age was the most predictive and significant factor in all sectors (coefficient = −3.091 to −4.091 and F value = 15.629 to 22.245), followed by axial length (coefficient = −10.428 to −23.458 and F value = 2.454 to 6.369). The central corneal thickness and MD values were not significant predictive factors in any of the sectors. No significant predictive factors were found for the differences in the choroidal thickness values observed between the superior and inferior field sectors.

Conclusions: Neither the glaucoma-related visual field damage nor glaucoma itself have any apparent associations with the whole macular choroidal thickness.

Trial Registration: Japan Clinical Trials Register (http://www.umin.ac.jp/ctr/ number, UMIN 000012527).

Editor: Demetrios Vavvas, Massachusetts Eye & Ear Infirmary, Harvard Medical School, United States of America

Funding: The authors have no support or funding to report.

Competing Interests: The authors have declared that no competing interests exist.

* Email: shunsukenakakura@yahoo.co.jp

Introduction

Whether the choroidal thickness is truly associated with the etiology or progression of glaucoma remains unknown. The uvea (choroid, iris and ciliary body) contains abundant large and small vessels, and utilizes more than 80% of the ocular blood flow [1]. The factors that influence the ocular blood flow, such as a low systolic perfusion pressure, low systolic blood pressure and history of cardiovascular disease, have been reported to be predictors of long-term glaucoma progression [2]. Recently, the development of enhanced-depth imaging optical coherence tomography (OCT) based on spectral-domain OCT has enabled clinicians to measure the choroidal thickness noninvasively. Previous studies have reported that a thinner choroidal thickness value at the fovea is associated with an older age [3–9], longer axial length [3–6,8,9] and thicker central corneal thickness (CCT) [6,9].

With respect to the association between glaucoma and the choroidal thickness, previous reports have shown no significant differences between glaucoma patients and normal subjects [5,7,9] or among individuals suspected of having glaucoma [6] based on the choroidal thickness value. However, Hirooka et al. reported that, in the setting of normal tension glaucoma (NTG), which was diagnosed when there was an untreated peak IOP≤21 mmHg, including the 24-h fluctuations, there was choroidal thinning 3 mm nasal from the fovea compared with that observed in normal subjects [10]. Meanwhile, Usui et al. reported that, in highly myopic eyes (with a spherical equivalent refractive error between -6 and -12 diopters, and an axial length greater than 26.5 mm), NTG patients exhibit thinner choroidal values at the fovea and around the optic disc than subjects without glaucoma [11]. However, even if the choroidal thinning or thickening is associated with glaucoma, whether such changes in the choroidal

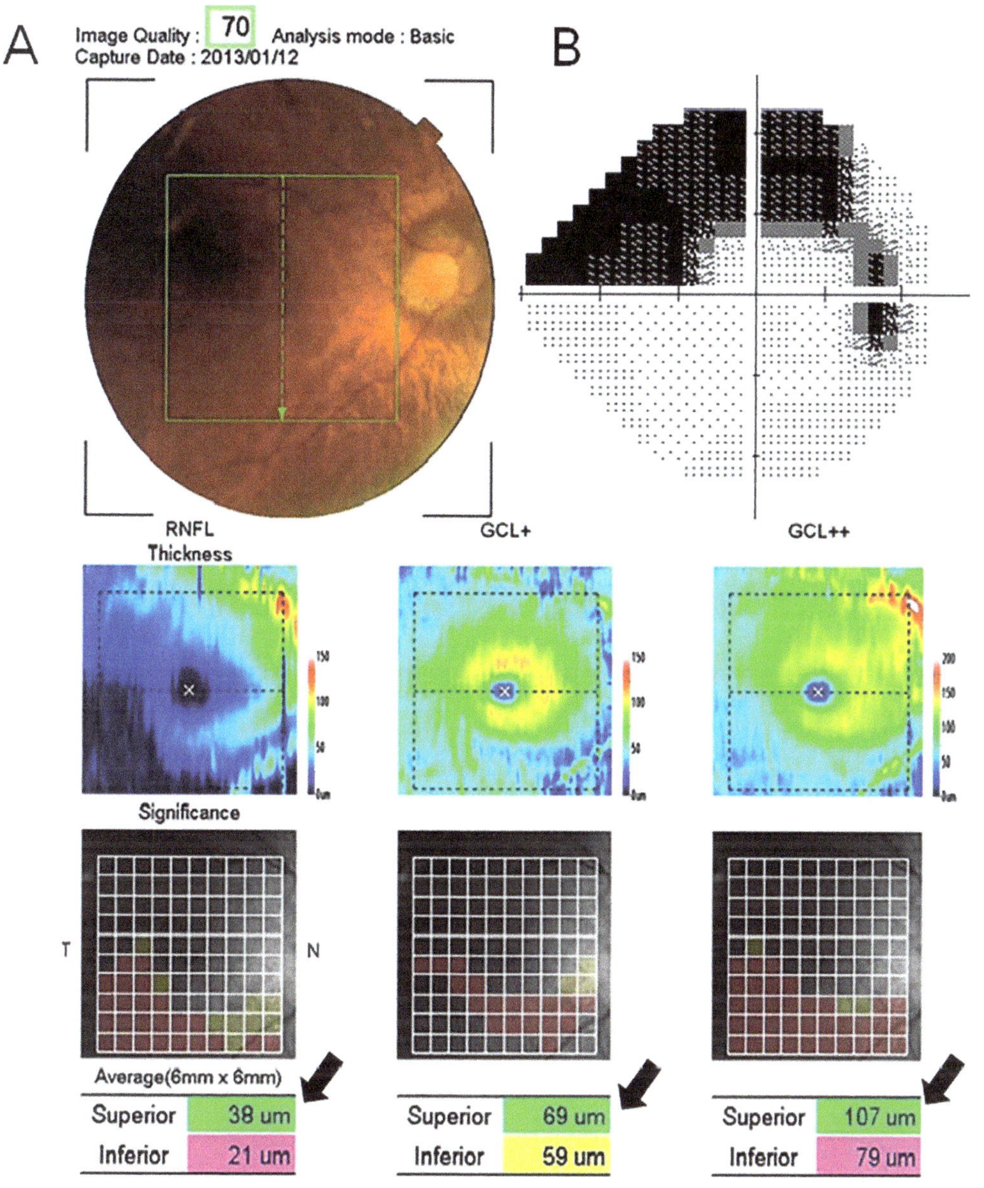

Figure 1. The 3D-OCT map and results of the HFA test in a 71-year-old male subject with glaucoma. (A) The 3D-OCT map provides a 10×10 grid map of the macular RNFL (GCL+), ganglion cell layer (GCL)/inner plexiform layer (IPL) thickness (GCL++) and macular RNFL+GCL+IPL. Upper panel: a pseudo-colored map of the measured thickness. Center panel: Each grid in the 10×10 grid was color-coded, with no color (within the normal limit), yellow (outside of the 95% normal limit) or red (outside of the 99% normal limit) used to indicate different values. Lower panel: the thicknesses of the total, superior and inferior hemiretinal sectors. The black arrows show the superior hemiretinal thickness, which is displayed as color-coded with green (within the normal limit), yellow (outside of the 95% normal limit) or red (outside of the 99% normal limit) based on the software program's normal built-in dataset. (B) The results of the HFA test. The MD was −9.38 dB ($P<0.5\%$) and the PSD was 14.54 dB ($P<0.5\%$). Superior glaucoma visual field damage corresponds to inferior optic disc rim thinning and the 3D-OCT data. The inferior visual field was intact.

thickness values are primary or occur secondarily due to the progression of glaucoma remains unknown.

Furthermore, most of the previous reports have focused on the subfoveal choroidal thickness and/or choroidal thickness values at +/− 3 mm nasal or temporal to the fovea. Glaucoma is generally characterized by optic disc changes with corresponding nerve fiver defects and visual field defects. The initial changes most frequently occur in the inferior optic disc rim, corresponding to a superior visual field defect, and it does not exceed the central line, since the normal retinal nerve fiber layers run symmetrically in the superior and inferior fields. However, the fovea is free of a nerve fiber layer, as the inner retina and ganglion cells are pushed away to the foveal slope. Therefore, the use of measurement points at the fovea or +/− 3 mm nasal or temporal to the fovea may not be appropriate for evaluating the relationship between glaucoma and the choroidal thickness.

Swept-source optical coherence tomography (SS-OCT) applies a swept wavelength laser as a light source [12,13], with a longer center wavelength that penetrates deeply into tissues. The longer wavelength (1,050 mm) of SS-OCT is attenuated by water absorption; however, SS-OCT can achieve much less roll-off, thus leading to retained sensitivity at increasing depths, and can

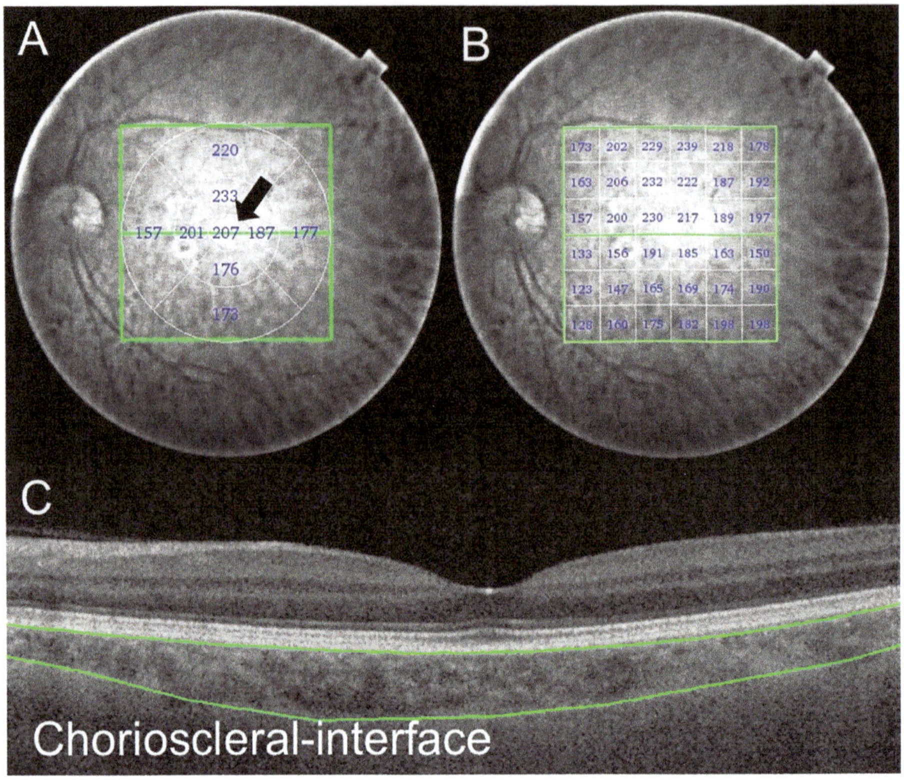

Figure 2. The choroidal thickness map of a 57-year-old normal male obtained using SS-OCT. The 3D raster scan protocol with 512A-scans ×256 B-scans was used to obtain the 3D imaging data for a 6×6-mm area. (A) The black arrow shows the central sector choroidal thickness as measured on the ETDRS grid within a 1×1-mm circular area. (B) The choroidal thickness values presented by the 6×6 rectangular grid map. Each value shows the mean choroidal thickness within a 1×1-mm square area. (C) Manual segmentation of the chorioscleral interface on the B-scan image. All 64 B-scan images were obtained for each subject.

operate at a higher speed than spectral domain OCT to obtain the choroidal thickness maps using the 3D raster scan protocol [14].

The aim of this study was to investigate the whole macular choroidal thickness (6×6 mm) in patients with superior glaucoma visual hemi-field defects in order to: 1) compare these values with those observed in normal subjects after adjusting for the previously identified factors associated with the choroidal thickness (age and axial length) and 2) to investigate whether the degree of glaucoma visual field damage is associated with the choroidal thickness and/

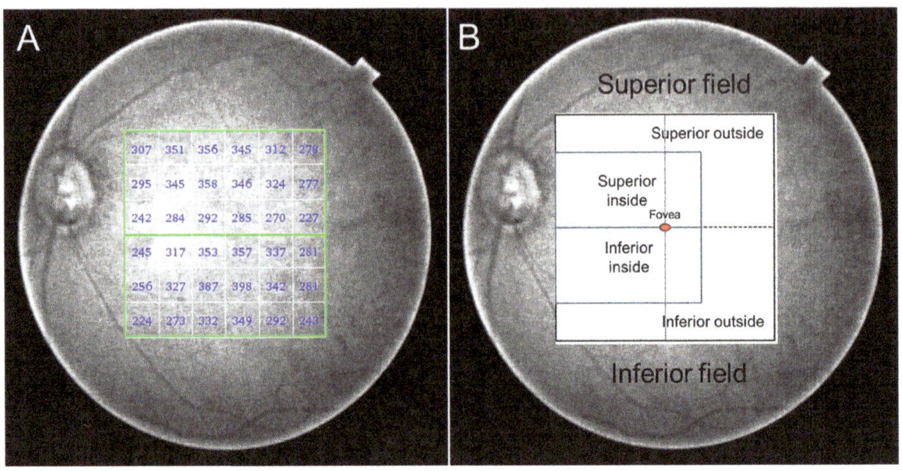

Figure 3. The choroidal thickness map of a 74-year-old female subject with glaucoma obtained using SS-OCT. (A) The choroidal thickness values presented on the 6×6 rectangular grid map. (B) The six sectors used in the present study. Each area was symmetrically divided between the superior and inferior sectors by a horizontal line.

or differences in the choroidal thickness values between the superior and inferior sectors.

Subjects and Methods

We studied 88 subjects (40 glaucoma patients and 48 normal subjects) treated at Saneikai Tsukazaki Hospital from October 2012 to December 2013. This study received approval from the Institutional Review Board of Saneikai Tsukazaki Hospital and was performed according to the tenets of the Declaration of Helsinki. Written informed consent was obtained from each participant prior to enrollment in this study. All subjects received a full ophthalmic examination (conducted by S.N. or T.N) and had a best-correlated visual acuity of more than 0.6, refractive errors (spherical equivalent) within ±6 diopters (D) and cylinder correction within ±3D. The refraction was measured using an autorefractor (KR-8800, Topcon Corporation, Japan). The axial length (AL) was measured using an IOLMaster, ver. 5.02 (Carl Zeiss Meditec, Jena, Germany), and the mean of five measurements was used in the subsequent analyses. The CCT values in the glaucoma subjects were measured with a specular microscope (SP-3000, Topcon Corporation, Japan). The intraocular pressure was measured using a Goldmann applanation tonometer with the subject in the sitting position.

All glaucoma patients had attended our clinic for at least one year and their disease was well controlled with topical anti-glaucoma eye drops. Each patient received a reliable visual field analysis (Humphry Visual Field Analyzer (HFA), Carl Zeiss Inc., Dublin, CA) according to the thresholding algorithm (SITA-standard) 30-2, and underwent HFA at four- to six-month intervals. The visual field test results used in the study were obtained within ± three months of the time when the choroidal thickness was measured, and which had fixation losses less than 20%, and the false-positive and false-negative errors were less than 15%. A glaucomatous visual field defect was defined as 1) a glaucoma hemifield test graded "outside the normal limits" and 2) a cluster of three contiguous points at the 5% level for the pattern deviation plot, with at least one point being P<1%. The mean deviation value (MD value) was used for the analysis. All patients had primary open angle glaucoma, as defined by 1) the results of a gonioscopic examination that revealed an open angle and 2) the presence of visual field defects in least one of the eyes whose locations corresponded to glaucomatous disc excavation, namely, the presence of a focal or diffuse defect of the optic disc rim with or without retinal nerve fiver layer (RNFL) defects.

In the present study, we recruited glaucoma patients who exhibited only focal or diffuse inferior optic rim thinning with corresponding superior visual field loss. Patients with a history of any previous glaucoma surgery or systemic diseases, such as diabetes mellitus or uncontrolled hypertension, the use of an oral carbonic anhydrase inhibitor (acetazolamide) and/or an unknown previous refraction before cataract surgery were excluded. Patients who displayed any optic disc changes suspected to be due to glaucoma at the superior optic disc rim confirmed based on the presence of ganglion cell-loss on three-dimensional OCT were also excluded (3D-OCT; Topcon, Inc., Tokyo, Japan). The 3D-OCT provides a 10×10 grid map of the macula RNFL and ganglion cell layer (GCL)/inner plexiform layer (IPL) thickness, and uses a software program that displays a deviation map indicating if there is a significant reduction of the total macular retinal thickness, superior hemiretinal thickness or inferior hemiretinal thickness compared to that observed in a built-in normal database in three areas (the mean macular RNFL, mean GCL/IPL and mean macular RNFL+ mean GCL/IPL), with a probability of less than 1% [15]. All glaucoma patients exhibited only inferior hemiretinal thickness abnormalities (displayed in yellow or red), with a normal superior hemiretinal thickness (displayed in green). Figure 1 shows the macular retinal thickness values in the glaucoma patients measured on 3D-OCT and the glaucoma visual field defects measured on HFA (The 3D-OCT data are provided in Table S1).

The inclusion criteria for normal subjects were 1) IOP ≤21 mm Hg 2) normal ophthalmoscopic appearance of the optic nerve (cup-to-disc ratio <0.5 in both eyes, cup-to disc ratio asymmetry <0.2, the absence of hemorrhage, or the presence of localized or diffuse rim thinning).[5] The exclusion criteria for the normal controls were as follows: 1) a history of intraocular surgery, 2) a history or evidence of chorioretinal or vitreoretinal disease and 3) systemic disease, such as diabetes mellitus or uncontrolled hypertension. Normal subjects did not undergo HFA testing.

Swept-source Optical Coherence Tomography (SS-OCT)

The macula area (6×6mm) of the eyes was examined with the SS-OCT instrument (DRI OCT-1; Topcon, Tokyo, Japan). The SS-OCT has an acquisition rate of 100,000 A-scans per second when operated with the 1-μm wavelength tunable laser centered at 1,050 nm, with an approximate 100-nm tuning range and a tissue imaging depth of 2.6 mm [14]. Following pupil dilation, the SS-OCT examinations were performed by experienced certified orthoptists (M.Y and E.T) from 1:00 PM to 5:00 PM to reduce the effects of diurnal fluctuations [16,17]. The 3D volumetric raster

Table 1. The patient demographics.

	Glaucoma N = 40		Normal N = 48		
	mean ±SD	range	mean ±SD	range	P value
Age (years)	65.2±11.8	40–85	66.4±11.8	31–87	0.631*
Sex/female (%)	31(78)		24(50)		0.007†
Right eye (%)	19(47)		27(56)		0.413†
IOP (mmHg)	15.8±2.6	12–21	15.6±2.8	9–21	0.832*
Axial length (mm)	23.7±1.2	20.6–26.0	23.9±1.1	21.8–27.6	0.514*
CCT (μm)	502.9±28.9	445–558	-	-	-
Mean deviation (dB)	−5.1±4.7	−19.64–0.24	-	-	-

*, Student's *t*-test
†, chi-square test.

Table 2. Comparisons among the sectors between the glaucoma and normal groups.

	Glaucoma	95% CI	Normal	95% CI	P value
The central sector	219.1±11.2	196.7–241.6	216.6±10.2	196.1–237.1	0.869
a: superior field ave	208.6±8.9	190.8–226.5	200.9±8.1	184.6–217.2	0.531
b: inferior field ave	193.2±9.1	174.9–211.5	185.4±8.3	168.8–202.1	0.536
c: superior inside ave	198.8±9.9	179.1–218.5	193.8±9.0	175.8–211.8	0.712
d: superior outside ave	216.7±8.5	199.7–233.6	206.6±7.7	191.1–222.1	0.390
e: inferior inside ave	188.0±10.1	167.8–208.1	183.0±9.2	164.7–201.4	0.720
f: inferior outside ave	197.3±8.7	179.8–214.7	187.4±8.0	171.4–203.3	0.408

Ave, average.
The data are presented as the age- and axial length-adjusted mean ± standard error of the mean (SEM) and 95% CI (confidence interval) (μm).
All P values were obtained with an ANCOVA using the age and axial length as covariates.

scan protocol was used, which covered an area measuring 6×6 mm centered on the fovea, with 512 A-scans × 256 B-scans. All images had image quality scores ≥45 (of 160), according to the manufacturer's recommendations.

Using a series of 64 B-scan images, each of which was created by averaging four consecutive B-scans, a choroidal thickness map was created via semiautomatic segmentation. The choroidal thickness was measured as the distance from the outer border of the retinal pigment epithelium to the inner surface of the chorioscleral interface. However, semiautomatic segmentation does not always provide the correct chorioscleral interface; therefore, manual segmentation using the built-in software program was performed on all 64 B-scan images in each patient by experienced certified orthoptists (M.Y and E.T). The interobserver reproducibility of the choroidal thickness values obtained using this manual segmentation method has previously been reported by our group, and the ICC for the choroidal thickness values between the two observers was very good (from 0.990 to 0.999) [14].

The central sector, the center of the 1.0-mm circle on the ETDRS grid (Figure 2) and the 6×6 rectangular grid (Figure 2) (1×1 mm for each section), was used for the subsequent sector analysis. The 6×6 rectangular grid (36 sections) was divided horizontally into the superior field (18 sections) and inferior field (18 sections). The superior field was divided superiorly inside (including the fovea, eight sections) and outside (the remaining 10 sections), and a similar partition was attempted on the inferior field (Figure 3). This deviation was developed for the present study based on the RNFL lanes.

Statistical Analysis

We used the JMP, version 10.0.0 software package (SAS Institute Inc., Cary, NC, USA) for the statistical analyses, and the data were expressed as the means ± standard deviation (SD). Values of $p<0.05$ were considered to be statistically significant. For comparisons of the demographic data between the glaucoma and normal subjects, we used Student's *t*-test for the age, IOP and axial length and the chi-square test for sex and the target eye.

We compared the macular choroidal thickness values between the glaucoma patients and normal subjects using an analysis of covariance, with covariance considered for age and the axial length. We used a stepwise regression analysis to evaluate the significant factors affecting the choroidal thickness and the differences in the choroidal thickness values between the sectors in the glaucoma patients based on the following representative factors: age, axial length, CCT and MD. The independent variable criterion of $P = 0.2$ was set for the analysis.

The sample size required to detect a 20% (approximately 40 μm) difference between the glaucoma and normal subjects with a significance level of 5% and a power of 80%, based on the

Table 3. The choroidal thickness values in the glaucoma group.

	mean ±SD	range
The central sector	222.6±71.7	77.0–397.0
a: superior field ave	210.4±57.1	103.7–346.8
b: inferior field ave	195.8±54.8	88.3–318.6
c: superior inside ave	202.3±64.1	90.0–359.6
d: superior outside ave	219.8±53.1	119.1–332.6
e: inferior inside ave	190.9±62.6	77.6–355.0
f: inferior outside ave	199.7±50.8	96.9–295.4
difference 1 (a-b)	14.5±29.6	−55.5–74.8
difference 2 (c-e)	11.4±24.6	−45.2–60.1
difference 3 (d-f)	20.0±33.2	−64.7–101.8

The values are presented as the means±SD (μm).
The values are slightly different from those in Table 2 because these are the raw data.

Table 4. The results of symmetrical comparisons between two sectors in the glaucoma group.

Comparison between two sectors	P value
superior vs inferior ave	0.001
superior inside vs inferior inside ave	<0.001
superior outside vs inferior outside ave	<0.001
superior inside vs outside ave	<0.001
inferior inside vs outside ave	0.004

Ave, average.
All p values were obtained using the paired t-test.

standard deviation of 54.8 μm in the inferior field choroidal thickness average in the glaucoma subjects, was estimated to be 30 patients per group.

Results

The patient demographics of the two groups and the MD values in the glaucoma patients are shown in Table 1. The glaucoma group consisted of more female patients than the normal group ($P<0.01$). No significant differences were found between the two groups in terms of the age, the target eye, IOP or axial length.

Table 2 shows the results of a comparison of the choroidal thickness values following adjustment for age and the axial length in all sectors, and the p values of the ANCOVA analysis. No significant differences were found between the glaucoma group and the normal group in any sector ($P>0.4$).

The raw data for the choroidal thickness values in the glaucoma group are shown in Table 3, and Table 4 shows a comparison between the superior field sectors and inferior field sectors (symmetrical comparison). The choroidal thickness values were significantly thinner in the inferior sectors in all symmetrical comparisons ($P<0.05$). We also compared the inside and outside choroidal thickness values, and found that the outside choroidal thickness values were significantly thicker in both the superior and inferior fields (all $P<0.05$). These data differ from the values in Table 2 because they were obtained without adjustment for age or the axial length.

The results of a stepwise regression analysis of independent predictors of the choroidal thickness, and the differences in the choroidal thickness values in all symmetrical sectors among the glaucoma subjects

Table 5 shows the results of the stepwise analyses to determine the predictors of the choroidal thickness using the previously reported factors; age, axial length, CCT and MD. According to these analyses, the age was found to be the most predictive and significant factor for the choroidal thickness in all seven sectors ($P<0.001$). The axial length was the second most predictive factor and was found to be a statistically significant predictor in almost all sectors. The CCT was identified as the only predictive factor in the symmetrical comparisons; however, all adjusted R2 values in the symmetrical comparison were low (0.037–0.063) and were not statistically significant (all $p>0.05$). The MD value was not identified as a significant factor in any sector or in the symmetrical comparisons.

Discussion

In the present study, we first reported that the whole macular choroidal thickness values in glaucoma subjects do not differ significantly from those of normal subjects. Previous reports have only shown pinpoint measurements of the choroidal thickness obtained using the enhanced-depth imaging method; however, by using SS-OCT, we were able to analyze the whole macular choroidal thickness and compare different sectors. The subjects evaluated in the present study exhibited only focal or diffuse inferior optic rim thinning with corresponding superior visual field damage. We first assumed that in such patients, the inferior macular choroidal thickness might be thinner due to the glaucoma-related damage compared with the superior macular choroidal thickness or the thickness in normal subjects.

However, no significant differences in the macular choroidal thickness were found between glaucoma patients and normal subjects in any of the sectors (All $p>0.4$). Furthermore, our results obtained by a stepwise regression analysis showed that the differences in the choroidal thickness values observed between the superior and inferior sectors had no association with glaucoma damage (MD value), suggesting that the secondary changes due to the progression of glaucoma may not extend to the choroid. This observation was also confirmed by the results of a comparison among sectors in the glaucoma patients (Table 4). The glaucoma patients had thicker values in the superior field than in the inferior field and in the temporal field (outside sector) compared to the nasal field (inside sector) in our study, similar to the findings observed in normal subjects [4,5,18]. The macular choroidal thickness value was affected by age and the axial length, but not the CCT or MD values, according to the stepwise regression analysis performed in this study. Therefore, this result suggests that the whole macular choroidal thickness values of our glaucoma patients were similar to those obtained in normal subjects, as demonstrated in previous reports [5,7,8]. Moreover, the values were not affected by either glaucoma itself or by glaucoma visual field progression.

Both glaucoma patients and normal subjects had a decreased choroidal thickness in inferior sections (Table 2), which is supported by the data form normal adults and children reported by Nagasawa et al. [12]. In addition, the initial changes in glaucoma frequently occur in the inferior optic disc rim, with superior visual field defects being found in glaucoma patients. It has been speculated that inferior choroidal thinning plus some other factors (not choroidal thinning alone) might be associated with the initial glaucomatous changes. However, no mechanism responsible for these changes has been proven. Ikuno et al., advocated two mechanisms underlying the inferior choroidal

Table 5. The results of the stepwise regression analyses of the choroidal thickness values using the age, axial length, CCT and MD as variables in the glaucoma group.

	Independent variables												
	Age			Axial length			CCT			MD value			
Dependent variables	Coefficient	F value	P value	Coefficient	F value	P value	Coefficient	F value	P value	Coefficient	F value	P value	Adjusted R^2
The central sector	**−4.091**	**17.718**	**<0.001**	**−23.458**	**5.646**	**0.022**	-			-			0.287
a: superior field average	**−3.309**	**18.515**	**<0.001**	**−16.963**	**4.715**	**0.036**	-			-			0.297
b: inferior field average	**−3.237**	**19.713**	**<0.001**	**−15.246**	**4.239**	**0.046**	-			-			0.313
c: superior inside average	**−3.568**	**16.545**	**<0.001**	**−22.536**	**6.369**	**0.015**	-			-			0.274
d: superior outside average	**−3.191**	**20.158**	**<0.001**	−13.531	3.510	0.069	0.325	1.753	0.193	-			0.318
e: inferior inside average	**−3.418**	**15.629**	**<0.001**	**−21.267**	**5.863**	**0.020**	-			-			0.261
f: inferior outside average	**−3.091**	**22.245**	**<0.001**	−10.428	2.454	0.125	-			-			0.355
Difference 1 (a-b)	-			-			0.275	3.631	0.064	-			0.063
Difference 2 (c-e)	-			-			0.212	2.533	0.119	-			0.037
Difference 3 (d-f)	-			-			0.329	3.395	0.073	-			0.057

-: excluded variables.
Statistically significant independent factors for the dependent variables are shown in bold.

thinning in normal subjects; one is the choroidal watershed, which isolates the choroidal circulation, and the other is the fetal choroidal fissure, which closes inferiorly at 16 weeks [19]. It also remains unclear as to why the initial changes due to glaucoma occur in the inferior rim; although gravity may be the simplest explanation.

In a comparison of the group characteristics, our glaucoma patients included more females than the normal control group ($P < 0.01$). This was likely due to patient selection, because typical notches or rim thinning are usually observed in patients with focal ischemic type discs, as classified by Nicolela and Drance [20]. They classified the glaucoma disc morphology into four subtypes: focal ischemic, myopic glaucomatous, senile sclerotic and generalized enlargement. The focal ischemic type is most commonly observed in female patients with primary open angle glaucoma [20], and similar findings have been noted in patients with normal tension glaucoma (NTG) [21].

However, Roberts et al. reported that there was a relationship between these glaucoma optic disc types and the peripapillary choroidal thickness values, in that patients with focal ischemic and generalized enlargement exhibited no statistically significant differences compared to healthy subjects [22]. No significant differences were found in the central sector choroidal thickness between the normal females and males (208.9 μm vs 218.6 μm, $P = 0.678$ by Student's *t*-test). Furthermore, no significant differences were found in the central sector choroidal thickness between female and male glaucoma patients (216.7 μm vs 242.6 μm, $P = 0.347$ according to Student's t-test). These data support our results, and previous reports have shown that sex is not a useful factor for predicting the choroidal thickness [6,8].

Other assessments to clarify the relationship between glaucoma and the choroidal thickness have been carried out by investigating the choroidal thickness values in peripapillary areas [6,22–24]. Because the blood supply of the prelaminar region of the optic nerve head is supplied by peripapillary choroidal vessels, and because the laminar cribrosa is supplied by the arterial circle of Zinn or the branches of the posterior ciliary arteries that supply the choroid [25], investigating the relationship between the peripapillary choroidal thickness and glaucoma is interesting. However, Maul et al. reported that the peripapillary choroidal thickness values were not significantly different between glaucoma and suspected glaucoma patients, and were not associated with glaucoma-related damage or the RNFL thickness [6]. Ehrlich et al. [23]. also reported that the peripapillary choroidal thickness values were not associated with the glaucoma damage, the RNFL thickness or the zone of β clock hours parapapillary choroidal atrophy, which are associated with glaucoma damage [26], in either glaucoma subjects or suspected cases. In addition, Suh et al. used spectral-domain OCT and reported that the peripapillary choroidal thickness values correlated with the subject age and axial length, but not with the CCT, MD, IOP or the presence of systemic disease [24].

These previous reports showed no apparent evidence of a relationship between glaucoma and the peripapillary choroidal thickness, which supports our results showing that neither glaucoma-related visual damage nor glaucoma itself have any apparent associations with the whole macular choroidal thickness.

Meanwhile, Usui et al. hypothesized that the 50% thinning in the choroidal thickness values observed in patients with highly myopic NTG results in reduced choroidal circulation, which may be associated with narrowing of the posterior ciliary arteries due to axial length elongation [11]. The differences in the anatomical structure caused by an abnormal refractive error may account for the differences in conclusions between the present and that study [11].

One limitation of the present study is that the adjusted R^2 values obtained in the stepwise analysis were <0.4. The age and axial length are representative predictive factors for the CT value. However, Aksoy et al. reported that the choroidal thickness is affected by more factors than was previously estimated; for example, the diurnal choroidal thickness changes occur at 30–60 μm, and the use of intravenous acetazolamide increases the CT values [27]. Therefore, we measured the choroidal thickness values during a limited time period (from 1:00 PM to 5:00 PM), and patients receiving an oral topical carbonic inhibitor (acetazolamide) were excluded. However, some patients use topical carbonic inhibitors, which can be absorbed through the mucous membranes in the nose, which then enter the intravenous circulation. In addition, topical prostaglandin analogues and beta blockers have the potential to affect the choroidal thickness. Furthermore, the systolic blood pressure values [16] and hypercholesterolemia [28] may also affect the choroidal thickness; however, these parameters were not examined in this study.

A second limitation is that this study included a relatively small number of subjects. However, it fulfilled a strict power analysis to detect a 20% difference in the choroidal thickness (40 μm) between glaucoma subjects and normal subjects compared with previous reports of 63 μm [5,8]. A third limitation is that whether the choroidal thickness truly represents the choroidal blood flow remains to be elucidated. In healthy younger subjects, the choroidal thickness was not associated with either the total choroidal blood flow or the subfoveal choroidal blood flow [29]. However, systemic administration of sildenafil citrate (Viagra, Pfizer, New York, NY) has been reported to increase the choroidal blood flow and the choroidal thickness in healthy subjects [30]. Further studies are therefore necessary to clarify the relationship between the choroidal thickness and the choroidal blood flow.

The fourth limitation is that we used manual segmentation techniques, according to previous reports. However, Mansouri et al. recently reported that the findings of automated segmentation obtained using SS-OCT are not affected by operator effects, and exhibit a high level of repeatability, and that the main artifact is blinking, not segmentation errors [31]. The fifth limitation associated with this study is that SS-OCT could cover only 20 degrees in the macula area which thus correlated with the first and second test-points in the 30-2 test program. The 10-2 test program was too small for the region and could not reflect the glaucoma visual field damage, therefore the 24-2 test program might closely correlate with the macula area obtained by SS-OCT. In summary, this study demonstrated that neither glaucoma-related visual damage nor glaucoma itself has any apparent association with the whole macular choroidal thickness.

Supporting Information

Table S1 The 3D-OCT values in the glaucoma group. All p values were obtained using the paired t-test. The values are presented as the mean±SD (μm).

Acknowledgments

The authors thank Hajime Yamakage for his advice on the statistical analyses performed in this study.

Author Contributions

Conceived and designed the experiments: SN TN HT YK. Performed the experiments: SN TN ET MY. Analyzed the data: SN HT. Contributed reagents/materials/analysis tools: SN. Wrote the paper: SN.

References

1. Alm A (1992) Ocular circulation. In: Moses R, Hart W (ed.) Adlerâ s physiology of the eye; clinical applications.9th ed.St Louis C.V Mosby; 198–227.
2. Leske MC, Heijl A, Hyman L, Bengtsson B, Dong L, et al (2007) Predictors of long-term progression in the early manifest glaucoma trial. Ophthalmology 114(11):1965–1972.
3. Ikuno Y, Kawaguchi K, Nouchi T, Yasuno Y (2010) Choroidal thickness in healthy Japanese subjects. Invest Ophthalmol Vis Sci 51(4):2173–2176.
4. Hirata M, Tsujikawa A, Matsumoto A, Hangai M, Ooto S, et al (2011) Macular choroidal thickness and volume in normal subjects measured by swept-source optical coherence tomography. Invest Ophthalmol Vis Sci 52(8):4971–4978.
5. Mwanza JC, Hochberg JT, Banitt MR, Feuer WJ, Budenz DL (2011) Lack of association between glaucoma and macular choroidal thickness measured with enhanced depth-imaging optical coherence tomography. Invest Ophthalmol Vis Sci 52(6):3430–3435.
6. Maul EA, Friedman DS, Chang DS, Boland MV, Ramulu PY, et al (2011) Choroidal thickness measured by spectral domain optical coherence tomography: factors affecting thickness in glaucoma patients. Ophthalmology 118(8):1571–1579
7. Rhew JY, Kim YT, Choi KR (2014) Measurement of subfoveal choroidal thickness in normal-tension glaucoma in Korean patients. J Glaucoma 23(1):46–49.
8. Mwanza JC, Sayyad FE, Budenz DL (2012) Choroidal thickness in unilateral advanced glaucoma. Invest Ophthalmol Vis Sci 53(10):6695–6701.
9. Arora KS, Jefferys JL, Maul EA, Quigley HA (2012) The choroid is thicker in angle closure than in open angle and control eyes. Invest Ophthalmol Vis Sci 53(12):7813–7818.
10. Hirooka K, Fujiwara A, Shiragami C, Baba T, Shiraga F (2012) Relationship between progression of visual field damage and choroidal thickness in eyes with normal-tension glaucoma. Clin Experiment Ophthalmol 40(6):576–582.
11. Usui S1, Ikuno Y, Miki A, Matsushita K, Yasuno Y, et al (2012) Evaluation of the choroidal thickness using high-penetration optical coherence tomography with long wavelength in highly myopic normal-tension glaucoma. Am J Ophthalmol 153(1):10–16.
12. Ohno-Matsui K, Akiba M, Moriyama M, Ishibashi T, Tokoro T, et al (2011) Imaging retrobulbar subarachnoid space around optic nerve by swept-source optical coherence tomography in eyes with pathologic myopia. Invest Ophthalmol Vis Sci 52(13):9644–9650.
13. Spaide RF, Akiba M, Ohno-Matsui K (2012) Evaluation of peripapillary intrachoroidal cavitation with swept source and enhanced depth imaging optical coherence tomography. Retina 2012:1037–44.
14. Nagasawa T, Mitamura Y, Katome T, Shinomiya K, Naito T, et al (2013) Macular choroidal thickness and volume in healthy pediatric individuals measured by swept-source optical coherence tomography. Invest Ophthalmol Vis Sci 54(10):7068–7074.
15. Kanamori A, Naka M, Akashi A, Fujihara M, Yamada Y, et al (2013) Cluster analyses of grid-pattern display in macular parameters using optical coherence tomography for glaucoma diagnosis. Invest Ophthalmol Vis Sci 54(9):6401–6408.
16. Usui S, Ikuno Y, Akiba M, Maruko I, Sekiryu T, et al (2012) Circadian changes in subfoveal choroidal thickness and the relationship with circulatory factors in healthy subjects. Invest Ophthalmol Vis Sci 53(4):2300–2307.
17. Tan CS, Ouyang Y, Ruiz H, Sadda SR (2012) Diurnal variation of choroidal thickness in normal, healthy subjects measured by spectral domain optical coherence tomography. Invest Ophthalmol Vis Sci 53(1):261–266.
18. Margolis R, Spaide RF (2009) A pilot study of enhanced depth imaging optical coherence tomography of the choroid in normal eyes. Am J Ophthalmol 147(5):811–815.
19. Ikuno Y, Kawaguchi K, Nouchi T, Yasuno Y (2010) Choroidal thickness in healthy Japanese subjects. Invest Ophthalmol Vis Sci 51(4):2173–2176.
20. Nicolela MT, Drance SM (1996) Various glaucomatous optic nerve appearances: clinical correlations. Ophthalmology 103(4):640–649.
21. Nakazawa T, Shimura M, Ryu M, Himori N, Nitta F, et al (2012) Progression of visual field defects in eyes with different optic disc appearances in patients with normal tension glaucoma. J Glaucoma 21(6):426–430.
22. Roberts KF, Artes PH, O'Leary N, Reis AS, Sharpe GP, et al (2012) Peripapillary choroidal thickness in healthy controls and patients with focal, diffuse, and sclerotic glaucomatous optic disc damage. Arch Ophthalmol 130(8):980–986.
23. Ehrlich JR, Peterson J, Parlitsis G, Kay KY, Kiss S, et al (2011) Peripapillary choroidal thickness in glaucoma measured with optical coherence tomography. Exp Eye Res 92(3):189–194.

24. Suh W, Cho HK, Kee C (2014) Evaluation of peripapillary choroidal thickness in unilateral normal-tension glaucoma. Jpn J Ophthalmol 58(1):62–67.
25. Hayreh SS (1969) Blood supply of the optic nerve head and its role in optic atrophy, glaucoma, and oedema of the optic disc. Br J Ophthalmol 53(11):721–748.
26. Manjunath V, Shah H, Fujimoto JG, Duker JS (2011) Analysis of peripapillary atrophy using spectral domain optical coherence tomography. Ophthalmology 118(3):531–536.
27. Aksoy Y, Çolakoglu K, Kar T, Sevinc MK, Eyi YE (2014) Choroidal thickness is affected by more factors than estimated. Invest Ophthalmol Vis Sci 55(3):1311.
28. Wong IY, Wong RL, Zhao P, Lai WW (2013) Choroidal thickness in relation to hypercholesterolemia on enhanced depth imaging optical coherence tomography. Retina 33(2):423–428.
29. Sogawa K, Nagaoka T, Takahashi A, Tanano I, Tani T, et al (2012) Relationship between choroidal thickness and choroidal circulation in healthy young subjects. Am J Ophthalmol 153(6):1129–1132.
30. Kim DY, Silverman RH, Chan RV, Khanifar AA, Rondeau M, et al (2013) Measurement of choroidal perfusion and thickness following systemic sildenafil (Viagra). Acta Ophthalmol 91(2):183–188.
31. Mansouri K, Medeiros FA, Tatham AJ, Marchase N, Weinreb RN (2014) Evaluation of retinal and choroidal thickness by swept-source optical coherence tomography: repeatability and assessment of artifacts. Am J Ophthalmol 157(5):1022–1032.

Neuroprotection of a Novel Cyclopeptide C*HSDGIC* from the Cyclization of PACAP (1–5) in Cellular and Rodent Models of Retinal Ganglion Cell Apoptosis

Huanhuan Cheng[1], Yong Ding[2]*, Rongjie Yu[3], Jiansu Chen[4], Chunyun Wu[5]

1 Department of Ophthalmology, The Third Affiliated Hospital of Sun Yat-sen University, Guangzhou, China, **2** Department of Ophthalmology, The First Affiliated Hospital of Jinan University, Guangzhou, China, **3** Bio-engineering Institute of Jinan University, Jinan University, Guangzhou, China, **4** Department of Ophthalmology, Medical College, Jinan University, Guangzhou, China, **5** Department of Parasitology, Medical College, Jinan University, Guangzhou, China

Abstract

Purpose: To investigate the protective effects of a novel cyclopeptide C*HSDGIC* (CHC) from the cyclization of Pituitary adenylate cyclase-activating polypeptide (PACAP) (1–5) in cellular and rodent models of retinal ganglion cell apoptosis.

Methodology/Principal Findings: Double-labeling immunohistochemistry was used to detect the expression of Thy-1 and PACAP receptor type 1 in a retinal ganglion cell line RGC-5. The apoptosis of RGC-5 cells was induced by 0.02 J/cm^2 Ultraviolet B irradiation. MTT assay, flow cytometry, fluorescence microscopy were used to investigate the viability, the level of reactive oxygen species (ROS) and apoptosis of RGC-5 cells respectively. CHC attenuated apoptotic cell death induced by Ultraviolet B irradiation and inhibited the excessive generation of ROS. Moreover, CHC treatment resulted in decreased expression of Bax and concomitant increase of Bcl-2, as was revealed by western-blot analysis. The in vivo apoptosis of retinal ganglion cells was induced by injecting 50 mM N-methyl-D-aspartate (NMDA) (100 nmol in a 2 μL saline solution) intravitreally, and different dosages of CHC were administered. At day 7, rats in CHC+ NMDA-treated groups showed obvious aversion to light when compared to NMDA rats. Electroretinogram recordings revealed a marked decrease in the amplitudes of a-wave, b-wave, and photopic negative response due to NMDA damage. In retina receiving intravitreal NMDA and CHC co-treatment, these values were significantly increased. CHC treatment also resulted in less NMDA-induced cell loss and a decrease in the proportion of dUTP end-labeling-positive cells in ganglion cell line.

Conclusions: C*HSDGIC*, a novel cyclopeptide from PACAP (1–5) attenuates apoptosis in RGC-5 cells and inhibits NMDA-induced retinal neuronal death. The beneficial effects may occur via the mitochondria pathway. PACAP derivatives like CHC may serve as a promising candidate for neuroprotection in glaucoma.

Editor: Rafael Linden, Universidade Federal do Rio de Janeiro, Brazil

Funding: This study was supported by National Natural Science Foundation of China (No. 31100545) (http://www.nsfc.gov.cn/nsfc/cen/daima/index.html) and the Science and Technology Bureau of Guangdong Province (2012B010300015) (http://pro.gdstc.gov.cn/stms/main.jsp). The funders had no role in study design, data collection and analysis, decision to publish, or preparation of the manuscript.

Competing Interests: The authors have declared that no competing interests exist.

* Email: dingyongjnu@163.com

Introduction

Glaucoma is conventionally defined as a chronic optic neuropathy characterized by the progressive loss of retinal ganglion cells (RGCs) and optic nerve fibers [1]. Given that glaucoma is essentially a neurodegenerative disorder, the development of neuroprotective therapeutic strategies that are based not only on intraocular pressure lowering is required [2]. Neuroprotectants such as neurotrophic factors represent an important candidate treatment for glaucoma neuropathy.

Pituitary adenylate cyclase activating polypeptide (PACAP) is an endogenous neuropeptide with highly potent neuroprotective and general cytoprotective effects [3]. PACAP belongs to the vasoactive intestinal peptide (VIP)/secretin/glucagon peptide superfamily and exists in two forms, PACAP27 and PACAP38, the latter being the more biologically active [4]. The receptors for PACAP can be basically divided into two main groups: PACAP receptor type 1 (PAC1), which binds PACAP with higher affinity than VIP, and VPAC receptors (VPAC1 and VPAC2), which bind PACAP and VIP with similar affinities [5]. As a PACAP preferring receptor, PAC1 which mediates the most effects of PACAP as a neurotransmitter, neuro-modulator, neurotrophic factor and neuro-protector has been demonstrated as the predominant receptor type of PACAP in RGCs, amacrine cells, inner nuclear layer and Muller cells [6]. PAC1 is currently considered as a potential target for the treatment of neurodegenerative and neuropathic diseases. Via the mediation of PAC1, PACAP has well-known neuroprotective effects in retinal neuronal cultures *in vitro* and against *in vivo* retinal degenerations including excitotoxic injury induced by glutamate and kainate, ischemic injury, degeneration caused by UV-A light, optic nerve transection and streptozotocin-induced diabetic retinopathy [7].

However, the use of native PACAP, which is the endogenous ligand of PAC1, as an efficient neuroprotective agent is limited by

PACAP's rapid degradation. PACAP can be easily hydrolyzed by the ubiquitous enzyme dipeptidyl-peptidase IV (DPP IV) to form, PACAP (3–38) or PACAP (5–38), an antagonist of PAC1 in most cases [8]. The degradation by DPP IV in the blood circulation also results in the poor metabolic stability with short half-life between 2 and 10 min while PACAP is injected into mice or human [9]. N-terminal truncation of PACAP by removal of the first five amino acids results in a potent PAC1 antagonist that retains the ability to bind PACAP binding sites, does not stimulate adenylate cyclase and inhibits the ability of PACAP to stimulate adenylate cyclase. The N-terminal domain of PACAP (His1–Ser2–Asp3–Gly4) is the key structure to activate PAC1 [10]. A novel cyclopeptide C*HSDGIC* (CHC) synthesized from the cyclization of the N-terminus of PACAP with disulfide has been revealed as a potent activator of PAC1 in our previous studies [11].As a synthetic derivative of PACAP, CHC was synthesized to overcome the poor stability of PACAP.

As is originally reported, RGC-5 is a clonal rat retinal cell line that displays RGC characteristics based on the expression of specific markers such as Thy-1, Brn-3c, Neuritin, N-methyl-D-aspartate (NMDA) and GABAb receptors, sensitivity to glutamate excitotoxicity and neurotrophin withdrawal [12]. RGC-5 cells constitute a widely used model for studying physiological and pathophysiological processes in retinal cells [13]; therefore we explored the effects of CHC on this cell line. To further evaluate the protective effects of CHC, retinal damage was induced by the intravitreal injection of NMDA into rat eyes. The cells in the ganglion cell layer (GCL) were exquisitely sensitive to both glutamate and its analog NMDA [14]. NMDA-induced reactive oxygen species (ROS)-production are well recognized to be mediators of ischemic retinal damage, and activation of NMDA receptors reportedly generated free radicals and reduced antioxidant ability in the rat hippocampus [15].Therefore, in the present study we investigated the protective effects of CHC against Ultraviolet B (UVB)-induced apoptosis in RGC-5 cells *in vitro* and NMDA-induced retinal degeneration *in vivo*.

Materials and Methods

Cell culture

RGC-5 cells (a generous gift from Zhongshan Ophthalmic Center, Sun Yat-sen University) was previously provided by Dr. Neeraj Agarwal (Department of Cell Biology and Genetics, UNT Health Science Center, Fort Worth, TX) [16]. The RGC-5 cells were cultured in Dulbecco's modified Eagle medium (DMEM, HyClone, USA) containing 1 g/L glucose, 10% fetal bovine serum (GibcoBRL, Invitrogen, Darmstadt), 100 U/mL penicillin, and 100 μg/mL streptomycin (HyClone, USA) under a humidified atmosphere of 95% air and 5% CO_2 at 37°C.

UVB irradiation

Exposure was produced by filtering banks of UVB fluorescence tubes (Spectronics, EB-260C, USA) at the wavelength of 312 nm. Exposure time was calculated with the formula: $H\lambda = t \cdot E\lambda$, where $H\lambda$ is the energy level indicated as exposure per unit area (J/cm^2), t is the exposure time (second), and $E\lambda$ is the irradiance (W/cm^2).

Immunocytochemistry staining for Thy-1 and PAC1

The cultured cells were fixed in 4% paraformaldehyde for 30 min. Following 3 washes with PBS, cells were permeabilized in 0.2% Triton X-100 for 30 min, blocked for 1 h in 10% FBS and 1% BSA in PBS, and then incubated overnight at 4°C with primary antibodies against PAC1 (1:200, sc-15964, Santa Cruz, USA) and Thy-1 (1:200, sc-19614, Santa Cruz, USA). For control experiments, primary antibodies were omitted. The next day, cells were washed 3 times with PBS and incubated with secondary FITC-conjugated donkey anti-goat IgG or DyLight 594-conjugated goat anti-mouse IgG (1:200, Santa Cruz, USA) for 1 h, and then counterstained with DAPI in 1% BSA in PBS at room temperature. Images were obtained with a fluorescence Olympus BX51 microscope (Olympus, Tokyo, Japan).

MTT assay

Cells were seeded in 96-well plates at a density of 5.0×10^3 cells per well until 70% confluent and then incubated with different concentrations of CHC or PACAP for 1 h. To minimize the absorption of phenol red, the medium above the cells was removed during UVB irradiation at the energy level of 0.02 J/cm^2. After incubation for another 24 h, cells were harvested and analyzed immediately for viability using the 3-(4, 5-dimethylthiazol-2-yl)-2, 5-diphenyltetrazolium bromide (MTT, Sigma, USA) assay. MTT was added at a final concentration of 0.5 mg/ml for 4 h at 37°C. Then the medium was removed and reduced MTT (blue formazan product) was solubilized by adding 100 μl of DMSO to each well. After agitation of the plates for 15 min, the optical density of the solubilized formazan in each well was measured on a spectrophotometer at a 490 nm test wavelength and a 630 nm reference wavelength.

Propidium Iodide (PI) and Hoechst 33342 Double Staining

Cells were stained with 10 μg/ml Hoechst 33342 and 10 μg/ml PI (Sigma, USA) for 30 min at 37°C. After being washed twice with serum free media, cells were imaged using fluorescence microscopy. PI positive cells were counted using a cell counter under a fluorescence microscope at 100 times magnification. The total number of PI positive cells in four different representative fields per well were quantified for each treatment group. Morphological changes of post UVB-radiated RGC-5 cells were also observed using bright-field phase contrast microscopy.

Assessment of ROS

Quantification of intracellular ROS accumulation was performed by flow cytometry using the fluorescent probe 2′,7′-dichlorofluorescein diacetate (DCFH-DA, KeyGEN, China). RGC-5 cells were subjected to the appropriate treatment and then incubated for 15 min in the dark at 37°C with DCFH-DA solution at a final concentration of 10 μM. After incubation, the cells were washed with PBS and analyzed within 30 min using a flow cytometry (BD FACSAria) equipped with an air-cooled argon laser tuned to 488 nm. To confirm intracellular localization of the fluorescent probe, RGC-5 cells on coverslips were stained with DCFH-DA (10 μg/ml) for 30 min at 37°C in culture medium in a humidified chamber and then fixed with 4% paraformaldehyde for 20 min. After washing in PBS, cells were observed under fluorescence microscope.

Western Blot Analysis

After pretreatment of 10 μM CHC or 100 nM PACAP and UVB exposure, RGC-5 cells were lysed with RIPA buffer containing a protease inhibitor cocktail (Bocai Biotechnology) and sonicated on ice. The sonicated material was centrifuged for 20 min at 15,000×rpm at 4°C, and then the supernatant was collected. Protein extracts (10 μg each sample as determined by BCA method) were separated on 10% SDS-PAGE gel and transferred onto a PVDF membrane (Bio-Rad). The membrane

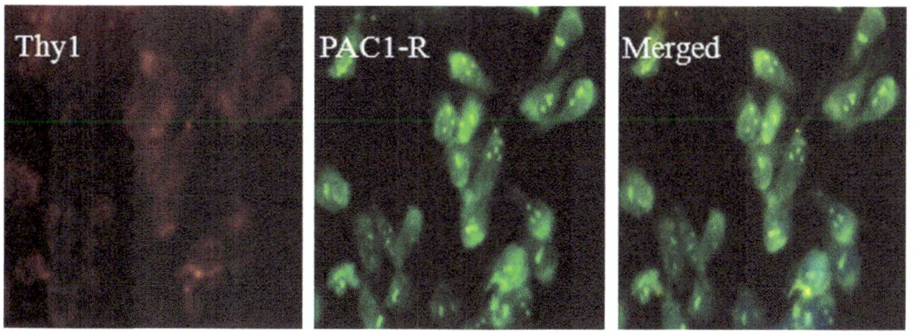

Figure 1. Immunolocalization studies for Thy-1(red) and PAC1 (green) with double staining. Evident labeling of the RGC marker Thy-1 was observed in RGC-5 cells. Immunostaining also showed diffuse expression of PAC1 in RGC-5 cells.

was incubated overnight at 4°C with primary antibodies that recognize: Bcl-2 (1:1000, Santa Cruz,USA), Bax (1:1000, Santa Cruz,USA) and β-actin (1:3000, Cell Signaling,USA). Horseradish peroxidase-conjugated secondary antibody (1:3000, Santa Cruz,USA) was used for 1 h at room temperature to detect the individual antigens and was enhanced by the use of ECL chemiluminescence reagent (Pierce). Protein expression levels were quantified by scanning the immunostaining band (Tanon2500) and analyzing the image with Image J 1.39 software.

Animals

The *in vivo* experiments were carried out on Sprague–Dawley rats at the age of 5–6 weeks old weighing 150–200 g. All animal procedures were performed in strict accordance with the recommendations in the Guide for the Care and Use of Laboratory Animals of the National Institutes of Health. The protocol was approved by the Jinan University Institutional Animal Care and Use Committee (IACUC). All efforts were made to minimize the suffering and number of animals used.

NMDA-Induced Retinal Injury Model

Rats were anesthetized by intraperitoneal injection of 10% chloral hydrate (4 ml/kg). The pupil was dilated with phenylephrine hydrochloride and tropicamide drops. The vitreous body was then injected with 50 mM NMDA (100 nmol; Sigma, St. Louis, MO, USA) in 2 µL saline solution. A 32G needle attached to a 10 µL microsyringe was used to deliver the solution 2 mm posterior to the temporal limbus to a depth of 1 mm. In the CHC-treated groups, CHC at a concentration of 10 pM to 100 nM was co-administered with NMDA in a total volume of 2 µL into the vitreous space. In the same manner, the eyes that received only an injection of saline were served as vehicle control.

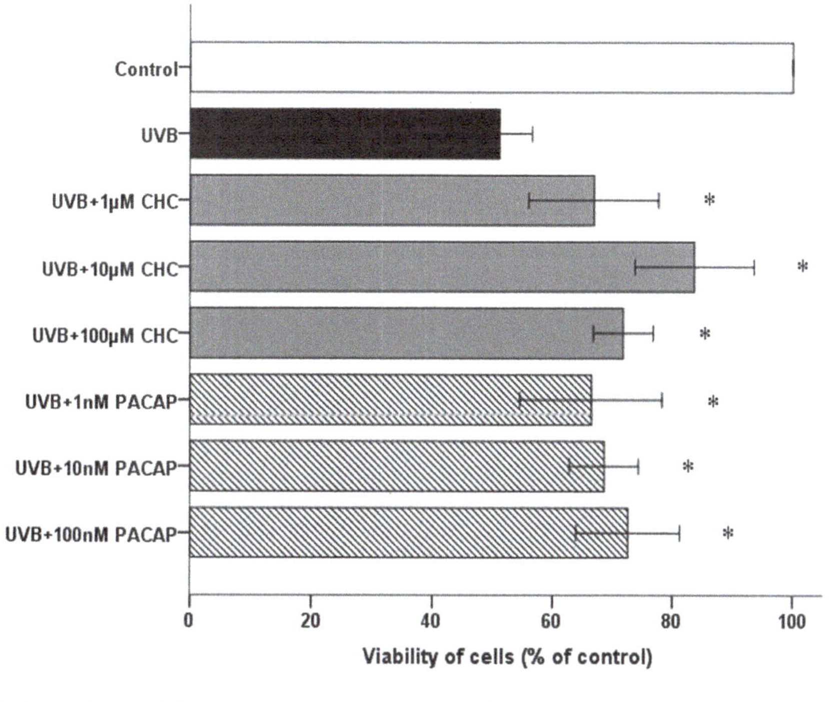

Figure 2. Viability of RGC-5 cells in different treatment groups at 24 h post UVB irradiation as measured by MTT assay. Co-administration of 10 µM CHC conferred the most significant protective effect compared with cells exposed to UVB only. The experiment was carried out three times independently and six replicate wells were set each time. *P<0.05, compared to UVB values.

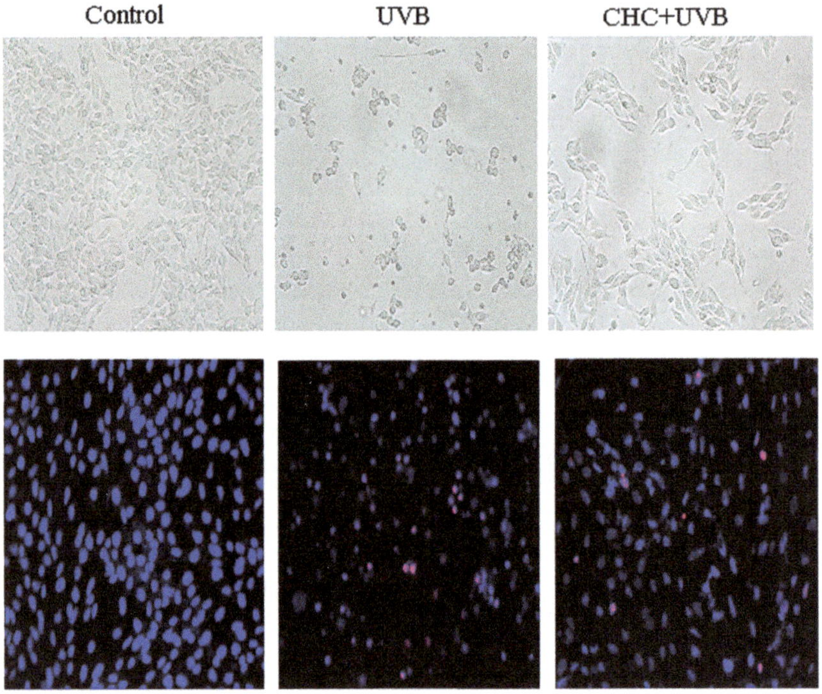

Figure 3. Representative light micrographs (A–C) and fluorescence micrographs of Hoechst33342 (blue)/PI (red) double staining (D–F) of normal RGC-5 cells, cells subjected to UVB irradiation and cells treated with 10 μM CHC and UVB irradiation. Normal control cells grew as an interconnected monolayer and exhibited axonal processes (A). Cells after UVB exposure became cuboidal and crenate in shape with the presence of vacuoles (B), which was markedly ameliorated with CHC pretreatment (C). Control cells showed normal nuclear morphology and are negatively stained for PI (D). UVB-irradiated cells including PI-positive cells, showed shrinkage and condensation of their nuclei (E). Treatment with 10 μM CHC reduced both nuclear shrinkage and PI-positive staining (F). Magnification is ×200.

Behavioral test

The light-dark test was carried out by standard techniques. The test box (custom-made by Metronet Technology Ltd) consisted of a dark compartment (30 cm×50 cm×50 cm) and a larger lit compartment (50 cm×50 cm×50 cm). A small opening in the center of the dividing wall at floor level allowed rats to move freely between the bright and dark chambers. Each rat was maintained in the box for 30 min and the time that different groups of rats (n = 5 for each group) spent in the dark area was recorded.

Electroretinography (ERG)

ERG was performed 7 days after the surgery. Rats (n = 6 for each group) were dark-adapted overnight and anesthetized with an intraperitoneal injection of 10% chloral hydrate (4 ml/kg). The pupil was dilated with 1% tropicamide and then the cornea anesthetized with 0.4% oxybuprocaine. Gold wire loop was placed on the cornea and two reference electrodes were inserted subcutaneously into the tissue behind earlobes. A steel needle was inserted into the subcutaneous tissue of the tail as the ground electrode.

The a-wave, b-wave, oscillatory potentials (OPs) and photopic negative responses (PhNR) were recorded using a Roland Consult electrophysiological diagnostic system (Brandenburg, Germany). Scotopic ERGs (a-wave, b-wave, OPs; 3.0 cds/m^2, white flash) were first recorded after dark adaptation. After light adaption under a continuous blue background (25 cds/m^2) for 5 min to suppress rod cell electrical activity, PhNR was recorded with red flashes (3.0 cds/m^2).

Histology

Histology was performed on the same rats as in the behavioral test to ensure the comparability of different research results. Rats were killed by pentobarbital overdose on the 7th day after NMDA or NMDA+CHC injection. The eyeballs (n = 6 per group) were fixed overnight in 10% formaldehyde and then embedded in paraffin. Three consecutive paraffin sections (thickness 4 μm) were used for the evaluation of neuronal cell death. Hematoxylin–eosin (HE) staining was performed according to the manufacturer's instruction. Six tissue blocks from six animals were prepared from each group. The number of cells/100 μm section length in the nasal and temporal sectors of the retina 375 to 625 μm from the optic nerve in the ganglion cell layer (GCL) was measured.

TUNEL staining

TUNEL (terminal deoxynucleotidyl transferase-mediated deoxyuridine triphosphate (UTP)-biotin nick end-labeling) staining (In Situ Cell Death Detection Kit; Roche Biochemicals, Mannheim, Germany) was performed to detect the internucleosomal DNA fragmentation that is characteristic of apoptosis. TUNEL staining was performed in addition to minor modification according to the instructional manual (n = 5 per group). Control sections were prepared with buffer solution without TdT and digoxigenin-labeled dUTP. Light-microscope images were photographed, and the labeled cells were counted in the GCL at a distance between 375 and 625 μm from the optic disc. The amount of cells staining positive for TUNEL was calculated as the percentage of the total cells in 200 μm of GCL.

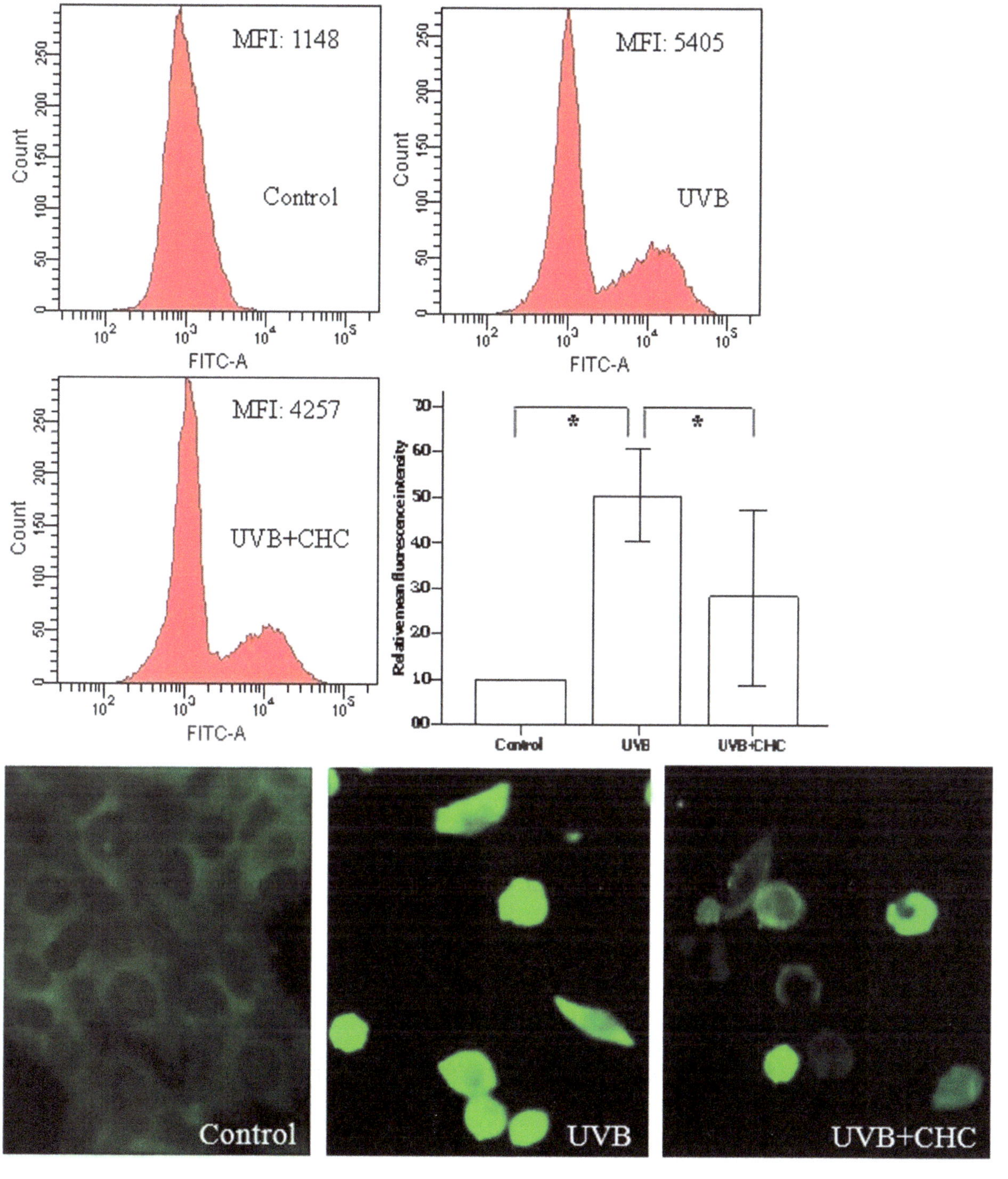

Figure 4. Effect of CHC on the ROS level in RGC-5 cells 24 h after UVB exposure as revealed by flowcytometry and fluorescence microscopy. RGC-5 cells exposed to UVB insult exhibited intense green fluorescent staining. 10 μM CHC clearly blunted the accumulation of ROS in UVB-exposed RGC-5 cells. Data were expressed as means±S.D. (*P<0.05).

Statistical analysis

Statistical comparisons were made by using an analysis of variance (ANOVA) followed by Student-Newman-Keuls or Tamhane's T2 test where appropriate. Data were presented as means ± S.E.M. A P value<0.05 was considered statistically significant.

Results

CHC attenuates the apoptosis of RGC-5 cells via the mitochondria pathway

Immunocytochemistry demonstrates strong staining for PAC1 in RGC-5 cells. Representative micrographs also showed discernible immunoreactivity for Thy-1 in all cells (Fig. 1). 0.02 J/cm^2 was identified as the ideal UVB energy level that reliably produced

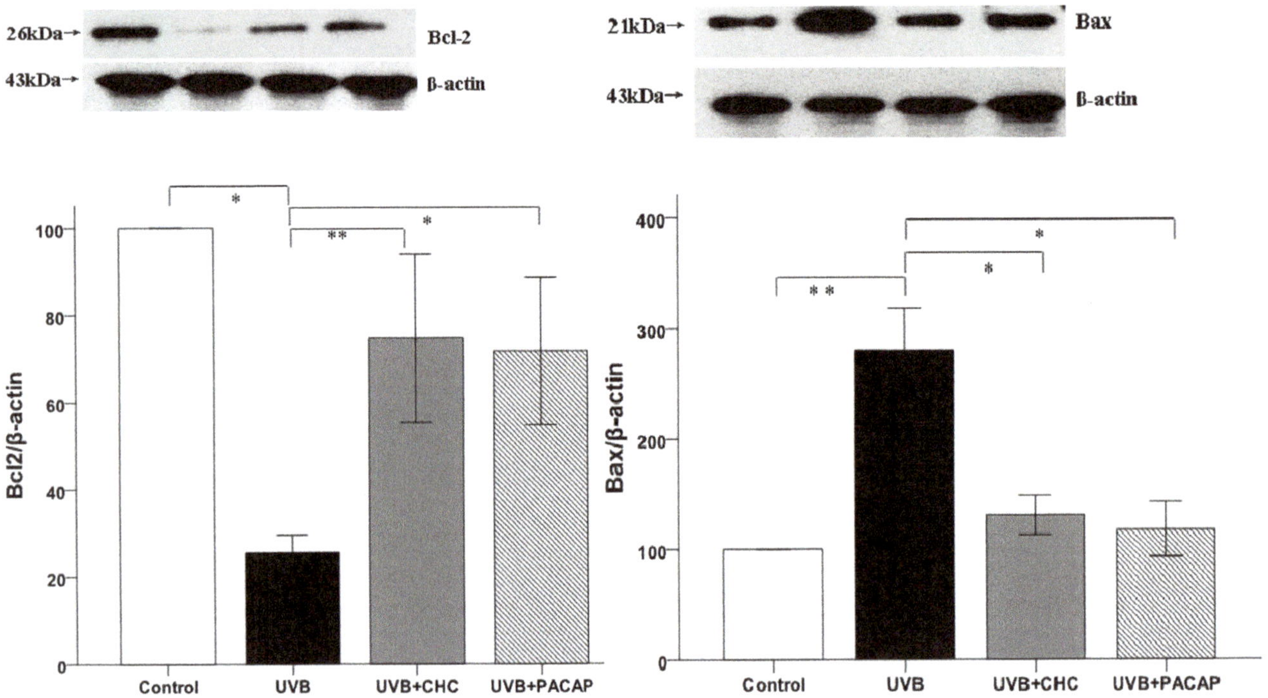

Figure 5. Western-blot analysis of RGC-5 cells exposed to UVB irradiation with or without the pretreatment of 10 μM CHC or 100 nM PACAP. UVB exposure caused a significant decrease in the protein level of Bcl-2 and a concomitant increase of Bax, while CHC significantly decreased the expression of apoptotic marker Bax and increased Bcl-2 expression. The results are expressed as means±S.D. (*P<0.01, **P<0.05).

an approximately 50% reduction in cell viability compared to the control. Viability of RGC-5 cells was reduced to 51.10±2.21% 24 h after 0.02 J/cm^2 UVB irradiation. This detrimental effect was markedly attenuated by the presence of CHC or PACAP (P< 0.05). 10 μM CHC afforded the greatest protection to the RGC-5 cells exposed to UVB damage, increasing viability to 80.3±2.35% (Fig. 2). Interesting discoveries were made by further distinguishing the viability of two different treatment groups. The viability of RGC-5 cells in the UVB+10 μM CHC treatment group was significantly higher than that treated with UVB and PACAP or other concentrations of CHC (P<0.05). The viability of cells with pretreatment of 1 μM CHC or 1 nM PACAP was significantly lower than that of those pretreated with CHC or PACAP at other concentrations (P<0.05), suggesting the limited protective effects CHC and PACAP at lower concentrations.

Normal control cells grew as an interconnected monolayer and exhibited axonal processes. Cells after UVB exposure became cuboidal and crenate in shape with the presence of vacuoles; while the structural morphology of RGC-5 cells was markedly maintained with CHC pretreatment, showing an elongated central axis (Fig. 3 A–C). Microscopic evaluation of apoptotic cells as a consequence of UVB exposure was determined by the Hoechst 33342 and PI double staining method. Control cells displayed normal nuclear morphology, while cells exposed to UVB

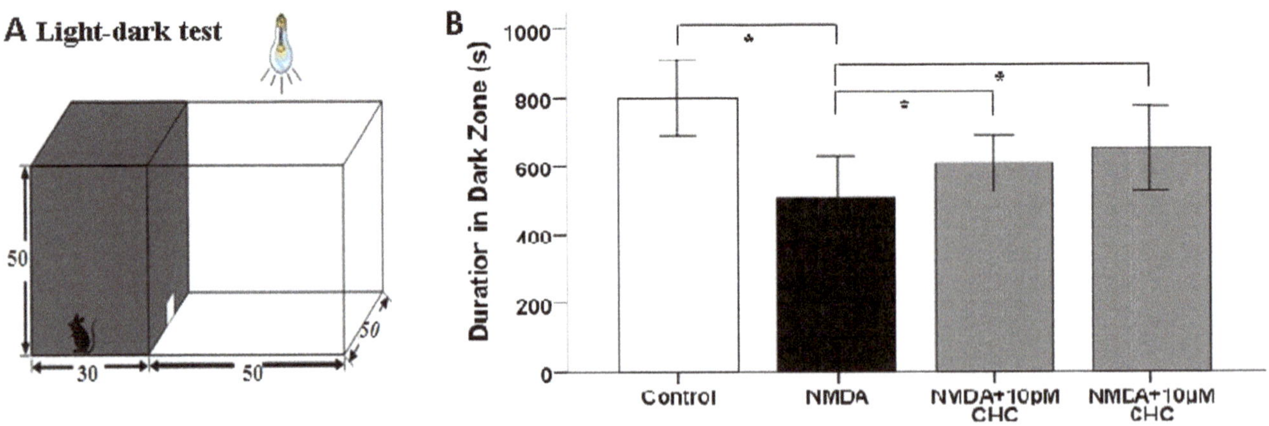

Figure 6. Enhancement of visual function in NMDA-injected SD rats with CHC co-application. (A) The light-dark test box consisting of a dark compartment and a larger lit compartment. (B) Time spent in the dark area by four groups of rats. The NMDA-CHC treated rats showed behavioral aversion to light. They spent significantly longer time in the dark chamber than rats injected with NMDA alone (*P<0.01).

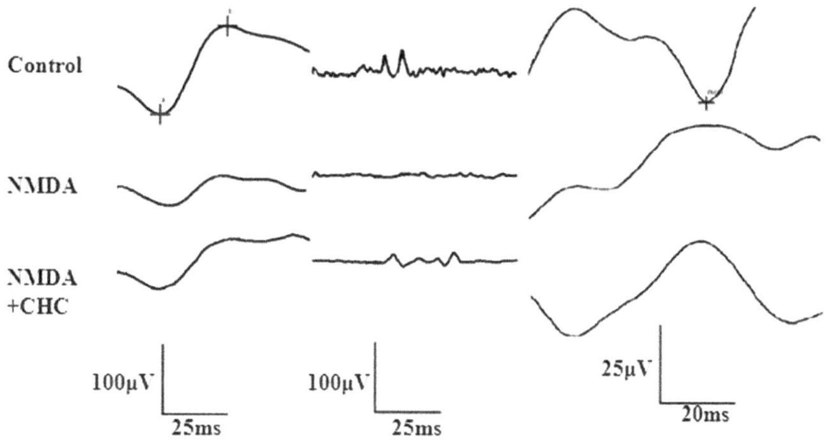

Figure 7. Different waves in ERG recordings of different treatment groups. Representative dark-adapted ERG components (a-wave, b-wave and OPs) and PhNR were recorded in control, NMDA and NMDA+CHC treatment groups. a-wave and b-wave are shown in the first column, while OPs and PhNR were shown in the second and third column respectively.

irradiation showed shrinkage and condensation of their nuclei with many red staining cells which were thought to be necrotic cells. CHC (10 μM) was significantly effective in blunting the cell death caused by UVB exposure (Fig. 3 D–F). UVB damage to RGC-5 cells elevated the percentage of PI positive cells (45.3±8.4%) relative to normal control cells. This increase was reduced by the pretreatment of 10 μM CHC (19.8±8.5%).

The measurement of ROS is based on the ability of the non-polar, non-fluorescent DCFH-DA to diffuse through the cell membrane and to be deacetylated by cytosolic esterases to form the polar, non-fluorescent dichlorodihydrofluorescein (DCFH), which is trapped inside the cell and gives rise to the formation of the fluorescent derivative dichlorofluorescein (DCF) by reacting with ROS [17]. ROS production is indicated by FITC fluorescence, and the mean intensity of fluorescence (MIF) was clearly enhanced in the cells subjected to UVB irradiation and up-regulated to over four-fold of control. Such enhancement was clearly reduced by the pretreatment of 10 μM CHC. Fluorescent microscopy examination of UVB-irradiated cells showed that the cells were strongly fluorescent, with a fairly uniform distribution of the dye indicating the spread of the oxidative burst within the cells, while cells protected with CHC showed a reduction in DCF accumulation (Fig. 4b).

The level of Bcl-2 and Bax protein relative to β-actin was investigated with western blot analysis. The result showed a marked decrease in the level of Bcl-2 with a concomitant increase in the level of Bax protein after UVB irradiation. In contrast, the effect of UVB irradiation on the expression of Bcl-2 and Bax was significantly attenuated by 10 μM CHC or 100 nM PACAP treatment. Furthermore, in terms of the expression level of these apoptosis-related markers, there was no significant difference between CHC and PACAP-treated cells, $P>0.05$ ((Fig. 5)).

Improvement of visual function and histology with CHC treatment

In the light-dark test, the total residence time in the test box for each rat was 30 min (1800 s). Time spent in the dark area by NMDA-treated rats was 505.27±50.19 s, significantly lower than that of normal control rats (799.95±69.34 s).With 10 pM or 10 μM CHC co-treatment, the duration in dark zone was increased to 608.43±50.88 s and 625.00±48.97 s respectively (Fig. 6).

The amplitudes of b-wave and PhNR were reduced in NMDA-injected rats compared with age-matched controls, whereas CHC co-administration markedly increased these amplitudes (Fig. 7). Amplitudes of OPs in NMDA-treated rats after 7 days were markedly lower than normal controls ($P<0.05$). 10 μM CHC co-administration slightly reversed NMDA-induced Ops reduction, but the difference was not statistically significant. As for the PhNR amplitudes, in NMDA group they were smaller than the control level, while with 10 μM CHC treatment the values were significantly increased,$P<0.05$ (Table 1).

In the intraocular NMDA-induced excitotoxicity model, a significant decrease was observed at day 7 in the number of cells in the GCL of vehicle-injected retina compared with the intact control (49.74±5.16/mm vs100.2±4.31/mm; $p<0.01$). In those groups in which CHC was injected into the vitreous body, the cell number in GCL was 53.94±3.0, 70.0±3.7, 62.9±4.54, 50.34±1.8 and 70.8±3.61/mm for CHC at concentrations of 100 fM, 10 pM, 1 nM, 100 nM and 10 μM respectively. The

Table 1. Amplitudes of ERG components in different groups.

Groups	N	b-wave (μV)	Ops (μV)	PhNR (μV)
Control	6	123.67±16.04	146.33±15.01	36.4±6.15
NMDA	6	44.83±2.75	42.93±15.00	12.74±5.05
NMDA+CHC	6	68.7±5.75*	58.83±4.18	22.57±0.87*

*$P<0.05$, compared with the NMDA group.

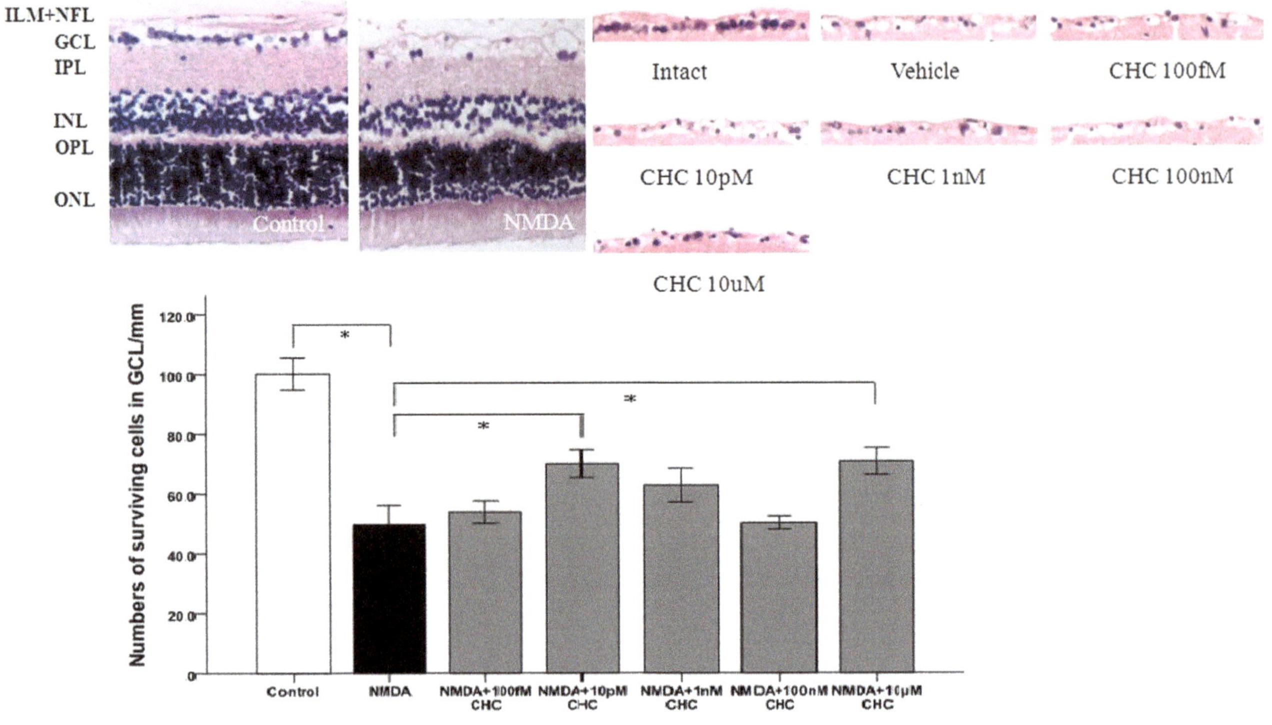

Figure 8. Representative photomicrograph showing HE staining of cell layers in the retina (100×). The number of cells per 100 μm in GCL decreased in NMDA-treated retinas but was increased by CHC treatment. The 10 pM and 10 μM CHC -treated groups are significantly different from the control vehicle group. *P<0.01 (ONL outer nuclear layer, OPL outer plexiform layer, INL inner nuclear layer, IPL inner plexiform layer, GCL ganglion cell layer, ILM inner limiting membrane).

increase was significant in the groups treated with 10 pM or 10 μM CHC compared with the vehicle-treated group, suggesting that the neuroprotective effect of CHC on RGCs was bimodal (Fig. 8).

In the case of TUNEL-positive cells, the percentage of TUNEL-positive cells in the intact control retina was 6.67±1.53%. After NMDA injection, a significant increase was recorded in the percentage of TUNEL-positive cells (66.67±6.11%), with CHC co-treatment the value dropped to 40.0±5.0% (Fig. 9).

Discussion

In the present study, we investigated the protective effects of a PACAP derivative in both *in vitro* and *in vivo* models of RGC apoptosis. To our knowledge, this is the first study investigating the anti-apoptotic effects and mechanism of a synthetic PACAP derivative in RGCs. These results are consistent with the large body of evidence demonstrating the retinoprotective action of PACAP in numerous models of retinal degeneration including excitotoxic retinal injury induced by NMDA in mice [18] and by monosodium glutamate in newborn rats [19]. PACAP treatment has also been shown to significantly attenuate the UVA-induced retinal damage [20], which was in accordance with our findings that PACAP and CHC inhibited UVB-induced apoptosis in RGC-5 cells.

Structural analysis has shown that the N-terminus of PACAP (HSDGI) is flexible and disordered [21], while C*HSDGIC* synthesized from cyclizing HSDGI and adding two Cys residues at both ends is more stable with a more fixed conformation. Furthermore, CHC has a small molecular weight (approximately 700 Da), which allows it to easily penetrate the blood-retina barrier. CHC is also a selective agonist of PAC1 without inducing side effects mediated through other receptors of PACAP [11].

PAC1 has gained considerable attention because it has been shown to mediate the anti-apoptotic and cytoprotective effects of PACAP [22] and accumulating studies have noticed the value of detecting PAC1 expression in retinal cells [23]. To confirm the results of western blot analysis in our previous studies [24], immunocytochemistry was performed on RGC-5 cells with Thy-1 and PAC1 antibodies. The RGC-5 cell line used in this study was positive for Thy-1, a specific marker for RGCs. Immunofluorescence also showed diffuse expression of PAC1 antigen, the putative target for PACAP analogs.

Currently there is controversy over the validity of RGC-5 cells. Recent publications emerged claiming that the RGC-5 cell line wasn't derived from rat but from mouse and was actually a photoreceptor cell line 661W. The antibodies against Thy-1 (HIS51) and PAC1 (K-20) used in our studies detect antigens of both mouse and rat origin, so we cannot exclude the possibility that the RGC-5 cell line is from mouse and not rat origin. However, we tend to be reticent about the opinion that RGC-5 cells are ganglion cell-like cells, because the RGC-5 cells used in our studies were positive for Thy-1 labeling, which is a RGC specific marker. In our experience, similar to RGCs, the RGC-5 cells used were sensitive to oxidative stress and neurtrophin withdrawal. 661W cells resemble neuronal cells, demonstrating cellular and biochemical characteristics exhibited by cone photoreceptor cells [25]. The authors deduced that the 661W cell line was also present in the RGC-5 originating laboratory, which probably resulted in cross contamination. If this is the reason, then we cannot help but wonder how the authors ensure that their conclusion wasn't also a mischaracterization due to cross

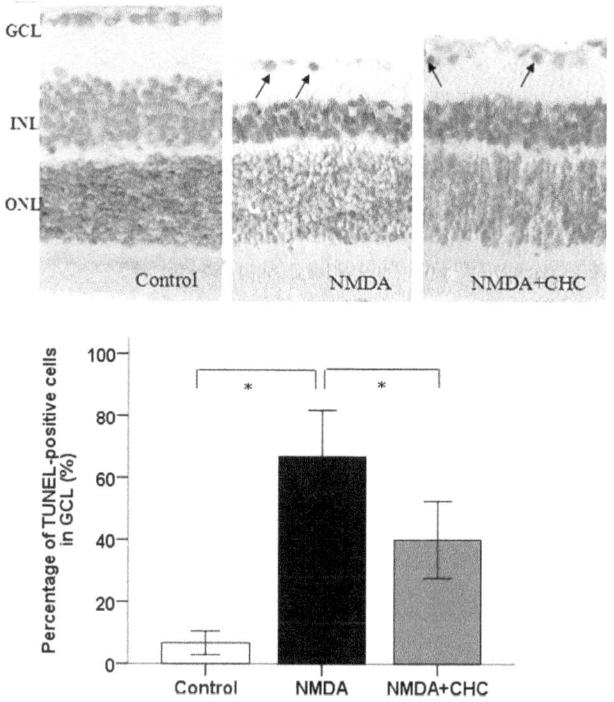

Figure 9. Representative photomicrogaphs illustrating the apoptosis of RGCs in response to NMDA (100×). Deep brown-stained cells indicate TUNEL-positive cells. The proportion of TUNEL-positive cells in the GCL of control SD rats, rats injected with NMDA alone or with NMDA+10 μM CHC were calculated. Data are shown as means±S.E.M. (n = 6). *P<0.05, comparing the NMDA and NMDA+CHC groups.

contamination since the phenotypic origin of RGC-5 was detected with 661W? Also the hypothesis of RGC-5 cells being photoreceptors cannot explain the evident labeling for Thy-1 in the current studies. As the two cell types are very different by molecular phenotyping, it is difficult to reconcile this discrepancy. In fact, the same group who published this recent report previously used RGC-5 cells for other studies, confirming their retinal ganglion cell origin [26]. Even though RGC-5 cells are not so ideal a model of RGCs as they were once considered, they still represent neuronal precursor cells which are useful for future neuroprotection type of investigations.

The effects of PACAP on apoptosis have been studied in numerous *in vitro* and *in vivo* models. PACAP influences apoptotic signaling at various levels from initiation to downstream cytosolic and mitochondrial pathways and finally affecting executor caspases [4]. Previous studies suggest that the protective effects of PACAP involve several mechanisms. Different apoptosis-related markers including p-Akt, extracellular signal-regulated kinase, PKC, Bcl-2, p-p38MAPK and activated caspases (8, 3, 12) [27], JNK, apoptosis inducing factor, cytochrome C, phospho-Bad [28] and p53 [29] have been investigated to demonstrate that inhibition of apoptosis is one of the PACAP-induced pathways with therapeutic potential. In the current studies, UVB-irradiation to RGC-5 cells results in ROS over-generation, with reduction of Bcl-2 and up-regulation of Bax, along with loss of mitochondria membrane potential loss and activation of caspase-3 as revealed in our previous studies [24]. This pathway represents the classic mitochondrial or intrinsic pathway to apoptosis. In agreement with previous studies about PACAP, CHC attenuates the apoptosis of RGC-5 cells by affecting the aforementioned central coordinators of mitochondria-mediated apoptosis pathway.

Oxidative stress plays an important role in the pathophysiology of glaucoma [30]. Because of the central role played by mitochondria as both a source and target of oxidative stress, therapeutic agents targeting mitochondria are proposed to protect RGCs from glaucomatous damage. Considering previous report that demonstrated oxidative stress in RGC-5 cells caused by UVB light [31], we adopted the UVB-irradiation paradigm to determine whether CHC provides protective effects via maintaining mitochondria function. Our study found that exposing RGC-5 cells to a small dose of UVB irradiation could lead to marked reduction in cell viability, which was attenuated by CHC at micro molar concentrations. Hoechst/PI staining also provided evidence for this finding.

Reactive oxygen species are formed in the eyes following a wide variety of stressors, and are largely implicated in glaucoma pathogenesis [32].

Mitochondria are the major source of superoxide production and are subject to the direct attack by ROS [33].Oxidative stress occurs when cellular production of ROS exceeds the capacity of anti-oxidant defenses. As proved by previous studies, mitochondria dysfunction could lead to increased production of ROS which could aggravate oxidative stress [34]. Neuroprotective candidates like sulbutiamine [35], isoquercitrin [36] and crocetin [37] have been demonstrated to exert ROS inhibitory effects on RGC-5 cells, but no study has investigated the ability of PACAP analogs to scavenge ROS in RGC-5 cells. Our study demonstrated for the first time that the increase in ROS due to UVB exposure was significantly reduced by the pretreatment of 10 μM CHC, indicating the inhibitory effect of CHC on mitochondria dysfunction and oxidative stress.

Additionally, the expression of Bcl-2 in UVB-exposed cells was decreased significantly compared to that of normal control cells (P<0.01). Bcl-2 family members like Bax promote apoptosis, whereas other members including Bcl-2 and Bcl-Xl exert anti-apoptotic effects [38]. In UVB+CHC group, Bcl-2 was up-regulated accompanied with the down-regulation of Bax. The execution of apoptosis is usually associated with an up regulation of Bax, which is a pro-apoptotic marker. The increased levels of Bax in the cell then combine with the Bcl-2 already present in the cell. This lowers the amount of free Bcl-2 in the cell, driving the cell toward apoptosis [39]. Bax and Bcl-2 proteins closely interact with the component forming the mitochondria permeability transition pore that allows proteins to escape from mitochondria into cytosol to initiate apoptosis [40]. In the current study, UVB irradiation resulted in ROS accumulation, an increase in Bax and a decrease in Bcl-2 besides mitochondrial membrane potential loss and caspase-3 activation as revealed by our previous findings [24].

Excessive activity of NMDA-type glutamatergic channels has been implicated as a mechanism for neuronal injury in neurologic disorders, including glaucoma [41]. Previous studies have demonstrated that intravitreal injection of NMDA resulted in significantly increased number of apoptotic RGCs and exogenous PACAP is able to counteract NMDA-induced toxicity [42]. Since neural retinal degeneration induced by NMDA has been well established as an experimental glaucoma model, we adopted this model to investigate the protective effects of CHC.

ERG has been considered as a more sensitive method to illustrate retinal injury than histology [43]. The amplitude of PhNR is well recognized as a marker to reflect the function of RGCs [44]. The b-wave mainly originates from bipolar cells that are post synaptic to photoreceptors [45]. Reduced amplitudes in b-wave and OPs are commonly seen in the early stage of retinopathy even before its onset [46]. With CHC administration, the amplitude of PhNR was increased from 1/3 to approximately 2/3 of the controls compared to eyes treated with NMDA only, suggesting marked recovery of RGC function. The functional outcomes, though not absolutely parallel with the morphological observation, was significantly improved after CHC treatment, indicating that, similar to PACAP [47], the protective effects of CHC could transfer to functional improvement.

Our morphometric analysis showed that intravitreal injection of CHC at different concentrations results in less cell loss in GCL. It was reported that the neuroprotection conferred by PACAP in NMDA-induced mice retinal damage was optimal at 100 pM increasing GCL cell number by about 16% of control, while no bimodal response was observed [42]. In our studies, the protective effect of CHC on the retina is not strongly dose-dependent, with optimal effects acquired at 10 μM and 10 pM respectively, increasing GCL cell number by around 20% of control. Similarly, it has been reported that in transient ischemia model induced by high ocular pressure in rats, the neuroprotective effect of PACAP is bimodal with a concentration peak of 10 fM related to the MAP kinase cascade and another peak of 10 to 100 pM reflecting the cAMP cascade [48]. The neuroprotective effect of PACAP in neuronal/astroglial cultures is also bimodal, with peak effects observed at a subpicomolar and a nanomolar concentration [49]. Emerging evidence suggests that nanomolar concentrations of PACAP affect neurons directly, while subpicomolar concentrations exert an indirect glial-cell-mediated protective effect [50]. Our results regarding the bimodal effect of CHC in the retina may suggest the involvement of two different pathways. Due to the difference in animal type and NMDA dosage, the results in the current studies aren't quite comparable to previous ones where NMDA amount ranged from 5 nmol to 200 nmol [51,52] and animal type varied between C57BL/6 mice and SD rats [53]. Besides, as is stated above, the results of previous studies aren't consistent either. The comparison of the protective mechanism and efficiency between the two different peptides will be further investigated in our future *in vivo* studies.

In conclusion, the present study demonstrates the neuroprotective effect of C*HSDGIC* from the cyclization of PACAP (1–5) against RGC apoptosis in both *in vitro* and *in vivo* models. CHC exerts protective effects through the mitochondria pathway. Analogs of PACAP, especially selective PAC1 agonists like CHC may have a therapeutic value in glaucoma as an adjuvant treatment modality.

Author Contributions

Conceived and designed the experiments: HHC RJY. Performed the experiments: HHC YD CYW. Analyzed the data: HHC JSC. Contributed reagents/materials/analysis tools: RJY YD CYW. Wrote the paper: HHC RJY.

References

1. Nucci C, Strouthidis NG, Khaw PT (2013) Neuroprotection and other novel therapies for glaucoma. Curr Opin Pharmacol 13:1–4.
2. Chang EE, Goldberg JL (2012) Glaucoma 2.0: neuroprotection, neuroregeneration, neuroenhancement, Ophthalmology 119: 979–986.
3. Yu R, Guo X, Zhong J, Li M, Zeng Z, et al. (2012) The N-Terminal HSDCIF Motif Is Required for Cell Surface Trafficking and Dimerization of Family B G Protein Coupled Receptor PAC1. PLoS ONE 7: e51811.
4. Vaudry D, Gonzales BJ, Basille M, Yon L, Fournier A, et al. (2000) Pituitary adenylate cyclase activating polypeptide and its receptors: from structure to function. Pharmacol Rev 52:269–324.
5. Vaudry D, Falluel-Morel A, Bourgault S, Basille M, Burel D,et al. (2009) Pituitary adenylate cyclase activating polypeptide and its receptors: 20 years after thediscovery. Pharmacol Rev 61: 283–357.
6. Seki T, Izumi S, Shioda S, Zhou CJ, Arimura A, et al. (2000) Gene expression for PACAP receptor mRNA in the rat retina by in situ hybridization and in situ RT-PCR. Ann N Y Acad Sci 921:366–9.
7. Atlasz T, Szabadfi K, Kiss P, Racz B, Gallyas F, et al. (2010) Pituitary adenylate cyclase activating polypeptide in the retina: focus on the retinoprotective effects, Ann N Y Acad Sci 1200:128–139.
8. Green BD, Irwin N, Flatt PR (2006) Pituitary adenylate cyclase-activating peptide (PACAP): assessment of dipeptidyl peptidase IV degradation, insulin-releasing activity and antidiabetic potential, Peptides 27:1349–1352.
9. Li M, Maderdrut JL, Lertora JJ, Batuman V (2007) Intravenous infusion of pituitary adenylate cyclase-activating polypeptide (PACAP) in a patient with multiple myeloma and myeloma kidney: a case study. Peptides 28:1891–1895.
10. Bourgault S, Vaudry D, Ségalas MI, Guilhaudis L, Couvineau A, et al. (2009) Molecular and conformational determinants of pituitary adenylate cyclase-activating polypeptide (PACAP) for activation of the PAC1 receptor, J Med Chem 52: 3308–3316.
11. Yu RJ, Wang JJ, Li J, Zhang H, Chen JS, et al. (2010) A novel cyclopeptide from the cyclization of PACAP (1–5) with potent activity towards PAC1 attenuates STZ-induced diabetes, Peptides 31:1062–1067.
12. Agarwal N, Agarwal R, Kumar DM, Ondricek A, Clark AF, et al. (2007) Comparison of expression profile of neurotrophins and their receptors in primary and transformed rat retinal ganglion cells. Mol Vis 13: 1311–1318.
13. Nieto PS, Valdez DJ, Acosta-Rodrı'guez VA, Guido ME (2011) Expression of Novel Opsins and Intrinsic Light Responses in the Mammalian Retinal Ganglion Cell Line RGC-5. Presence of OPN5 in the Rat Retina. PLoS ONE 6: e26417.
14. Shimazaki H, Hironaka K, Fujisawa T, Tsuruma K, Tozuka Y, et al. (2011) Edaravone-loaded liposome eyedrops protect against light-induced retinal damage in mice.Invest Ophthalmol Vis Sci 52:7289–7297.
15. Ueda Y, Doi T, Nagatomo K, Nakajima A (2007) In vivo activation of N-methyl-Daspartate receptors generates free radicals and reduces antioxidant ability in the rat hippocampus: experimental protocol of in vivo ESR spectroscopy and microdialysis for redox status evaluation, Brain Res 1178:20–27.
16. Li J, Dong Z, Liu B, Zhuo Y, Sun X, et al. (2011) Hypoxia induces beta-amyloid in association with death of RGC-5 cells in culture. Biochem Biophys Res Commun 410:40–44.
17. Carini M, Aldini G, Piccone M, Facino RM (2000) Fluorescent probes as markers of oxidative stress in keratinocyte cell lines following UVB exposure. Farmaco 55:526–534.
18. Wada Y, Nakamachi T, Endo K, Seki T, Ohtaki H, et al. (2013) PACAP attenuates NMDA-induced retinal damage in association with modulation of the microglia/macrophage status into an acquired deactivation subtype, J Mol Neurosci 51:493–502.
19. Atlasz T, Szabadfi K, Reglodi D, Kiss P, Tamás A, et al. (2009) Effects of pituitary adenylate cyclase activating polypeptide (PACAP1–38) and its fragments on retinal degeneration induced by neonatal MSG treatment. Ann N Y Acad Sci 1163:348–352.
20. Atlasz T, Szabadfi K, Kiss P, Marton Z, Griecs M, et al. (2011) Effects of PACAP in UV-A radiation-induced retinal degeneration models in rats, J Mol Neurosci 43:51–57.
21. Corcho FJ, Mokoena P, Bisetty K, Perez JJ (2009) Molecular dynamics (MD) simulations of VIP and PACAP27, Biopolymers 91:391–400.
22. Delcourt N, Thouvenot E, Chanrion B, Galéotti N, Jouin P, et al. (2007) PACAP type I receptor transactivation is essential for IGF-1 receptor signalling and antiapoptotic activity in neurons, EMBO J 26: 1542–1551.
23. Szabadfi K, Atlasz T, Kiss P, Reglodi D, Szabo A, et al. (2012) Protective effects of the neuropeptide PACAP in diabetic retinopathy. Cell Tissue Res 348: 37–46.
24. Ding Y, Cheng H, Yu R, Tang C, Liu X, et al. (2012) Effects of cyclopeptide C*HSDGIC* from the cyclization of PACAP (1–5) on the proliferation and UVB-induced apoptosis of the retinal ganglion cell line RGC-5. Peptides 36:280–285.
25. Tan E, Ding XQ, Saadi A, Agarwal N, Naash MI, et al. (2004) Expression of cone-photoreceptor-specific antigens in a cell line derived from retinal tumors in transgenic mice. Invest Ophthalmol Vis Sci 45:764–768.
26. Agarwal N (2013) RGC-5 cells. Invest Ophthalmol Vis Sci 54: 7884.
27. Szabadfi K, Szabo A, Kiss P, Reglodi D, Setalo G Jr,et al. (2014) PACAP promotes neuron survival in early experimental diabetic retinopathy. Neurochem Int 64:84–91.
28. Rácz B, Gallyas F Jr, Kiss P, Tóth G, Hegyi O, et al. (2006) The neuroprotective effects of PACAP in monosodium glutamate-induced retinal lesion involve inhibition of proapoptotic signaling pathways. Regul Pept 137:20–26.
29. Giunta S, Castorina A, Bucolo C, Magro G, Drago F, et al. (2012) Early changes in pituitary adenylate cyclase-activating peptide, vasoactive intestinal peptide and related receptors expression in retina of streptozotocin-induced diabetic rats. Peptides 37:32–39.

30. Osborne NN (2008) Pathogenesis of ganglion "cell death" in glaucoma and neuroprotection: focus on ganglion cell axonal mitochondria. Prog Brain Res 173: 339–352.
31. Balaiya S, Murthy RK, Brar VS, Chalam KV (2010) Evaluation of ultraviolet light toxicity on cultured retinal pigment epithelial and retinal ganglion cells. Clin Ophthalmol 4: 33–39.
32. Pinazo-Durán MD, Zanón-Moreno V, García-Medina JJ, Gallego-Pinazo R (2012) Evaluation of presumptive biomarkers of oxidative stress, immune response and apoptosis in primary open-angle glaucoma. Curr Opin Pharmacol 13:98–107.
33. Orrenius S (2007) Reactive oxygen species in mitochondria-mediated cell death, Drug Metab Rev 39: 443–455.
34. Jezek P, Hlavatá L (2005) Mitochondria in homeostasis of reactive oxygen species in cell, tissues, and organism. Int J Biochem Cell Biol 37: 2478–2503.
35. Kang KD, Majid AS, Kim KA, Kang K, Ahn HR, et al. (2010) Sulbutiamine counteracts trophic factor deprivation induced apoptotic cell death in transformed retinal ganglion cells. Neurochem Res 35: 1828–1839.
36. Jung SH, Kim BJ, Lee EH, Osborne NN (2010) Isoquercitrin is the most effective antioxidant in the plant Thuja orientalis and able to counteract oxidative-induced damage to a transformed cell line (RGC-5 cells). Neurochem Int 57:713–721.
37. Yamauchi M, Tsuruma K, Imai S, Nakanishi T, Umigai N, et al. (2011) Crocetin prevents retinal degeneration induced by oxidative and endoplasmic reticulum stresses via inhibition of caspase activity. Eur J Pharmacol 650: 110–119.
38. Jurgensmeier JM, Xie Z, Deveraux Q, Ellerby L, Bredesen D, et al. (1998) Bax directly induces release of cytochrome c from isolated mitochondria, Proc Natl Acad Sci U S A 95: 4997–5002.
39. Charles I, Khalyfa A, Kumar DM, Krishnamoorthy RR, Roque RS, et al. (2005) Serum deprivation induces apoptotic cell death of transformed rat retinal ganglion cells via mitochondrial signaling pathways. Invest Ophthalmol Vis Sci 46: 1330–1338.
40. Desagher S, Martinou JC (2000) Mitochondria as the central control point of apoptosis, Trends Cell Biol 10: 369–377.
41. Hironaka K, Inokuchi Y, Fujisawa T, Shimazaki H, Akane M, et al. (2011) Edaravone-loaded liposomes for retinal protection against oxidative stress-induced retinal damage. Eur J Pharm Biopharm 79: 119–125.
42. Endo K, Nakamachi T, Seki T, Kagami N, Wada Y, et al. (2010) Neuroprotective Effect of PACAP Against NMDA-Induced Retinal Damage in the Mouse. J Mol Neurosci 43: 22–29.
43. Osborne NN, Casson RJ, Wood JP, Chidlow G, Graham M, et al. (2004) Retinal ischemia: mechanisms of damage and potential therapeutic strategies. Prog Retin Eye Res 23: 91–117.
44. Chen H, Zhang M, Huang S, Wu D (2008) The photopic negative response of flash ERG in nonproliferative diabetic retinopathy. Doc Ophthalmol 117: 129–135.
45. Weymouth AE, Vingrys AJ (2008) Rodent electroretinography: methods for extraction and interpretation of rod and cone responses. Prog Retin Eye Res 27: 1–44.
46. Zhu B, Wang W, Gu Q, Xu X (2008) Erythropoietin protects retinal neurons and glial cells in early-stage streptozotocin-induced diabetic rats. Exp Eye Res 86: 375–382.
47. Varga B, Szabadfi K, Kiss P, Fabian E, Tamas A, et al. (2010) PACAP Improves Functional Outcome in Excitotoxic Retinal Lesion: An Electroretinographic Study. J Mol Neurosci 43: 44–50.
48. Li M, David C, Kikuta T, Somogyvari-Vigh A, Arimura A (2005) Signaling cascades involved in neuroprotection by subpicomolar pituitary adenylate cyclase-activating polypeptide 38. J Mol Neurosci 27: 91–105.
49. Onoue S, Endo K, Ohshima K, Yajima T, Kashimoto K (2002) The neuropeptide PACAP attenuates b-amyloid (1–42)-induced toxicity in PC12 cells. Peptides 23:1471–1478
50. Seki T, Itoh H, Nakamachi T, Endo K, Wada Y, et al.(2010) Suppression of Rat Retinal Ganglion Cell Death by PACAP Following Transient Ischemia Induced by High Intraocular Pressure. J Mol Neurosci 43:30–34.
51. Hironaka K, Inokuchi Y, Fujisawa T, Shimazaki H, Akane M, et al. (2011) Edaravone-loaded liposomes for retinal protection against oxidative stress-induced retinal damage. Eur J Pharm Biopharm 79:119–125.
52. Kido N, Tanihara H, Honjo M, Inatani M, Tatsuno T,et al. (2000) Neuroprotective effects of brain-derived neurotrophic factor in eyes with NMDA-induced neuronal death. Brain Res 884:59–67.
53. Wada Y, Nakamachi T, Endo K, Seki T, Ohtaki H,et al. (2013) PACAP attenuates NMDA-induced retinal damage in association with modulation of the microglia/macrophage status into an acquired deactivation subtype. J Mol Neurosci 51:493–502.

Outcomes in Cochrane Systematic Reviews Addressing Four Common Eye Conditions: An Evaluation of Completeness and Comparability

Ian J. Saldanha*, Kay Dickersin, Xue Wang, Tianjing Li

Department of Epidemiology, Johns Hopkins Bloomberg School of Public Health, Baltimore, Maryland, United States of America

Abstract

Introduction: Choice of outcomes is critical for clinical trialists and systematic reviewers. It is currently unclear how systematic reviewers choose and pre-specify outcomes for systematic reviews. Our objective was to assess the completeness of pre-specification and comparability of outcomes in all Cochrane reviews addressing four common eye conditions.

Methods: We examined protocols for all Cochrane reviews as of June 2013 that addressed glaucoma, cataract, age-related macular degeneration (AMD), and diabetic retinopathy (DR). We assessed completeness and comparability for each outcome that was named in ≥25% of protocols on those topics. We defined a completely-specified outcome as including information about five elements: *domain*, *specific measurement*, *specific metric*, *method of aggregation*, and *time-points*. For each domain, we assessed comparability in how individual elements were specified across protocols.

Results: We identified 57 protocols addressing glaucoma (22), cataract (16), AMD (15), and DR (4). We assessed completeness and comparability for five outcome domains: quality-of-life, visual acuity, intraocular pressure, disease progression, and contrast sensitivity. Overall, these five outcome domains appeared 145 times (instances). Only 15/145 instances (10.3%) were completely specified (all five elements) (median = three elements per outcome). Primary outcomes were more completely specified than non-primary (median = four versus two elements). Quality-of-life was least completely specified (median = one element). Due to largely incomplete outcome pre-specification, conclusive assessment of comparability in outcome usage across the various protocols per condition was not possible.

Discussion: Outcome pre-specification was largely incomplete; we encourage systematic reviewers to consider all five elements. This will indicate the importance of complete specification to clinical trialists, on whose work systematic reviewers depend, and will indirectly encourage comparable outcome choice to reviewers undertaking related research questions. Complete pre-specification could improve efficiency and reduce bias in data abstraction and analysis during a systematic review. Ultimately, more completely specified and comparable outcomes could make systematic reviews more useful to decision-makers.

Editor: Kypros Kypri, University of Newcastle, Australia, Australia

Funding: This project was funded by the National Eye Institute, grant number 1U01EY020522 (http://www.nei.nih.gov/). The funder had no role in study design, data collection and analysis, decision to publish, or preparation of the manuscript.

Competing Interests: All authors are affiliated with the US Satellite of the Cochrane Eyes and Vision Group (the group responsible for producing the Cochrane Reviews evaluated as part of this work): Drs. Kay Dickersin and Tianjing Li are Faculty members; Dr. Xue Wang is a Methodologist; and Dr. Ian Saldanha is a Research Assistant. Drs. Kay Dickersin, Tianjing Li, and Xue Wang have authored several Cochrane systematic reviews that are assessed as part of this study.

* Email: isaldan1@jhmi.edu

Introduction

In clinical trials, an outcome is an event or measure in study participants that is used to assess the effectiveness and/or safety of the intervention being studied [1]. Choosing relevant outcomes is a critical early step in the design of clinical trials and systematic reviews for a number of reasons [2]. In clinical trials, expected effect sizes on critical outcomes are used to determine sample size [3]. In addition, there is general agreement that by pre-specifying the primary and secondary outcomes and limiting the number of statistical analyses, clinical trialists reduce the likelihood of Type I error (i.e., finding a statistically significant treatment effect just by chance, in the absence of a true treatment effect) and outcome reporting bias (i.e., selectively reporting outcomes based on the strength and/or direction of the findings). Although satisfactory solutions have not yet been developed, there is growing recognition that these issues also apply to systematic reviews [4]–[5]. Indeed, the Cochrane Collaboration recommends that systematic reviewers limit the number of and pre-specify all outcomes for their systematic review [6]–[7].

The process of conducting a systematic review of intervention effectiveness begins with formulating a research question, and then, finding and synthesizing the evidence from studies that address the question. In formulating the question, the systematic reviewer defines the population, intervention, comparison, and outcomes (PICO) to be examined. Studies that address the review question, typically clinical trials, should be broadly similar on the population, intervention and comparison groups, but frequently report different outcomes from those chosen by the systematic reviewer. Clinical trialists typically measure numerous outcomes, sometimes in the hundreds [8]. It is likely that these outcomes are different from those chosen by the systematic reviewer; overlap of the chosen outcomes can vary from none to complete (Figure 1). In many cases, the primary outcome of interest to the systematic reviewers may not have been an outcome of interest to the clinical trialists [9], or may not be reported clearly or consistently in the clinical trial reports or associated documents [10]. Systematic reviewers thus face an important decision: should they choose outcomes to be examined based on what they believe to be important outcomes ("systematic review author judgment") or based on what they know is reported in the relevant clinical trials ("clinical trialist judgment")?

How systematic reviewers choose outcomes and pre-specify them in systematic review protocols is currently unclear. One view is that, unlike clinical trialists, systematic reviewers should not base outcome choice on sample size/power calculations and Type I error rates. Instead, the objective of medical research should be to draw conclusions based on all sources of available evidence [11]. Systematic reviews, which are often used to inform clinical practice guidelines and policy, could and even should include all the outcomes that patients, clinicians, and policy-makers need to know about. Systematic reviews also allow elucidation of existing research gaps in a given field [12], for example, when outcomes are not examined in trials and should be.

In our view, regardless of who chooses the outcomes to be assessed in a systematic review and how those outcomes are chosen, all outcomes need to be specified completely and clearly if they are to be of use to decision-makers.

The objective of our study was to assess the completeness of pre-specification and comparability of outcomes in all Cochrane reviews addressing four common eye conditions. Our purpose is not to hold systematic review protocols to a standard that may not have been described at the time they were published, rather it is to initiate a discussion on important questions for systematic reviewers: how should systematic reviewers choose outcomes to address in the review; how should these outcomes be reported (i.e., which elements are necessary for complete reporting) by systematic reviewers; and if outcomes are pre-specified in systematic review protocols, should these protocols be formally updated with amendments to reflect changing outcome specification?

Methods

Review protocols examined

The Cochrane Collaboration publishes and archives all its systematic review protocols, completed reviews, and updates in *The Cochrane Database of Systematic Reviews*. Protocols for systematic reviews, hereafter referred to as 'protocols', were eligible for our study if they were published by the Cochrane Eyes and Vision Group (CEVG) in *The Cochrane Database of Systematic Reviews* in or before June 2013 (Issue 6), and if they addressed any of the following four eye conditions: glaucoma, age-related macular degeneration (AMD), cataract, and diabetic retinopathy (DR). We selected these four conditions because of their high disease burden across populations and the range of interventions addressing them [13]. For each eligible review, we identified the oldest available protocol and, when no protocol could be found for a review, we contacted CEVG editors and review authors via email to ask whether they had a copy. When these efforts were not successful, we used the most recent version of the completed review in place of the protocol.

Five elements of a completely specified outcome

We used an outcome definition that includes five elements: (1) the *domain* or outcome title (e.g., visual acuity); (2) the *specific measurement* or technique/instrument used to make the measurement (e.g., Snellen chart); (3) the *specific metric* or format of the outcome data from each participant that will be used for analysis (e.g., value at a time-point, change from baseline); (4) the *method of aggregation* or how data from each group will be summarized (e.g., mean, percent/proportion); and (5) the *time-points* that will be used for analysis (e.g., 3 months) (Figure 2). Whereas Zarin et al. specify these same elements [8], they define the first four elements and consider time-points related to each of those four.

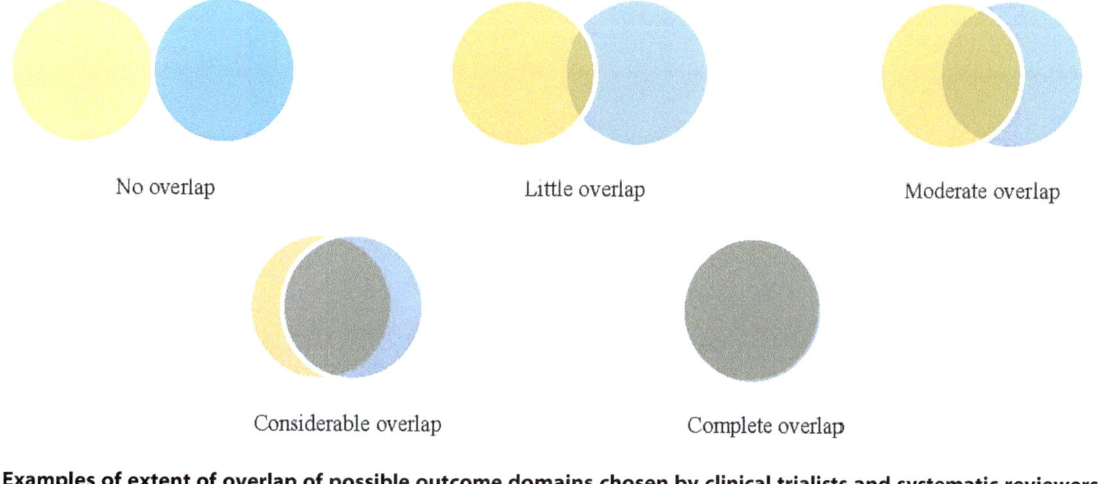

Figure 1. Examples of extent of overlap of possible outcome domains chosen by clinical trialists and systematic reviewers. Yellow - Outcomes chosen by clinical trialists. Blue - Outcomes chosen by systematic reviewers. Grey - Outcomes chosen by BOTH clinical trialists and systematic reviewers.

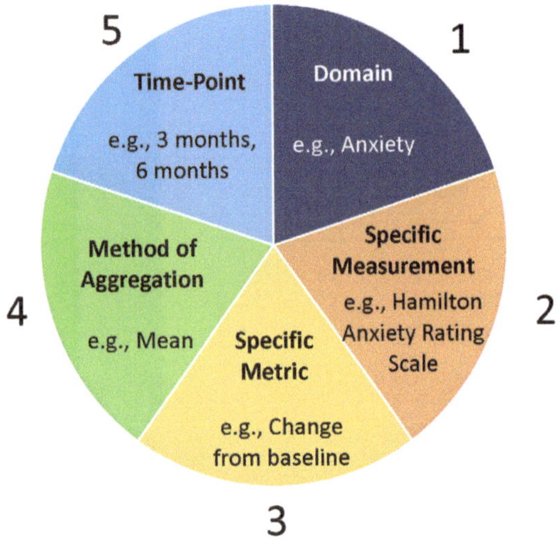

Figure 2. Five elements of a completely specified outcome, with anxiety as an example.

Selecting outcome domains for data extraction

Before beginning data extraction, one investigator (IS) identified all outcome domains in the Methods sections of included protocols. We then selected for data extraction those outcome domains appearing in at least 25% of eligible protocols. Then, for those eligible protocols with published completed reviews, we compared the Methods section of the protocol with the Methods section of the most recent version of the corresponding completed review, noting any differences in the specified outcome domains. We did this step to evaluate whether focusing on the protocols, some of which were published a while ago, would mean that we were assessing a different set of outcome domains than those currently being evaluated by the review authors.

Data extraction

We designed, tested, and finalized a data extraction form using Google Forms©. Two investigators (IS and XW) extracted data independently and resolved discrepancies through consensus or discussion with a third author (TL). We extracted data about the eye condition and year of publication of each protocol. We extracted from the Methods section the following data pertaining to each eligible outcome: type of outcome (primary, non-primary, or unclear [if not specified]) and each of the five outcome elements described earlier. For element 2, we extracted all specific measurements that were specified, or classified the specific measurement as unclear (if not specified). We classified element 3 (specific metric) into one or more of the following categories: (i) value at a time-point, (ii) time-to-event, (iii) change from baseline, and (iv) unclear (if not specified). We classified element 4 (method of aggregation) into one or more of the following categories: (i) mean, (ii) median, (iii) percent/proportion, (iv) absolute number, and (v) unclear (if not specified). For element 5, we extracted all time-points that were specified, or classified the time-points as unclear (if not specified).

Data analysis

We assessed the extent of completeness using the number of elements specified out of five possible, and considered an outcome specified in the Methods section as "complete" if all five elements were specified. For each outcome, we calculated median, interquartile range (IQR), and proportion of outcome elements specified. We performed Kruskal-Wallis tests for nonparametric comparisons of medians and distributions of extent of completeness by condition addressed, year of protocol publication, type of outcome, and outcome domain.

We assessed the frequency and comparability of outcome elements (i.e., similarity of categories for each element) for elements 3 and 4 across protocols addressing each of the four eye conditions. Protocols could specify more than one category for a given element. Comparability was therefore assessed as the distribution of those categories across protocols. As an example, if one protocol specified visual acuity at a time-point as well as change in visual acuity from baseline, we counted both categories for specific metric (element 3). In another example, protocols addressing cataract and assessing the outcome of visual acuity were considered to be comparable in method of aggregation (element 4) if they all specified mean or all specified median or both. However, they would not be comparable in element 4 if some specified mean and others specified median.

Statistical significance was defined at the 5% level. All data were analyzed using STATA© version 12 (College Station, TX).

Results

Characteristics of protocols examined

Our search identified 57 eligible systematic reviews (Table 1). We were able to find protocols for 54 reviews (94.7%), and used the Methods section of completed reviews for the remaining three (5.3%). An updated protocol was published for one of the 54 protocols. Glaucoma was the most frequently addressed condition (22 protocols), followed by cataract (16 protocols), AMD (15 protocols), and DR (4 protocols). Approximately half of the protocols (29/57; 50.9%) were published between 2006 and 2010. Thirty-four protocols were associated with a completed review, the most recent version of which was published a median of five (IQR 4–8, range 0–15) years after publication of the protocol.

Outcome domains used in protocols

We examined five outcome domains named in at least 25% of the eligible protocols (Table 2): quality-of-life (47/57 protocols; 82.5%), visual acuity (47/57; 82.5%), intraocular pressure (21/57; 36.8%), disease progression (15/57; 26.3%), and contrast sensitivity (15/57; 26.3%). One protocol did not name any of these five outcome domains. For most completed systematic reviews (30/34; 88.2%), these five outcome domains were similar to what was named in their corresponding protocols. Compared to their protocols, two completed systematic reviews dropped quality-of-life while one completed review added it. One completed systematic review dropped contrast sensitivity.

Completeness of outcome pre-specification

Across the 57 protocols, the five most frequent outcome domains appeared 145 times ('instances'); however, only 15/145 instances (10.3%) involved complete pre-specification (i.e., where all five elements of the outcome were specified). Overall, a median of three (IQR 2–4) elements were specified per outcome (Table 3). Extent of completeness was not statistically significantly different by condition. Completeness of outcome specification may be better in protocols published later compared to earlier, (median of three [IQR 2–4] elements specified in 2006–2010 versus one [IQR 1–3] in 2000 or earlier), although the difference was not statistically significant ($p = 0.1635$).

Fifty-four of 57 protocols (94.7%) specified at least one primary outcome. Among the five outcome domains evaluated in our

Table 1. Number of protocols and outcome domains by condition, year published, and whether specified as primary outcome.

Characteristic	Number (%) of protocols	Number (%) of outcomes
All	57[1] (100)	145[2] (100)
Condition addressed		
Glaucoma	22 (38.6)	51 (35.2)
Cataract	16 (28.1)	35 (24.1)
Age-related macular degeneration (AMD)	15 (26.3)	47 (32.4)
Diabetic retinopathy (DR)	4 (7.0)	12 (8.3)
Year of protocol publication		
2000 or earlier	6 (10.5)	13 (9.0)
2001 to 2005	15 (26.3)	37 (25.5)
2006 to 2010	29 (50.9)	76 (52.4)
2011 or later	7 (12.3)	19 (13.1)
Type of outcomes domain specified	Not applicable	
Outcomes specified as primary		48 (33.1)
Outcomes specified as non-primary		88 (60.7)
Type of outcome unclear		9 (6.2)

[1] 54 protocols and 3 completed reviews; One protocol did not include any of the outcome domains selected for detailed data extraction.
[2] 139/145 of the outcomes were described in the 54 protocols.

study, at least one was a primary outcome in 48/57 (84.2%) protocols. Extent of completeness appeared to differ by outcome type, with primary outcomes being most completely specified and outcomes with type unclear being least completely specified (median four versus one respectively, $p = 0.0001$). Intraocular pressure was the most completely specified outcome in our sample, with a median of four (IQR 3–4) elements specified (Table 2). Quality-of-life was least completely specified, with a median of one (IQR 1–2) element specified. The patterns of completeness of individual elements were similar across outcomes (Figure 3). Method of aggregation was specified least often, while domain and time-points were specified more often than other elements. The completeness of individual elements for the quality-of-life outcome was less than for other outcomes, overall. Although intraocular pressure was the most completely specified outcome, only 24% of protocols assessing it specified the specific measurement. Patterns of completeness of individual outcome elements also appeared to be similar across conditions, except for outcomes in DR protocols, where there were only four protocols and so the percentages are unlikely to be reliable (Figure 4).

Table 4 provides some examples of incomplete specification of outcomes in our sample of systematic reviews.

Comparability of outcome elements

Table 5 shows the distribution of specific metrics (element 3) and methods of aggregation (element 4) across instances of usage of outcome domain, by condition. The specific metric was unclear for large proportions of individual instances (often as high as 100% for the 16 instances of usage of quality-of-life in protocols addressing glaucoma and for the four instances of usage of contrast sensitivity in protocols addressing cataract). For instances where the specific metric was specified, the most frequent specific metrics were 'value at a time-point' and 'change from baseline'.

The method of aggregation was unclear for large proportions of individual instances (often as high as 100% for the 16 instances of usage of quality-of-life in protocols addressing glaucoma and for the four instances of usage of visual acuity in protocols addressing DR). For instances where the method of aggregation was specified, the most frequent methods of aggregation were 'mean' and 'percent/proportion'.

Table 2. Completeness (number of completely-specified elements out of five possible) by outcome domain.

Characteristic	Number (%) of protocols	Median (IQR) number of completely-specified elements per outcome	p-value
All	57[1] (100)	3.0 (2.0–4.0)	-
Outcome domain			
Quality-of-life	47 (82.5)	1.0 (1.0–2.0)	0.0001
Visual acuity	47 (82.5)	3.0 (2.0–4.0)	
Intraocular pressure	21 (36.8)	4.0 (3.0–4.0)	
Disease progression	15 (26.3)	3.0 (2.0–4.0)	
Contrast sensitivity	15 (26.3)	2.0 (1.0–3.0)	

[1] One protocol did not include any of the outcome domains selected for detailed data extraction.

Table 3. Completeness (number of completely-specified elements out of five possible) by type of protocol/outcome.

Characteristic	Median (IQR) number of completely specified elements per outcome	p-value
All[1]	3.0 (2.0–4.0)	NA
Condition addressed		
Glaucoma	3.0 (2.0–4.0)	0.1218
Cataract	3.0 (2.0–4.0)	
Age-related macular degeneration (AMD)	2.0 (1.0–3.0)	
Diabetic retinopathy (DR)	3.0 (1.5–4.0)	
Year of protocol publication		
2000 or earlier	1.0 (1.0–3.0)	0.1635
2001 to 2005	2.0 (2.0–4.0)	
2006 to 2010	3.0 (2.0–4.0)	
2011 or later	2.0 (2.0–3.0)	
Type of outcome domain specified		
Outcomes specified as primary	4.0 (3.0–4.0)	0.0001
Outcomes specified as non-primary	2.0 (1.0–3.0)	
Type of outcome not specified	1.0 (1.0–2.0)	

[1] 54 protocols and 3 completed reviews; Median 3.0 (2.0–4.0) for outcomes in the 54 protocols and 1.5 (1.0–2.0) for outcomes in the 3 reviews (p = 0.0627); One protocol did not include any of the outcome domains selected for detailed data extraction.

Discussion

Summary of main findings

We have shown that, if outcome pre-specification in systematic review protocols is judged using recommended standards for clinical trials, then it is largely incomplete. Although completeness appears to have improved somewhat over time, on average, only three of five standard elements of an outcome were pre-specified. Due to largely incomplete outcome pre-specification, a conclusive assessment of comparability in outcome elements across the various protocols per condition was not possible. However, we observed variation in specific metrics and methods of aggregation.

Completeness of outcome pre-specification

There are some reasons that might explain why outcomes were not completely specified in our study of systematic review protocols. First, although we believe complete specification of all five elements is necessary for a number of reasons, the idea is new to the systematic review community. This is demonstrated by the fact that the Cochrane Handbook states only that the name of the

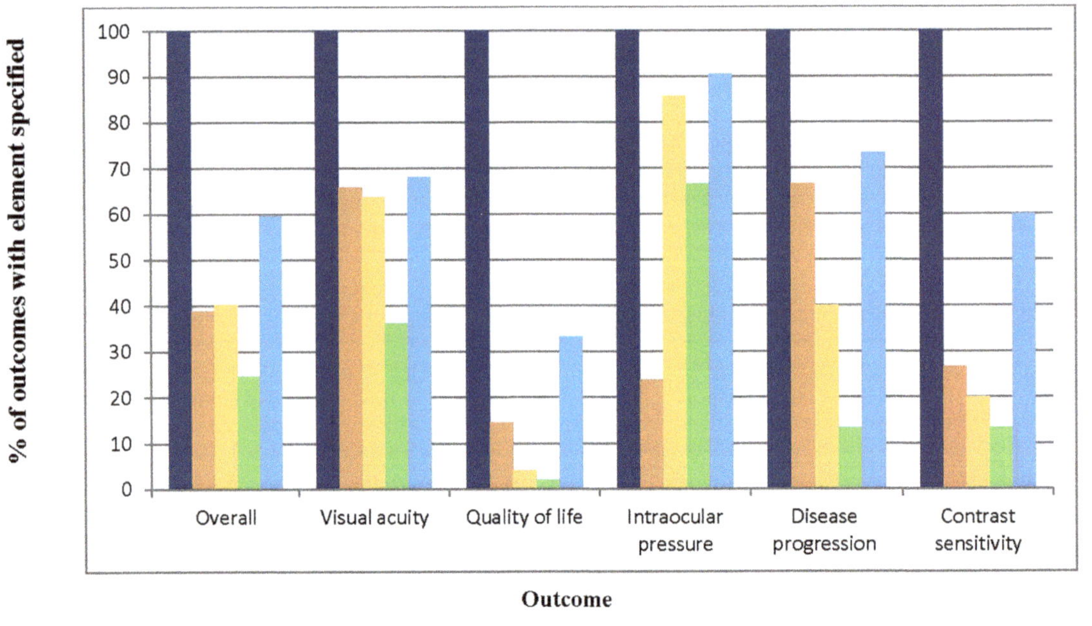

Figure 3. Completeness of specification of outcome elements, by outcome. Navy blue - Domain. Orange – Specific measurement. Yellow – Specific metric. Green – Method of aggregation. Blue – Time-point(s).

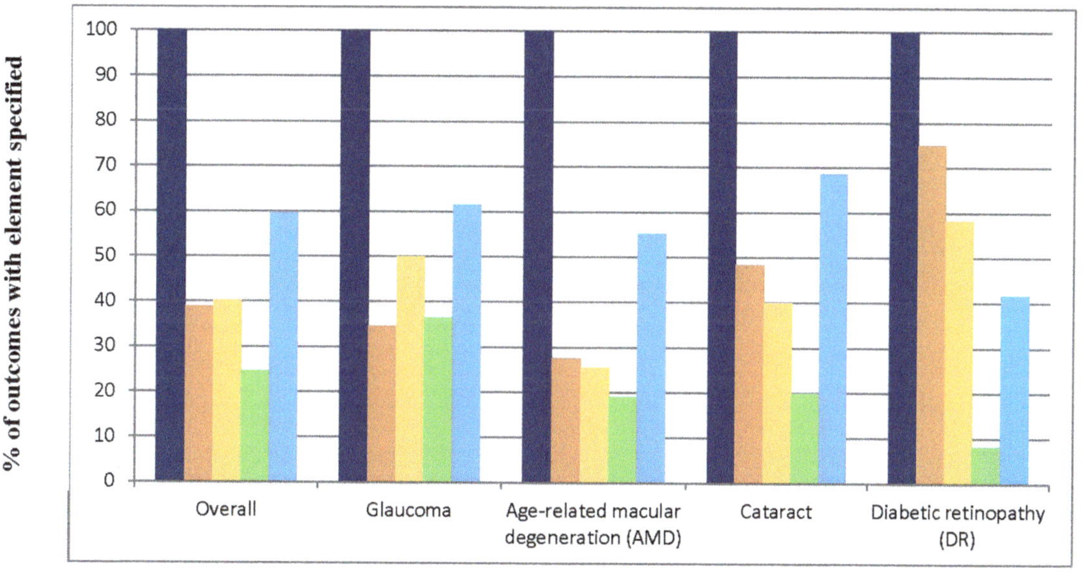

Figure 4. Completeness of specification of outcome elements, by condition. Navy blue - Domain. Orange – Specific measurement. Yellow – Specific metric. Green – Method of aggregation. Sky blue – Time-point(s).

outcome (equivalent to *domain* [element 1]), type of scale (equivalent to *specific measurement* [element 2]), and timing of measurement (equivalent to *time-points* [element 5]) must be pre-specified[6]; and there is no explicit mention of pre-specification of *specific metric* (element 3) or *method of aggregation* (element 4). Indeed, elements 1 and 5 were the most often-specified elements in our sample of protocols, though element 2 was frequently not specified (70% of the time) (Figure 3).

Another possible explanation for incomplete pre-specification of outcomes is that choice of outcomes could be influenced by the findings of (and outcomes examined in) the clinical trials that would be included in the review. We did not assess the outcomes examined at the level of the clinical trials to determine the likelihood that this occurred, but suggest that doing so may contribute to a better understanding of how review outcomes are chosen. Are they chosen because systematic reviewers consider them the most important outcomes to examine, because they are the outcomes that have been examined in clinical trials, or both? If the review outcomes were chosen purely because they were the outcomes that have been reported in clinical trials, this is troubling because of the possibility of "meta-bias". We know, for example, that outcomes reported in clinical trials could have been selectively reported because of desirable or undesirable findings [14]–[15]. By pre-specifying in the protocol the outcomes to be examined in the review, systematic reviewers minimize the potential for bias [5], [16], and reassure readers that the choice of outcomes was not influenced by the results of individual clinical trials. That said, systematic reviewers are usually familiar with their field and *a priori* aware of potentially eligible clinical trials and/or how the outcome in question is frequently measured. Complete pre-specification also could improve efficiency in data abstraction and analysis during a systematic review.

Systematic reviewers may also anticipate potential variation in outcomes across included clinical trials, and may allow for this by pre-specifying the elements of the outcome domain of interest in broad rather than specific terms (e.g., "visual acuity" versus "change in visual acuity from baseline to 1 year, as measured using a Snellen chart"). If such variation is suspected, systematic reviewers could explicitly state that all variations of a given element(s) will be included. This could minimize the occurrence of what Page et al. refer to as "selective inclusion" in systematic reviews [5].

Table 4. Examples of incomplete outcome pre-specification.

Exact text from methods section of protocol	Number of completely-specified elements (out of five possible)
"The primary outcome for the review will be visual acuity."	1
"When available quality of life data will be described for those with operated and unoperated cataract."	1
"Postoperative visual acuity"	1
"Quality of life"	1
"Contrast sensitivity"	1
"Vision-related quality of life at one year"	2
"Mean IOP"	2

Table 5. Frequency of categories of specific metric (element 3) and method of aggregation (element 4) across instances of usage of outcome domains by condition.

Condition/Outcome domain (Number of protocols/Number of instances)	Categories of specific metric (element 3) (% of instances)				Categories of method of aggregation (element 4) (% of instances)			
	Value at a time-point	Time-to-event	Change from baseline	Unclear	Mean	Percent/proportion	Absolute number	Unclear
Glaucoma (22 protocols)								
Quality-of-life (16 instances)	-	-	-	100	-	-	-	100
Visual acuity (13 instances)	31	-	31	46	8	39	-	54
Intraocular pressure (20 instances)	55	10	25	15	50	10	-	40
Disease progression (2 instances)	-	50	50	-	-	-	-	100
Cataract (16 protocols)								
Quality-of-life (12 instances)	17	-	-	83	-	8	-	92
Visual acuity (15 instances)	53	-	20	33	-	33	-	67
Intraocular pressure (1 instance)	100	-	-	-	100	100	-	-
Disease progression (3 instances)	-	-	33	67	-	-	-	100
Contrast sensitivity (4 instances)	-	-	-	100	-	-	-	100
Age-related macular degeneration (15 protocols)								
Quality-of-life (15 instances)	-	-	-	100	-	-	-	100
Visual acuity (15 instances)	47	-	33	40	20	13	13	60
Disease progression (6 instances)	-	-	-	100	-	-	17	83
Contrast sensitivity (11 instances)	18	-	9	73	18	18	-	82
Diabetic retinopathy (4 protocols)								
Quality-of-life (4 instances)	-	-	-	100	-	-	-	100
Visual acuity (4 instances)	100	-	25	-	-	-	-	100
Disease progression (4 instances)	50	25	-	25	25	-	-	75

Notes:
- If there was no instance of usage of a certain outcome domain across all reviews addressing a given condition, the above table does not include a row for that outcome domain for that condition.
- Percentages are row percentages (adding up individual categories within an element). Percentages sometimes total more than 100% for an element because some protocols used more than one category for that element.
- No reviews used "median" as a method of aggregation (element 4).

We assume that primary outcomes for both clinical trials and systematic reviews are chosen based on perceived clinical importance and/or importance to patients; and that they are usually measured and reported more thoroughly than non-primary outcomes [17]. Not surprisingly, in our study, primary outcomes were more completely specified than other outcome types. Our estimate of 94.7% protocols pre-specifying a primary outcome is somewhat higher than the 88% that has been reported as pre-specified in clinical trial protocols [18], and this could be related to the fact that we were examining protocols entered into software that requests the domain names of the pre-specified outcomes.

In our study, the most incompletely pre-specified outcome was quality-of-life, a key patient-important outcome. This finding is concordant with other studies that have found that outcome reporting in clinical trials is a bigger problem for patient-important outcomes than other types of outcomes [19]–[20]. Further, when patient-important outcomes are not primary outcomes in clinical trials, the likelihood that reporting is complete is further reduced [20]. Our study aimed to evaluate the completeness and comparability of all outcomes, both patient-important and not.

Our recommendation is that systematic reviewers should engage in discussion about and strongly consider pre-specifying all five elements of each outcome they wish to examine. When explicit pre-specification of all five elements of a given outcome is not possible, for example when all possible options for a given outcome element are not known or are too numerous, the systematic reviewers should enumerate all known acceptable options for each element and explicitly state that all options for that element would be accepted, or provide rationale for why it is impossible to completely pre-specify an element.

The Preferred Reporting Items for Systematic Reviews and Meta-analyses Protocols (PRISMA-P) is currently under development [21]. We hope that the availability of reporting guidelines (including details about outcome specification) will improve the completeness of specification of outcomes. Assuming that the Cochrane Collaboration recognizes the importance of completeness of pre-specification, there are some possible ways to ensure that review authors are aware of the five elements of a completely specified outcome. First, editorial teams at Cochrane Review Groups (CRGs) should make all review authors aware of the five outcome elements early in the process (no later than the protocol development stage). Second, peer reviewers should be directed to consider whether the outcomes are completely pre-specified and not likely to have been chosen based on the strength and direction of the findings for those outcomes. Third, the Cochrane Handbook and other systematic review guidance materials, in addition to training workshops and other educational avenues, should incorporate explicit descriptions of all five outcome elements. Other organizations producing guidance on systematic review methodology (e.g., Agency for Healthcare Research and Quality [AHRQ], the Centre for Reviews and Dissemination [CRD]) should also incorporate descriptions of the five outcome elements in their guidance materials.

Organizations such as the Cochrane Collaboration suggest limiting the number of outcomes examined in a systematic review [6]. However, in order to evaluate whether the effect of an intervention persists over time, an otherwise identical outcome (i.e., identical in the other four elements) is often measured at a number of time-points. For the purpose of counting the number of outcomes measured, we recommend that these repeated measurements be counted as one outcome regardless of the number of time-points at which the outcome is assessed.

Comparability of outcome elements

In the era of evidence-based medicine, decision-makers in healthcare (e.g., patients, clinicians, and policy-makers) increasingly rely on systematic reviews. It is important that decision-makers have access to high quality and up-to-date individual systematic reviews as well as are able to compare results across systematic reviews. Cochrane "overviews" (Cochrane reviews which compile evidence from related reviews of interventions into a single accessible and usable document) [6], and network meta-analyses (analyses of three or more interventions for a given condition in one meta-analysis) [22]–[23] are examples of formal comparisons across systematic reviews. To better feed into these formal comparisons and clinical practice guidelines, the elements of outcomes used in the various systematic reviews addressing a given condition should be comparable. In our study, the largely incomplete pre-specification of outcomes in protocols restricted our ability to assess comparability in outcome elements across protocols. In cases where the various elements were specified, however, we observed variation in specific metrics and methods of aggregation. An example of such variation is: one protocol pre-specified that the outcome domain of visual acuity would be measured as mean change in visual acuity (number of letters) from baseline to one year, while another protocol pre-specified that visual acuity would be measured as percent of participants with improvement in visual acuity of at least three letters at one year. While both protocols specified the same outcome domain at the same time-point, differences in the specific metric (mean change versus value at a time-point) and method of aggregation (mean versus percent) would preclude a direct comparison of the visual acuity results.

Efforts to promote comparability of outcomes across related clinical trials have led to the creation of core outcome measures within research fields [24]–[26]. One such effort is the Core Outcome Measures in Effectiveness Trials (COMET) Initiative [27], whose investigators have produced guidance on methods for identifying core outcome sets [28]. Because the issue of comparability of outcomes across systematic reviews is complex, we recommend that researchers within a field (e.g., systematic reviewers, Cochrane review group editors, clinical trialists) and patients consider developing comparable outcomes across systematic reviews, adding to a core list over time as appropriate.

There are pros and cons of establishing comparability in outcomes across reviews, however. Increased comparability will likely facilitate formal comparisons across systematic reviews and development of clinical practice guidelines. In addition, decision-makers would be better able to compare more directly the effectiveness of treatment options. For example, hundreds of measurement scales (*specific measurements*) have been used to assess mental status in schizophrenia [29] and quality-of-life [30], making comparability across clinical trials very challenging. Finally, use of comparable outcomes could discourage authors from 'cherry-picking' outcomes to be used in their studies [31].

On the other hand, comparability across reviews is not always possible or desirable. Limiting outcomes to those used by previous researchers risks excluding an outcome that is in fact important, or authors may be compelled to include an outcome that they do not consider important. Additionally, it might not be possible to identify *a priori* all relevant outcomes and outcome elements for a rapidly evolving field or for a field with a large number of relevant outcomes.

Availability of protocols and amendments to protocols

We were unable to obtain 3/57 (5.3%) protocols associated with our sample of Cochrane reviews. This poses a concern for investigators conducting methodological research in systematic reviews, and for users of systematic reviews generally. Although we do not believe that relying on the Methods sections of three completed Cochrane reviews in the cases where we could not find the protocols is likely to have influenced our findings, we believe that all protocols and previous versions of completed systematic reviews should be made available to researchers. Furthermore, an updated protocol was published for only one of the protocols we examined. The Cochrane Collaboration should consider keeping all protocols up-to-date by publishing updated versions of protocols or publishing protocol amendments for all its reviews. In this way, Cochrane review protocols would be formally amended in the same way that clinical trial protocols are amended and made available, providing an accessible audit trail. This practice will facilitate Cochrane's contribution of its protocols and updates to PROSPERO [32]–[33], an international database of prospectively registered systematic reviews.

Our focus on Cochrane reviews is both a strength and a limitation. Assuming that Cochrane reviews are among the most rigorously conducted and reported systematic reviews [34]–[35], it is likely that completeness and comparability of outcomes are higher in our sample of reviews than in other reviews. It would be useful to know how others producing systematic reviews (e.g., AHRQ, CRD, independent authors) choose and describe outcomes in their systematic reviews.

As discussed, we did not examine the individual clinical trials examined by each Cochrane review in our sample to learn more about the source of non-comparability in outcome elements. Nor did we test for empirical evidence of outcome reporting bias on the part of the systematic reviewers. Because our assessments of completeness and comparability were based on what was reported in the protocols (and some completed reviews), it is possible that our findings were a consequence of unsatisfactory reporting and that the rationale for the outcomes chosen could not be determined without asking the systematic review authors directly.

Our study should be replicated in other disease areas and on a larger scale to assess the applicability of our findings to other fields. Although we have compared the outcomes pre-specified in the protocol with what is in the corresponding completed review's Methods section, a next step would be to compare the outcomes in the Methods with those in the Results section. This would allow a confirmation of the potential bias by systematic reviewers that has been demonstrated by Kirkham et al. using a cohort of Cochrane reviews [36] and by various investigators studying this issue in clinical trials [14], [17], [37]–[38].

Conclusions

We recommend that systematic review authors strongly consider pre-specifying all outcomes of interest using the five elements of a completely specified outcome (domain, specific measurement, specific metric, method of aggregation, and time-points), amending the protocol formally, as needed. We further suggest that researchers and other stakeholders, such as patients, carefully consider the pros and cons of establishing comparability in outcomes across systematic reviews addressing a given condition.

Acknowledgments

We acknowledge the contributions of Deborah Zarin, MD; Karen Robinson, MA, PhD; Swaroop Vedula, MD, MPH, PhD; and Evan Mayo-Wilson, MSc, MPA, DPhil for their comments on previous versions of this manuscript. We also acknowledge the contributions of Michael Marrone, MPH, Kristina Lindsley, MS, and James Heyward, BA for their help with data abstraction and locating systematic review protocols for this study.

Author Contributions

Conceived and designed the experiments: IJS KD XW TL. Performed the experiments: IJS KD XW TL. Analyzed the data: IJS KD XW TL. Contributed reagents/materials/analysis tools: IJS KD XW TL. Wrote the paper: IJS KD XW TL.

References

1. Meinert CL (2012) Clinical trials dictionary: Terminology and usage recommendations. 2nd edition. Wiley. Hoboken, NJ.
2. Institute of Medicine (2011) Finding what works in health care: standards for systematic reviews. Available: http://www.iom.edu/Reports/2011/Finding-What-Works-in-Health-Care-Standards-for-Systematic-Reviews.aspx. Accessed 2014 September 12.
3. Campbell MJ, Julious SA, Altman DG (1995) Estimating sample sizes for binary, ordered categorical, and continuous outcomes in two group comparisons. BMJ 311(7013): 1145–1148.
4. Bender R, Bunce C, Clarke M, Gates S, Lange S, et al. (2008) Attention should be given to multiplicity issues in systematic reviews. J Clin Epidemiol 61(9): 857–865.
5. Page MJ, McKenzie JE, Forbes A (2013) Many scenarios exist for selective inclusion and reporting of results in randomized trials and systematic reviews. J Clin Epidemiol 66(5): 524–537.
6. Higgins JPTGreen S, (editors) (2011) Cochrane Handbook for Systematic Reviews of Interventions Version 5.1.0 [updated March 2011]. The Cochrane Collaboration. Available: www.cochrane-handbook.org. Accessed 2014 September 12.
7. Chandler J, Churchill R, Higgins J, Tovey D (2012) Methodological standards for the conduct of new Cochrane Intervention Reviews. Version 2.2. 17, December 2012. Available: http://www.editorial-unit.cochrane.org/sites/editorial-unit.cochrane.org/files/uploads/MECIR_conduct_standards%202.2%2017122012.pdf. Accessed 2014 September 12.
8. Zarin DA, Tse T, Williams RJ, Califf RM, Ide NC (2011) The ClinicalTrials.gov results database–update and key issues. N Engl J Med 364(9): 852–860.
9. Singh S, Loke YK, Enright PL, Furberg CD (2011) Mortality associated with tiotropium mist inhaler in patients with chronic obstructive pulmonary disease: systematic review and meta-analysis of randomised controlled trials. BMJ 14; 342:d3215. doi: 10.1136/bmj.d3215
10. Jefferson T, Jones MA, Doshi P, Del Mar CB, Heneghan CJ, et al. (2012) Neuraminidase inhibitors for preventing and treating influenza in healthy adults and children. Cochrane Database Syst Rev (1):CD008965.
11. Goodman SN (1989) Meta-analysis and evidence. http://www.ncbi.nlm.nih.gov/pubmed/2666026Control Clin Trials 10(2): 188–204.
12. Robinson KA, Saldanha IJ, Mckoy NA (2011) Development of a framework to identify research gaps from systematic reviews. J Clin Epidemiol 64(12): 1325–1330.
13. National Eye Institute (2010) Statistics and Data Available: http://www.nei.nih.gov/eyedata. Accessed 2014 September 12.
14. Vedula SS, Bero L, Scherer RW, Dickersin K (2009) Outcome reporting in industry-sponsored trials of gabapentin for off-label use. N Engl J Med 361(20): 1963–1971.
15. Dwan K, Altman DG, Cresswell L, Blundell M, Gamble CL, et al. (2011) Comparison of protocols and registry entries to published reports for randomised controlled trials. Cochrane Database Syst Rev Issue 1. Art. No.: MR000031. doi: 10.1002/14651858.MR000031.pub2
16. Stewart L, Moher D, Shekelle P (2012) Why prospective registration of systematic reviews makes sense. Syst Rev 1: 7. doi:10.1186/2046-4053-1-7
17. Kirkham JJ, Dwan KM, Altman DG, Gamble C, Dodd S, et al. (2010) The impact of outcome reporting bias in randomised controlled trials on a cohort of systematic reviews. BMJ 340: c365. doi: 10.1136/bmj.c365
18. Mathieu S, Boutron I, Moher D, Altman DG, Ravaud P (2009) Comparison of registered and published primary outcomes in randomized controlled trials. JAMA 302(9): 977–984.
19. Wieseler B, Kerekes MF, Vervolgyi V, Kohlepp P, McGauran N, et al. (2012) Impact of document type on reporting quality of clinical drug trials: a comparison registry reports, clinical study reports, and journal publications. BMJ 344 d8141 doi: 10.1136/bmj.d8141
20. Wieseler B, Wolfram N, McGauran N, Kerekes MF, Vervolgyi V, et al. (2013) Completeness of reporting of patient-relevant clinical trial outcomes: comparison

of unpublished clinical study reports with publicly available data. PLOS Med 10 (10) e1001526. doi: 10.1371/journal.pmed.1001526

21. EQUATOR Network (2014) Reporting Guidelines under development. Available: http://www.equator-network.org/library/reporting-guidelines-under-development/#99. Accessed 2014 September 12.
22. Caldwell DM, Ades AE, Higgins JP (2005) Simultaneous comparison of multiple treatments: combining direct and indirect evidence. BMJ 331(7521): 897–900.
23. Li T, Puhan M, Vedula SS, Singh S, Dickersin K for the Ad Hoc Network Meta-analysis Methods Meeting Working Group (2011) Network meta-analysis – highly attractive and more methodological research is needed. BMC Medicine 9(1): 79. doi:10.1186/1741-7015-9-79
24. Miller AB, Hoogstraten B, Staquet M, Winkler A (1981) Reporting results of cancer treatment. Cancer 47(1): 207–214.
25. Tugwell P, Boers M, Brooks P, Simon LS, Strand V (2007) OMERACT: An international initiative to improve outcome measures in rheumatology. Trials 8: 38.
26. Dworkin RH, Turk DC, Farrar JT, Haythornthwaite JA, Jensen MP, et al. (2005) Core outcome measures for chronic pain trials: IMMPACT recommendations. Pain 113(1–2): 9–19.
27. COMET Initiative (2014) Overview. Available: http://www.comet-initiative.org/about/overview. Accessed 2014 September 12.
28. Williamson PR, Altman DG, Blazeby JM, Clarke M, Devane D, et al. (2012) Developing core outcome sets for clinical trials: issues to consider. Trials 13(132). doi: 10.1186/1745-6215-13-132
29. Thornley B, Adams C (1998) Content and quality of 2000 controlled trials in schizophrenia over 50 years. BMJ 317(7167): 1181–1184.
30. Salek S (1999) Compendium of Quality of Life Instruments. Wiley. ISBN: 0-471-98145-1.
31. Clarke M (2007) Standardising outcomes for clinical trials and systematic reviews. Trials 8: 39.
32. Booth A, Clarke M, Dooley G, Ghersi D, Moher D, et al. (2012) The nuts and bolts of PROSPERO: an international prospective register of systematic reviews. Sys Rev 1: 2. doi: 10.1186/2046-4053-1-2
33. Booth A, Clarke M, Dooley G, Ghersi D, Moher D, et al. (2013) PROSPERO at one year: an evaluation of its utility. Sys Rev 2: 4. doi: 10.1186/2046-4053-2-4
34. Jadad AR, Cook DJ, Jones A, Klassen TP, Tugwell P, et al. (1998) Methodology and reports of systematic reviews and meta-analyses: A comparison of Cochrane reviews with articles published in paper-based journals. JAMA 280(3): 278–280.
35. Moher D, Tetzlaff J, Tricco AC, Sampson M, Altman DG (2007) Epidemiology and reporting characteristics of systematic reviews. PLoS Med 4(3): e78.
36. Kirkham JJ, Altman DG, Williamson PR (2010) Bias due to changes in prespecified outcomes during the systematic review process. PLoS One 5(3): e9810. doi: 10.1371/journal.pone.0009810
37. Chan AW, Altman D (2005) Identifying outcome reporting bias in randomized trials on PubMed: review of publications and survey of authors. BMJ 330(7494): 753.
38. Chan AW, Hrobjartsson A, Haahr MT, Gøtzsche PC, Altman DG (2004) Empirical evidence for selective reporting of outcomes in randomized trials: comparison of protocols to published articles. JAMA 291(20): 2457–2465.

16

Characterization of a New Epidemic Necrotic Pyoderma in Fur Animals and Its Association with *Arcanobacterium phocae* Infection

Heli Nordgren[1*¤a], Kirsi Aaltonen[2,3], Tarja Sironen[2,3], Paula M. Kinnunen[2¤b], Ilkka Kivistö[3], Mirja Raunio-Saarnisto[4], Anna-Maria Moisander-Jylhä[5], Johanna Korpela[5], Ulla-Maija Kokkonen[6], Udo Hetzel[2¤c], Antti Sukura[2], Olli Vapalahti[2,3,7]

1 Production Animal Section, Finnish Food Safety Authority (Evira), Seinäjoki, Finland, **2** Department of Veterinary Biosciences, Faculty of Veterinary Medicine, University of Helsinki, Helsinki, Finland, **3** Department of Virology, Haartman institute, University of Helsinki, Helsinki, Finland, **4** Seinäjoki Laboratory Section, Finnish Food Safety Authority (Evira), Seinäjoki, Finland, **5** Finnish Fur Breeders Association (FFBA), Vantaa and Vaasa, Finland, **6** Section for Poultry, Wild and Laboratory Animals, Finnish Food Safety Authority (Evira), Helsinki, Finland, **7** Department of Virology and Immunology, HUSLAB, Hospital district of Helsinki and Uusimaa, Helsinki, Finland

Abstract

A new type of pyoderma was detected in Finnish fur animals in 2007. The disease continues to spread within and between farms, with severe and potentially fatal symptoms. It compromises animal welfare and causes considerable economic losses to farmers. A case-control study was performed in 2010–2011 to describe the entity and to identify the causative agent. Altogether 99 fur animals were necropsied followed by pathological and microbiological examination. The data indicated that the disease clinically manifests in mink (*Neovison vison*) by necrotic dermatitis of the feet and facial skin. In finnraccoons (*Nyctereutes procyonoides*), it causes painful abscesses in the paws. Foxes (*Vulpes lagopus*) are affected by severe conjunctivitis and the infection rapidly spreads to the eyelids and facial skin. A common finding at necropsy was necrotic pyoderma. Microbiological analysis revealed the presence of a number of potential causative agents, including a novel *Streptococcus* sp. The common finding from all diseased animals of all species was *Arcanobacterium phocae*. This bacterium has previously been isolated from marine mammals with skin lesions but this is the first report of *A. phocae* isolated in fur animals with pyoderma. The results obtained from this study implicate *A. phocae* as a potential causative pathogen of fur animal epidemic necrotic pyoderma (FENP) and support observations that the epidemic may have originated in a species - shift of the causative agent from marine mammals. The variable disease pattern and the presence of other infectious agents (in particular the novel *Streptococcus* sp.) suggest a multifactorial etiology for FENP, and further studies are needed to determine the environmental, immunological and infectious factors contributing to the disease.

Editor: Glenn Francis Browning, The University of Melbourne, Australia

Funding: Co-authors Anna-Maria Moisander-Jylhä and Johanna Korpela are employed by the Finnish Fur Breeders' association. The funder provided support in the form of salary for authors Anna-Maria Moisander-Jylhä and Johanna Korpela, but did not have any additional role in the study design, data collection and analysis, decision to publish, or preparation of the manuscript. The specific roles of these authors are articulated in the 'author contributions' section.

Competing Interests: Finnish Fur Breeders' association supported the work. Co-authors Anna-Maria Moisander-Jylhä , DVM and Johanna Korpela, DVM are employed by the Finnish Fur Breeders' association. There are no patents, products in development or marketed products to declare.

* Email: heli.nordgren@profur.fi

¤a Current address: Department of Veterinary Biosciences, Faculty of Veterinary Medicine, University of Helsinki, Helsinki, Finland and Finnish Fur Breeders Association (FFBA), Vantaa and Vaasa, Finland
¤b Current address: Plans and Policy Division, Defense Command, Finnish Defense Forces, Helsinki, Finland
¤c Current address: Vetsuisse Faculty, Institute of Veterinary Pathology, University of Zürich, Zürich, Switzerland

Introduction

In 2007, Finnish fur farmers and the industry were affected by a new type of disease pattern in fur animals characterized by severe suppurative skin inflammation (pyoderma), affecting all major fur animal species in the country: captive mink (*Neovison vison*), foxes (*Vulpes lagopus*) and finnraccoons (*Nyctereutes procyonoides*, a raccoon dog bred in Finland for the fur industry). The disease manifests slightly differently in each species, but pyoderma is the common feature. The disease causes significant economic losses for the fur industry and affects animal wellbeing. Similar signs were documented in farmed mink in Canada in 1996 and also in USA in 1970 [1]. According to the Canadian farmers, the occurrence of the clinical signs was linked to the feeding of the mink with byproducts of seal. The Canadian study suggested that the cause of pododermatitis in mink was an unidentified infectious agent with secondary bacteriologic pyoderma. Similar signs have, to the best of our knowledge, never been described in foxes and finnraccoons. The disease pattern has been detected in fur animals in Denmark, Poland, The Netherlands, Spain, Iceland, and most recently in Sweden and Norway (personal communication from veterinarians treating fur animals, Nordic Association of Agricultural Scientists, NJF, Fur animal veterinarian meeting, Levi, Finland, 2014).

In mink, bacterial dermatitis is a relatively common finding and often associated with biting wounds. Only a few young individuals are usually affected [2]. The most common bacteria found on infected skin are *Staphylococcus* spp. and *Streptococcus* spp. These infections are less common in finnraccoons and foxes. The new deep pyoderma differs from previous disease patterns by spreading within the farm, and in the worst case affecting the entire pack.

In 1997, a novel bacterium, *Arcanobacterium phocae*, was isolated from gray seals (*Halichoerus grypus*) and common seals (*Phoca vitulina*) around Scotland, UK [3]. Skin lesions associated with *A. phocae* were first described in a study analyzing samples gathered between 1994 and 2000; *A. phocae* isolates were recovered from 141 marine mammals, stranded along the central California coast (USA). *A. phocae* was cultured from 66 California sea lions (*Zalophus californianus*), 50 Pacific harbor seals (*Phoca vitulina richardii*), 19 northern elephant seals (*Mirounga angustirostris*), five southern sea otters (*Enhydra lutris nereis*), and one common dolphin (*Delphinus delphis*). In marine mammals, *A. phocae* isolates are most commonly obtained from superficial pyogenic infections such as abscesses, wounds and exudates. However, some cases with deep-seated and systematic infections have also been documented. Many of the infections are associated with bite and bullet wounds or other kinds of traumatic skin injury. *A. phocae* isolates from marine mammals are often present in mixed bacterial infections [4].

Arcanobacterium phocae is a Gram-positive coccobacillus that occasionally morphs into a short rod. The bacteria are non-motile and beta-hemolytic on blood agar. *A. phocae* is catalase positive and oxidase negative and in the CAMP reaction test, a reverse CAMP reaction with *Staphylococcus aureus* and a positive CAMP reaction with *Rhodococcus equi* are typical. It has also been found to be susceptible to all tested antibiotics including aminoglycosides, β-lactams, bacteriostatic and bacterisidal antibiotics, fluoroquinolones, macrolides, rifamycins, and polyketides [4].

A. phocae belongs to the genus *Arcanobacterium* first described by Collins *et al.* in 1982 [5]. This genus is currently under taxonomic revision [6]: the genus *Arcanobacterium sensu stricto* has been suggested to contain the species *A. haemolyticum*, *A. phocae*, *A. pluranimalium*, and *A. hippocoleae*. In addition, the recently discovered *A. canis* [7] and *A. phocisimile* [8] have been suggested to belong to this genus. Five previous members of the genus *Arcanobacterium* have been proposed to form a new genus, *Trueperella* [6]: *T. bernardiae*, *T. pyogenes*, *T. bialowiezense*, *T. bonasi*, and *T. abortisuis*. These bacteria may be recovered from various organs such as the respiratory and digestive tracts, abscesses and systemic infections. *Arcanobacterium* spp. and *Trueperella* spp. have also been reported from other infections and colonization of both healthy and diseased humans and animals [3,9–11].

In 2010, the Finnish Fur Breeders association (FFBA), Finnish Food Safety Authority Evira and University of Helsinki (UH) started a collaborative project to describe the clinical signs, gross and histological lesions, epidemiological aspects, as well as the etiological agent(s) of the disease. Here, we describe the manifestation and pathology of the fur animal epidemic necrotic pyoderma (FENP) and provide microbiological evidence for *Arcanobacterium phocae* as its candidate etiological agent.

Materials and Methods

Ethics statement

The Animals investigated here were culled for pelting as part of normal procedures in fur animal husbandry, and thus no ethical permission was required in any of the organizations or institutions involved. The carcasses of all included individuals (99) were obtained as donations from 13 fur animal farms. No animals were culled for research purposes. The mink were euthanized on the farm using CO or CO_2 gas, and foxes and finnraccoons using electricity by the methods described in legislation concerning culling of the animals ((EU) N: o 1099/2009). The animal welfare is secured on the farms by a Certification Program, created and managed by the Finnish Fur Breeders Association. The certification program means continuous development in the farms, strict monitoring and documentation of all activities. The samples used in this study came from certified farms, and the farms voluntarily sent the samples to Evira.

Sampling

Between November 2010 and January 2011, 21 mink, 19 foxes and 21 finnraccoons exhibiting typical signs were gathered from 10 farms with a history of disease. Furthermore, 11 mink and finnraccoons and 12 foxes were taken from three farms where the disease had never been detected, and a further four clinically healthy mink were collected from two diseased farms (altogether 99 animals). A complete necropsy with histological and microbiological examination was performed on all animals. The animals were gathered at pelting time, when mostly young animals (average seven months) are kept on the farms with equal numbers of both sexes. The animals used in the study were not treated with any medication.

The 21 diseased mink were collected from two (17+4) farms. Both sexes were represented (nine females and 12 males). Sampled mink were under one year of age. Both diseased and healthy mink had been vaccinated against virus enteritis caused by mink enteritis parvovirus (MEV), botulism caused by *Clostridium botulinum* and hemorrhagic pneumonia caused by *Pseudomonas aeruginosa*.

The 19 diseased foxes were collected from three farms (11+5+3), and healthy controls (12) from one farm. Most of the foxes were less than one year old, but some lacked anamnestic information. Both sexes were represented but diseased females predominated (16) and healthy controls were all male. None of the farms had vaccinated the foxes against parvovirus.

The 21 diseased finnraccoons originated from five farms (2+12+4+2+1) and healthy controls (11) from one farm. Most of the diseased finnraccoons were female (13) and most of the healthy controls were male (7). All these finnraccoon farms vaccinated the animals against parvovirus with the mink enteritis vaccine.

Gross pathology

The gross lesions were described by the location, width and severity (mild, moderate, severe) of the lesion and the duration (acute, chronic) of the process. Any lesions in the internal organs were also recorded.

Histopathology

Samples of brain, heart, lung, trachea, spleen, liver, kidney, bladder, duodenum, jejunum, ileum, colon, local lymph nodes, and skin (mink, finnraccoon) and eyes (fox) were fixed in 10% phosphate buffered formalin for at least 24 h, embedded in paraffin and sectioned at 4 μm. All tissues were stained with hematoxylin and eosin (H&E), and selected tissues with special stains (Gomori Methenamine Silver (GMS), Zieh-Neelsen (ZN), and Warthin Starry silver stain (WS)).

Bacteriological studies

Bacteriological investigations were performed in the Seinäjoki unit of Evira. Samples of brain, heart, lung, spleen, liver, kidney, duodenum, jejunum, ileum, colon, local lymph nodes, and skin (mink, finnraccoon) and eyes (fox) were cultured on blood agar plates containing 5% defibrinated bovine blood and incubated aerobically at 37°C for 24–48 hours. Skin and eye samples were also cultured anaerobically at 37°C for 4–7 days. Earlier investigations found no yeast, fungi, *Salmonella*, *Campylobacter* spp., other anaerobic pathogens or mycoplasma in the diseased animals, so these tests were excluded from this study. Bacterial species were confirmed either by biochemical methods or 16S RNA PCR and sequencing. Three isolates were tested for antibiotic susceptibility with VetMIC-panels for Gram-positive bacteria (VetMIC GP mo) and for small animals (VetMIC smådjur) (The National Veterinary Institute, SVA, Sweden).

PCR detection of *Arcanobacterium phocae*

Due to the relatively low sensitivity of bacterial cultures and the nature of the sample material, with the potential loss of bacterial cultivability, a PCR -method was developed for the detection of *A. phocae*. Tissue biopsy samples (third eyelid and tissue samples from affected paws or face) were homogenized by mortar and pestle or by cutting with scalpel. DNA was extracted from these homogenates as well as from the eye swabs using a DNA blood and tissue kit (Qiagen) according to the manufacturer's instructions, with tissue lysis overnight. PCR primers Forw-5′-TGGCATGCTGTTGGGGTGT-3′ and Rev-5′-TCGGCTCCGTATGCCAAGGC-3′ were designed to amplify a 182-nt product from the 16S–23S intergenic region. Real-time PCR was performed using the MAXIMA SYBR Green kit (Thermo Fisher Scientific) in a StrataGene Mx3005p thermocycler. The program contained a preliminary denaturation step of 10 minutes at 95°C followed by 40 cycles of denaturation at 95°C for 15 s, annealing at 65°C for 60 s and extension at 72°C for 60 s, with measurement after the annealing step. The specificity of the products was checked by running a melting curve analysis and by direct sequencing of the products. The analytical sensitivity of the PCR assay was estimated by a dilution series of DNA extracted from a pure culture of *A. phocae*, and was determined to be one bacterial genome per reaction. The sensitivity in sample matrix was assayed by spiking negative tissue samples with the same extraction, and was shown to be ten bacterial copies per reaction. The copy number was estimated using the genomic size of the closest known relative, *Arcanobacterium haemolyticum* and a copy number counter (Thermo Fisher Scientific). The analytical specificity of the assay was estimated using DNA extracted from *Escherichia coli*, *Staphylococcus pseudintermedius*, *Streptococcus halichoeri*, *Streptococcus canis*, *Streptococcus pyogenes*, *Arcanobacterium haemolyticum* and the novel *Streptococcus* found in this study. These all remained negative, except in extremely high concentrations of pure bacterial cultures. This led to the definition of a diagnostic cut-off for the cycle threshold value (Ct) set to 31 approximately corresponding to 50 copies (Table S1). For samples above this cut-off, but with the correct melting temperature, sequencing was performed to confirm the specificity of each positive result.

Virological studies

Serum and tissue samples (lung, trachea, bladder and rectum) were collected and sent to the Helsinki unit of Evira for virological studies. Canine distemper virus (CDV) was tested from the lung, trachea, and bladder samples, and mink enteritis parvovirus (MEV) from the rectum samples, both by PCR modified from [12] and [13], respectively. Antibodies against CDV and MEV were measured from the serum collected from the necropsied animals. The serum neutralization test was used for the detection of antibodies to CDV [14], and the hemagglutination inhibition test for antibodies to MEV [15]. Pieces of the affected skin and eyes were frozen in Universal Transport Medium (UTM) -tubes (Copan, USA) at −70°C and sent to the University of Helsinki to further investigations. From these samples, positivity for herpesvirus DNA was tested with PCR [16]. All mink were tested against plasmacytosis (Aleutian Mink Disease virus) in the laboratory of the Finnish Fur Breeders Association in Vaasa with an ELISA-test [17].

Virus isolation trials

Tissue samples from infected animals were homogenized by manual grinding with mortars and pestles over dry ice. Dulbecco's modified phosphate buffered saline solution with 0.2% bovine serum albumin, 10 U/ml penicillin, 0.1 mg/ml streptomycin, and 0.25 µg/ml amphotericin B (Fungizone, Invitrogen) was used in the homogenizing with 700 µl of D-PBS added to approximately 10–50 mg of tissue. Swabs taken from infected eyes were vortexed and 100 µl of the medium was diluted with 400 µl of D-PBS. Samples of the homogenate and transport medium were collected for nucleic acid extraction and electron microscopy (EM), for which samples were negatively stained with uranyl acetate and the potential presence of viruses studied using a JEOL 1400 transmission electron microscope at 80 kV.

A preliminary isolation test was performed using Madin-Darby canine kidney epithelial (MDCK, ATCC CCL-34), Mink Lung epithelial (Mv1Lu, ATCC CCL-64), canine tumor fibroblast (A-72, ATCC CRL-1542), and feline kidney epithelial (CRFK, ATCC CCL-94) cell lines. Based upon the cell type and species match, and tolerance of long growth times, MDCK and Mv1Lu cell lines were chosen for the main experiment. The MDCK cells were propagated in Eagle's minimum essential medium (MEM) with 10% fetal bovine serum (FBS), 0.3 mg/ml glutamine, 10 U/ml penicillin, and 0.1 mg/ml streptomycin and the Mv1Lu cells in Dulbecco's modified minimum essential medium (D-MEM) with added glucose and 7% fetal bovine serum (FBS), 0.3 mg/ml glutamine, 10 U/ml penicillin, and 0.1 mg/ml streptomycin. The cells were incubated at 37°C with 5% CO_2, and were grown to approximately 75% confluence on six well plates before infection. After washing the cells with PBS, 300 µl of homogenate was pipetted onto them and incubated for 1 hour with gentle shaking every 15 minutes. One milliliter of the cell-specific growth medium with only 2% FBS was added onto the cells and they were incubated over night, after which another milliliter of this medium was added.

Cell cultures were followed for signs of cytopathic effect (CPE) daily, and samples of the medium and cells were collected when CPE was detected. The culture medium was changed once a week and the cells were allowed to grow for approximately 3 weeks. Samples of the medium containing cells were also collected when the medium was changed. Selected samples showing possible CPE were assessed by EM as described earlier in this section.

Results

Clinical signs of fur animal epidemic necrotic pyoderma

The disease was found in all three species of fur animals: mink (*Neovison vison*), foxes (*Vulpes lagopus*), and finnraccoons

(*Nyctereutes procyonoides*). However the clinical manifestation differed in each of them. Commonly observed signs in affected mink included skin inflammation on the paws and the facial skin. Any paw could be affected, but inflammation was usually first noted on the front paws. Lesions on the head were usually around the eyes, ears, or nose. In foxes, the first clinical sign detected was anorexia, followed by serous discharge from the eyes, which rapidly turned purulent. In some cases, the suppurative inflammation spread to the eyelids and the facial skin. In finnraccoons, the infection was usually limited to the paws. Paws were swollen, and in severe cases deep abscesses formed and the infection could proceed proximally along the limbs. Poor appetite was observed in prolonged cases.

Gross lesions in the study animals

The mink typically (15/21) had chronic severe necrotic pyoderma in the facial skin. Crust formation was detected with brownish exudate and attached bedding material (Fig. 1a). Lesions ranged from 2 cm×2 cm to 8 cm×8 cm and often covered the nose, eyes, and ears. Beneath the crust tissue, necrosis and hyperemia were observed. Some mink (3) had an alopecic ring around the lesion. Similar but smaller-sized lesions were seen on the legs in five out of 21 necropsied mink (Table 1). One mink had lesions on a hind leg, and others on their front legs (4/21). Lesions were observed on the footpads, nail beds, or dorsal skin of the paw. Two mink had a nail missing and the inflammation had spread to the bone structures. One mink only had alopecia in the dorsal skin of the paw, with no ulcer or crust formation. The exact progression of the disease could not be recorded, as all samples represented chronic inflammation. Splenomegaly was seen in 10/21 of the diseased mink, and 7/21 had swollen and enlarged local axillary or popliteal lymph nodes (Table 1). One mink had fatty liver, considered as an incidental finding, and two were extremely cachectic. Congestion in internal organs was seen in 4/21 animals.

Samples of foxes (19) represented a variety of the stages of the disease and it was therefore possible to describe the presumptive disease progression. An early sign of the disease was serous discharge from the eyes followed by the third eyelid becoming hyperemic, with vesicle development. The discharge turned purulent as the disease progressed. The purulent inflammation spread from the eye to the eye lids (Fig. 1b) and sometimes to the entire skin of the face. Entropion was noted in the eyelids of 3/19 of the animals (Table 1). Three foxes had enlarged and swollen local lymph nodes, and two had a fatty liver. In the internal organs no other significant findings were recorded.

Diseased finnraccoons had abscesses between the toes (Fig. 1c), 17/21 had lesions on the front paws, and both front and hind paws were affected in 4/21 (Table 1). The abscesses were intact, but one also had fistulae. One control animal had abscesses between the toes. Altogether, 10/21 of the diseased finnraccoons had splenomegaly and 10/21 had enlarged local lymph nodes (axillary and/or popliteal).

Histopathology

Skin samples from 19/21 mink displayed severe chronic necrotic pyoderma with ulceration and crusting, and 11/19 had coccoid bacteria in the epidermal layer (Fig. 2a). Severe necrosis (11/21) and vasculitis (8/21) that had led to thrombosis were detected. The inflammation appeared to spread to hair follicles in 4/21 cases (perifolliculitis/folliculitis). Hyperkeratosis (10/21) and parakeratosis (8/21) were observed in the samples (Fig. 2b). Some vacuolated keratinocytes (4/21) as well as hypergranulosis (4/21) were occasionally seen. Perivascular and periadnexal lympho-plasmacytic inflammation was noted in 9/21 cases. In two samples, eosinophilic material resembling inclusion bodies was detected. Special stains (GMS and ZN) were used, but no evidence of parasites, fungi, or mycobacteria was seen. WS staining revealed no silver stain-positive organisms. The samples represented chronic inflammation, and it is possible that the first insults of infection could no longer be detected in these samples. The healthy controls had no inflammatory changes, but slight hyper- and parakeratosis in the footpads was seen in 2/11 of the healthy controls from the uninfected farm, as well as in two out of the four healthy controls from the diseased farms.

Diseased mink had histologically reactive changes in the spleen (9/12) and in the local lymph nodes (3/12), as well as perivascular or peribronchial lymphocytosis in lung specimens (4). One diseased mink had severe pneumonia with Langerhans cells, syncytia, and alveolar histiocytosis. In the lungs of the healthy controls, varying degrees of perivascular and peribronchial lymphocytosis were detected (4/11). In two healthy individuals, gathered from a diseased farm, perivascular and peribronchial lymphocytosis was observed in the lung samples (2/4). No specific changes were detected in the other internal organs of any of the mink.

The foxes displayed conjunctivitis which spread from the limbus to the corneal center, progressing centrally to an ulcerative keratitis. Occasional findings were made of phtisis, hypopyon, and conjunctival inflammation extending into the retrobulbar/peri-scleral tissues, and chronic, purulent pustular dermatitis in the eyelids. These findings were not consistent. The inflammation was chronic, lympho-plasmacytic conjunctivitis with mild to moderate, predominantly neutrophilic inflammation. In severe cases, lympho-plasmacytic keratitis and serocellular crusts with coccoid bacteria were present. Hypereosinophilia of basal epithelia, corneal edema and activation of keratocytes was also detected. No specific changes were observed in the internal organs of any of the foxes.

Finnraccoons had varying degrees of chronic deep diffuse neutrophilic inflammation that also involved the subcutis (18/21) (Fig. 2d and e). In many samples, severe furunculosis (13/21) was detected. In 8/21 of the samples there was hyperkeratosis in the epidermis, with ulceration, hemorrhage, and necrosis with coccoid bacteria. Samples were seen with marked eosinophilia in the lesion (5), as well as lympho-plasmacytic inflammation (3), in addition to purulent inflammation. The samples from finnraccoons represented chronic cases. On necropsy, one of the individuals submitted to the study as a healthy control was observed to exhibit the typical lesions of FENP. The histopathological changes were also similar to the changes in the diseased animals. No specific changes were detected in the internal organs of any of the finnraccoons.

Bacteriology

The main finding in bacteriological cultures was *Arcanobacterium phocae*, identified by sequencing of the 16S RNA gene. It was cultured from a total of 16/21 of the diseased mink skin samples and 6/19 of the diseased fox eye samples. In the fox samples with purulent discharge, *A. phocae* was cultured from 5/11 samples. In the fox samples with serous discharge, *A. phocae* was only cultured in one sample (1/8). *A. phocae* was cultured from 8/21 of diseased finnraccoon samples. Furthermore the finnraccoon submitted to the study as a healthy control, but exhibiting the typical lesions, was positive for *A. phocae*. The difference between detecting *A. phocae* in primarily diseased mink and foxes but not healthy ones was statistically clearly significant (Table 2, Table S1).

On blood agar, *A. phocae* grew in 24 hours as very small, pinpoint-like colonies with a strong hemolytic zone around the colonies. A CO_2-enriched atmosphere or anaerobic conditions did

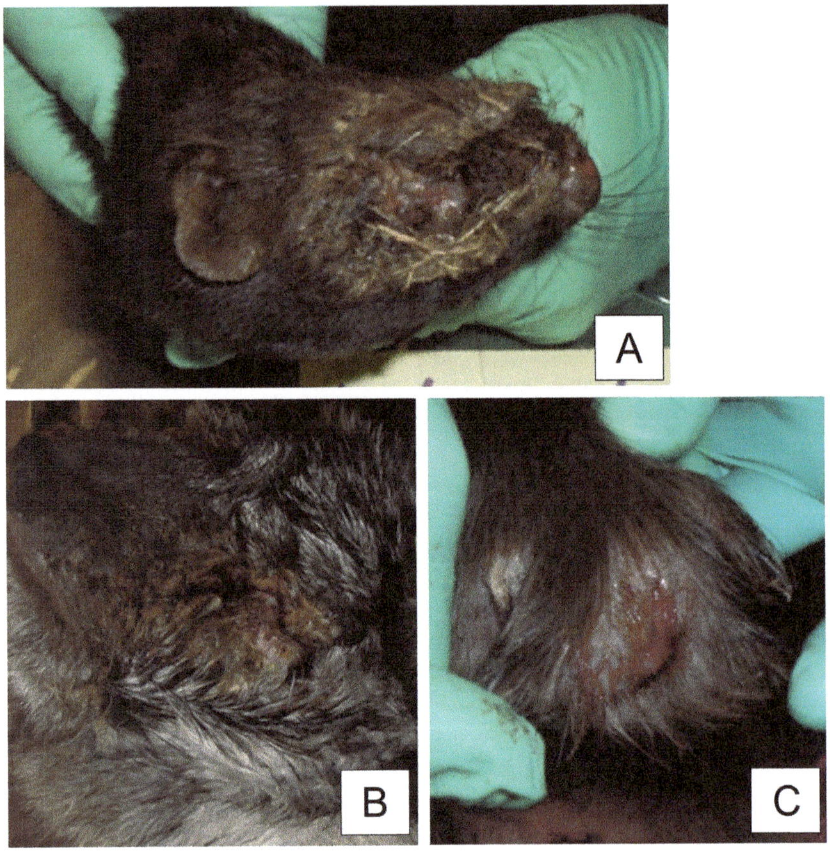

Figure 1. Macroscopic changes in FENP in mink, foxes and finnraccoons. A typical macroscopic finding in a mink with FENP is severe necrotic pyoderma with crust formation around the eyes and nose. Some bedding material is detached in the exudate (A). A typical lesion in foxes with FENP is observed around the eyes. The eyelids clot together due to the purulent inflammation (B). Finnraccoons with FENP have painful abscesses between the toes (C).

not enhance their growth. They were small, pleomorphic rods and they stained unevenly Gram-positive. They were catalase- positive, oxidase-negative, and they gave a positive CAMP-reaction to *Rhodococcus equi* and *Streptococcus agalactiae* (synergistic hemolysis), and an inverse CAMP -reaction to *Staphylococcus aureus*.

A. phocae was most commonly (26/31) isolated as a mixed culture, together with bacteria belonging to the genus *Streptococcus* or *Staphylococcus*. In five diseased cases, however, *A. phocae* was the only isolate (Table 2). All the tested isolates of *A. phocae* were susceptible to all the antibiotics available for treatment.

Some of the *Streptococcus* isolates (28/38) were determined to represent a previously unknown *Streptococcus* based on the 16S RNA gene sequence. The sequence showed the novel *Streptococcus* to be closely related, but not identical, to streptococci of marine origin, such as *Streptococcus halichoeri*. They also grew on blood agar in 24 hours as very small, pinpoint-like colonies, and CO_2 -enrichment or anaerobic conditions did not enhance their growth. They were Gram-positive cocci, but they stained unevenly. The colonies were nonhemolytic. They were catalase-positive, oxidase-negative, and were categorized as group B by the

Table 1. Gross pathology of the study animals.

Macroscopic change	Mink (n = 21)	Foxes (n = 19)	Finnraccoons (n = 21)
Enlarged local lymph node	5 (22%)	3 (16%)	10 (48%)
Splenomegaly	10 (48%)	0	10 (48%)
Pyoderma in facial skin	15 (71%)	3 (16%)	0
Pyoderma/abscess in paws	6 (29%)	0	21 (100%)
Bilateral conjunctivitis	0	17 (89%)	0
Unilateral conjunctivitis	0	2 (11%)	0
Purulent discharge from eyes	0	11 (58%)	0
Serous discharge from eyes	0	8 (42%)	0

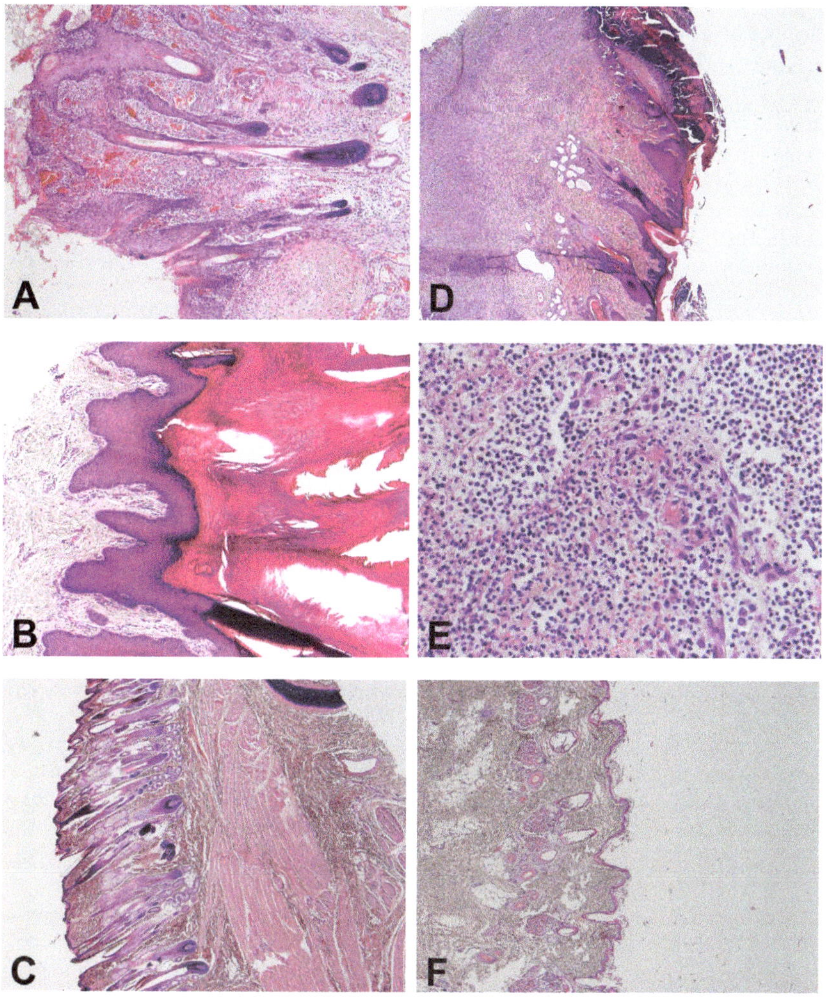

Figure 2. Histopathological findings in FENP in mink and finnraccoons. A facial skin section from mink shows chronic, deep, and diffuse neutrophilic inflammation with hemorrhage, ulceration, and crusting (A). Severe orthokeratotic hyperkeratosis detected in a skin section from a mink foot (B). A sample of a section from the skin of the eyelid of a healthy control mink is shown in (C). A section from a diseased finnraccoon paw with abscess between the toes shows chronic, deep and diffuse neutrophilic inflammation with ulceration and crusting (D). Necropurulent inflammation in the subcutis is demonstrated in (E), and a section from the skin of a paw of a healthy control finnraccoon in (F). All sections are stained with hematoxylin and eosin, and the respective objectives used in A to F were 10×, 10×, 4×, 4×, 40× and, 4×.

Table 2. Detection of *Arcanobacterium phocae* and *Streptococcus* spp. in fur animals, and their association to disease signs of FENP.

	PCR positive for *A. phocae*		Positive for *A. phocae* in culture		Positive for *Streptococcus* spp in culture	
		p-values*		*p*-values		*p*-values
Diseased mink	21 (21)	<0.001	16 (21)	<0.001	16 (21)	<0.001
Healthy mink	1 (11)		0 (11)		0 (11)	
Healthy mink on a diseased farm	3 (4)		0 (4)		0 (4)	
Diseased finnraccoons	20 (20)	<0.01	8 (20)	0.068	10 (20)	<0.01
Healthy finnraccoons	6 (11)		1 (11)		0 (11)	
Diseased foxes	19 (19)	<0.001	6 (19)	0.036	2 (19)	0.3677
Healthy foxes	0 (12)		0 (12)		0 (12)	
All diseased animals	60 (60)	<0.001	30 (60)	<0.001	28 (60)	<0.001
All healthy animals	10 (38)		1 (38)		0 (38)	

The table shows the probabilities of getting a positive result from diseased animals as opposed to healthy animals.
* Calculated from Fisher's exact test.

Lancefield test. In addition, the finding of the cultivable streptococcal species in diseased mink and finnraccoons, but not foxes, was statistically significant (Table 2).

PCR studies on *A. phocae*

All the diseased animals of all three species were positive for *A. phocae* DNA (Table 2). Furthermore, most of these had relatively high amounts of bacteria as indicated by the Ct-values in real-time PCR. Most of the samples from the healthy controls of mink and foxes were negative, although some weak positive reactions were detected, indicating very low amounts of bacteria (Table 2). The finnraccoons displayed a somewhat different result: six out of the 11 healthy finnraccoons were positive in PCR for *A. phocae*. The bacterial load was rather low in these negative samples, but some of the diseased finnraccoons had comparable, low, DNA levels. However, the statistical difference in detecting *A. phocae* by PCR in all diseased but only 6/11 healthy finnraccoons was clearly significant ($p = 0.003$, Fisher's exact test) (Table 2). Evidently, the difference between detecting *A. phocae* in primarily diseased mink and foxes but not healthy ones by PCR was also statistically very highly significant (Table 2). When all animals were pooled together, the statistical significance of finding *A. phocae* DNA predominantly in animals with FENP (Table 2) had a p value of 1.8×10^−16 (Fisher's exact test).

Virology

Canine distemper virus or antibodies against it were not detected in any species. Herpesviruses were not detected by PCR, virus culture, or EM. All mink were negative in an ELISA-test for AMDV and for MEV antibodies. In foxes and finnraccoons, antibodies against MEV were detected in both diseased and healthy animals. MEV DNA was detected in a rectal sample from one healthy fox.

Virus isolations were attempted from the affected tissue samples and eye swabs, and as a control, from corresponding samples of healthy animals. Occasionally, unspecific CPE was observed, and samples of supernatant as well as original tissues were analyzed by electron microscopy. However, no viral agents were detected.

Discussion

In this study we described a novel disease, fur animal epidemic necrotic pyoderma (FENP), which appeared in Finland in 2007. The clinical signs appeared to be distinct for each fur animal species: necrotic skin inflammation affecting both the head and paws in mink, severe eye inflammation in foxes that spreads to the eyelids and facial skin, and abscesses in the paws of finnraccoons. The disease mostly affected young animals of both sexes. It appeared to have spread within and between farms, and was evidently a severe and painful disease that caused - and still causes - economic losses to farmers. No effective treatment has been available. Dermatitis in general has poor prognosis with the need for prolonged treatments. Antibiotic therapy (penicillin, tetracycline, and Trimethoprim-sulphamethoxazole) administered via feed has been attempted, mostly with no effect. If antibiotics (penicillin, amoxicillin, and amoxicillin clavulanate) are administered as injections in the early stage of the disease with a large dosage, clinical signs and morbidity may decrease although relapses are common. When treating tens or hundreds of thousands of semi-wild animals, long term administration of injections is impractical. The housing system also makes it difficult to detect the early signs of the disease thus critically delaying the onset of treatment. Current recommendation is to euthanize the first infected animals, when detected, and then disinfect the cages.

Here, we describe the clinical signs and the gross- and histopathology of the disease in three species. We also describe the major microbiological findings. We found *Arcanobacterium phocae* in all of the diseased animals, which was confirmed both by sequencing and phenotypic characterization. Initially, *A. phocae* was cultured from 50% of the diseased individuals and none of the healthy animals. Notably, all the diseased animals were further confirmed as *A. phocae* positive by rtPCR. Furthermore, necrosis is one of the typical changes that were observed in the diseased fur animals, and it is known that bacteria belonging to the genus *Arcanobacterium* produce toxins with dermonecrotic activity [18]. In some healthy controls, low amounts of *A. phocae* were detected by PCR. These individuals were either healthy mink from an affected farm or finnraccoons, of which half were from a supposedly disease-free farm. Later, the disease was reported to affect animals on this farm. Statistical analysis revealed a significant correlation for all species between FENP and *Arcanobacterium phocae* when detected by PCR, and culturing results gave a strong correlation for mink and foxes.

The samples of mink and finnraccoons presented with chronic inflammation that may have influenced the results. During the study period it was difficult to obtain lesions of the early stages, because the signs and lesions appeared to develop rapidly. Due to the housing system of fur animals, the farmers do not handle the animals individually, which makes it difficult to detect early signs of the disease. Although infection by *A. phocae* may indeed be the primary cause of the disease, it is also possible that the onset of the disease could have been covered by a secondary bacterial infection caused by *A. phocae*. Some of the findings suggest that *A. phocae* can be naturally found on the skin of fur animals, and therefore might not be able to cause the disease alone. Thus, another factor, such as a bite wound, a scratch, a mechanical injury, or another microbial agent, might be required for the disease to proceed.

With histopathology, hyperkeratosis and ulceration of the epidermis were detected, which could be caused by trauma. However, especially in the samples from mink, the inflammation was mainly deep diffuse purulent infection with prominent vasculitis. Vasculitis causes thrombosis, which leads to necrosis of the skin tissue. The pathogenesis of vasculitis generally varies between animal diseases. It is seen in viral diseases such as feline infectious peritonitis, as well as in bacterial infections such as erysipelas in swine. In cats and dogs, similar skin lesions are detected in mycobacterial infections. Most of the infections are due to penetrating injury through skin to the subcutis with soil or dirt contamination. These infections can, with time, become deep-seated and extensive [19]. However, the histopathological pattern of the fur animal samples was atypical to mycobacterial infections and ZN stains did not demonstrate any acid fast bacteria. Parasitic agents, immune-mediated disease and toxins are also known to cause vasculitis and otherwise predispose animals to infection. However, no parasites were detected in this study.

A viral pathogen was considered, since early-onset signs in foxes included serous discharge from the eyes, usually associated with viral infections. Furthermore, with histology, occasional inclusion body -like structures were noted. However, viral cultures from the affected tissue samples did not reveal any viral agents, although this does not exclude a viral cause of the disease. Distemper could manifest as skin changes seen in the mink, and also conjunctivitis in foxes, but, no CDV or antibodies against it were detected in any studied animals. MEV DNA was detected in one healthy fox. Both healthy and diseased foxes and finnraccoons had antibodies against MEV, partly due to vaccinations. All the mink were tested against AMDV, another parvovirus affecting fur animals, with negative results. Furthermore, a screen for herpesviruses using a broadly-reactive PCR protocol also yielded negative results.

Bacterial cultures and subsequent sequencing also revealed a novel *Streptococcus* sp. of probable marine origin. This could reinforce the suggested connection between *A. phocae*-caused pyoderma and the feeding of fur animals with marine mammal byproducts [1]. Alternatively, this novel *Streptococcus* could just be a previously undetected member of the normal flora of the fur animals. The novel *Streptococcus* was not detected as frequently as *A. phocae*, and thus it is not as likely as *A. phocae* to be the main etiological agent. Statistical analysis did show a correlation between FENP and the novel *Streptococcus* sp., and thus indicates its role as a significant cofactor, warranting further studies for its basic characterization. Interestingly the novel *Streptococcus* was found less frequently in foxes than in mink and finnraccoons, which could contribute to the differences in the manifestation of the disease.

This study demonstrated that the bacterium *Arcanobacterium phocae* is associated with the new disease, FENP, seen in fur animals, and suggests that it plays an important role in the pathogenesis of the disease. In further studies, the pathogenicity of *Arcanobacterium phocae* to mink, foxes, and finnraccoons should be investigated by experimental infections to clarify whether Koch's postulates can be fulfilled, i.e. whether it is capable of causing the described disease, or whether other environmental, immunological, or infectious factors are necessary. In conclusion, this study described a new, economically important, and potentially lethal disease of fur animals that severely compromises animal welfare on farms. The study also revealed its likely etiological agent, *A. phocae*, suggesting a potential species shift from marine mammals as the origin of this epidemic.

Acknowledgments

We thank the staff of Evira, Seinäjoki and Professor Marjukka Anttila for expert assistance and Katariina Vapalahti for the statistical analysis.

Author Contributions

Conceived and designed the experiments: HN KA TS PMK MRS AS OV. Performed the experiments: HN KA TS IK MRS AMMJ JK UMK UH. Analyzed the data: HN KA TS MRS UH AS OV. Contributed reagents/materials/analysis tools: MRS OV. Wrote the paper: HN KA TS PMK IK MRS AMMJ JK UMK UH AS OV.

References

1. Bröjer C (2000) Pododermatitis in farmed mink in Canada. M.Sc. Thesis, The University of Guelph, Canada. Available: http://www.collectionscanada.gc.ca/obj/s4/f2/dsk3/ftp04/MQ56305.pdf, Accessed 2013 September 12.
2. Onderka D (1996) Integument of Mink. In: Hunter, D.B and Lemieux, N., editors. Mink: biology, health and disease. Guelph: Graphic and Print Services. pp. 15.1–15.8.
3. Ramos CP, Foster G, Collins MD (1997) Phylogenetic analysis of the genus *Actinomyces* based on 16S rRNA gene sequences: description of *Arcanobacterium phocae* sp. nov., *Arcanobacterium bernardiae* comb. nov., and *Arcanobacterium pyogenes* comb. nov. Int J Syst Bacteriol 32:419–429.
4. Johnson SP, Jang S, Gulland FM, Miller MA, Casper DR, et al. (2003) Characterization and clinical manifestations of *Arcanobacterium phocae* infections in marine mammals stranded along the central California coast. J Wildl Dis 39:136–44.
5. Collins MD, Jones D, Schofield GM (1982) Reclassification of '*Corynebacterium haemolyticum*' (MacLean, Liebow & Rosenberg) in the genus Arcanobacterium gen.nov. as *Arcanobacterium haemolyticum* nom.rev., comb.nov. J Gen Microbiol 128: 1279–81.
6. Yassin AF, Hupfer H, Siering C, Schuman P (2011) Comparative chemotaxonomic and phylogenetic studies on the genus *Arcanobacterium* Collins et al. 1982 emend. Lehnen et al. 2006: proposal for *Trueperella* gen. nov. and emended description of the genus *Arcanobacterium*. Int J Syst Evol Microbiol 61: 1265–1274.
7. Hijazin M, Prenger-Berninghoff E, Sammra O, Alber J, Lämmler C, et al. (2012) *Arcanobacterium canis* sp. nov., isolated from otitis externa of a dog, and emended description of the genus *Arcanobacterium* Collins et al. 1983 emend. Yassin et al. 2011. Int J Syst Evol Microbiol 62:2201–5.
8. Hijazin M, Sammra O, Ülbegi-Mohyla H, Nagib S, Alber J, et al. (2013) *Arcanobacterium phocisimile* sp. nov. isolated from harbor seals. Int J Sys Evol Microbiol 63: 2019–2024.
9. Funke GA, von Graevenitz A, Clarridge JE III, Bernard KA (1997) Clinical microbiology of coryneform bacteria. Clin Microbiol Rev 10: 125–159.
10. Mackenzie A, Fuite LA, Chan FT, King J, Allen U, et al. (1995) Incidence and pathogenicity of *Arcanobacterium haemolyticum* during a 2-year study in Ottawa. Clin Infect Dis 21: 177–181.
11. Skov RL, Sanden AK, Danchell VH, Robertsen K, Ejlertsen T (1998) Systemic and deep-seated infections caused by *Arcanobacterium haemolyticum*. Eur J Clin Microbiol Infect Dis 17: 578–582.
12. Barret T, Visser KG, Mamaev L, Goatley L, van Bressem MF, et al. (1993) Dolphin and porpoise morbilliviruses are genetically distinct from phocine distemper virus. Virology 193: 1010–1012.
13. Uwatoko K, Michio S, Nakajima M, Yamaura K (1995) Rapid method utilizing the polymerase chain reaction for detection of canine parvovirus in feces of diarrheic dogs. Vet Microbiol 43: 315–323.
14. Ek-Kommonen C, Sihvonen L, Pekkanen K, Rikula U, Nuotio L (1997) Outbreak of canine distemper in vaccinated dogs in Finland (1997) Vet Rec, October 11, 383.
15. Carmichael LE, Joubert JC, Pollock RVH (1980) Hemagglutination by canine parvovirus: serologic studies and diagnostic applications. Am J Vet Res 41: 784–791.
16. VanDevanter DR, Warrener P, Bennet L, Schultz ER, Coulter S, et al. (1996) Detection and analysis of diverse herpesviral species by consensus primer PCR. J Clin Microbiol 34:1666–1671.
17. Knuuttila A, Aronen P, Saarinen A, Vapalahti O (2009) Development and evaluation of an enzyme-linked immunosorbent assay based on recombinant VP2 capsids for the detection of antibodies to Aleutian mink disease virus. Clin Vaccine Immunol 16:1360–5.
18. Wagner DC (1991) *Arcanobacterium haemolyticum*: biology of the organism and diseases in man. Ped Inf Dis J 10:933.
19. Malik R (2004) Mycobacterial diseases affecting the skin or subcutis of cats and dogs. Vet Dermatol 15: doi: 10.1111/j.1365-3164.2004.00410_5-1.x

17

Low Birth Weight Is a Risk Factor for Severe Retinopathy of Prematurity Depending on Gestational Age

Pia Lundgren[1]*, Anna Kistner[1,2], Eva M. Andersson[3], Ingrid Hansen Pupp[4], Gerd Holmström[5], David Ley[4], Aimon Niklasson[6], Lois E. H. Smith[7], Carolyn Wu[7], Ann Hellström[1¶], Chatarina Löfqvist[1¶]

1 Institute of Neuroscience and Physiology, Sahlgrenska Academy at University of Gothenburg, Gothenburg, Sweden, **2** Institution of Molecular Medicine and Surgery, Karolinska Institutet, Stockholm, Sweden, **3** Department of Occupational and Environmental Medicine, Sahlgrenska Academy at University of Gothenburg, Gothenburg, Sweden, **4** Department of Pediatrics, Institute of Clinical Sciences, Lund University and Skane University Hospital, Lund, Sweden, **5** Department of Neuroscience, Ophthalmology, Uppsala University, Uppsala, Sweden, **6** Department of Pediatrics, Institute of Clinical Sciences, Sahlgrenska Academy at University of Gothenburg, Gothenburg, Sweden, **7** Department of Ophthalmology, Boston Children's Hospital, Harvard Medical School, Boston, Massachusetts, United States of America

Abstract

Objective: To evaluate the impact of low birth weight as a risk factor for retinopathy of prematurity (ROP) that will require treatment in correlation with gestational age at birth (GA).

Study design: In total, 2941 infants born <32 weeks GA were eligible from five cohorts of preterm infants previously collected for analysis in WINROP (Weight IGF-I Neonatal ROP) from the following locations: Sweden (EXPRESS) ($n=426$), North America ($n=1772$), Boston ($n=338$), Lund ($n=52$), and Gothenburg ($n=353$). Data regarding GA at birth, birth weight (BW), gender, and need for ROP treatment were retrieved. Birth weight standard deviation scores (BWSDS) were calculated with Swedish as well as Canadian reference models. Small for gestational age (SGA) was defined as BWSDS less than −2.0 SDS using the Swedish reference and as BW below the 10th percentile using the Canadian reference charts.

Results: Univariate analysis showed that low GA ($p<0.001$), low BW ($p<0.001$), male gender ($p<0.05$), low $BWSDS_{Canada}$ ($p<0.001$), and SGA_{Canada} ($p<0.01$) were risk factors for ROP that will require treatment. In multivariable logistic regression analysis, low GA ($p<0.0001$), male gender ($p<0.01$ and $p<0.05$), and an interaction term of BWSDS*GA group ($p<0.001$), regardless of reference chart, were risk factors. Low BWSDS was less important as a risk factor in infants born at GA <26 weeks compared with infants born at GA ≥26 weeks calculated with both reference charts ($BWSDS_{Sweden}$, OR = 0.80 vs 0.56; and $BWSDS_{Canada}$, OR = 0.72 vs 0.41).

Conclusions: Low BWSDS as a risk factor for vision-threatening ROP is dependent on the infant's degree of immaturity. In more mature infants (GA ≥26 weeks), low BWSDS becomes a major risk factor for developing ROP that will require treatment. These results persist even when calculating BW deficit with different well-established approaches.

Editor: Kypros Kypri, University of Newcastle, Australia, Australia

Funding: This work was supported by the Swedish Medical Research Council (grant numbers 2011-2432 and 2008-2842), government grants (grant numbers ALFGB-137491 and ALFGB-21611), VINNOVA (grant numbers 2009-01152 and 2009-00221), the Torsten and Ragnar Söderberg Foundation, the Skåne Council Foundation for Research and Development, the Linnéa and Josef Carlsson Foundation, and, in part, by the NIH/NEI (EY022275, EY017017, P01 HD18655), Research to Prevent Blindness Senior Investigator Award, Alcon Research Institute Award, Lowy Medical Foundation, Herman Svensson Foundation and V. Kann Rasmussen Foundation and European Commission FP7 project 305485 PREVENT-ROP. The funders had no role in study design, data collection and analysis, decision to publish, or preparation of the manuscript.

Competing Interests: The authors have declared that no competing interests exist.

* Email: pia.lundgren@gu.se

¶ These authors are last authors on this work.

Introduction

Retinopathy of prematurity (ROP) is a disease affecting very preterm infants that can potentially result in blindness. Timely detection and treatment of ROP is crucial. It is important to determine all risk factors in order to improve the identification of infants at greatest risk for severe ROP.

The most important risk factors for ROP are the degree of prematurity [1] and low birth weight (BW) [2], but there are other risk factors associated with infant postnatal morbidity such as days of ventilation [3], sepsis [4], hyperglycemia [5], blood transfusions [6], and bronchopulmonary dysplasia [7].

In recent years, studies have consistently identified poor postnatal weight gain as a strong predictor of ROP [8–12]. Study findings have, however, been contradictory as to whether or not prenatal growth restriction is a risk factor for ROP. Prenatal growth restriction can be defined as the infant's deficit from normal birth weight standard deviation score (BWSDS). The term small for gestational age (SGA), defined as BW per GA below a certain percentile or confidence interval based on growth charts, is also frequently used to describe infants' prenatal growth restriction. SGA was found to be a risk factor for ROP in some studies [2,13–15]. However, in other studies no significant differences were found between infants born SGA and those with a BW appropriate for their gestational age and the risk of developing ROP [3,16–18]. A possible explanation for these inconsistent results may be differences in the characteristics of the study populations and study designs. The definition of SGA has varied in previous studies where it has been defined as a BW ranging from below the 3rd (approximately corresponding to 2 SD below the gestational-age related mean) to below the 10th percentile. Furthermore, the definition of normal BW in relation to GA varies according to different growth charts. Growth charts used throughout the world vary in design; some are based on longitudinal fetal ultrasound weight estimations and thereby aim to reflect undisturbed intrauterine growth [19,20], some are based on live births [21,22], and others on live as well as still births [23].

Therefore, the aim of this study was to clarify the association between low BW and the development of ROP that will require treatment in a large cohort of very preterm infants. Calculation of BW deficit and definition of SGA was performed according to different reference models of GA-related growth to determine if this would affect the results.

Our major findings were that low BWSDS is a risk factor for preterm infants who will require treatment for ROP and that the impact of low BWSDS in more mature infants who will require ROP treatment is greater. The results persisted independent of differences in the growth charts applied.

Study Population and Methods

Study population

For this study, data from five cohorts enrolled in the WINROP (Weight IGF-1 Neonatal ROP) studies were retrospectively reviewed. These were: the *EXPRESS cohort*, extremely preterm (GA <27 weeks, $n = 707$) infants born in Sweden between 2004 and 2007 [24]; *North American multicenter cohort*, preterm infants ($n = 1965$) born at ten level III neonatal intensive care units in the USA and Canada between 2006 and 2009 [25]; *Boston cohort*, preterm infants ($n = 374$) born at Brigham and Women's Hospital, Boston (USA) between 2005 and 2008 [26]; *Lund cohort*, preterm infants ($n = 60$) born at Skane University Hospital, Lund (Sweden) between 2005 and 2007 [11]; and *Gothenburg cohort*, preterm infants ($n = 354$) screened and/or treated for ROP at Sahlgrenska University Hospital, Gothenburg (Sweden) between 2004 and 2007 [10]. Comprehensive descriptions of all infants and data collected in each cohort have been reported previously [10,11,24–26].

Data regarding correlations between ROP requiring treatment and GA, BW, and gender were retrieved retrospectively from each original study. In the current analysis, infants were excluded if they were born after 32 week GA. Infants who died before 40 weeks postmenstrual age were also excluded since ROP grading may have been incomplete. Due to different inclusion criteria in the cohorts, the number of infants excluded due to death before 40 weeks postmenstrual age differed. The number of infants excluded in each cohort is presented in Figure 1.

ROP screening and treatment

ROP screening examinations were conducted according to current national guidelines for each cohort. The revisited International Classification of Retinopathy of Prematurity was used for ROP classification in all cohorts [27]. Details on current ROP screening guidelines and schedules and the performance of the ROP examinations are described in each previous publication [1,10,11,24–26]. The recommendations of the Early Treatment for Retinopathy of Prematurity Cooperative Group were followed for treatment [28].

Statistical analysis

Birth weight standard deviation scores (BWSDS) were calculated using two well-established growth charts, both developed for infants born after 22 weeks GA. The Swedish gender-specific reference is considered to reflect undisturbed intrauterine growth [19], and the Canadian gender-specific reference is based on live as well as still births [23]. SGA was defined as BW less than −2.0 BWSDS based on the Swedish growth reference and as BW below the 10th percentile based on the Canadian growth reference. We further defined severe growth restriction as a BW below the 3rd percentile using the Canadian growth reference.

The outcome indicator variable was whether or not the infants required ROP treatment. Logistic regression was used to analyze risk factors. Infants were divided into five GA week groups; infants born at GAs of 22–23 weeks, 24–25 weeks, 26–27 weeks, 28–29 weeks, and 30–31 weeks. For infants born GA ≥26 weeks, all variables reflecting prenatal growth restriction, regardless growth reference or definition, were highly significant as risk factors as follows: $BWSDS_{Sweden}$ for GA 26–27 weeks and for GA 28–29 weeks (*p-values* <0.01); SGA_{Sweden} for GA 26–27 weeks ($p<0.001$); $BWSDS_{Canada}$ for GA 26–27 weeks and for GA 28–29 weeks (*p-values*<0.01); SGA_{Canada} for GA 26–27 weeks and for GA 28–29 weeks (*p-values*<0.01); severe growth restriction (Canada) for GA 26–27 weeks and for GA 28–29 weeks ($p<0.001$). To assess whether BWSDS had a different impact on ROP requiring treatment for infants born at GA <26 weeks compared with infants born at GA ≥26 weeks, we allowed for different associations with BWSDS by including an interaction term (BWSDS*GA group, where GA group = 1 if GA ≥26 weeks and 0 if GA <26 weeks). The multivariable logistic regression analysis included GA, gender, BWSDS, the indicator variable GA group, and the interaction term BWSDS*GA group. Two different BWSDS were calculated; one using the Swedish growth reference and one using the Canadian growth reference. Hence, two multivariable logistic regression models were estimated.

IBM SPSS Statistics 20 for Microsoft Windows (IBM Corporation, Armonk, NY) was used for statistical analysis as well as SAS version 9.3. Mann-Whitney U test was used for group comparisons. Correlations were assessed using the Spearman correlation coefficient (r_S). Wilcoxon Signed Rank test was used to compare the two BWSDS references. The association with the outcome (ROP requiring treatment or no ROP treatment) is expressed as the odds ratios (OR) with 95% confidence intervals (CI). The Hosmer and Lemeshow test was used to assess the goodness-of-fit for the multivariable logistic regression model [29].

Ethics statement

The Swedish studies were approved by the Regional Ethical Review Board of Gothenburg, Sweden. The American studies were retrospective chart reviews; hence no consent for data retrieval was needed.

Results

Study population

For this study, 2941 infants were eligible. Infants were from the EXPRESS cohort (426 infants), North American cohort (1772 infants), Boston cohort (338 infants), Lund cohort (52 infants), and the Gothenburg cohort (353 infants) (Figure 1). The birth

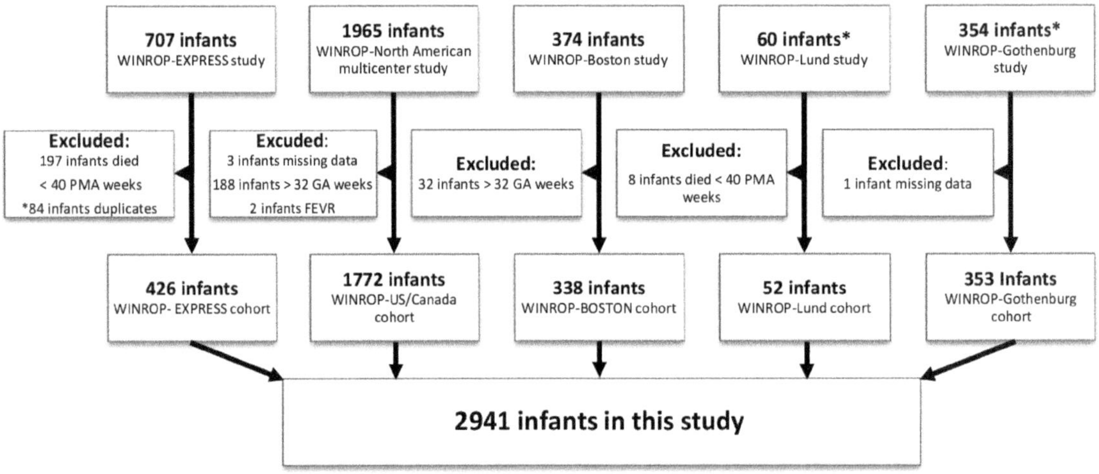

Abbreviations: FEVR indicates familial exudative vitreoretinopathy; GA, gestational age; PMA, postmenstrual age; WINROP, weight IGF 1 neonatal retinopathy of prematurity.

*84 infants in the EXPRESS study were also included in the Lund and Gothenburg cohort; hence, these infants were excluded from the EXPRESS study.

Figure 1. Flowchart of the study population.

characteristics of infants in each cohort/GA group are described in Table 1.

BWSDS and GA groups

A negative correlation between BWSDS and GA was found regardless of growth reference; low BWSDS was associated with higher GA (Swedish reference: $r_S = -0.25$, $p<0.001$, Canadian reference $r_S = -0.12$, $p<0.001$). Median BWSDS, regardless definition, was lower in infants treated for ROP compared with infants not treated for ROP between GA 24–29 weeks (Mann-Whitney U test, $p<0.05$, Figure 2).

Prevalence of SGA

The prevalence of SGA, regardless of definition, increased with GA. The prevalence of SGA_{Sweden} was 5.6% (7/126) in the 22–23 weeks GA group, and increased to 40.4% (289/716) in the 30–31 weeks GA group. The prevalence of SGA_{Canada} was 4.0% (5/126) in the 22–23 weeks GA group and increased to 17.6% (126/716) in the 30–31 weeks GA group (Table 1).

Prevalence of infants treated for ROP

The prevalence of infants treated for ROP was 45.2% (57/126) in the 22–23 weeks GA group. The prevalence decreased to 0.1% (1/716) in the 30–31 weeks GA group. The prevalence of infants treated for ROP varied from 17.1% (73/426) in the EXPRESS cohort to 4.1% (14/338) in the Boston cohort (Table 1).

Risk factors for ROP that will require treatment

Possible risk factors for an infant who will require ROP treatment were as follows: GA (weeks at birth), BW (50-g increments), gender, BWSDS and SGA calculated and defined by both the Swedish and Canadian growth references, and severe growth restriction calculated by the Canadian growth reference. First, each risk factor was evaluated separately using logistic regression. For the whole cohort, low GA at birth ($p<0.001$), low BW ($p<0.001$), and male gender ($p<0.05$) were significant risk factors. Neither low $BWSDS_{Sweden}$ nor SGA_{Sweden} were significant risk factors for ROP that will require treatment. However, low $BWSDS_{Canada}$ ($p<0.001$), SGA_{Canada} ($p<0.01$), and severe growth restriction ($p<0.001$) were risk factors. When dividing the infants into GA groups, BWSDS, SGA, and severe growth restriction were significant risk factors for infants born at GA 26–27 weeks independent of whether these were defined according to the Swedish or Canadian growth references (Table 2).

In the next step, multivariable logistic regression analysis was used. Low GA ($p<0.0001$), male gender ($p<0.01$ and $p<0.05$), and the interaction term (BWSDS*GA group) ($p<0.001$), regardless of BWSDS growth reference, were risk factors for ROP that will require treatment. The multivariable logistic regression analysis was performed with the Swedish as well as the Canadian growth references (Hosmer-Lemeshow test did not indicate any lack of fit for either model, $p_{Swe} = 0.67$, $p_{Can} = 0.53$). Independent of which growth reference was used, BWSDS was less important as a risk factor in infants born at GA <26 weeks compared with infants born at GA ≥26 weeks ($BWSDS_{Sweden}$; OR = 0.80, 95% CI 0.70–0.91 *vs* OR = 0.56, 95% CI 0.47–0.68 and $BWSDS_{Canada}$; OR = 0.72 95% CI 0.60–0.87 *vs* OR = 0.41, 95% CI 0.31–0.55) (Table 3 and Figure 3). Consequently, infants born at GA < 26 weeks had reduced odds of requiring treatment by 20–28% for every 1 SD increase in BWSDS compared with infants born at GA ≥26 weeks who had a 44–59% reduction for every 1 SD increase in BWSDS.

Table 1. Birth characteristics of infants enrolled in the study by cohort and GA group.

COHORT	No. infants	GA weeks+days median (range)	BW grams median (range)	Swedish reference BWSDS median (range)	SGA BWSDS <−2.0 SDS Swedish reference	Canadian reference BWSDS median (range)	SGA BW <10th percentile Canadian reference	Severe growth restriction BW <3rd percentile Canadian reference	Male gender % (*n*)	ROP requiring treatment % (*n*)
EXPRESS	426	25+4/7	780	−0.68	16.9%	0.13	9.4%	2.1%	54.0%	17.1%
		(22+1/7 to 26+6/7)	(361–1315)	(−5.18 to 3.88)	(72/426)	(−2.69 to 2.87)	(40/426)	(9/426)	(230/426)	(73/426)
North	1772	28+0/7	1010	−1.34	31.6%	−0.20	13.7%	3.8%	52.5%	9.8%
American		(22+5/7 to 31+6/7)	(378–2240)	(−6.62 to 3.35)	(560/1772)	(−3.27 to 2.87)	(242/1772)	(67/1772)	(931/1772)	(173/1772)
Boston	338	28+5/7	1050	−1.31	34.0%	−0.11	13.9%	4.7%	54.7%	4.1%
		(23+1/7 to 31+6/7)	(450–2400)	(−5.18 to 4.47)	(115/338)	(−2.58 to 3.07)	(47/338)	(16/338)	(185/338)	(14/338)
Lund	52	26+1/7	850	−0.77	25.0%	−0.01	7.7%	3.8%	51.9%	17.3%
		(23+0/7 to 30+5/7)	(448–1716)	(−5.00 to 0.89)	(13/52)	(−3.07 to 1.30)	(4/52)	(2/52)	(27/52)	(9/52)
Gothenburg	353	29+4/7	1290	−1.04	22.4%	0.02	11.0%	2.3%	59.2%	7.4%
		(23+3/7 to 31+6/7)	(425–2210)	(−5.59 to 2.50)	(79/353)	(−2.88 to 2.47)	(39/353)	(8/353)	(209/353)	(26/353)
GA GROUP										
GA 22–23	126	23+4/7	582	−0.46	5.6%	0.13	4.0%	0%	52.4%	45.2%
wk		(22+1/7 to 23+6/7)	(361–925)	(−3.27 to 3.88)	(7/126)	(−1.56 to 2.87)	(5/126)		(66/126)	(57/126)
GA 24–25	690	25+0/7	720	−0.84	18.0%	−0.06	10.6%	2.9%	55.2%	24.8%
wk		(24+0/7 to 25+6/7)	(348–1154)	(−5.00 to 2.49)	(124/690)	(−3.07 t0 2.41)	(73/690)	(20/690)	(381/690)	(171/690)
GA 26–27	714	26+6/7	920	−1.16	26.5%	−0.03	11.3%	3.8%	51.4%	8.1%
wk		(26+0/7 to 27+6/7)	(398–1430)	(−5.43 to 2.27)	(189/714)	(−2.87 to 2.28)	(81/714)	(27/714)	(367/714)	(58/714)
GA 28–29	695	29+0/7	1180	−1.36	33.1%	−0.07	12.5%	3.2%	56.0%	1.2%
wk		(28+0/7 to 29+6/7)	(410–2095)	(−5.89 to 3.34)	(230/695)	(−3.09 to 2.87)	(87/695)	(22/695)	(389/695)	(8/695)
GA 30–31	716	30+6/7	1422	−1.67	40.4%	−0.32	17.6%	4.6%	52.9%	0.1%
wk		(30+0/7 to 31+6/7)	(378–2400)	(−6.62 to 4.47)	(289/716)	(−3.27 to 3.07)	(126/716)	(33/716)	(379/716)	(1/716)
Total	**2941**	**27+5/7**	**980**	**−1.2**	**28.5%**	**−0.11**	**12.6%**	**3.5%**	**53.8%**	**10.0%**
		(22+1/7 to 31+6/7)	(348–2400)	(−6.62–4.47)	(839/2941)	(−3.27 to 3.07)	(372/2941)	(102/2941)	(1582/2941)	(295/2941)

Abbreviations: BW, indicates birth weight; BWSDS, birth weight standard deviation score; GA, gestational age; ROP, retinopathy of prematurity; SGA, small for gestational age.; wk, weeks.

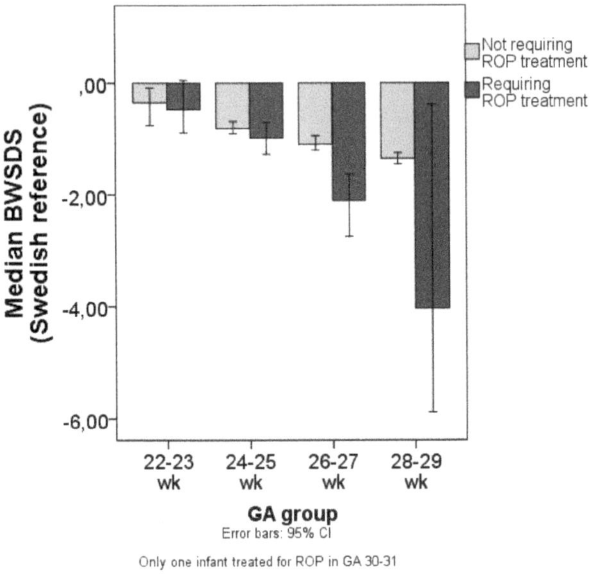

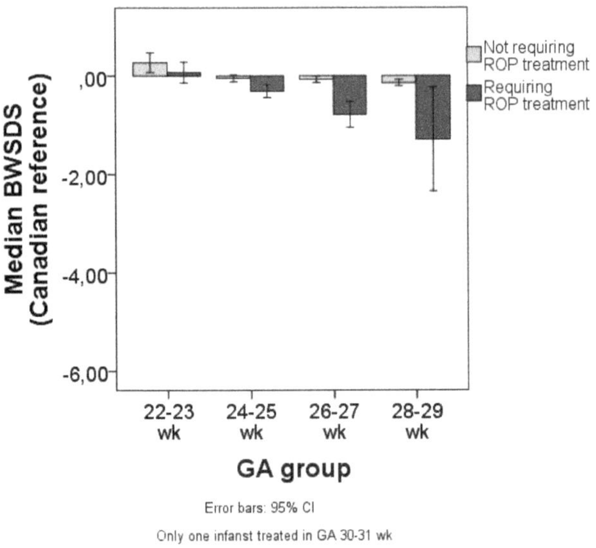

Figure 2. The median BWSDS of infants treated for ROP. The BWSDS was calculated according to the Swedish or Canadian growth reference within each GA group.

Discussion

In this study, we established that the impact of low BWSDS and SGA as risk factors for severe ROP requiring treatment is dependent on GA at birth. This result persisted even when we used two different growth charts to calculate BWSDS and define SGA. GA at birth is a strong predictor of ROP and a low BWSDS may enforce the power of this predictor in more mature infants. These findings may help to explain the inconclusive results of previous studies. The risk of developing severe ROP that requires treatment is increased for the most immature infants; growth restriction is less of a risk factor. If born at a more mature age, the preterm infant's risk is minor for severe ROP unless the infant is born growth restricted. Our new finding that low BWSDS and SGA increases the risk significantly in more mature infants will be of value when counseling parents regarding their infant's risk of developing severe ROP and planning for ROP screening. Our findings could improve the ability to identify those more mature infants at greater risk for ROP who may require treatment, and spare mature infants at minor risk at least some of the painful and stressful eye examinations.

In previous studies concerning low BWSDS as a risk factor for ROP, infants were grouped differently. This could explain why the results have been inconclusive [2,3,13,14,16–18]. However, Qui et al. [15] reported that the impact of SGA as a risk factor for severe ROP varies for infants born ≤26, 27–28, 29–30, or 31–32 weeks GA. Consequently, differences among study results concerning low BWSDS as a risk factor for ROP may depend on the infants' GA at birth. An additional difference in these reports is the degree of ROP investigated, which varied from "any ROP" to "severe ROP".

Variability among the study results may also arise from the different growth charts used for calculating BWSDS, and in the definition of SGA. In the studies noted above, SGA was defined as a BW deficit of less than the 3rd to below the 10th percentile. In the present study, we chose to use two well-established but different growth references, both of which were developed for preterm infants from GA of 22 weeks, but constructed differently regarding the included infants. We defined SGA as less than −2 SDS of GA-appropriate BW with the Swedish reference, and SGA defined as BW below the 10th percentile with the Canadian reference. We found a significantly lower median BWSDS and higher prevalence of SGA in the cohort when we used the Swedish growth reference to calculate BWSDS compared with results calculated with the Canadian growth reference. This finding is not unexpected since the Swedish reference is based on fetal ultrasound, which is considered to reflect undisturbed intrauterine growth, and the Canadian reference which is based on live and still born preterm infants, regardless cause of preterm birth or death. One must question whether strict cutoffs for prenatal growth restriction, such as SGA, are the preferred choice when estimating an infant's risk of developing severe ROP.

In univariate logistic regression for the whole cohort, $BWSDS_{Sweden}$ and SGA_{Sweden} were not significant risk factors, whereas $BWSDS_{Canada}$ and SGA_{Canada} were risk factors. These results show that when estimating prenatal growth restriction, the choice of the growth chart reference may affect the results. Subgroup analysis showed that SGA and BWSDS were variable risk factors dependent on GA at birth. Low BWSDS, as well as SGA, regardless of definition, had the same impact. The more mature the infant, the greater the impact of low BWSDS as a risk factor for severe ROP that will require treatment.

In multivariable logistic regression analysis, we confirmed that the odds of requiring treatment for ROP were reduced with higher BWSDS. As we designed an interaction term, the product of relevant BWSDS and GA group, we established that BWSDS (regardless of growth reference) was dependent on GA at birth. Infants born at GA <26 weeks had reduced odds of requiring treatment for ROP by 20–28% for every 1 SD increase in BWSDS compared with infants born at GA ≥26 weeks, who had a 44–59% reduction for every 1 SD increase in BWSDS ($BWSDS_{Sweden}$; OR = 0.80 vs 0.56 and $BWSDS_{Canada}$; OR = 0.72 vs 0.41). To our knowledge, no previous study has evaluated BWSDS in preterm infants as a risk factor for severe ROP while taking into account the interaction with GA at birth, and considering different BW deficit references.

The underlying reason for the observed shift in the impact of BWSDS as a risk factor for ROP that will require treatment should

Table 2. Association between infant natal characteristics and ROP that required treatment (analyzed using univariate logistic regression analysis).

Clinical characteristics	Whole cohort	GA groups			
	GA 22–32 wk	GA 22–23 wk	GA 24–25 wk	GA 26–27 wk	GA 28–29 wk
	(*n* = 2941)	(*n* = 126)	(*n* = 690)	(*n* = 714)	(*n* = 695)
Variable					
Male gender					
OR	1.30	NS	1.50	NS	NS
95% CI	1.02–1.67*		1.05–2.13*		
GA, wk					
OR	0.47	NS	0.44	NS	NS
95% CI	0.43–0.52***		0.31–0.63***		
BW (50 g increments)					
OR	0.74	NS	0.86	0.79	0.80
95% CI	0.72–0.77***		0.80–0.92***	0.73–0.85***	0.69–0.93**
BWSDS, Swedish reference					
OR	NS	NS	0.86	0.56	0.44
95% CI			0.75–0.99*	0.46–0.69***	0.27–0.73**
SGA, Swedish reference					
OR	NS	NS	NS	3.62	NS
95% CI				2.10–6.25***	
BWSDS, Canadian reference					
OR	0.78	NS	0.70	0.40	0.24
95% CI	0.68–0.89***		0.57–0.86**	0.29–0.54***	0.10–0.54**
SGA, Canadian reference					
OR	1.60	NS	1.80	4.67	12.30
95% CI	1.16–2.20**		1.08–3.01*	2.54–8.57***	2.88–52.41**
Severe growth restriction, Canadian reference					
OR	2.43	–	NS	7.83	21.10
95% CI	1.48–3.99***	–		3.40–18.04***	4.70–94.75***

Abbreviations: BW indicates birth weight; BWSDS, birth weight standard deviation score; GA, gestational age; NS, not significant; OR, odds ratio; ROP, retinopathy of prematurity; SGA, small for gestational age; wk, weeks.
*$p<0.05$,
**$p<0.01$,
***$p<0.001$.

be discussed. A confounding factor of this finding may be the increasing prevalence of infants born with low BWSDS with increasing GA at birth. Infants born with low BWSDS or SGA have an increased risk for perinatal death, both fetal and neonatal [30–32]. Moreover, when low BWSDS and SGA is associated with additional prematurity, the perinatal mortality rates increase [33]. Stoll et al. [34] suggested that the increased survival rates with increasing GA partly reflect physicians' attitudes towards providing intensive care, as measured by the frequent use of antenatal corticosteroids as well as the frequency of active resuscitation in the delivery room [34,35]. Consequently, more aggressive lifesaving interventions are initiated for infants born at an older GA, even for severely growth-retarded fetuses. Thus, the increasing impact of low BWSDS as a risk factor for ROP that will require treatment may be a reflection of the increasing number of surviving infants born with low BWSDS with additional GA weeks at birth. Regardless of the reason behind the finding that low BWSDS is a risk factor for ROP depending on GA, the result remains the same; infants who are born more mature but that are growth restricted should receive adequate attention from the screening ophthalmologist.

Today, most current ROP screening guidelines, which primarily use GA and BW as screening criteria, are vague about the selection of which infants should be screened. Prenatal as well as postnatal growth restriction can be identified by utilizing web-based systems such as WINROP [10,11] and CHOP [36]. By improving the identification of infants at greatest risk for ROP that will require treatment, ophthalmological interventions can focus on those infants at greatest risk, sparing those at minor risk from at least some stressful and painful eye examinations.

In our study, male gender was a significant risk factor for ROP that will require treatment according to univariate logistic regression analysis in the whole cohort (OR = 1.30, 95% CI 1.02–1.47, $p<0.05$) and for infants born during GA 24–25 week (OR = 1.50, 95% CI 1.16–2.20, $p<0.05$). In the earliest descriptions of ROP in the 1940s, male preterm infants were described as

Table 3. Association between infant natal characteristics and ROP that required treatment (according to multivariable logistic regression analysis).

Variable	OR	P	95% CI
BWSDS for Infants with GA <26 weeks at birth (Swedish reference)	0.80	0.0007	0.70–0.91
BWSDS for Infants with GA ≥26 weeks at birth (Swedish reference)	0.56	<0.0001	0.47–0.67
GA	0.41	<0.0001	0.35–0.48
Male gender	1.45	0.0085	1.10–1.91
OR variable	**OR**	*p*	**95% CI**
BWSDS for Infants with GA <26 weeks at birth (Canadian reference)	0.72	0.0008	0.60–0.87
BWSDS for Infants with GA ≥26 weeks at birth (Canadian reference)	0.41	<0.0001	0.31–0.55
GA	0.44	<0.0001	0.38–0.51
Male gender	1.32	0.0463	1.00–1.74

Abbreviations: BWSDS indicates birth weight standard deviation score; GA, gestational age; OR, odds ratio; ROP, retinopathy of prematurity.

more frequently affected by ROP than female ones [37]. A few subsequent reports have supported these findings [2,38]. In the multivariable logistic regression analysis, male gender persisted as a risk factor. Whether or not male gender is also a risk factor for severe ROP dependent on GA will require further investigation.

A major strength of this study is that we calculated BWSDS using two different, well-established growth reference charts; one based on undisturbed intrauterine growth, and the other based on live as well as still born preterm infants. Using both reference models, low BWSDS as well as SGA were risk factors for ROP that will require treatment depending on the infants' immaturity at birth.

Another major strength is the large size of the cohort eligible for assessment, which included 2941 infants from three countries; Canada, Sweden, and the USA. With this constellation of study cohorts, we successfully enrolled almost 700 infants in each pairwise GA group, with the exception of the most preterm group, GA 22–23 weeks.

A limitation of this study is that other established risk factors were not considered when calculating the risk of ROP that will require treatment such as genetic disorders, twin situation, race, and other postnatal morbidities such as days of ventilation, bronchopulmonary dysplasia, septicemia, and necrotizing enterocolitis. Further studies of BWSDS and other postnatal morbidities as risk factors for severe ROP, with special attention to correlations with the infants' GA at birth, would be of great interest.

In summary, growth restriction at birth, calculated using two differently defined well-established growth references, is an important risk factor for ROP that will require treatment, and was dependent on the infants' degree of immaturity. ROP screening criteria need to be continually revised according to new findings in order to focus attention on those infants at greatest risk for severe ROP, and to spare infants at reduced risk from at least some of the stressful eye screening examinations.

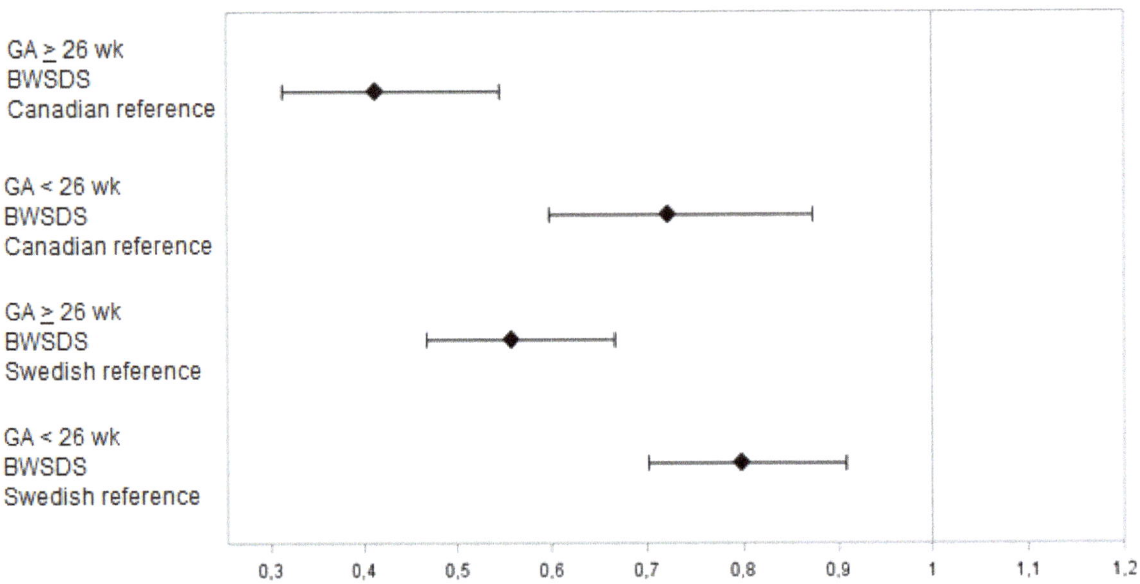

Figure 3. BWSDS odds ratio for infants for ROP requiring treatment in relation to immaturity. The BWSDS was calculated using the Swedish or Canadian growth chart reference for different GA cut-offs.

Author Contributions

Conceived and designed the experiments: PL CL AH. Performed the experiments: PL CL AH. Analyzed the data: PL EA CL. Contributed reagents/materials/analysis tools: GH CW LES IHP AH DL AN AH. Wrote the paper: PL CL AH. Reviewed the manuscript and contributed with constructive comment: AK EA IHP GH AN DL LES CW.

References

1. Austeng D, Kallen KB, Ewald UW, Jakobsson PG, Holmstrom GE (2009) Incidence of retinopathy of prematurity in infants born before 27 weeks' gestation in Sweden. Arch Ophthalmol 127: 1315–1319.
2. Darlow BA, Hutchinson JL, Henderson-Smart DJ, Donoghue DA, Simpson JM, et al. (2005) Prenatal risk factors for severe retinopathy of prematurity among very preterm infants of the Australian and New Zealand Neonatal Network. Pediatrics 115: 990–996.
3. (2010) Incidence of and risk factors for neonatal morbidity after active perinatal care: extremely preterm infants study in Sweden (EXPRESS). Acta Paediatr 99: 978–992.
4. Klinger G, Levy I, Sirota L, Boyko V, Lerner-Geva L, et al. (2010) Outcome of early-onset sepsis in a national cohort of very low birth weight infants. Pediatrics 125: e736–740.
5. Kaempf JW, Kaempf AJ, Wu Y, Stawarz M, Niemeyer J, et al. (2011) Hyperglycemia, insulin and slower growth velocity may increase the risk of retinopathy of prematurity. J Perinatol 31: 251–257.
6. Fortes Filho JB, Eckert GU, Valiatti FB, Dos Santos PG, da Costa MC, et al. (2010) The influence of gestational age on the dynamic behavior of other risk factors associated with retinopathy of prematurity (ROP). Graefes Arch Clin Exp Ophthalmol 248: 893–900.
7. Holmstrom G, Broberger U, Thomassen P (1998) Neonatal risk factors for retinopathy of prematurity–a population-based study. Acta Ophthalmol Scand 76: 204–207.
8. Allegaert K, Vanhole C, Casteels I, Naulaers G, Debeer A, et al. (2003) Perinatal growth characteristics and associated risk of developing threshold retinopathy of prematurity. Journal of Aapos 7: 34–37.
9. Binenbaum G, Ying GS, Quinn GE, Dreiseitl S, Karp K, et al. (2011) A clinical prediction model to stratify retinopathy of prematurity risk using postnatal weight gain. Pediatrics 127: e607–614.
10. Hellstrom A, Hard AL, Engstrom E, Niklasson A, Andersson E, et al. (2009) Early Weight Gain Predicts Retinopathy in Preterm Infants: New, Simple, Efficient Approach to Screening. Pediatrics 123: E638–E645.
11. Loqvist C, Hansen-Pupp I, Andersson E, Holm K, Smith LEH, et al. (2009) Validation of a New Retinopathy of Prematurity Screening Method Monitoring Longitudinal Postnatal Weight and Insulinlike Growth Factor I. Archives of Ophthalmology 127: 622–627.
12. Wallace DK, Kylstra JA, Phillips SJ, Hall JG (2000) Poor postnatal weight gain: A risk factor for severe retinopathy of prematurity. Journal of Aapos 4: 343–347.
13. Bardin C, Zelkowitz P, Papageorgiou A (1997) Outcome of small-for-gestational age and appropriate-for-gestational age infants born before 27 weeks of gestation. Pediatrics 100: E4.
14. Zaw W, Gagnon R, da Silva O (2003) The risks of adverse neonatal outcome among preterm small for gestational age infants according to neonatal versus fetal growth standards. Pediatrics 111: 1273–1277.
15. Qiu X, Lodha A, Shah PS, Sankaran K, Seshia MM, et al. (2012) Neonatal outcomes of small for gestational age preterm infants in Canada. Am J Perinatol 29: 87–94.
16. Allegaert K, de Coen K, Devlieger H (2004) Threshold retinopathy at threshold of viability: the EpiBel study. Br J Ophthalmol 88: 239–242.
17. Woo SJ, Park KH, Ahn J, Oh KJ, Lee SY, et al. (2011) A co-twin study of the relative effect of birth weight and gestational age on retinopathy of prematurity. Eye (Lond) 25: 1478–1483.
18. Fortes Filho JB, Valiatti FB, Eckert GU, Costa MC, Silveira RC, et al. (2009) Is being small for gestational age a risk factor for retinopathy of prematurity? A study with 345 very low birth weight preterm infants. J Pediatr (Rio J) 85: 48–54.
19. Marsal K, Persson PH, Larsen T, Lilja H, Selbing A, et al. (1996) Intrauterine growth curves based on ultrasonically estimated foetal weights. Acta Paediatr 85: 843–848.
20. Niklasson A, Albertsson-Wikland K (2008) Continuous growth reference from 24(th) week of gestation to 24 months by gender. Bmc Pediatrics 8.
21. Roberts CL, Lancaster PA (1999) Australian national birthweight percentiles by gestational age. Med J Aust 170: 114–118.
22. Usher R, McLean F (1969) Intrauterine growth of live-born Caucasian infants at sea level: standards obtained from measurements in 7 dimensions of infants born between 25 and 44 weeks of gestation. J Pediatr 74: 901–910.
23. Kramer MS, Platt RW, Wen SW, Joseph KS, Allen A, et al. (2001) A new and improved population-based Canadian reference for birth weight for gestational age. Pediatrics 108: E35.
24. Lundgren P, Stoltz Sjostrom E, Domellof M, Kallen K, Holmstrom G, et al. (2013) WINROP identifies severe retinopathy of prematurity at an early stage in a nation-based cohort of extremely preterm infants. PLoS One 8: e73256.
25. Wu C, Lofqvist C, Smith LEH, VanderVeen DK, Hellstrom A, et al. (2012) Importance of Early Postnatal Weight Gain for Normal Retinal Angiogenesis in Very Preterm Infants A Multicenter Study Analyzing Weight Velocity Deviations for the Prediction of Retinopathy of Prematurity. Archives of Ophthalmology 130: 992–999.
26. Wu C, VanderVeen DK, Hellstrom A, Lofqvist C, Smith LEH (2010) Longitudinal Postnatal Weight Measurements for the Prediction of Retinopathy of Prematurity. Archives of Ophthalmology 128: 443–447.
27. Gole GA, Ells AL, Katz X, Holmstrom G, Fielder AR, et al. (2005) The international classification of retinopathy of prematurity revisited. Archives of Ophthalmology 123: 991–999.
28. Good WV, Hardy RJ, Dobson V, Palmer EA, Phelps DL, et al. (2003) Revised indications for the treatment of retinopathy of prematurity - Results of the early treatment for retinopathy of prematurity randomized trial. Archives of Ophthalmology 121: 1684–1696.
29. Hosmer DW, Lemeshow S (2000) Applied Logistic Regression. New York: John Wiley and Sons, Inc.
30. Piper JM, Xenakis EMJ, McFarland M, Elliott BD, Berkus MD, et al. (1996) Do growth-retarded premature infants have different rates of perinatal morbidity and mortality than appropriately grown infants? Reply. Obstetrics and Gynecology 87: 1064–1064.
31. McIntire DD, Bloom SL, Casey BM, Leveno KJ (1999) Birth weight in relation to morbidity and mortality among newborn infants. New England Journal of Medicine 340: 1234–1238.
32. Gardosi J, Madurasinghe V, Williams M, Malik A, Francis A (2013) Maternal and fetal risk factors for stillbirth: population based study. BMJ 346: f108.
33. Kamoji VM, Dorling JS, Manktelow BN, Draper ES, Field DJ (2006) Extremely growth-retarded infants: Is there a viability centile? Pediatrics 118: 758–763.
34. Stoll BJ, Hansen NI, Bell EF, Shankaran S, Laptook AR, et al. (2010) Neonatal Outcomes of Extremely Preterm Infants From the NICHD Neonatal Research Network. Pediatrics 126: 443–456.
35. Smith PB, Ambalavanan N, Li L, Cotten CM, Laughon M, et al. (2012) Approach to Infants Born at 22 to 24 Weeks' Gestation: Relationship to Outcomes of More-Mature Infants. Pediatrics 129: E1508–E1516.
36. Binenbaum G, Ying GS, Quinn GE, Huang J, Dreiseitl S, et al. (2012) The CHOP Postnatal Weight Gain, Birth Weight, and Gestational Age Retinopathy of Prematurity Risk Model. Arch Ophthalmol 130: 1560–1565.
37. Kinsey VE, Zacharias L (1949) Retrolental fibroplasia; incidence in different localities in recent years and a correlation of the incidence with treatment given the infants. J Am Med Assoc 139: 572–578.
38. Nodgaard H, Andreasen H, Hansen H, Sorensen HT (1996) Risk factors associated with retinopathy of prematurity (ROP) in northern Jutland, Denmark 1990–1993. Acta Ophthalmol Scand 74: 306–310.

18

Exploring Combinations of Auditory and Visual Stimuli for Gaze-Independent Brain-Computer Interfaces

Xingwei An[1,2]*, Johannes Höhne[2,3], Dong Ming[1]*, Benjamin Blankertz[2]

1 Department of Biomedical Engineering, Tianjin University, Tianjin, China, **2** Neurotechnology Group, Berlin Institute of Technology, Berlin, Germany, **3** Machine Learning Group, Berlin Institute of Technology, Berlin, Germany

Abstract

For Brain-Computer Interface (BCI) systems that are designed for users with severe impairments of the oculomotor system, an appropriate mode of presenting stimuli to the user is crucial. To investigate whether multi-sensory integration can be exploited in the gaze-independent event-related potentials (ERP) speller and to enhance BCI performance, we designed a visual-auditory speller. We investigate the possibility to enhance stimulus presentation by combining visual and auditory stimuli within gaze-independent spellers. In this study with N = 15 healthy users, two different ways of combining the two sensory modalities are proposed: simultaneous redundant streams (Combined-Speller) and interleaved independent streams (Parallel-Speller). Unimodal stimuli were applied as control conditions. The workload, ERP components, classification accuracy and resulting spelling speed were analyzed for each condition. The Combined-speller showed a lower workload than uni-modal paradigms, without the sacrifice of spelling performance. Besides, shorter latencies, lower amplitudes, as well as a shift of the temporal and spatial distribution of discriminative information were observed for Combined-speller. These results are important and are inspirations for future studies to search the reason for these differences. For the more innovative and demanding Parallel-Speller, where the auditory and visual domains are independent from each other, a proof of concept was obtained: fifteen users could spell online with a mean accuracy of 87.7% (chance level <3%) showing a competitive average speed of 1.65 symbols per minute. The fact that it requires only one selection period per symbol makes it a good candidate for a fast communication channel. It brings a new insight into the true multisensory stimuli paradigms. Novel approaches for combining two sensory modalities were designed here, which are valuable for the development of ERP-based BCI paradigms.

Editor: Virginie van Wassenhove, CEA.DSV.I2BM.NeuroSpin, France

Funding: This work was supported by the China Scholarship Council and National Natural Science Foundation of China (Grant No. 81222021). Furthermore, the authors acknowledge financial support by the BMBF Grant Nos. 16SV5839 and 01GQ0850, by the European ICT Programme Project FP7-224631. This paper only reflects the authors' views and funding agencies are not liable for any use that may be made of the information contained herein. The funders had no role in study design, data collection and analysis, decision to publish, or preparation of the manuscript.

Competing Interests: The authors have declared that no competing interests exist.

* Email: xing-wei.an@hotmail.com (XA); richardming@tju.edu.cn (DM)

Introduction

Brain-computer interfaces (BCIs) can provide direct communication by non-muscular methods for people with severe motor impairments [1,2]. Most BCI systems either are based on modulations of local brain oscillations (mostly sensorimotor rhythms (SMRs)) that are induced by certain voluntary control strategies such as Motor Imagery based techniques [3,4], or they exploit event-related potentials (ERPs) that are modulated according to the allocation of attention to selected stimuli. While SMR-based BCIs have the advantage of providing a continuous control signal (in time and magnitude), ERP-based BCIs are commonly considered to be more stable [5] and more efficient for selection tasks, such as mental typewriting. In ERP-based spellers, users can select symbols by directing their attention to stimuli, from the visual, auditory or tactile domain.

The Matrix Speller designed by Farwell and Donchin [6] was the first approach to provide communication to users with severe motor disabilities based on ERPs. It is remarkable that this early approach is still popular, and many novel variants have been devised that still follow the original idea quite closely. Some of these approaches have optimized the exploitation of visual evoked potentials (VEPs) that are elicited by stimuli within the foveal field [7,8]. Also, it is the Matrix Speller that is employed in one of the rare cases of 'home use' BCIs by a paralyzed user [9]. However, it was shown in [10,11] that the performance of the Matrix Speller depends critically on the user's ability to fixate the target character which limits its applicability to users with a certain degree of oculomotor control. To also accommodate users with impaired ocular motor control, recent studies proposed alternative paradigms to implement gaze-independent visual BCI spellers, see [12,13,14,15,16]. For an overview of gaze-independent spellers see [17].

As an alternative paradigm for users with limited or even no vision several research groups investigate spellers based on tactile or somatosensory [18,19] and auditory [20,21,22] stimuli. Paradigms with somatosensory stimuli were considered as a suitable alternative for vision and/or hearing impaired BCI users. Studies about auditory stimuli [20,21,22] examined approaches similar to the visual matrix speller, mapping different sounds to rows and/or columns of the symbol matrix, such as the words from 1 to 10 (for a 5*5 matrix), and 6 environmental sounds (for 6*6 matrix). A novel approach that allowed considerably higher transmission rates was proposed by Schreuder and colleagues [23,24]. The key idea was to employ spatially distributed auditory stimuli, which allowed a fast presentation speed and an easier allocation of attention. Höhne et al. [25,26] introduced a variant of that approach that uses less spatial directions but adds pitch or just the sound of the letters as independent features. More recently, it was shown that the use of syllables as natural stimuli not only improved the users' ergonomic ratings but also increased the classification accuracy [27]. Klobassa et al. [21] used a multimodal audio-visual speller paradigm to provide a better 'training' in initial sessions to finally use mono-auditory speller.

Instead of uni-modal stimuli paradigms, researchers started to focus on using bimodal stimuli [18,28,29,30,31]. Talsma and colleagues [32] reviewed the developments in the understanding of the interaction between attention and multi-sensory processing, focusing on studies using audio-visual stimulus material. Their review also identified several important directions and challenges for future research in this field. Teder-Sälejärvi et al. [28] used randomized sequences of unimodal (auditory (**A**) or visual (**V**)) and simultaneous bimodal (**AV**) stimuli presented to right- or left-field locations. The results in that study showed overlapping but distinctive patterns of multisensory integration for spatially congruent and incongruent **AV** stimuli. Belitski and his colleagues [30] presented an extension of the matrix speller using a so-called 'visual+auditory' paradigm as a transient process for best performance and moved smoothly to purely auditory. Results demonstrated the effectiveness of this approach with this transient process. It was also found that the 'visual + auditory' stimuli increased the average strength of the stimulus response in matrix-speller style BCIs, when compared to unimodal stimuli. However, this study refers only to gaze-dependent visual spellers. Though it was not designed for ERP spelling, Thurlings and her team [31] investigated the effect of bimodal visual-tactile stimulus presentation on the ERP components, BCI performance and participants' task performance. Results of this study showed enhanced early components (N1), which may enhance the BCI performance, while also showed reduced late ERP components (P300).

We live in a multisensory world in which we are continuously deluged with stimulus input through multiple sensory pathways [32]. Therefore it is important to address the following questions: (1) Can multi-sensory integration be exploited in a gaze-independent ERP speller in order to enhance BCI performance? (2) Is there any difference of brain response between single and multi-sensory stimuli? (3) Is it possible to use a BCI paradigm with two independent channels, coding different information?

To answer these questions, we designed a visual-auditory speller (called Combined-Speller, denoted as **AV**) by simultaneous presentation of visual stimuli and auditory stimuli. To enable a comparison with the uni-modal speller paradigms, the mono-visual (denoted as **V**) and mono-auditory (denoted as **A**) spellers are also studied in addition. For answering the third question, we propose a new and truly multi-modal BCI approach (called Parallel-Speller, denoted as **V*A**). In the Parallel-Speller, the visual and auditory stimuli are coded independently.

Material and Methods

Participants

Fifteen healthy subjects (8 female) aged 24-34 (mean 26.9±2.63 years) participated in this study. Two of the participants had already participated in earlier BCI experiments. Each participant did not suffer from a neurological disease and had normal hearing. They also provided written informed consent confirming the notification of the experimental process, the using of the data and the personal right of themselves. Subjects were paid for their participation with 8€/hour, and the entire experiment lasted 3 to 4 hours. The study was approved by the Ethics Committee of the Charité University Hospital (number EA4/110/09).

Stimuli

This study compares four different conditions related to sensory modalities that can be used to drive a BCI speller. Two conditions use stimuli in one sensory modality only, labeled **V** for visual speller and **A** for auditory speller. These experimental settings are similar to existing speller paradigms and have been used for comparison with the novel multimodal spellers. The speller of the **AV** condition (Combined-Speller) uses simultaneous auditory and visual stimuli as redundant information, while the Parallel-Speller (**V*A** condition) exploits alternating auditory and visual cues as independent streams. Figure 1 and Figure 2 show the course of the experiment. The three conditions **V**, **A**, and **AV** used a vocabulary of thirty symbols and a two periods selection procedure as explained below (Figure 1), while condition **V*A** allows to select one out of thirty six symbols within a single selection period (Figure 2). The thirty-symbol alphabet comprised the standard Latin alphabet, punctuation marks '.' and ',', a space symbol '_' and a backspace symbol '<' that could be used to erase the previous symbol. The thirty six-symbol alphabet extended the thirty-symbol alphabet by additional control keys (lower cases 's' for 'Shift', 'c' for 'Ctrl', 'A' for 'Alt', 'p' for 'Space') and punctuation marks ('-' and '?').

In all conditions, the selection of one symbol is coded by two selection steps of one out of six targets each. In the first selection step, a group of symbols (e.g., 'ABCDE') is selected, while in the second selection step one symbol of that group is selected. In the condition **V*A** both steps are performed at the same time (one by each modality), while in the other speller they are performed subsequently. For the serial selection, each group contains five characters (or symbols) and one symbol ('^') that serves as a backdoor to return to the group selection step that can be used in case of an erroneous group selection. In the concurrent selection of group and symbol in condition A*V, the backdoor functionality makes no sense. Therefore, additional symbols were used as replacement. (A different option would have been to have only five symbols per group such that the symbol stage would only be a five class selection. This would have been an advantage with respect to the accuracy of the Parallel-Speller. However, as the focus of this study was the comparison of the multimodal speller with the unimodal spellers, the preference was given to keep the complexity of the selections constant.).

It is important to note that before each selection period, a countdown was launched. It included the intensification of the visual and (or) auditory target stimuli for three times. This was followed by the pre-flashing of the last 3 digits (3, 2, 1) synchronized with the subsequent stimulus sequence. The design of the countdown part did not only provide a cue for the targets but also helped the participant to get used to the flashing frequency.

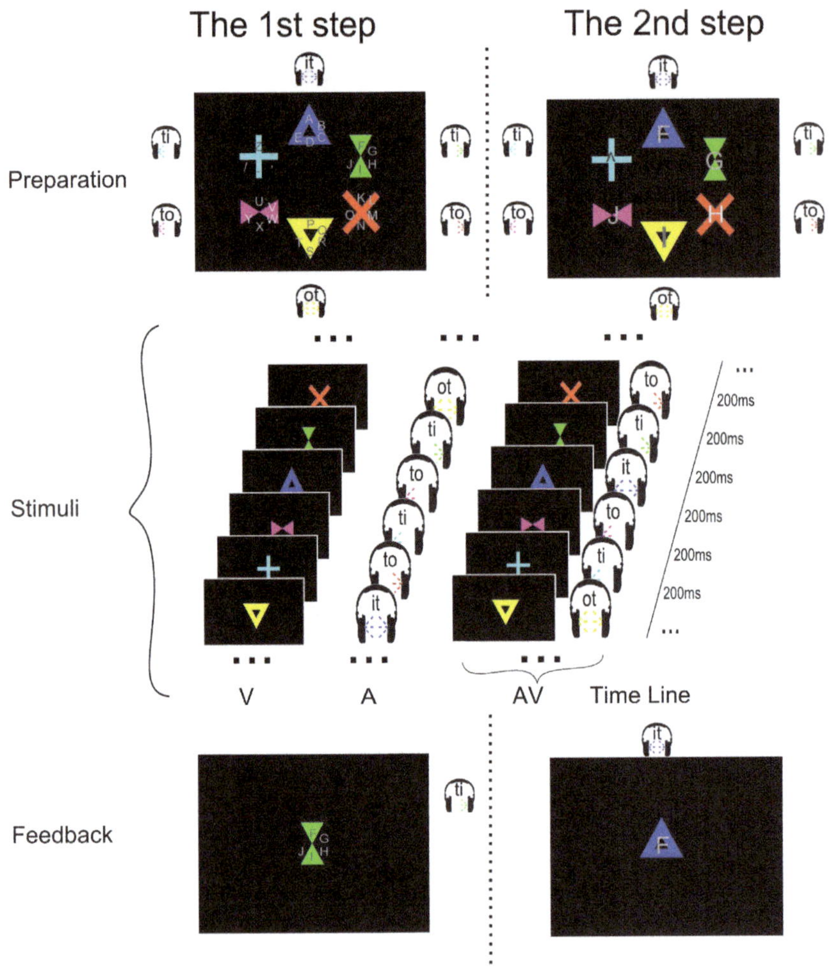

Figure 1. Visualization of the experimental design of the experiment for unimodal speller (Visual: V and Auditory: A) and Combined-Speller (AV). The left column shows the first selection period for group selection. The right column shows the second selection period for symbol selection. The upper channel shows the 'target cue' part before stimuli start, including the cue for showing the position (or voice) of the target and the countdown part for hint of the start. The middle panel shows the time sequence of each stimuli paradigm. The lower panel shows the feedback after each selection period. For the first selection period, the group of the target symbol was chosen, and the symbols in that group will re-distributed into these six visual shapes (the last shape, light blue cross, was left blank as the 'backdoor' symbol) according to their position in the chosen group.

In condition **V**, visual stimuli were presented as in the Center Speller [12]. The Center Speller is a gaze-independent speller, where participants attend to the center of the screen at which the 6 stimuli are presented in a pseudo-random sequence. Six different stimuli were designed such that they had a unique geometrical shape and color (Figure 1), providing two distinct features for visual discrimination. During the presentation of the stimuli, the geometrical shapes were presented centrally in a sequential fashion. The duration of each stimulus was 130 ms and the stimulus onset asynchrony (SOA) was kept at 200 ms. The reason for choosing 130 ms as the duration of the visual stimuli was to match the duration of the auditory stimuli (see below).

In condition **A**, auditory stimuli were presented in a similar fashion as in [25]. We used only 6 stimuli in this study (Figure 1). Short spoken syllables (left 'ti', left 'to', middle 'it', middle 'ot', right 'ti', right 'to') were sung with different pitches by three speakers (bass, tenor and soprano human voices) as stimuli. Every speaker was presented only from one fixed direction (bass: from the left, tenor: from the middle, soprano: from the right). For each direction we recorded 2 stimuli (stimuli with vowel 'i' and stimuli with vowel 'o'). The stimuli with the vowel 'i' (left 'ti', middle 'it' and right 'ti') were recorded with high pitch (A#) and the stimuli with vowel 'o' (left 'to', middle 'ot' and right 'to') were recorded with comparatively low pitch (C#). All of the auditory stimuli were kept within 130 ms as the duration of the visual stimuli. The SOA was also chosen to be 200 ms, such that conditions **V** and **A** were the analog in most aspects but used different sensory modalities.

In condition **AV**, corresponding visual and auditory stimuli were presented simultaneously, while those two concurrent streams coded the same information, see Figure 1. Therefore, targets in the visual sequence always appear at the very same time as targets in the auditory sequence. Senkowski et al. reported the timing of multimodal stimuli to be a crucial aspect [33]. Thus, we investigated the optimal delay in a pilot experiment and finally set the timing that auditory stimuli were presented about 17 ms (1 fame of a 60 Hz monitor) earlier than the corresponding visual stimuli. Participants were instructed to concentrate on the combined visual and auditory stimuli at the same time.

During conditions **V**, **A**, and **AV**, the order of stimuli was randomized within each repetition with the constraint that the

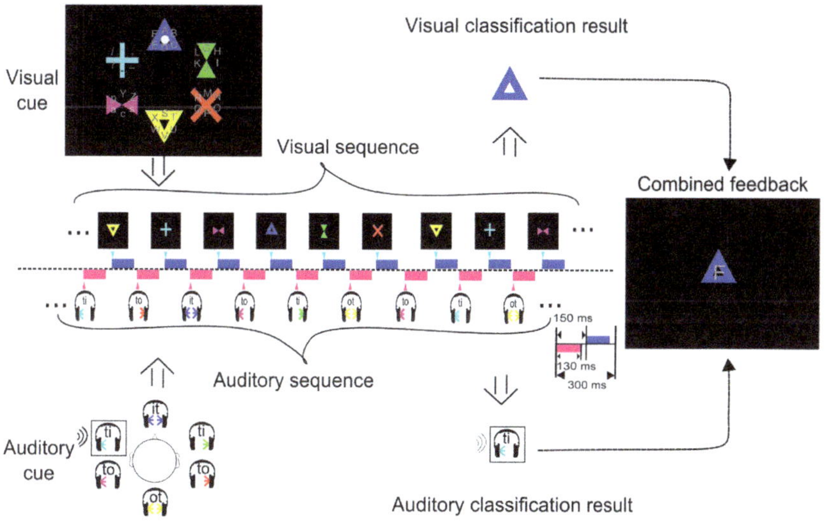

Figure 2. Visualization of the experimental design of the experiment for Parallel-Speller (V*A). Six symbols locate in each group, making a total of thirty-six symbols. The presentation of the visual stimuli was used to choose the group the symbol was in. The position of the symbol in the group was selected through the auditory domain. The upper panel shows the sequence of visual target selection, and the lower panel shows that of the auditory target selection.

same stimulus could not appear with less than two different stimuli in between. Participants were instructed to count the number of target occurrences to help them focus on the stimuli.

In condition **V*A**, the same visual and auditory stimuli have been used, but they were presented as independent sequences. The SOA in each sequence was 300 ms and the onset between auditory and visual cues was 150 ms, with 130 ms duration of each stimuli, see Figure 2. To spell a letter, the group was selected through visual stream, while the within-group selection was done via the auditory domain. That way, two independent decisions are made parallel. For example, to select the symbol 'F', which is the sixth symbol in the first group (cf. Figure 2 visual cue), the target in the visual sequence is the blue triangle and in the auditory sequence the base 'ti' (cf. Figure 2 auditory cue). As it was described above selections of visual and auditory targets were made simultaneously and independently. However those two channels stimuli were alternatively presented in a rapid sequence (see Figure 2 visual and auditory sequences). After several presentations of each stimulus (10 repetitions were used in this experiment), the binary classification and multiclass selection was performed independently for each stimulus domain – resulting in a visual and an auditory output. Combining the visual and auditory output, the final symbol was spelled (see Figure 2).

Note that due to the independence of the two streams, targets in the visual and in the auditory sequence occur at different times in both sequences. The minimum inter-target distance within each modality (visual target to visual target or auditory target to auditory target, cf. Figure 2) is three stimuli and equivalently 900 ms. However, it may happen that two target presentations are only 150 ms apart (e.g. the time between a visual target and auditory target). This cannot be circumvented, as any combination of group and symbol-with-group can be the pair of targets.

Procedure

Visual stimuli were presented on a 19' TFT screen with a refresh rate of 60 Hz and a resolution of 1280*1024 px^2. Auditory stimuli were presented through a light neckband headphone (Sennheiser PMX 200) that was positioned comfortably. Participants were seated in a comfortable chair at a distance of about 1 m from the screen. During the preparation of the EEG, the written and verbal instructions were provided. Thereafter, subjects were instructed to sit still, relax and try to minimize eye movements (try not to blink, though it is inevitable) during the course of a trial.

There were 2 offline calibration runs for each the conditions **V**, **A**, and **AV**. In each calibration run, participants are provided with a sequence of 6 symbols for which they have to perform the 'selections' by allocating attention to the corresponding target stimuli. In total, there were 12 symbols (6 symbols * 2 calibration runs) for each condition in the calibration phase. The sequence of symbols to spell was randomly selected from all available symbols, and this differed between subjects. The 6 runs of the 3 conditions (**V**, **A**, **AV**) were conducted in pseudo-randomly order.

After the calibration phase, offline analysis was conducted to train a classifier (see [34] and Section 2.4) on the collected data of condition **AV**. After a short pause, participants were instructed to complete one self-conceived word (without telling the experimenter) in free spelling mode comprising 6–10 symbols with condition **AV**. During free spelling, participants could use the backdoor symbol '^' (which is contained in every group) to cancel the selection of the group and use the backspace symbol ('<') to erase the previous symbol, if a wrong group or symbol was selected. Free-spelling was conducted as motivation and for getting familiar with online spelling. Thereafter, participants were asked to spell twenty predefined symbols in the so-called copy-spelling mode (again condition **AV**). In contrast to free-spelling, erroneously selected symbols needed not to be deleted as in the free spelling part. As a two-period spelling paradigm, the spelling in condition **AV** faces the problem that the first period (group selection) could be wrong, which will definitely lead to wrong symbol selection. In this study, the default visual and auditory targets in the second period were the same as the correct target should be, no matter the correct group was selected or not. From the symbols the participants selected, it is easy to analyze the accuracy in each period.

Condition **V*A** was conducted after a short break. The reason for having this condition always at the end was that participants should have experienced the simpler conditions first in order to be able to cope with this more demanding condition. This training effect was conjectured to outweigh the possible detrimental effect of fatigue that may occur at the end of the experiment. Participants underwent a calibration of 4 runs (6 symbols in each run), a free spelling phase where self-chosen words could be spelled, and finally the copy spelling of a predefined sentence.

In the calibration phase, there were similar countdown and feedback parts for each trial to select the target symbol. The intensification of the target in the countdown part was a flashing circle in the center of the target visual shape with the target auditory stimuli presented through the earphone (both for three times), followed by the pre-flashing of the last 3 digits (3, 2, 1) synchronized with the subsequent stimulus sequence. Only one selection period was needed to choose the target symbol. The visual stimuli and auditory stimuli were presented independently and alternatively as described in Section 2.2. Considering the complexity of the task, it is difficult to quickly count the number of targets occurrences. There were 20 target occurrences in 18 s. It is possible that visual target and auditory target may occur consequently. In this circumstance, participants need to count two numbers in 600 ms. Thus participants were not asked to count the number target occurrences, but just to pay attention to the target stimuli in the auditory as well as in the visual stream. After the presentation of 10 repetitions of the stimuli (since the task is difficult than other paradigms, more repetitions were used here), the outputs of the visual and auditory classification were made according to these two stimuli streams.

The offline analysis for condition **V*A** were conducted after the calibration phase, followed by free spelling and copy spelling runs. During free spelling, the participants could spell any word without telling the experimenter, and could use the backspace symbol ('/') to erase the previous symbol, if a wrong symbol was selected. Thereafter, twenty predefined symbols (the same as in condition **AV**) in the so-called copy-spelling mode without erasing the wrong symbols selected.

For this whole experiment, we have ten calibration runs in total. Each calibration run lasts for less than 3 minutes, while 6 symbols are spelled. For conditions **V**, **A** and **AV**, there are 2 selection periods for choosing a symbol, compared to only one selection period for per symbol in condition **V*A**. Besides the calibration runs, for condition **AV** and **V*A**, free spelling and copy spelling runs were also conducted after their calibration runs. Neither copy spelling nor free spelling was done with unimodal stimuli (condition **V** and **A**). Between each run, participants could rest for 2–5 min. There is no break within runs.

Data acquisition and analysis

Electroencephalogram (EEG) signals were acquired using a Fast'n Easy Cap (EasyCap GmbH, Munich, Germany) with 63 Ag/AgCl electrodes placed at the standard positions of the international 10–20 system. Channels were referenced to the nose, with the Ground electrode located at the front (at position AFz). Electrooculogram (EOG) signals were recorded additionally. Signals were amplified using two 32-channel amplifiers (Brain Amp by Brain Products, Munich, Germany), sampled at 1 kHz. Further online and offline analysis was performed in Matlab. Statistical analysis was performed with both IBM SPSS statistics 20 and MATLAB. The visual and auditory feedback was implemented using the open source framework PyFF (Venthur et al., 2010).

To evaluate the workload of each condition, participants were asked to fill in the NASA TLX questionnaire (NASA Human Performance Research Group, 1987) after the calibration phase of each condition. It was introduced as a measure of usability in BCI by Pasqualotto et al. [35] and Riccio et al. [36], and it has been used to compare the workload for a visual and an auditory speller by Käthner et al. [37]. It was used here as a multidimensional rating procedure to derive an overall workload score based on a weighted average of ratings on six sub-scales (Mental workload, Physical workload, Temporal workload, Performance, Effort needed and Frustration) for each condition. There were fifteen pair-wise comparisons of each two of the six subscales (Mental vs. Physical, Mental vs. Temporal, and Physical vs. Temporal, et al.) for the participants to choose the subscale in the comparison which weighs more for the whole workload. The subscale wins in each pair-wise comparison will count 1. So the sum score of the weightings is fifteen. A high score reveals an increased importance for workload.

Generally, EEG is prone to various sources of noise arising from factors such as 50 Hz power noise or ECG artifacts. Moreover, the discriminative components of the ERP are mainly found below 40 Hz. A Chebychev filter was therefore applied for offline analysis, using a passband up to 40 Hz and a stopband starting at 49 Hz and then down sampled to 100 Hz. It removes particularly well the line noise and other high-frequency noise [12,23]. For online classification, signals were subsampled to 100 Hz without prior filtering. The continuous signals were then segmented into epochs between -150ms and 800 ms relative to each stimulus onset, using the first 150ms as a baseline.

Classification was based on spatio-temporal features [34] and preceded as in [12] and [16]. For each condition, the sample-wise r^2 coefficients (augmented with the sign of the difference) were calculated for *targets* vs. *nontargets*. Five time intervals in which those coefficients indicated highly discriminative information were generally determined heuristically [34] but sometimes manually adjusted by the experimenter (for example when the time intervals were chosen before the onset of the stimuli, the experimenter should choose one after the onset instead). Spatio-temporal features were determined from single-trials by averaging all samples within those intervals for each channel. This provides feature-vectors with dimensionality 63 (number of EEG channels) times 5 (number of time intervals), i.e. 315. For classification, regularized Linear Discriminant Analysis (LDA) with shrinkage regularization of the covariance matrix was used, see [34] for details. Classification was done for each stimulus, as a binary task to distinguish the *target* sub-trials from the *non-target* sub-trials. For online classification, in each selection period, one out of six stimuli had to be chosen (the one that was attended by the participant with highest probability). To that end, real-valued classifier outputs (distance to the separating hyperplane) were averaged for each of the six stimuli across all available repetitions and the stimulus with the highest scores was selected. In this study the number of repetitions was six for condition **AV** and ten for condition **V*A**.

In an offline analysis, the temporal distribution as well as the spatial distribution class discriminative information was investigated for each participant and condition. Therefore, the accuracy of a classifier was estimated which was trained either on all channels and sliding time intervals (window size = 20 ms, step size = 5 ms) or only one channel and heuristically determined time intervals.

As Schreuder et al. [38] has shown that the number of repetitions can significantly impact BCI performance, the BCI performance when using smaller numbers of repetitions was also estimated in offline analysis. Cross-validation was used to evaluate the classification performance based on the calibration data, also for the unimodal conditions with which no online spelling has been performed.

Though in general context the Information Transfer Rate (ITR) is a reasonable performance measure text, we consider the actual symbols per minute (SPM) for spelling applications is more straightforward and realistic [38]. For single level interfaces, a correct selection counts as +1 symbol. An erroneous selection counts as -1 symbol, to account for the added effort of performing a backspace. We used the formula described in [38] to investigate the SPM for each speller:

$$\text{symbols per minute} = 60/\text{time per symbol} \quad (1)$$

$$E = \text{Percent correct-Percent erroneous} \quad (2)$$

$$\text{SPM} = \text{symbols per minute} * E \quad (3)$$

Need to notice that the *time per symbol* includes all the necessary overhead including countdown part, classification and feedback time.

Results

In this study, we investigate and compare workload, ERP components, classification accuracy and spelling speed in each speller. We compare all of these features among condition **V**, **A**, and **AV** to investigate whether multi-sensory stimuli enhance BCI performance in the gaze-independent speller and to find the difference among brain response. We also present those results for condition V*A to study the possibility to use a BCI paradigm with two independent channels coding different information.

Behavioral data

The subjective workload that was imposed in each spelling condition was estimated based on the NASA TLX questionnaire. The left column of Figure 3 shows the mean rating with SD (standard deviation, stands for the standard deviation of the sampling distribution of the rating score) for each subscale and the overall weighted workload with SEM (standard error of the mean) for each condition. Also the grand averaged weights of the subscales were plotted on the right of the figure.

Results show that condition **AV** has the lowest, while condition **V*A** has the highest subjective workload for each sub-scale and overall. The data of workload has an approximate Gaussian distribution (K-S test, $p>0.05$), and they have equal sample variances (Levene tests, $p> 0.05$). Univariate ANOVA of the workload with factor *condition* and *subscale* was conducted. The results show significant effects of factors *condition* ($p <.001$) and *subscale* ($p <.001$), but no significant effects on *condition*subscale* ($p =.967$). Pairwise comparison was also conducted on *conditions*. Significant differences were found for each comparison of conditions **A**, **AV**, and **V*A** ($p <.050$). Condition V and V*A also have significant difference ($p <.001$). The overall workload of all 4 conditions follow an approximate Gaussian distribution (K-S test, $p =.980$).The results do not show significant difference among conditions **V**, **A**, and **AV** ($p>.01$), but significant difference ($p <.01$) between condition A*V and the other three conditions (**V, A, AV**). Moreover, the pie chart plot of weightings for the subscales reveals the subscale *Mental* (*30.3%*) to be the most important factor of workload, followed by *Effort* (*17.0%*).

Event-related potentials

Figure 4 depicts the grand-average (N = 15 participants) of the event-related potentials (ERPs) and spatial-temporal diversities of the class-discriminative information of the first 3 conditions (left: **V**, middle: **A**, right: **AV**). FC5 electrode was used in [27] for the early negative auditory ERP components. In visual P3-speller literatures, PO7, P7 and (or) P8 were used to check the early negative ERP components. Also concerning the ERP scalp maps in Figure 4, we choose the three channels (Cz, FC5 and P7) to analysis. These three channels of grand averaged ERPs are plotted on the top of the figure. The matrix plots under the ERPs show the spatial-temporal discriminative information (signed r^2) of *targets* vs. *non-targets* in each condition. To compare each component across different conditions, scalp maps of the class-discriminative information (r^2) are shown for 4 fixed time intervals, which are marked in the ERP plots. The components shown in this 4 time intervals are denoted as 'N1', 'N2', 'P3' and 'P4', according to the polarity and the order of the components.

In condition **V**, there is a prominent negative component 250-350 ms after stimulus onset located at lateral parieto-occipital electrodes (P7, P9) with higher amplitudes on the left hemisphere. This component is referred to as N2. The ERPs at P7 in Figure 4.1a depicts the difference of grand average ERPs between *targets* and *nontargets*. As expected, a positive component is observed approximately 350-560 ms (channel Cz) after the stimulus onset (referred to as P3 components). As seen from the spatial-temporal distribution matrix plot (Figure 4.1b), the positive component starts from the centro-parietal area and extends to the surrounding electrodes. The decay of the discriminative information of this component progresses from occipital to frontal electrodes, see Figure 4.1b.

In condition **A**, all components have lower amplitudes compared to the corresponding components in condition **V**, which is in agreement with existing literature. An early negative component observed at approximately 150-230 ms (referred as N1 component) occurs at fronto-central areas. As already observed by Höhne et al. [27], this component is stronger on the left hemisphere than on the right hemisphere. The P3 component starts at around 360 ms with a focus in the central area.

Figure 4.3 depicts the ERPs and topographies of the class-discriminative information in condition **AV**. The N1 component in condition **AV** occurs around the frontal area with a higher amplitude on the left hemisphere, which is similar to condition **A**. The N2 component observed at parieto-occipital electrodes shows a similar but weaker response compared with that in condition **V**. The P3 component starts from the fronto-central area between 350 ms and 500 ms, showing an earlier discriminative response than that in condition **V** similar as in condition **A**. Surprisingly, the decay of the P3 component progresses from the front to the occipital area (Figure 4.3b) vary much in contract to the condition **V**.

Figure 5 shows the ANOVA (using Matlab) results of ERP response for conditions **V**, **A**, and **AV** (Left: Targets, right: Non-Targets). The ERP response has significant differences of 3 conditions were marked light blue ($p <.05$). Light pink marked time-zones show the significant difference between condition **V** and **AV** ($p <.05$). The early components of the ERP response after stimulus onset show significant differences both for Targets and Non-Targets, which might indicate that those difference was influenced by the stimuli properties of different stimuli. Light pinked zones could indicate the influence of auditory stimuli to visual stimuli response. No obvious significant difference was found for P300 components during 250–450 ms. Thus, the characteristics of the individual auditory stimuli influence rather

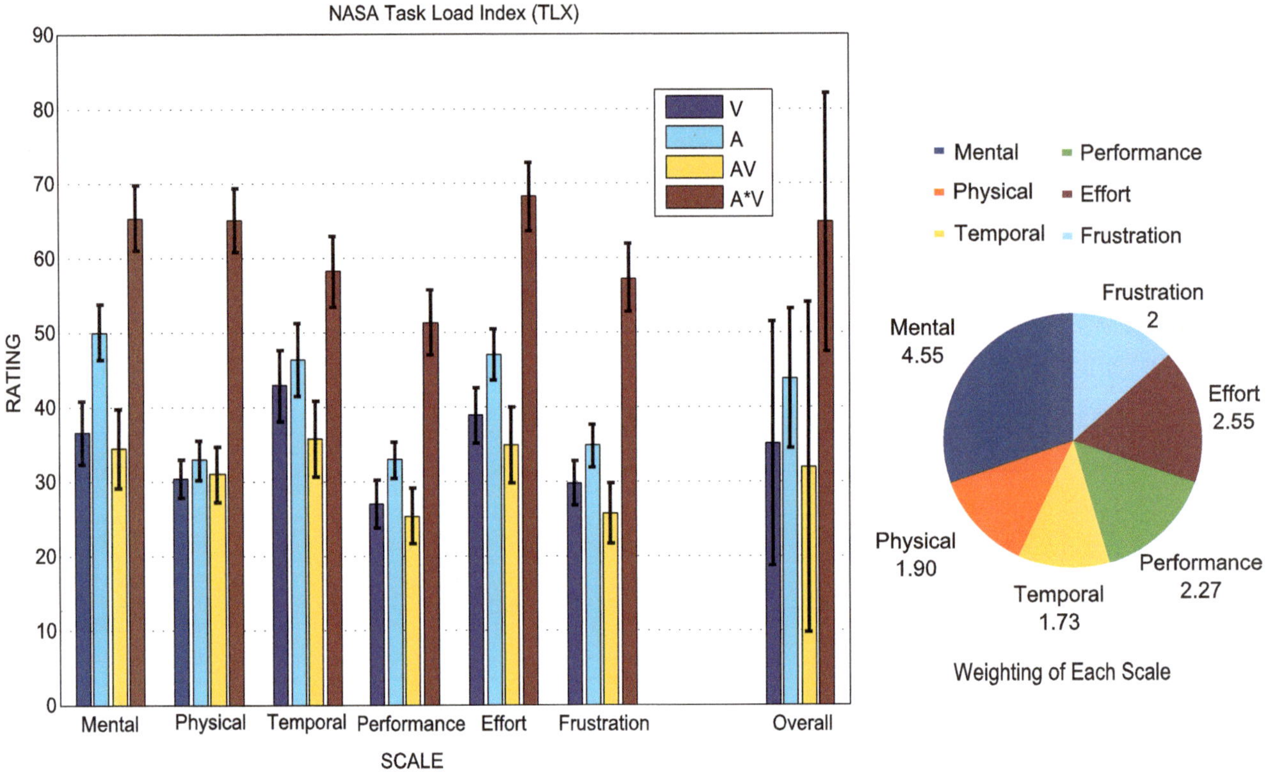

Figure 3. The NASA TLX workload and the overall weighted score of different conditions. The left column shows the mean rating with the standard deviation (SD) for each subscale and the overall weighted workload for each condition. The pie chart shows the grand-averaged weighting for each subscale. The total weighting is 15, due to 15 pair-wise comparisons of the sub-scales (see section 2.4).

the early ERP components, while later components are not affected.

Figure 6 show the ERPs (as well as the ANOVA results) and class-discriminative information (signed r^2) separately for visual and auditory stimuli in condition **V*A** (left: visual; right: auditory). The upper two subfigures show the ANOVA results of Targets versus Non-Targets for visual and auditory stimuli independently. Significant differences are found at large time zones for Target versus Non-Target ERP response. For the grand averaged visual response, the negative component at occipital area is observed at 250–380 ms after the visual stimulus onset, and the positive component at the central area occurs at 450 ms. The auditory negative component is observed at frontal areas from 100 to 250 ms and the positive response appears at the central area between 400 and 500 ms.

Offline binary accuracy

The single trial classification accuracies for each condition, which have an approximate Gaussian distribution (K-S test, $p > 0.05$) and equal sample variances (Levene tests, $p = .875$), were estimated and depicted in Figure 7. ANOVA of the accuracies with the factor condition was conducted. As expected, the classification accuracies in condition **V** and **AV** are significantly better than that in condition **A** ($p < .001$). However, there is no significant difference between condition **V** and condition **AV** ($p = 1$). No significant differences were found between V and V|A*V as well as between A and A|A*V ($p > .05$).

Figure 8.a depicts the grand average temporal distribution of discriminative information. To investigate which time intervals contribute most to classification success, a time window of 20 ms and time step of 5 ms were used to calculate the temporal distribution of the classifications. Cross-validation results of those features for each time point provide a temporal distribution of the multivariate discriminative information. The curve for condition **A** shows lower classification accuracy compared to condition **V** for the whole time period except for the early interval 200–260 ms. Condition **AV** effectively exploits the early components of both modalities with accuracies above both unimodal conditions between 200 and 300 ms. However, starting from about 380 ms the results of **AV** are inferior to those of **V**, which is in line with the observation of the earlier decay of the P3 component in the bimodal condition (see Figure 4).

Analogously to Figure 8.a, Figure 8.b shows the temporal evolution of the discriminative information for condition **V*A**. It is quite similar to the results for the unimodal conditions in Figure 8.a. However, surprisingly, for the auditory stimuli in the Parallel-Speller (**V*A**), the discriminative information starts earlier than in the unimodal condition **A**, which may be due to an increased level of attention.

Complementary to Figures 8, the spatial distribution of the discriminative information is displayed in Figure 9. The top row shows the results of the first 3 conditions (**V**, **A**, **AV**). In condition **V**, higher accuracies of the occipital electrodes suggest that visual and visual-attentional components are essential ingredients for classification. Discriminative information from cognitive processes as reflected in the P3 is spatially more wide spread and therefore not so prominent is this display of single channel analysis. Classification accuracies for condition **A** show the importance of fronto-central electrodes in particular on the left hemisphere,

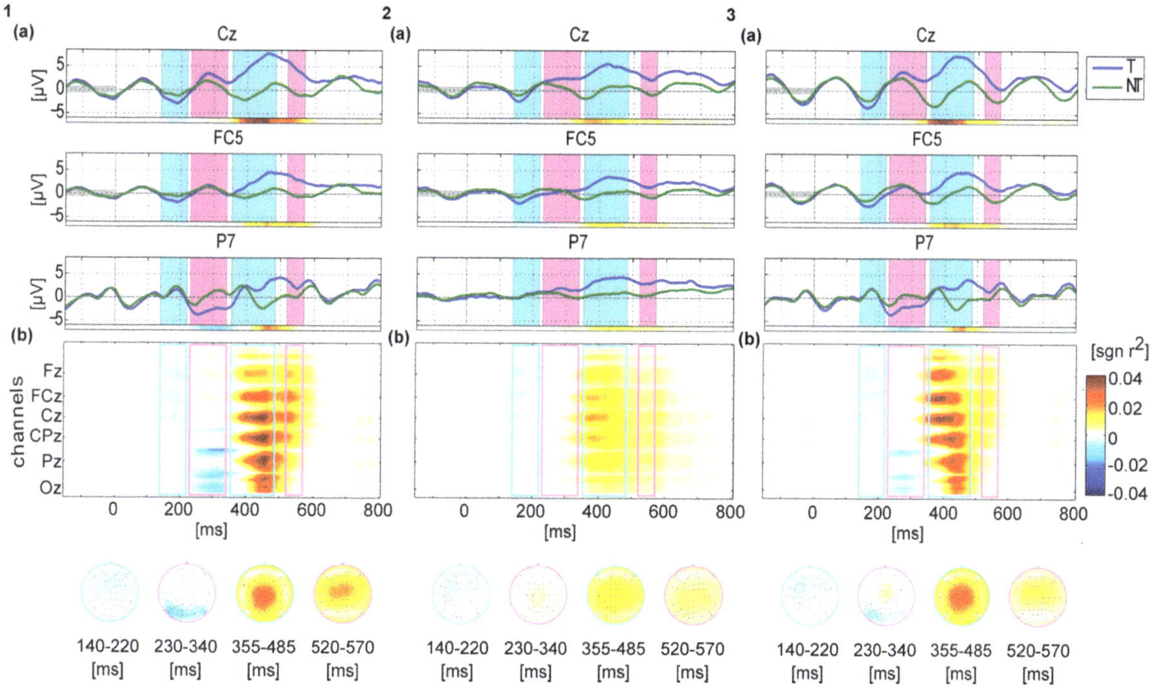

Figure 4. Grand averaged ERP and spatio-temporal diversity of the class-discriminative information for the first 3 conditions. Conditions are arranged in columns (left: **V**, middle: **A**, right: **AV**). All plots share the same color scale. The top row shows the ERPs for targets and non-targets of three selected electrodes Cz, FC5 and P7. The pink and green shade areas in each plot marked the time intervals, for which the scalp maps are shown at the bottom also colored accordingly. The colored bar underneath of each plot gives the signed correlation coefficient (sign r^2). It indicated the difference between target and non-target classes for the chosen channel. In the middle, the spatio-temporal distribution of class-discriminative information was shown as a matrix plot, under which also the scalp maps of the chosen intervals were shown depicting the averaged r^2 values within the time intervals. The matrix plot shows the signed r^2 values for each EEG channel and for each time point. The light-blue and light-magenta rectangles depicted the chosen time interval as the shaded area in the top rows.

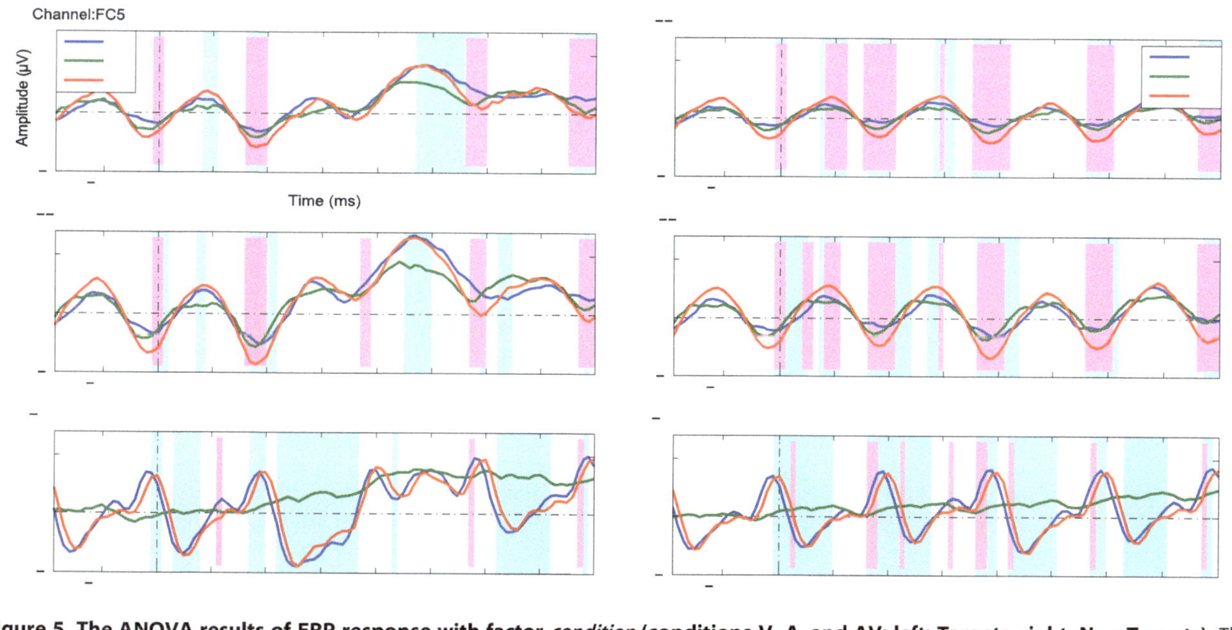

Figure 5. The ANOVA results of ERP response with factor *condition* (conditions V, A, and AV; left: Targets, right: Non-Targets). The time intervals with significant difference of ERP response for conditions **V**, **A**, and **AV** was marked light blue ($p < .05$). The pink-marked time-zones show the time intervals that have significant difference of conditions **V** and **AV** ($p < .05$).

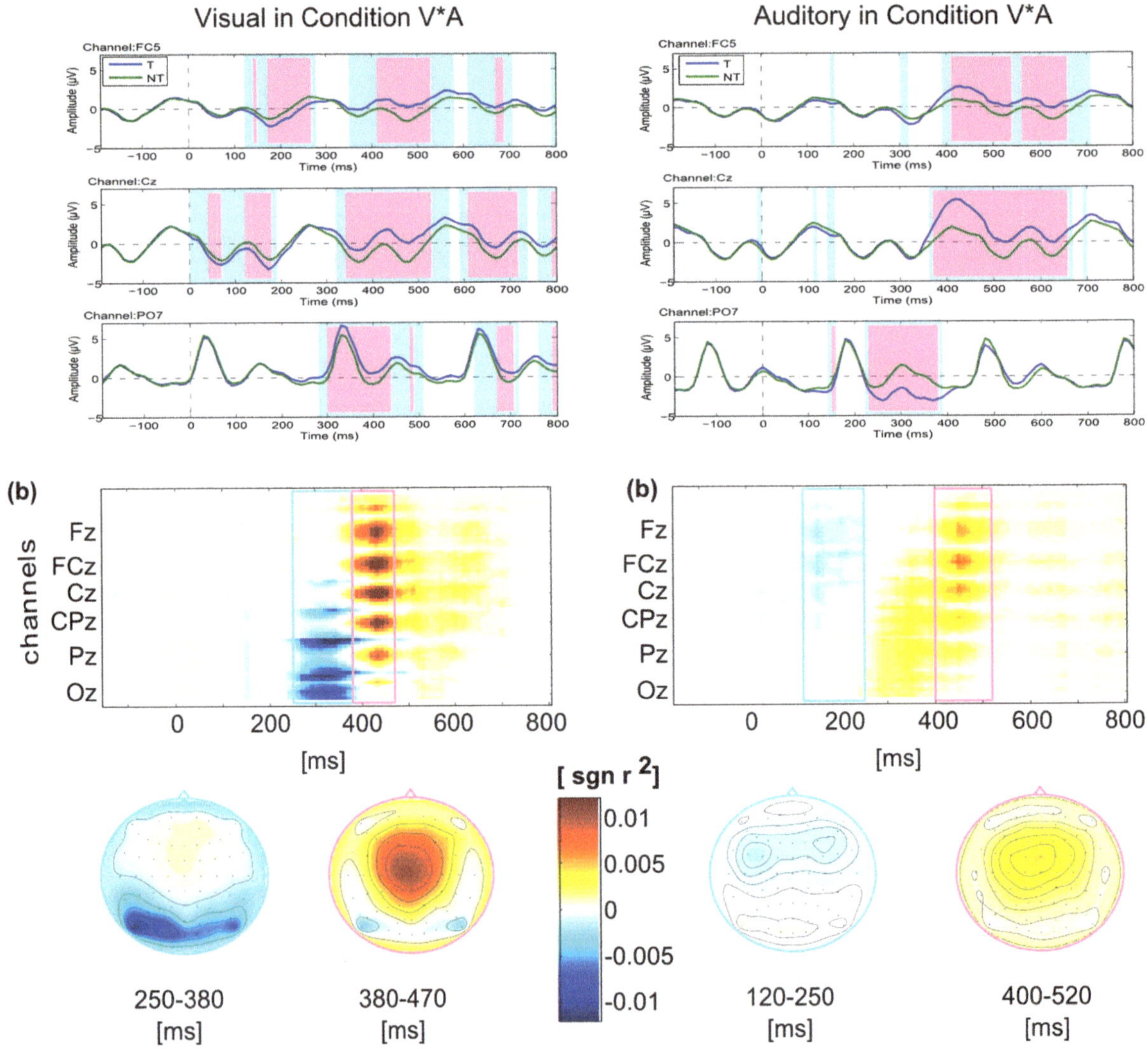

Figure 6. The ANOVA results of ERP response and class-discriminance (signed r^2) maps of Targets versus Non-Targets in condition V*A. The two columns show the ERP responses for visual (left) and auditory (right) stimuli independently in condition **V*A**. The first row shows the ERP responses for the three selected electrodes FC5, Cz and PO7. The time intervals with significant difference of ERP response for Targets and Non-Targets was marked light blue ($p < .05$). The pink-marked time-zones show the time intervals that have more significant difference with $p < .01$. Spatio-temporal diversities of the class-discriminative information are shown in the second row. All plots share the same color scale (different scale in the colorbar compared to Figure 4). The spatial distribution of class-discriminant information is depicted with scalpmaps for two time intervals.

which is in line with the ERP results shown in Figure 4. The asymmetry also exists in condition **AV**.

The classification accuracies in condition **V*A** are lower than in the other conditions. Therefore, in the second row a different scale for the colormap is used for better display. Apart from the lower absolute value, the maps of classification accuracy look similar to the maps for the corresponding uni-modal conditions in the row above. The occipital area of the map for V|V*A seems to show a stronger lateralization to the left side than the maps of the visual-only condition.

Online Spelling Results

Figure 10 depicts the results of conditions **AV** and **V*A** in the online copy-spelling mode of this study. Each participant had to spell 20 symbols ('AUDIO_VISUAL_SPELLER') in both paradigms.

For condition **AV** (Combined-Speller), 6 repetitions of the stimuli were used for each selection, and two selection periods (group selection and symbol selection) have been conducted for each symbol. The blue bar in Figure 10 shows the symbol accuracies in condition **AV**. More than *73.3%* participants (11 in 15 participants) could get accuracy over *90%*. Only 2 of all the participants got accuracy under *80%*. The mean accuracy is *92.0%* (chance level *<3%*) with a speed of more than 2 symbols per minute.

In the Parallel-Speller (condition **V*A**) 10 repetitions of the stimuli have been used. The visual stimuli coded the group and the auditory stimuli coded the position of the symbol in the visual group. Since there is no pause or the need for correcting selection errors during copy-spelling, all of the participants finished this part within 10 min. The red and green bars in Figure 10 shows the visual (**V**) and auditory (**A**) selection accuracies separately. The visual selections for thirteen participants are over 90.0%, while

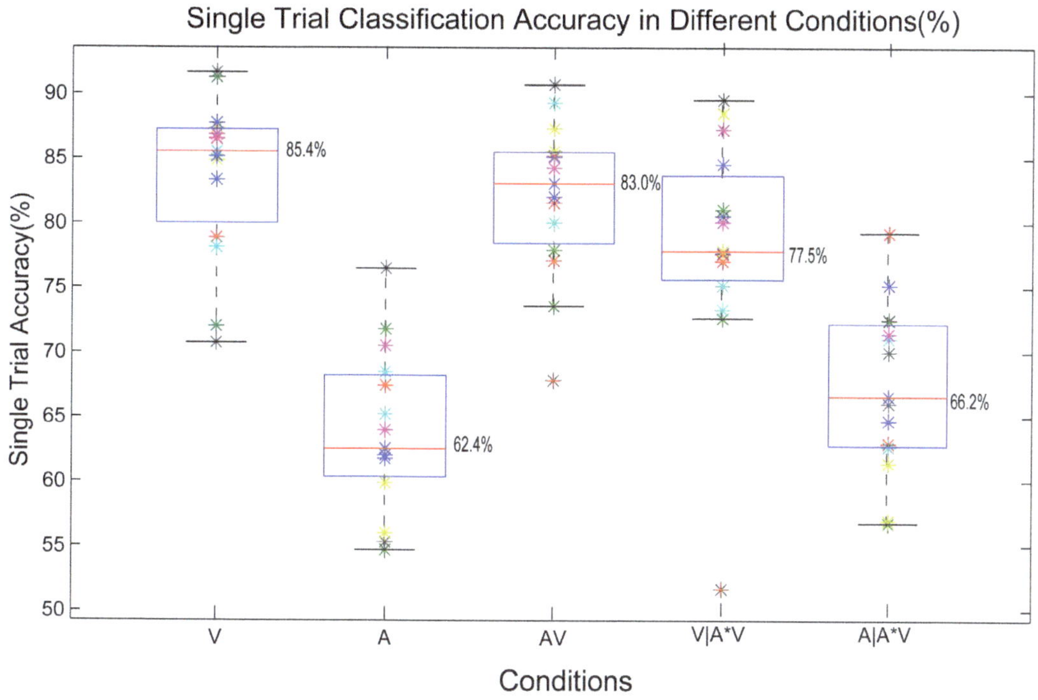

Figure 7. Single trial classification accuracies in different conditions for the binary *target* vs *non-target* discrimination. Accuracies are estimated by cross-validation on the calibration data using class-wise normalized loss function (chance level = 0.5). Each colored '*' represents the accuracy for each participant in giving conditions. The edges of the blue box in each column reveal the 25% and 75% data range. The central red mark is the median accuracy overall the participants in the giving condition.

only six participants could get accuracies over 90.0% for the auditory condition. Thus, the selection errors of the symbols are mostly due to an error of the auditory-based selection. Eleven of the participants achieved at least *80.0%* accuracy. Four participants spelled less than 16 correct symbols, thus displaying a selection accuracy of below 80%. All users could spell online with a mean accuracy of 87.7% (chance level <3%) showing a competitive average speed of 1.65 symbols per minute.

We also performed offline simulations where we determined the spelling speed (symbols/minute) as a function of the number of the sequences using the calibration data. Figure 11 shows the results for different conditions. ANOVA measures with factors *condition* and *number of repetitions* was conducted to investigate the significance of each factor for the first 3 conditions. The results show significant effects of factors *condition* ($p < .001$), *number of repetitions* ($p < .001$) but no significant effect of the factor

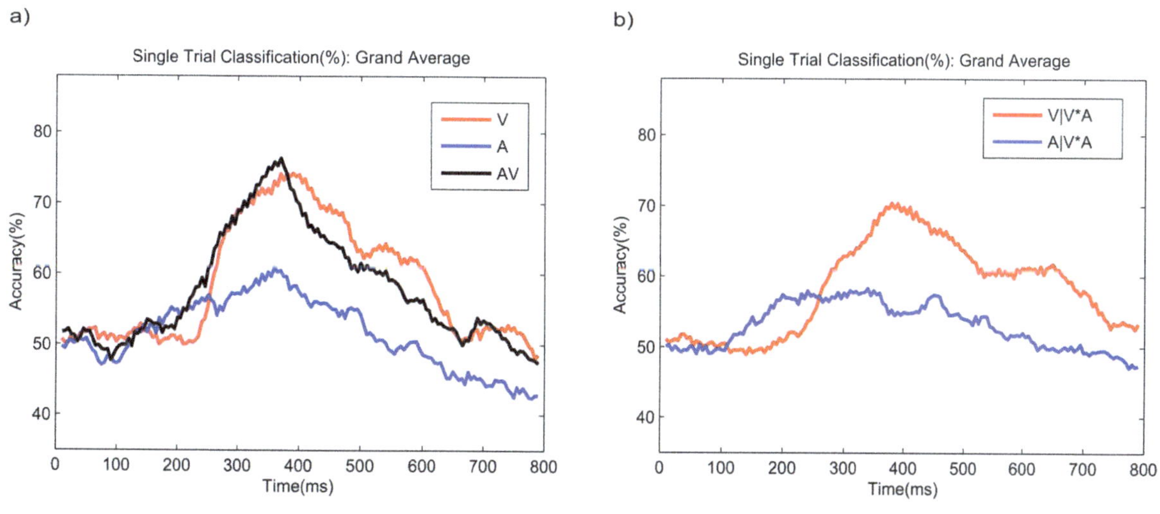

Figure 8. The grand averaged temporal distribution of discriminative information for each condition. a) The single trial classification for the unimodal spellers and Combined Speller (red: condition **V**; blue: condition **A**; black: condition **AV**). b) The temporal distribution of the single trial classification accuracy for condition **V*A** (red: visual classification; blue: auditory classification). The time window used in this study is 20 ms with a time step of 5 ms.

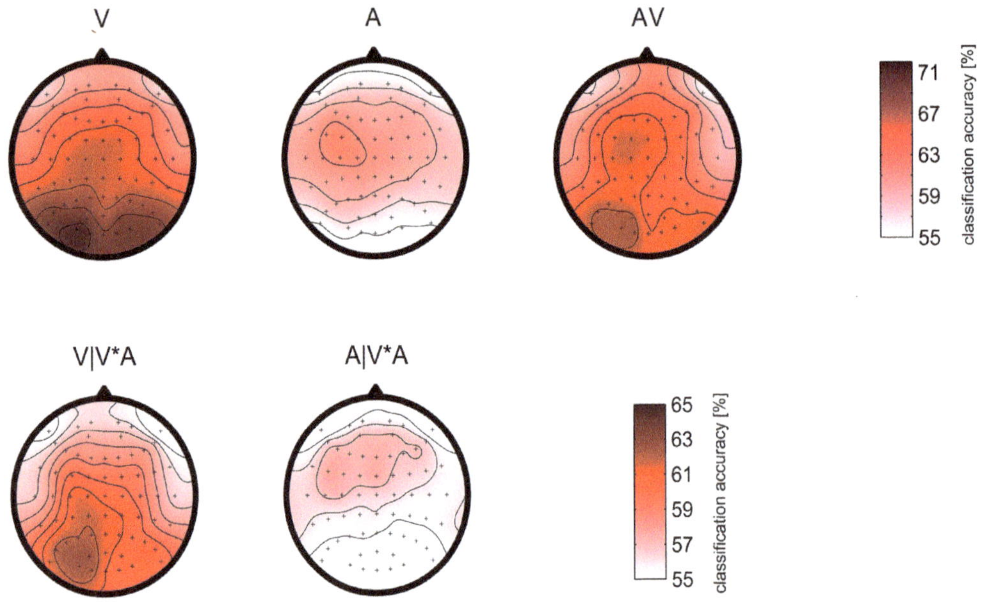

Figure 9. Spatial distribution of classification performance. Classification was made for each electrode individually. The time intervals were chosen by a heuristic between [0 800] after the stimulus onset. The grand average for each of the condition is shown and the binary classification accuracies are indicated by color gradients. The plots in the first row use the same color scale as shown on the right of that row. The figures in the second row use a different color bar as shown on the right of the second row.

condition * *repetition* (p = *.210*). However, concerning only the offline stimulation results of the spelling speed for conditions **V** and **AV**, there were significant effects of the *repetition* (F = *21.996*, p = *0*) factor, but no significant effect of the *condition* (F = *3.125*, p = *0.079*) and the *condition* * *repetition* (F = *.067*, p = *.997*) factors.

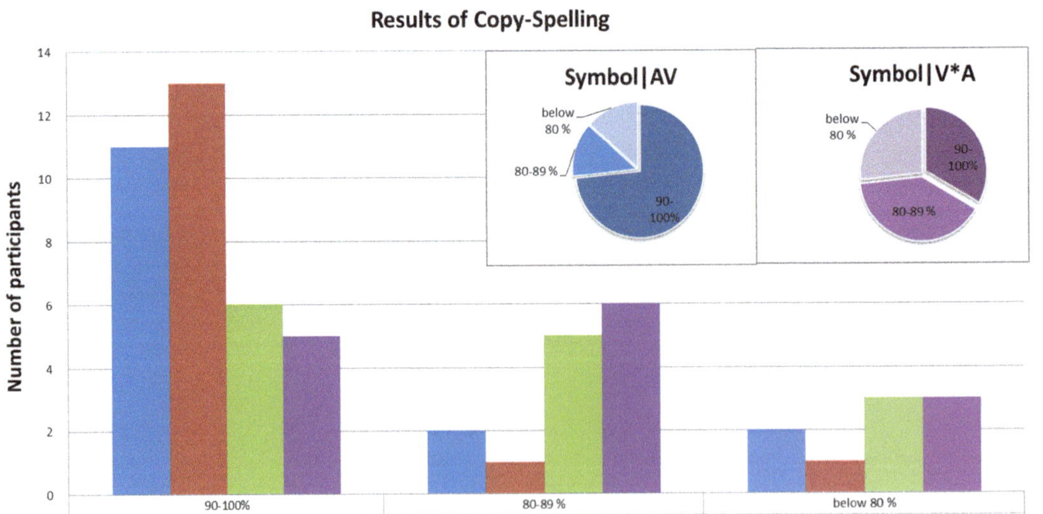

	90-100%	80-89 %	below 80 %
Symbol|AV	11	2	2
Visual|V*A	13	1	1
Auditory|V*A	6	5	3
Symbol|V*A	5	6	3

Figure 10. The distribution results of online copy spelling. The histogram shows the number of participants, whose classification accuracies were located in each accuracy scale. The accuracies were separated into 7 scales. 'Symble|AV' stands for the symbol selection accuracies in condition **AV**, and 'Symbol|V*A' stands for the symbol selection accuracies in condition **V*A**. The red bar, which is noted as 'Visual|V*A', represents the visual selection accuracies in condition **V*A**. The green bar, denoted as 'Auditory|V*A', shows the auditory selection accuracies distribution. The blue-dominant pie chart shows the proportion of each accuracy scale for the symbol selection accuracies in condition AV. The purple-dominant pie chart shows the proportion in condition **V*A**.

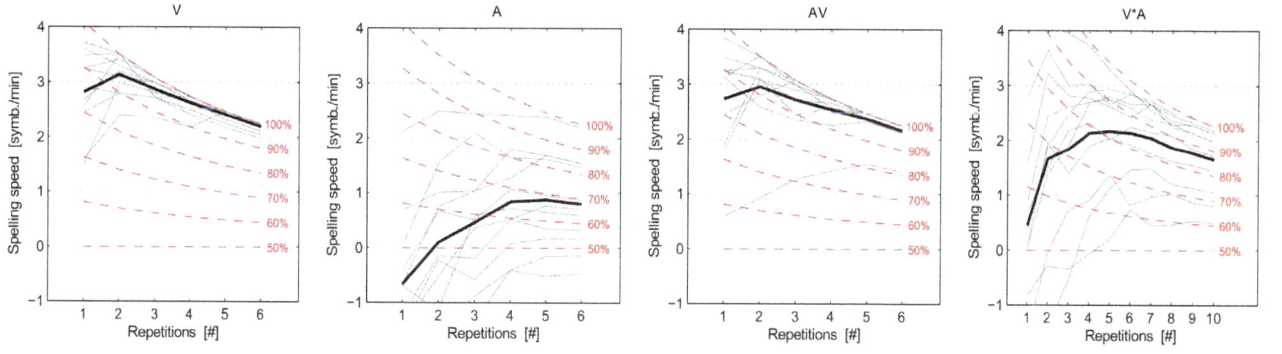

Figure 11. Spelling speed for each of the 4 conditions plotted against the number of repetitions. Thin gray lines depict results for single participants and the solid black line depicts the mean. Red dashed lines represent the spelling speed for fixed levels of symbol selection accuracy. Spelling accuracy for the empirical data (solid black line) can be deduced by comparing the black solid line to the red dashed lines. The accuracy is based on the calibration data for each condition.

Discussion

To answer the questions mentioned in section 1, two ways of combining visual and auditory stimuli were investigated: the first one employed simultaneous visual and auditory stimuli which represent the same information (called Combined-Speller, denoted as AV). The second one used two independent streams of visual and auditory stimuli which allow integrating two selection periods into a single one (called Parallel-Speller, denoted as V*A). There were two central goals in this study: first, to evaluate the advantages and disadvantages of the Combined-Speller and to compare it with the uni-modal paradigms (comparing workload, ERP response and discrimination information); second, to demonstrate the feasibility and usability of the Parallel-Speller (discussing the ERP response, spelling speed and so on), in which two independent decisions are made parallel.

Comparing the Combined-Speller with uni-modal paradigms

Workload. In our study, workload was used as a measure of usability of a system. Mental demand is the major factor for the weighted overall workload. Thus it is important to reduce the mental workload when operating a BCI system. It was reported in [36] that the workload for an auditory speller was significant higher than that for a (gaze-dependent) visual speller. Similar result but not significant difference was obtained here for an auditory compared with a gaze-independent visual paradigm. In particular, participants mentioned the difficulty of ignoring the non-targets, which had the same syllables or came from the same speakers as the target stimuli. However, when being asked after the whole experiment, some participants felt it was easier to attend uni-modal auditory speller compared with uni-modal visual speller, especially after having to focus on the center of the screen for such long time. The workload for the Combined-Speller (condition AV) was insignificantly lower than that for the mono-visual and mono-auditory paradigms. However, Participants (except one) mentioned that they were more relaxed during the Combined-Speller without always intensively focusing to either the visual stimuli or the auditory stimuli. Some participants regarded the target auditory stimuli as cues for the coming visual target, while others regarded the visual stimuli as cues instead. Thus, one can get to the conclusion that with an increasing runtime of the experiment, the Combined-Speller is the best choice with respect to workload, not only because the low workload it needs during spelling, but also the changing of modality to release the mental workload.

The ERP and class-discrimination information. Belitski et al. [30] reported that multi-modal (audio+visual) stimulation increased the average strength of the stimulus response in matrix speller style BCIs, when compared to either visual or auditory stimulation in isolation. Thurling et al. [31], however, reported an enhanced N1 and reduced P300 in bimodal visual-tactile paradigm.

Detailed results were derived in our study. From Figure 4, we could find that the peak of the visual N1 component of Combined-Speller is shifted to the left hemisphere. This might be due to the evoked responses of the auditory stimulation. The discriminability of the N2 component is reduced compared to the uni-modal visual speller, with a possible explanation that the positive response caused by the auditory stimuli affected the negative response for visual stimuli at the same time. Focusing on the following positive components, we find that the P3 component in the Combined-Speller had a shorter latency than in the mono-visual paradigm. While the P3 component in the unimodal visual speller featured a second component with more frontal focus, this sub-component was absent in the bimodal condition. However, the exact mechanism of the response in the Combined-Speller remains to be investigated in further studies.

From the statistical analysis of the ERPs (Figure 5) for 3 channels, we could find that the early ERP components show significant improvements (i.e. increased discriminability) in the Combined-Speller compared to the uni-modal visual and auditory spellers. The time intervals marked in light blue and pink show the significant difference amongst the three conditions. Thus, the bimodal stimulation in condition **AV** mainly impacts the early ERP components such as P1 and N1. No obvious significant difference were found during P300 component from 250 – 450 ms between conditions **V** and **AV**. However, both conditions yield to significantly higher P300 amplitude than condition A. Since channel PO7 reflects mostly on the visual processing, conditions **V** and **AV** don't show significant differences at that channel.

The spatial information of the discriminant information shown in Figure 9 reveals two important findings: the visual response area was affected by the auditory stimuli, with the central higher classification area shifting left as the auditory stimuli; the occipital electrodes featured less classification accuracies in Combined-Speller than that in the uni-modal visual speller. As possible reason, it can be speculated that less attention was allocated to the visual stimuli due to the concurrent auditory stimulation.

Thus, visual stimuli with concurrent auditory stimuli have significant difference between single modal visual and auditory stimuli. ERP difference was mostly on early exogenous components during 0 – 200 ms after stimuli onset and in frontal and central electrodes.

Parallel-Speller

In previous studies [21,30,31], multi-modal spelling paradigms all used visual and auditory stimuli to convey the same information. Our study used for the first time visual and auditory stimuli to convey different information in parallel. The workload of the parallel speller is considerably higher than for the other three spellers.

Figure 6 provides an overview over the class-discriminative information for the Parallel-Speller. The negative and positive components occurred at specific area were clearly found for visual and auditory stimuli respectively in Parallel-Speller. It shows that the visual and auditory stimuli could work independently, though having a higher workload used (according to Figure 3).

Besides, the temporal and spatial distribution of single trial classification accuracy also showed a possible classifier for visual and auditory stimuli respectively, similar though lower accuracies and tightened response area as uni-modal visual and auditory stimuli.

Performances of Combined-Speller and Parallel-Speller

Riccio et al. [17] provides a comparison of most BCI spellers with visual and (or) auditory stimuli. The comparison was discussed and depicted in a table (Table 1 in [17]) through the accuracy, bits per symbol, symbols per minute and bits per minute of the BCIs. Most spellers using auditory or visual + auditory stimuli have accuracies less than 70% and ITR less than 1.9 bits per minute if the total number of selections is more than twenty. Concerning the visual stimuli, only one (out of thirteen) speller has an ITR up to 10 bits per minute. We describe the Combined-Speller and the Parallel-Speller. Compared to the gaze-independent spellers reviewed by Riccio et al. [17], our paradigms featured competitive selection accuracies (94.9% for Combined-Speller and 85.9% for Parallel-Speller) and overall BCI performances (ITR of 10.01 and 8.85 bits per minute respectively).

The spelling speed (symbols per minute), which is one of the evaluation of the feasibility of spelling system, shows that for the Parallel-Speller most participants could spell 2 symbols per minute when 5 repetitions were used. Two participants could even spell about 3.5 symbols per minute when 2 repetitions were used, which is comparable even better than other paradigms. All of the above results prove the feasibility and usability of the Parallel-Speller.

Furthermore, slower spelling speeds have been obtained with the parallel speller. Apart from the slower spelling speed, several participants indicated a preference for the Parallel-Speller, due to the fact that there is only one period to select a symbol. Several measures to be taken in future developments can be expected to give improvement in this respect: (a) Due to the more difficult task, some training might be required. (b) Given the difference in detectability in the sensory domains, an uneven distribution of the auditory and visual stimuli might be beneficial. For example, if symbols are distributed in eight groups of four each, double the number of repetitions for auditory stimuli can be collected. (c) The current study used a considerable 'overhead' for the selection procedure in the Parallel-Speller. The 'overhead' contains the countdown part (hint for the target stimuli or a blank period for remember the targets, and the pre-flashing of the last digits), the classification time (to compute the result selections) and feedback (to show the selected group or symbols on the screen), more information was described in section 2.3. In this study, the stimulation time for each symbol in Parallel-Speller was about 18 s, while the 'overhead' (the countdown, classification and feedback) occupied about 10 s. For Combined-Speller, the stimulation time for each symbol was 2*7.2 s, while the 'overhead' was about 2*6.1 s. We assume that after practicing with the Parallel-Speller, the assistant time could reduce to 6.1 s as in Combined-Speller. (d) An optimal stopping method (Schreuder et al, 2013) could be employed to enhance the performance for the Parallel-Speller.

The Parallel-Speller is a novel approach for an ERP speller, which provides new insight into multisensory processing. Moreover, it represents a way to practice these two human sensory channels.

Conclusions

In a multisensory world, it might be advisable to also use multisensory stimulation for BCI applications. We approached this topic by comparing unimodal stimuli (from either visual or auditory domain), with multisensory stimuli from both domains. We studies two kinds of multisensory integration in an ERP-based BCI speller: the Combined-Speller and the Parallel-Speller.

For the Combined-Speller, most participants pointed out the positive aspect that it is not necessary to continuously locate attention to a fixed modality. The ERP response as well as the distribution of discriminative information was observed to be different for combined-speller compared to unimodal stimuli. It remains an area of future research to exploit such differences. Comparing the Combined-Speller to uni-modal paradigms we found shorter latencies, lower amplitudes, as well as a shift of the temporal and spatial distribution of discriminative information. As it was already suggested in this study, the Combined-Speller is a good choice for BCI speller with a low workload.

Moreover, a novel multimodal stimulus paradigm, called 'Parallel-Speller', was introduced. The Parallel-Speller combines two independent streams of stimuli, enabling a 1-out-of-36 decision with a single step. However, the workload is increased compared to all other conditions. The results for its classification and brain response showed that it is possible to apply such a truly multimodal paradigm. We hope that the new way of combining sensory modalities could stimulate further discussions and novel applications.

Author Contributions

Conceived and designed the experiments: XWA JH BB DM. Performed the experiments: XWA JH. Analyzed the data: XWA JH. Contributed reagents/materials/analysis tools: BB. Wrote the paper: XWA JH BB DM.

References

1. Wolpaw JR, Wolpaw EW (2012) Brain-Computer Interfaces: Principles and Practice. Oxford University Press.
2. Dornhege G (2007) Toward Brain-Computer Interfacing. MIT Press.
3. Wolpaw JR, McFarland DJ (2004) Control of a two-dimensional movement signal by a noninvasive brain-computer interface in humans. Proc Natl Acad Sci USA 101: 17849–54.
4. Blankertz B, Dornhege G, Krauledat M, Müller KR, Curio G (2007) The non-invasive Berlin brain-computer interface: fast acquisition of effective performance in untrained subjects. Neuroimage 37: 539–50.
5. Mak JN, Wolpaw JR (2009) Clinical applications of brain-computer interface: current state and future prospects. IEEE Rev Biomed Eng 2: 187–99.

6. Farwell LA, Donchin E (1988) Talking off the top of your head: toward a mental prosthesis utilizing event-related brain potentials. Electroencephalogr Clin Neurophysiol 70: 510–23.
7. Zhang D, Song H, Xu H, Wu W, Gao S, et al. (2012) An N200 speller integration the spatial profile for the detection of the non-control state. J.Neural Eng 9: 026016.
8. Bin G, Gao X, Wang Y, Li Y, Hong B, et al. (2011) A high-speed BCI based on code modulation VEP. J Neural Eng 8: 025015.
9. Sellers EW, Vauqhan TM, Wolpaw JR (2010) A brain-computer interface for long-term independent home use. Amyotroph Lateral Scler 11 (5): 449–55.
10. Brunner P, Joshi S, Briskin S, Wolpaw JR, Bischof H, et al. (2010) Does the 'P300' speller depend on eye gaze?. J Neural Eng7: 056013.
11. Treder MS, Blankertz B (2010) (C)overt attention and visual speller design in an ERP-based brain-computer interface. Behavioral and Brain Function 6: 28.
12. Treder MS, Schmidt NM, Blankertz B (2011) Gaze-independent brain–computer interfaces based on covert attention and feature attention. J Neural Eng 8: 066003.
13. Schaeff S, Treder MS, Venthur B, Blankertz B (2012) Exploring motion VEPs for gaze-independent communication. J Neural Eng 9: 045006.
14. Liu Y, Zhou Z, Hu D (2011) Gaze-independent brain-computer speller with covert visual search tasks. Clin Neurophysiol 122(6): 1127–36.
15. Aloise F, Aricò P, Schettini F, Riccio A, Salinari S, et al. (2012) A covert attention P300-based brain-computer interface: Geospell. Ergonomics 55(5): 538–551.
16. Acqualaqna L, Blankertz B (2013) Gaze-independent BCI-spelling using rapid serial visual presentation (RSVP). Clin Neurophysiol 124(5): 901–8.
17. Riccio A, Mattia D, Simione L, Olivetti M, Cincotti F (2012) Eye-gaze independent EEG-based brain-computer interfaces for communication. J Neural Eng 9(4): 045001.
18. Brouwer A-M, van Erp JBF, Aloise F, Cincotti F (2010) Tactile, Visual, and Bimodal P300s: Could Bimodal P300s Boost BCI Performance? SRX Neuroscience 2010: 1–9.
19. Van der Waal M, Severens M, Geuze J, Desain P (2012) Introducing the tactile speller: an ERP-based brain–computer interface for communication. Journal of Neural Engineering 9: 045002.
20. Kübler A, Furdea A, Halder S, Hammer EM, Nijboer F, et al. (2009) A brain-computer interface controlled auditory event-related potential (p300) spelling system for locked-in patients. Annals of the New York Academy of Sciences 1157: 90–100.
21. Klobassa DS, Vaughan TM, Brunner P, Schwartz NE, Wolpaw JR, et al. (2009) Toward a high-through put auditory P300-based brain-computer interface. Clin Neurophysiol 120(7): 1252–61.
22. Halder S, Hammer EM, Kleih SC, Bogdan M, Rosenstiel W, et al. (2013) Prediction of auditory and visual p300 brain-computer interface aptitude. PloS one 8: e53513.
23. Schreuder M, Blankertz B, Tangermann M (2010) A New Auditory Multi-Class Brain-Computer Interface Paradigm: Spatial Hearing as an Informative Cue. PloS One 5: e9813.
24. Schreuder M, Rost T, Tangermann M (2011) Listen, you are writing! Speeding up online spelling with a dynamic auditory BCI. Front Neuroscience 5: 112.
25. Höhne J, Schreuder M, Blankertz B, Tangermann M (2011) A Novel 9-Class Auditory ERP Paradigm Driving a Predictive Text Entry System. Front Neurosci 5: 99.
26. Höhne J, Tangermann M (2014) Towards user-friendly spelling with an auditory brain-computer interface: the CharStreamer paradigm. PloS One 9: e98322.
27. Höhne J, Krenzlin K, Dähne S, Tangermann M (2012) Natural stimuli improve auditory BCIs with respect to ergonomics and performance. J Neural Eng 9: 045003.
28. Teder-Sälejärvi WA, Di Russo F, McDonald JJ, Hillyard SA (2005) Effects of spatial congruity on audio-visual multimodal integration. Journal of Cognitive Neuroscience 17: 1396–409. doi:10.1162/0898929054985383.
29. Campanella S, Bruyer R, Froidbise S, Rossignol M, Joassin F, et al. (2010) Is two better than one? A cross-modal oddball paradigm reveals greater sensitivity of the P300 to emotional face-voice associations. Clincal Neurophysiology 121: 1855–1862.
30. Belitski A, Farquhar J, Desain P (2011) P300 audio-visual speller. J Neural Eng 8: 025022.
31. Thurling ME, Brouwer Am, Van Erp JBF, Blankertz B, Werkhoven PJ (2012) Does bimodal stimulus presentation increase ERP components usable in BCIs? J Neural Eng 9: 045005.
32. Talsma D, Senkowski D, Soto-Faraco S, Woldorff MG (2010) The multifaceted interplay between attention and multisensory integration. Trends Cogn Sci 14: 400–10.
33. Senkowski D, Talsma D, Grigutsch M (2007) Good times for multisensory integration: effects of the precision of temporal synchrony as revealed by gamma-band oscillations. Neuropsychologia 45: 561–571.
34. Blankertz B, Lemm S, Treder MS, Haufe S, Müller KR (2011) Single-trial analysis and classification of ERP components-a tutorial. Neuroimage 56: 814–825.
35. Pasqualotto E, Simonetta A, Gnisci V, Federici S, Olivetti M (2011) BelardinelliToward a usability evaluation of BCIs. Int J Bioelectromagn 13: 121–22.
36. Riccio A, Leotta F, Bianchi L, Aloise F, Zickler C, et al. (2011) Workload measurement in a communication application operated through a P300-based brain-computer interface. J Neural Eng 8: 025028.
37. Käthner I, Ruf CA, Pasqualotto E, Braun C, Birbaumer N, et al. (2013) A po auditory P300 brain-computer interface with directional cues. Clin Neurophyisol 124: 327–38.
38. Schreuder M, Höhne J, Blankertz B, Haufe S, Dickhaus T, et al. (2013) Optimizing event-related potentail based brain-computer interface: a systematic evaluation of dynamic stopping methods. J Neural Eng 10: 036025.

19

Systemic Adverse Events after Intravitreal Bevacizumab versus Ranibizumab for Age-Related Macular Degeneration

Wei Wang, Xiulan Zhang*

Zhongshan Ophthalmic Center, State Key Laboratory of Ophthalmology, Sun Yat-Sen University, Guangzhou, People's Republic of China

Abstract

Objective: To assess whether the incidence of systemic adverse events differs between those who used bevacizumab and those who used ranibizumab in the treatment of age-related macular degeneration (AMD).

Methods: A systematic literature search was conducted to identify randomised controlled trials (RCTs) comparing the use of intravitreal bevacizumab with the use of ranibizumab in AMD patients. Results were expressed as risk ratios (RRs) with accompanying 95% confidence intervals (CIs). The data were pooled using the fixed-effect or random-effect model according to the heterogeneity present.

Results: Four RCTs were included in the final meta-analysis. Overall, the quality of the evidence was high. There were 2,613 treated patients: 1,291 treated with bevacizumab and 1,322 treated with ranibicizumab. No significant differences between bevacizumab use and ranizumab use were found in terms of the incidence of death from all causes, arteriothrombotic events, stroke, nonfatal myocardial infarction, vascular death, venous thrombotic events, and hypertension, with the pooled RRs being 1.11 (0.77, 1.61), 1.03 (0.69,1.55), 0.84 (0.39,1.80), 0.97 (0.48, 1.96), 1.24 (0.63, 2.44), 2.38 (0.94, 6.04), and 1.02 (0.29, 3.62), respectively.

Conclusions: The meta-analysis shows that both treatments are comparably safe. However, the findings from our study must be confirmed in future research via well-designed cohort or intervention studies because of the limited number of studies.

Editor: Andreas Wedrich, Medical University Graz, Austria

Funding: This research was supported by the National Natural Science Foundation of China (81371008). No additional external funding was received. The funders had no role in study design, data collection and analysis, decision to publish, or preparation of the manuscript.

Competing Interests: The authors have declared that no competing interests exist.

* Email: zhangxl2@mail.sysu.edu.cn

Introduction

Age-related macular degeneration (AMD) is the most common cause of blindness in individuals over 50 years of age [1–3]. Although an estimated 80% of patients with AMD have the non-neovascular (dry) form, the neovascular (wet) form is responsible for almost 90% of severe visual losses resulting from AMD [4–6]. Vascular endothelial growth factor-A (VEGF-A) has been proven to play a major role in the pathogenesis of wet AMD [7,8]. Since the mid-2000s, antivascular endothelial growth factor (anti-VEGF) therapy has become the mainstay of treatment for wet AMD [9].

Ranibizumab (Lucentis, Genentech, Inc., South San Francisco, CA, USA) is a recombinant humanized immunoglobulin G1κ isotype monoclonal antibody fragment directed toward all isoforms of VEGF-A [7]. It has been approved for the treatment of wet AMD by the food and drug administration (FDA) in the US (2006), Europe (2007), Japan (2009), and many other countries. However, the cost of ranibizumab is immense: monthly injections at a dose of 0.5 mg result in an annual cost greater than US $23,000 per patient [10].

Similar to ranibizumab, bevacizumab (Avastin, Genentech, Inc., South San Francisco, CA, USA) is a recombinant humanized full-length antibody that can inhibit all isoforms of VEGF-A [11]. In 2004, it was approved for the treatment of metastatic cancer of the colon or rectum, but it has not gained FDA approval for intravitreal use. Therefore, it can be utilized only in an off-label setting. For the past several years, it has been used off-label to treat wet AMD with very encouraging results. Bevacizumab has attracted more and more interest because of its low cost, which is especially important considering the number of injections that are necessary at 4- to 6-week intervals. A report suggested that the US medicare system could save more than US$1 billion within 2 years if bevacizumab replaced ranibizumab [7,10].

Although anti-VEGF agents are injected in small quantities into the eye, concerns about systemic safety have been raised, especially for the off-label use of bevacizumab. Research has shown that the systemic administration of bevacizumab, along with chemotherapeutic agents, can increase the risk of thromboembolic events two-fold over chemotherapy alone [12]. Many recently published randomized clinical trials (RCTs) have evaluated intravitreal bevacizumab and ranibizumab for the treatment of wet AMD. The results of the comparison of the AMD Treatments Trial (CATT) and the Age-related Choroidal Neovascularization Trial (IVAN) demonstrated that bevacizumab was not inferior to ranibizumab in the treatment of wet AMD [13,14]. However, these studies were not sufficiently powerful to detect drug-specific differences in the rates of systemic adverse events. Hence, the crucial question of whether adverse effects differ between off-label bevacizumab and licensed ranibizumab has not yet been answered [15].

To determine whether the intravitreal injection of bevacizumab creates a higher risk of systemic adverse events than ranibizumab injection does, we undertook a systematic review and meta-analysis of all relevant head-to-head RCTs.

Methods

This study was reported in accordance with the Preferred Reporting Items for Systematic Reviews and Meta-Analyses (PRISMA) statement (Checklist S1) [16]. All stages of study selection, data extraction, and quality assessment were performed independently by two reviewers (W.W. and X.Z.). Any disagreement was resolved via discussion and consensus.

1. Literature Search

Studies were identified through a systematic search of Pubmed, Embase, the Chinese Biomedicine Database, and the Cochrane library from inception up to December 2013. The initial search terms were (Ranibizumab or Lucentis) AND (Bevacizumab or Avastin) AND ("Macular degeneration" or AMD), which were filtered by "Humans" and "Randomized Controlled Trial." In addition, the reference lists of identified studies were manually checked to include other potentially eligible trials. This process was performed iteratively until no additional articles could be identified.

2. Study Selection

Studies were considered acceptable for inclusion in the meta-analysis if they met the following criteria: (1) the study design included randomized clinical trials; (2) the population was patients with wet AMD; (3) the interventions were intravitreal bevacizumab and intravitreal ranibizumab, which were directly compared in head-to-head design; (4) the incidence of systemic adverse events was reported; (5) there was a follow-up time of at least 1 year; and (6) there were at least ten patients in each arm. If there were multiple reports for a particular study, the most recent publication was included. Trials were excluded if they (1) were abstracts, letters, or meeting proceedings; (2) had repeated data or did not report outcomes of interest; or (3) included patients with other indications than wet AMD, patients previously treated with VEGF inhibitors, or patients receiving systemic anti-VEGF therapy.

3. Data Extraction

The following information was extracted from each study: first author; year of publication; study design; inclusion and exclusion criteria; number of patients in each group; characteristics of the study population; adverse events; the period, and number of injections preceding an adverse event. A Thromboembolic Event (TEE) was defined as any arteriothrombotic or venous thrombotic event [17].

4. Quality Assessment

The methodological quality of each trial was evaluated using the Jadad scale [18]. The scale consists of three items describing randomization (0–2 points), blinding (0–2 points), and dropouts and withdrawals (0–1 points) in the reporting of a randomized controlled trial. A score of 1 is given for each of the points described. A further point is awarded when the method of randomization and/or blinding is given and is appropriate, whereas when it is inappropriate, a point is deducted. The quality scale ranges from 0 to 5 points. Higher scores indicate better reporting. The studies are said to be of low quality if the Jadad score is ≤ 2 and of high quality if the score is ≥ 3.

5. Statistical Analysis

All outcomes were expressed as risk ratios (RRs) with accompanying 95% confidence intervals (CIs). Outcome measure was assessed on an intent-to-treat (ITT) basis, the ITT population being comprised of all randomized patients who received the study medication and provided a valid baseline measurement. The cochrane Q test was used to detect the heterogeneity of the effects. Significant heterogeneity was defined as a P value of <0.05. A fixed-effects model or random-effects model was used, depending on the presence or absence of heterogeneity. The I^2 value was used to demonstrate the percentage of the variability attributable to heterogeneity rather than to sampling error. Studies with an I^2 statistic of $<25\%$ are considered to have no heterogeneity, those with an I^2 statistic of 25% to 50% are considered to have low heterogeneity, those with an I^2 statistic of 50% to 75% are considered to have moderate heterogeneity, and those with an I^2 statistic of $>75\%$ are considered to have high heterogeneity [19]. Sensitivity analyses were performed by investigating the influence of a single study on the overall pooled estimate via omitting one study at a time. Potential publication bias was assessed by using Begg's and Egger's tests [20,21]. A P value <0.05 was judged to be statistically significant, except when otherwise specified. All statistical analyses were performed using Stata version 12.0 (Stata Corp, College Station, TX).

Results

1. Literature Search

The selection process and reasons for exclusion are detailed in Figure 1. The initial search identified 125 potentially relevant articles, of which 71 were excluded based on the titles and abstracts. The remaining 54 were retrieved for a full-text review, and 40 of them were excluded because 38 included unqualified patients, two involved unqualified interventions, eight contained duplicated data [22–29], one did not report outcomes of interest [30], and one contained only one patients (<10) in the ranibizumab arm [31]. Thus, four RCTs [13,14,32,33] were included in the final meta-analysis.

2. Study Characteristics and Quality

The main characteristics of the four RCTs included in the meta-analysis are presented in Table 1, and the outcome data of each included trial are described in Table 2. These studies were published between 2012 and 2013. The sizes of the RCTs ranged from 317 to 1,185 patients (a total of 2,613; 1,291 with bevacizumab and 1,322 with ranibicizumab). Of the four trials, one was done in the USA [14], one in the UK [13], one in France [33], and one in Australia [32]. The trials included in this

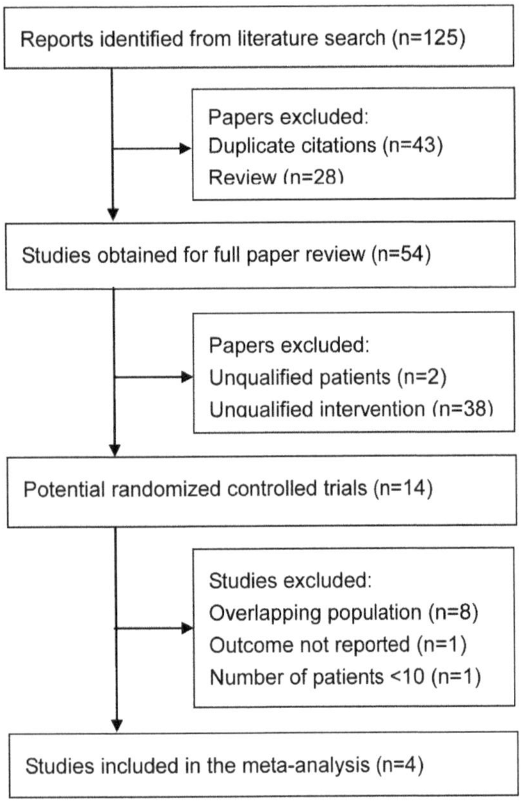

Figure 1. Flowchart of studies included in meta-analysis. RCT, randomized controlled trial.

meta-analysis appeared to have been reasonably designed and conducted. All studies had a statement regarding randomization and double-blindness. Four trials described the methods of randomization. Four trials reported withdrawals and dropouts. All trials described the main outcome, and no missing data seemed to influence the results. The Jadad score of the studies included was 5.

3. Risk of Systemic Adverse Events

The risk estimates for systemic adverse events associated with intravitreal bevacizumab, as compared with ranibizumab, were summarized in Table 3. No significant differences between bevacizumab and ranizumab were found in terms of the incidence of death from all causes, arteriothrombotic events, stroke, nonfatal myocardial infarction, vascular death, venous thrombotic events, and hypertension, with the pooled RRs being 1.11 (0.77, 1.61), 1.03 (0.69,1.55), 0.84 (0.39,1.80), 0.97 (0.48, 1.96), 1.24 (0.63, 2.44), 2.38 (0.94, 6.04), and 1.02 (0.29, 3.62), respectively. When any arteriothrombotic or venous thrombotic events, such as TEE, were combined, no significant difference was detected (RR, 1.22; 95% CI: 0.85 to 1.75; $P=0.292$) (Figure 2). Furthermore, when adverse events were divided by MedDRA system organ class, there was also no significant difference between bevacizumab and ranibizumab injections. The tests for heterogeneity were all non-significant (all $P>0.1$). We tested the robustness of our analyses by performing sensitivity analyses excluding the CATT study (largest trial). Excluding this study did not change our final results.

Table 1. Baseline characteristics of the head-to-head studies comparing ranibizumab with bevacizumab.

Study	Location	Center	Blind	Duration	Intervention	No. of eyes	Age (years)	Male (%)	Visual acuity (letters)	Foveal thickness (mm)
CATT	USA	44	double	2 years	Ranibizumab Monthly	301	79.2±7.4	39.2%	60.1±14.3	458±184
					Bevacizumab Monthly	286	80.1±7.3	37.1%	60.2±13.1	463±196
					Ranibizumab as Needed	298	78.4±7.8	37.9%	61.5±13.2	458±193
					Bevacizumab as Needed	300	79.3±7.6	38.7%	60.4±13.4	461±175
IVAN	UK	23	double	2 years	Ranibizumab	314	77.8±7.6	41%	67·8±17·0	471.6±192.5
					Bevacizumab	296	77.7±7.3	39%	66·1±18·4	465.6±183.1
GEFAL	France	38	double	1 year	Ranibizumab	129	78.68±7.27	31.21%	55.78±13.99	354.75±109.90
					Bevacizumab	119	79.62±6.90	35.82%	54.62±14.07	359.21±120.72
MANTA	Austria	10	double	1 year	Ranibizumab	163	77.6±8.1	36.20%	56.4±13.5	365.0±8.1
					Bevacizumab	154	76.7±7.8	36.36%	57.0±13.0	374.6±8.4

CATT = The Comparison of Age-related macular degeneration Treatments Trials; IVAN = The Alternative treatments to Inhibit VEGF in Age-related choroidal Neovascularization study; MANTA = The Multicenter Anti-VEGF Trial; GEFAL = The Groupe d'Etude Français Avastin versus Lucentis dans la DMLA néovasculaire (The French Study Group Avastin versus Lucentis for neovascular AMD).

Table 2. Outcome data of randomized controlled trials included in the meta-analysis.

Adverse events	CAAT		IVAN		GEFAL		MANTA	
	Ranibizumab (N = 599)	Bevacizumab (N = 586)	Ranibizumab (N = 314)	Bevacizumab (N = 296)	Ranibizumab (N = 246)	Bevacizumab (N = 255)	Ranibizumab (N = 163)	Bevacizumab (N = 154)
Systemic adverse event								
Death-all causes	32	36	15	15	3	2	2	3
Arteriothrombotic events	28[*]	29	13	10	1	1	3	5
Stroke	8	8	6	3	0	0	1	1
Nonfatal myocardial infarction	9	7	4	4	1	1	2	3
Vascular death	12	14	3	4	0	0	0	0
Venous thrombotic events	3	10	3	4	0	1	0	0
Hypertension	3	4	0	0	2	1	0	0
MedDRA system organ class								
Cardiac disorders	47	62	20	19	5	2	1	1
Infections	41	54	9	12	2	4	3	3
Nervous system disorders	34	36	9	8	0	3	1	2
Injury and procedural complications	23	35	12	10	2	4	3	2
Neoplasms benign and malignant	27	22	11	14	1	1	2	1
Surgical and medical procedures	0	0	16	14	0	5	0	1
Gastrointestinal disorders	11	28	3	9	5	3	0	0
Any other system organ class	81	104	25	27	11	10	2	3

Table 3. Risk ratio of systemic adverse events associated with intravitreal bevacizumab compared with ranibizumab.

Avastin vs Lucentis	Study(n)	RR (95%CI)			Heterogeneity		Overall Effect	
		Estimate	Lower	Up	P	I^2(%)	Z	P
Death-all causes	4	1.11	0.77	1.61	0.907	0.00%	0.56	0.572
Arteriothrombotic events	4	1.03	0.69	1.55	0.828	0.00%	0.15	0.879
Stroke	3	0.84	0.39	1.80	0.737	0.00%	0.46	0.649
Nonfatal myocardial infarction	4	0.97	0.48	1.96	0.925	0.00%	0.09	0.928
Vascular death	2	1.24	0.63	2.44	0.842	0.00%	0.61	0.541
Venous thrombotic events	3	2.38	0.94	6.04	0.676	0.00%	1.83	0.067
Hypertension	2	1.02	0.29	3.62	0.471	0.00%	0.03	0.977
MedDRA system organ class								
Cardiac disorders	4	1.20	0.88	1.62	0.460	0.00%	1.16	0.245
Infections	4	1.36	0.97	1.91	0.965	0.00%	1.79	0.074
Nervous system disorders	4	1.11	0.75	1.66	0.606	0.00%	0.52	0.602
Injury and procedural complications	4	1.31	0.87	1.98	0.578	0.00%	1.30	0.194
Neoplasms benign and malignant	4	0.96	0.62	1.48	0.743	0.00%	0.18	0.854
Surgical and medical procedures	3	1.75	0.43	7.16	0.222	33.60%	0.78	0.434
Gastrointestinal disorders	3	1.90	0.78	4.62	0.141	49.00%	1.41	0.158
Any other system organ class	4	1.25	0.99	1.56	0.803	0.00%	1.90	0.058

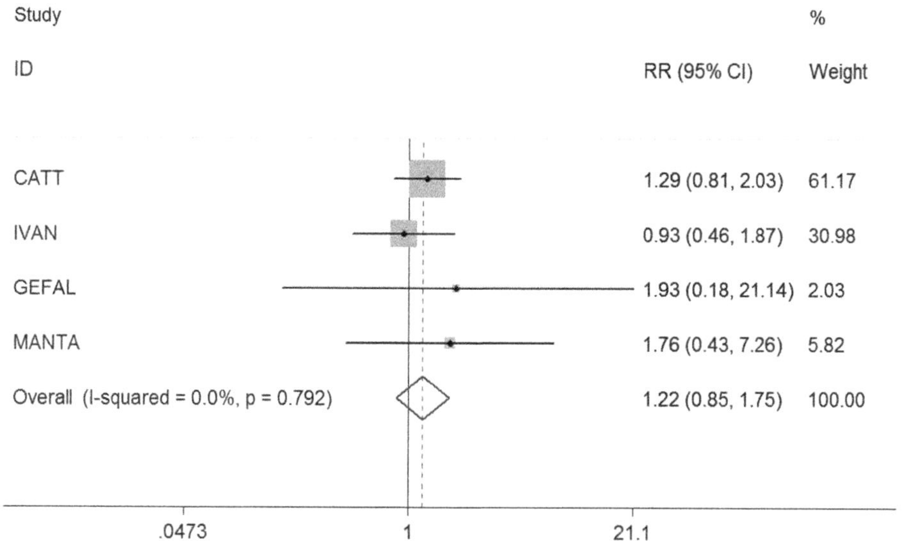

Figure 2. Risk ratio of thromboembolic events associated with intravitreal bevacizumab compared with ranibizumab. Each study is shown by the point estimate of relative risk "risk ratio" (RR) - the size of the square is proportional to the weight of the study - and 95%confidence interval for the RR (lines extending from the squares); the pooled RR and 95%confidence interval are shown as a diamond.

4. Publication Bias

Due to the limited number (<10) of studies included in each analysis, publication bias was not assessed.

Discussion

The development of VEGF inhibitors has revolutionized the treatment of AMD. Bevacizumab and ranibizumab are the two most common VEGF inhibitors in ophthalmic practice [34]. Although anti-VEGF agents are injected into the eye in small quantities, concerns about systemic safety have been raised [35]. Until relatively recently, high-quality data comparing the efficacy and safety of ranibizumab and bevacizumab in AMD were lacking. Because many adverse events are relatively uncommon, clinical trials often lack the power to detect small but clinically important risk differences. Hence, meta-analyses pooling data from multiple studies provide important insights [15,36]. The main aim of this study is to provide an evidence-based analysis of the safety profile for bevacizumab versus that of intravitreal ranibizumab injections in patients with AMD. In the present meta-analysis, we have reviewed the literature regarding the safety of intravitreal bevacizumab as compared with that of ranibizumab. The pooled results suggest that the incidence of specific systemic complications did not differ significant between bevacizumab and ranibizumab. Also, no heterogeneity was observed across the studies.

Several high-quality non-randomized studies [37–40] focusing on adverse effects for bevacizumab versus ranibizumab are summarized in Table 4. All of them reported that the rates of specific systemic adverse events, such as all-cause mortality, stroke, acute myocardial infarction, and venous thromboembolism during the bevacizumab and ranibizumab periods were not different. However, the limitation of these studies was that a non-randomized study design was used (case control or cohort study). The principal finding of our meta-analysis is consistent with the aforementioned studies on the topic.

Thus far, ranibizumab and bevacizumab have been evaluated in several systematic reviews [11,17,34,41]. However, the published reviews focused on the beneficial effects and clinical effectiveness of VEGF inhibitors, without adequately addressing their adverse effects. Furthermore, they are mainly based on indirect comparative studies; this may lower the evidence level. In Schmucker and colleagues' report [41], only one multiple-center, head-to-head RCT (CATT) was included; it had relatively modest sample sizes. In another meta-analysis by Chakravarthy et al. [13], no difference in the frequency of death, arterial thrombotic events, or hospital admission for heart failure was recorded between the drugs. Their study is limited by the fact that only 1-year CATT data were included. In our study, we incorporated the 2-year CATT data and two other well-designed RCTs. We found a similar risk of specific adverse events between the bevacizumab and ranibizumab groups. From a theoretical viewpoint, the risk of the development of systemic adverse events may be higher with bevacizumab than with ranibizumab [10]. Bevacizumab is more likely to induce immunologic activation and will remain in systemic circulation than ranibizumab. Thus, bevacizumab administration may create a higher risk of systemic adverse events. These highlight the need for ongoing surveillance and large population-based studies to investigate these outcomes [15].

The results of this meta-analysis must be interpreted cautiously in light of the strengths and limitations of the included trials. A key strength of this study is the fact that all the studies included in this meta-analysis were published by established centers of excellence using a randomized controlled design and all of them were well-performed and of high quality. In addition, with the enlarged sample size, we have enhanced statistical power to provide more precise and reliable effect estimates. Despite our rigorous methodology, some limitations of the current study should not be ignored. First, we cannot fully exclude publication bias. The number of included studies is insufficient to carry out further statistical testing to detect publication bias through an asymmetry plot. In addition, we did not attempt to gain access to unpublished results. More RCTs are warranted to confirm or refute our finding in the future update meta-analysis. Second, all studies have come from western populations with predominately Caucasian participants. The relatively good distribution of the study population makes findings from this meta-analysis a fair representation of the general population. The safety of these drugs for other ethnicities,

Table 4. Summary of high-quality non-randomized studies comparing ranibizumab with bevacizumab.

Author, country	Design	Population	Method	Results
Campbell et al., 2012, Canada	Population based nested case-control study	Older adults with a history of physician diagnosed retinal disease identified between 1 April 2006 and 31 March 2011.	Cases were patients admitted to hospital for ischaemic stroke, acute myocardial infarction, venous thromboembolism, for congestive heart failure. Event-free controls were matched to cases on the basis of year of birth, sex, history of the outcome in the previous 5 years, and diabetes	Adjusted odds ratios for bevacizumab relative to ranibizumab were 1.03 (0.67 to 1.60) for ischaemic stroke, 1.23 (0.85 to 1.77) for acute myocardial infarction, 0.92 (0.51 to 1.69) for venous thromboembolism, and 1.35 (0.93 to 1.95) for congestive heart failure. Results showed these risks did not differ significantly between bevacizumab and ranibizumab injections.
Campbell et al., 2012, Canada	Population-based, time series analysis	All patients aged 66 years or older with physician-diagnosed retinal disease between 2002 and 2010 (N = 116 388).	Segmented regression analysis was used to evaluate changes in the rate of hospitalization for ischemic stroke associated with the introduction of bevacizumab and ranibizumab.	Bevacizumab trend change coefficient: -0.0026 stroke hospitalizations/1000 subjects/month (P = 0.20); Ranibizumab trend change coefficient: -0.0011 stroke hospitalizations/1000 subjects/ month (P = 0.78). Results showed that stroke rates in the bevacizumab and ranibizumab periods were not different.
French et al., 2011, USA	Cohort study	Beneficiaries of the Veterans Health Administration aged ≥55 years with AMD in fiscal years 2007-2009 were included.	Anti-vascular endothelial growth factor exposure was identified through pharmacy records. Cox proportional hazard model was adjusted for age, gender, number of injections, and ocular and medical comorbidities.	The adjusted HR for all-cause mortality were 0.94 (95%CI: 0.72 to 1.22) for bevacizumab and 0.85 (95%CI: 0.67 to1.08) for ranibizumab. Results showed lack an association between the use of either ranibizumab or bevacizumab and mortality.
Curtis et al., 2010, USA	Cohort study	Medicare beneficiaries 65 years or older with a claim for AMD in fiscal years 2005-2006 were included.	When the patients received a therapy different from the initial therapy, the data were censored. The associations between anti-VEGF therapies and the risks of all-cause mortality, incident myocardial infarction, bleeding, and incident stroke were calculated.	Adjusted HRs for ranibizumab relative to bevacizumab were 0.90 (0.79-1.02) for all-cause mortality, 0.84 (0.66-1.06) for myocardial infarction, 1.03 (0.93-1.15) for bleeding, 0.81 (0.68-0.98) for stroke. Results showed these risks did not differ significantly between bevacizumab and ranibizumab injections.

such as Asians, must be tested. Furthermore, patients enrolled in RCTs meet strict eligibility criteria, which may exclude many patients at a higher risk for systemic adverse events. These limitations likely resulted in an underestimation of the incidence of systemic adverse events. However, the determination of the risk of systemic adverse events associated with bevacizumab versus ranibizumab was not likely affected, because this underestimation should have had similar impacts on both arms. Finally, given that the treatment of wet AMD is not limited to 2 years, more data from studies of longer durations are needed to determine the relative safety of each anti-VEGF agent over the long term.

In conclusion, there is no difference between bevacizumab and ranibizumab in terms of the risk of specific systemic adverse events. However, the results should be interpreted cautiously because the relevant evidence remains limited, and the findings must be confirmed through future research involving well-designed cohort studies or RCTs.

Author Contributions

Conceived and designed the experiments: WW XZ. Performed the experiments: WW XZ. Analyzed the data: WW XZ. Contributed reagents/materials/analysis tools: WW XZ. Wrote the paper: WW XZ.

References

1. Owen CG, Jarrar Z, Wormald R, Cook DG, Fletcher AE, et al. (2012) The estimated prevalence and incidence of late stage age related macular degeneration in the UK. Br J Ophthalmol 96: 752–756.
2. Rudnicka AR, Jarrar Z, Wormald R, Cook DG, Fletcher A, et al. (2012) Age and gender variations in age-related macular degeneration prevalence in populations of European ancestry: a meta-analysis. Ophthalmology 119: 571–580.
3. Kawasaki R, Yasuda M, Song SJ, Chen SJ, Jonas JB, et al. (2010) The prevalence of age-related macular degeneration in Asians: a systematic review and meta-analysis. Ophthalmology 117: 921–927.
4. Schmier JK, Jones ML, Halpern MT (2006) The burden of age-related macular degeneration. Pharmacoeconomics 24: 319–334.
5. Brown MM, Brown GC, Sharma S, Stein JD, Roth Z, et al. (2006) The burden of age-related macular degeneration: a value-based analysis. Curr Opin Ophthalmol 17: 257–266.
6. Ferris FR, Wilkinson CP, Bird A, Chakravarthy U, Chew E, et al. (2013) Clinical classification of age-related macular degeneration. Ophthalmology 120: 844–851.
7. Frampton JE (2013) Ranibizumab: a review of its use in the treatment of neovascular age-related macular degeneration. Drugs Aging 30: 331–358.
8. Ambati J, Fowler BJ (2012) Mechanisms of age-related macular degeneration. Neuron 75: 26–39.
9. Lally DR, Gerstenblith AT, Regillo CD (2012) Preferred therapies for neovascular age-related macular degeneration. Curr Opin Ophthalmol 23: 182–188.
10. Campbell RJ, Bell CM, Campbell EL, Gill SS (2013) Systemic effects of intravitreal vascular endothelial growth factor inhibitors. Curr Opin Ophthalmol 24: 197–204.
11. Schmucker C, Ehlken C, Hansen LL, Antes G, Agostini HT, et al. (2010) Intravitreal bevacizumab (Avastin) vs. ranibizumab (Lucentis) for the treatment of age-related macular degeneration: a systematic review. Curr Opin Ophthalmol 21: 218–226.
12. Hurwitz HI, Tebbutt NC, Kabbinavar F, Giantonio BJ, Guan ZZ, et al. (2013) Efficacy and safety of bevacizumab in metastatic colorectal cancer: pooled analysis from seven randomized controlled trials. Oncologist 18: 1004–1012.
13. Chakravarthy U, Harding SP, Rogers CA, Downes SM, Lotery AJ, et al. (2013) Alternative treatments to inhibit VEGF in age-related choroidal neovascularisation: 2-year findings of the IVAN randomised controlled trial. Lancet 382: 1258–1267.

14. Martin DF, Maguire MG, Fine SL, Ying GS, Jaffe GJ, et al. (2012) Ranibizumab and bevacizumab for treatment of neovascular age-related macular degeneration: two-year results. Ophthalmology 119: 1388–1398.
15. Cheung CM, Wong TY (2013) Treatment of age-related macular degeneration. Lancet 382: 1230–1232.
16. Moher D, Liberati A, Tetzlaff J, Altman DG (2009) Preferred reporting items for systematic reviews and meta-analyses: the PRISMA statement. J Clin Epidemiol 62: 1006–1012.
17. Abouammoh MA (2013) Ranibizumab injection for diabetic macular edema: meta-analysis of systemic safety and systematic review. Can J Ophthalmol 48: 317–323.
18. Jadad AR, Moore RA, Carroll D, Jenkinson C, Reynolds DJ, et al. (1996) Assessing the quality of reports of randomized clinical trials: is blinding necessary? Control Clin Trials 17: 1–12.
19. Higgins JP, Thompson SG, Deeks JJ, Altman DG (2003) Measuring inconsistency in meta-analyses. BMJ 327: 557–560.
20. Egger M, Davey SG, Schneider M, Minder C (1997) Bias in meta-analysis detected by a simple, graphical test. BMJ 315: 629–634.
21. Begg CB, Mazumdar M (1994) Operating characteristics of a rank correlation test for publication bias. Biometrics 50: 1088–1101.
22. Ying GS, Huang J, Maguire MG, Jaffe GJ, Grunwald JE, et al. (2013) Baseline predictors for one-year visual outcomes with ranibizumab or bevacizumab for neovascular age-related macular degeneration. Ophthalmology 120: 122–129.
23. Jaffe GJ, Martin DF, Toth CA, Daniel E, Maguire MG, et al. (2013) Macular morphology and visual acuity in the comparison of age-related macular degeneration treatments trials. Ophthalmology 120: 1860–1870.
24. DeCroos FC, Toth CA, Stinnett SS, Heydary CS, Burns R, et al. (2012) Optical coherence tomography grading reproducibility during the Comparison of Age-related Macular Degeneration Treatments Trials. Ophthalmology 119: 2549–2557.
25. Chakravarthy U, Harding SP, Rogers CA, Downes SM, Lotery AJ, et al. (2012) Ranibizumab versus bevacizumab to treat neovascular age-related macular degeneration: one-year findings from the IVAN randomized trial. Ophthalmology 119: 1399–1411.
26. Grunwald JE, Daniel E, Ying GS, Pistilli M, Maguire MG, et al. (2012) Photographic assessment of baseline fundus morphologic features in the Comparison of Age-Related Macular Degeneration Treatments Trials. Ophthalmology 119: 1634–1641.
27. Martin DF, Maguire MG, Ying GS, Grunwald JE, Fine SL, et al. (2011) Ranibizumab and bevacizumab for neovascular age-related macular degeneration. N Engl J Med 364: 1897–1908.
28. Donahue SP, Recchia F, Sternberg PJ (2010) Bevacizumab vs ranibizumab for age-related macular degeneration: early results of a prospective double-masked, randomized clinical trial. Am J Ophthalmol 150: 287, 287.
29. Subramanian ML, Ness S, Abedi G, Ahmed E, Daly M, et al. (2009) Bevacizumab vs ranibizumab for age-related macular degeneration: early results of a prospective double-masked, randomized clinical trial. Am J Ophthalmol 148: 875–882.
30. Biswas P, Sengupta S, Choudhary R, Home S, Paul A, et al. (2011) Comparative role of intravitreal ranibizumab versus bevacizumab in choroidal neovascular membrane in age-related macular degeneration. Indian J Ophthalmol 59: 191–196.
31. Subramanian ML, Abedi G, Ness S, Ahmed E, Fenberg M, et al. (2010) Bevacizumab vs ranibizumab for age-related macular degeneration: 1-year outcomes of a prospective, double-masked randomised clinical trial. Eye (Lond) 24: 1708–1715.
32. Krebs I, Schmetterer L, Boltz A, Told R, Vecsei-Marlovits V, et al. (2013) A randomised double-masked trial comparing the visual outcome after treatment with ranibizumab or bevacizumab in patients with neovascular age-related macular degeneration. Br J Ophthalmol 97: 266–271.
33. Kodjikian L, Souied EH, Mimoun G, Mauget-Faysse M, Behar-Cohen F, et al. (2013) Ranibizumab versus Bevacizumab for Neovascular Age-related Macular Degeneration: Results from the GEFAL Noninferiority Randomized Trial. Ophthalmology.
34. Mitchell P (2011) A systematic review of the efficacy and safety outcomes of anti-VEGF agents used for treating neovascular age-related macular degeneration: comparison of ranibizumab and bevacizumab. Curr Med Res Opin 27: 1465–1475.
35. Aujla JS (2012) Replacing ranibizumab with bevacizumab on the Pharmaceutical Benefits Scheme: where does the current evidence leave us? Clin Exp Optom 95: 538–540.
36. Torjesen I (2013) Avastin is as effective as Lucentis in treating wet age related macular degeneration, study finds. BMJ 347: f4678.
37. Campbell RJ, Gill SS, Bronskill SE, Paterson JM, Whitehead M, et al. (2012) Adverse events with intravitreal injection of vascular endothelial growth factor inhibitors: nested case-control study. BMJ 345: e4203.
38. Campbell RJ, Bell CM, Paterson JM, Bronskill SE, Moineddin R, et al. (2012) Stroke rates after introduction of vascular endothelial growth factor inhibitors for macular degeneration: a time series analysis. Ophthalmology 119: 1604–1608.
39. French DD, Margo CE (2011) Age-related macular degeneration, anti-vascular endothelial growth factor agents, and short-term mortality: a postmarketing medication safety and surveillance study. Retina 31: 1036–1042.
40. Curtis LH, Hammill BG, Schulman KA, Cousins SW (2010) Risks of mortality, myocardial infarction, bleeding, and stroke associated with therapies for age-related macular degeneration. Arch Ophthalmol 128: 1273–1279.
41. Schmucker C, Ehlken C, Agostini HT, Antes G, Ruecker G, et al. (2012) A safety review and meta-analyses of bevacizumab and ranibizumab: off-label versus goldstandard. PLoS One 7: e42701.

20

Grasping without Sight: Insights from the Congenitally Blind

Kayla D. Stone*, Claudia L. R. Gonzalez

The Brain in Action Laboratory, Department of Kinesiology, University of Lethbridge, Lethbridge, Alberta, Canada

Abstract

We reach for and grasp different sized objects numerous times per day. Most of these movements are visually-guided, but some are guided by the sense of touch (i.e. haptically-guided), such as reaching for your keys in a bag, or for an object in a dark room. A marked right-hand preference has been reported during visually-guided grasping, particularly for small objects. However, little is known about hand preference for haptically-guided grasping. Recently, a study has shown a reduction in right-hand use in blindfolded individuals, and an absence of hand preference if grasping was preceded by a short haptic experience. These results suggest that vision plays a major role in hand preference for grasping. If this were the case, then one might expect congenitally blind (CB) individuals, who have never had a visual experience, to exhibit no hand preference. Two novel findings emerge from the current study: first, the results showed that contrary to our expectation, CB individuals used their right hand during haptically-guided grasping to the same extent as visually-unimpaired (VU) individuals did during visually-guided grasping. And second, object size affected hand use in an opposite manner for haptically- versus visually-guided grasping. Big objects were more often picked up with the right hand during haptically-guided, but less often during visually-guided grasping. This result highlights the different demands that object features pose on the two sensory systems. Overall the results demonstrate that hand preference for grasping is independent of visual experience, and they suggest a left-hemisphere specialization for the control of grasping that goes beyond sensory modality.

Editor: Cristina Becchio, University of Turin and the Italian Institute of Technology, Italy

Funding: The current study was funded by the Natural Sciences and Engineering Research Council of Canada (NSERC Fund # 14367) and the University of Lethbridge. The funders had no role in study design, data collection and analysis, decision to publish, or preparation of the manuscript.

Competing Interests: The authors have declared that no competing interests exist.

* Email: kayla.stone@uleth.ca

Introduction

We execute hundreds of reaching and grasping movements a day. Both vision and hapsis (i.e. sense of touch) play an integral role in guiding these movements. For example, when reaching for an object, such as an apple, both visual and haptic cues are needed to successfully complete the movement. Initially vision is used to identify the apple (e.g. shape, size, colour) and hapsis is used to assess properties such as object weight, temperature, and texture [1–3]. Numerous studies have reported a preference to use the right hand during visually-guided grasping [4–11], so it is likely one would choose this hand to pick up the apple. However, suppose you are searching for your keys in a bag, or a glass of water in the middle of the night. In these scenarios, only haptic cues would be used and essential to locate, recognize, and grasp the objects. Would the right-hand preference seen during visually-guided grasping persist in the absence of vision? To answer this question, Stone and Gonzalez [12] asked sighted and blindfolded participants to reach for and grasp blocks scattered on a tabletop in order to construct 3D models. The results showed that participants used their right hand significantly more to grasp the blocks while sighted, but even so, a preference to grasp with the right hand persisted during the blindfolded trials. However, if these blindfolded trials were preceded by five minutes of haptic experience (without vision), equal use of the right and left hands was observed [12]. This finding suggests that hapsis significantly influences hand preference for grasping and raises the possibility that individuals who have never had a visual experience (but a lifetime of haptic experience) would exhibit little to no hand preference.

A population absent of any visual experience are congenitally blind (CB) individuals. CB refers to an individual who was born without vision (or lost vision shortly thereafter) thus resulting in no recollection of a visual experience [13]. These individuals use their sense of touch hundreds of times per day to identify, manipulate, and pick up objects, and therefore have had extensive experience using haptically-guided grasping. Hand preference for grasping in CB individuals, however, has only been reported anecdotally in children [14–17] and these studies have shown mixed results. Hand preference for grasping in an adult CB population remains unknown. Based on the results of Stone and Gonzalez [12] in which a brief haptic experience equalized hand use, one would predict no hand preference for grasping in CB individuals. Or perhaps, even a left-hand preference as several studies have shown a left-hand advantage during the haptic discrimination of objects [1,18–22]. In the present study we investigated these speculations. The *first goal* therefore, was to document hand preference for grasping in an adult CB population.

Hand preference for reaching and grasping is also influenced by the different motor programs that mediate these movements. It has been proposed that planning to reach for an object is guided by its spatial attributes (distance, position), whereas planning to grasp an object is guided by its intrinsic properties (size, shape; [23]). With respect to grasping for example, when picking up the aforementioned apple, the motor program that mediates the grasp would assess its size and shape and transform this information into the appropriate grip type. In this case, most likely a grip that requires all five fingers (i.e. a power grasp) would be used. In contrast, if one were to pick up a grape, its small size would prompt the use of only the thumb and index finger (i.e. a precision grasp). That is, previous research has shown that object size significantly affects hand preference during visually-guided grasping. For example, Vainio et al. [24] found a right-hand preference for precision grips and a left-hand preference for power grips. Similarly, other studies have shown that individuals will use their right hand more often to grasp small as opposed to big objects [4,25]. It remains to be shown if this pattern persists for grasping without vision. Kinematic studies have shown that, in the absence of vision, visually-unimpaired individuals display disruptions in their movement including larger maximum grip apertures [26–29] and slower movement times [30,31]. Interestingly, this does not seem to be the case for blind individuals. Kinematic analyses have shown that when reaching for an object, blind individuals *do* display differences in movement (i.e. a double opening and closing of the hand towards the target), but they still accurately scale to the size of the unseen object (in a manner similar to sighted individuals) [32,33]. In light of this evidence, we investigated if object size affects hand *preference* for those with lifelong deprivation of visual experience (CB individuals). Addressing this possibility was the *second goal* of the current study.

CB and visually unimpaired (VU) individuals were tested on the block building task (see [4,10,12]). Participants were asked to replicate models from a tabletop of evenly distributed building blocks. Participants built three models using small blocks and three models using big blocks to assess the effect of object size on hand preference. In Experiment One, CB and a group of age- and gender-matched VU participants (VU-Matched controls) were assessed for haptically-guided grasping (all participants were blindfolded). In Experiment Two, visually- and haptically-guided grasping were directly compared in two groups of VU students (VU-Sighted, VU-Blindfolded). In both experiments, hand preference for grasping was documented in ipsilateral (same side as the hand) and contralateral (opposite side of the hand) space as studies have found that reaching across the midline is a powerful indicator of hand preference [6,8,34].

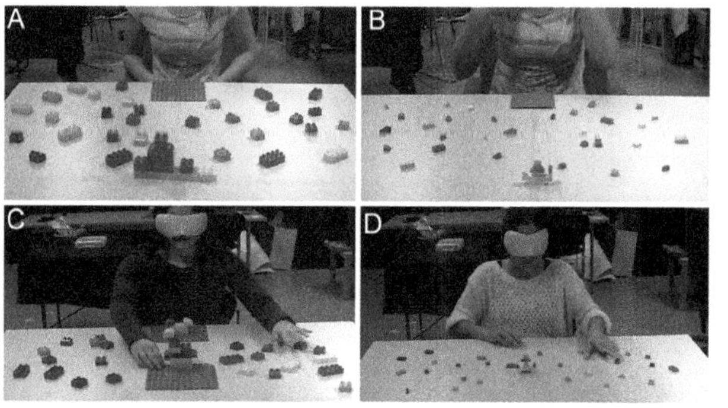

Figure 1. Experimental setup with big blocks (A). Photograph of experimental setup with big blocks scattered across the tabletop. **Experimental setup with small blocks (B).** Photograph of experimental setup with small blocks scattered across the tabletop. **Power grasp formation for big blocks (C).** Photograph of blindfolded participant exhibiting an extension of all five fingers (resembling a power grasp) while reaching for a big block. **Power grasp formation for small blocks (D).** Photograph of blindfolded participant exhibiting an extension of all five fingers (resembling a power grasp) while reaching for a small block.

Experiment One

Methods and Procedures

Participants. With respect to the photographs of participants in Figure 1, each individual signed a consent form that read: "The results from this study will be reported in general terms in the form of speech, writing, photograph or video that may be presented in manuscripts submitted for publication in scientific journals, or oral and/or poster presentations at scientific meetings, seminars, and/or conferences." Participants were therefore aware that their photograph may be used for a published manuscript when their signature was given on the consent form for the current experiment.

A priori power analysis suggested that with power at 0.95, effect size of 0.7, and statistical significance set at 0.05, the current study would require a total sample size of 16 participants (G*Power 3.1.9.2). A total of 24 participants were recruited for this experiment. Furthermore, it should be noted that participant's gender was not balanced, as gender differences have not been reported in earlier studies involving a similar task [25].

Congenitally blind (CB) participants: Ten self-reported right-handed CB individuals (8 males) and two late blind individuals (1 female) were recruited from the Canadian National Institute for the Blind (CNIB) in Lethbridge, Edmonton, Medicine Hat and Calgary (Alberta). These participants were between the ages of 20 and 76 years of age. The two late blind individuals suffered from retitinitis pigmentosa. One had been totally blind for over 50 years and the other for 10 years, although this individual reported suffering from visual deprivation since childhood. Visually-unimpaired (VU)-Matched controls: Twelve self-reported right-handers (9 males) recruited from the Lethbridge area between the ages of 20 and 73 participated. For each CB participant, we tested one VU participant of the same gender and approximately the same age (±3 years). The study was approved by the University of Lethbridge Human Subjects Research Committee (protocol #2011–22) and all participants gave written informed consent in accordance with the Declaration of Helsinki. Participants were naïve to the purposes of the study.

Apparatus and Stimuli. *Handedness Questionnaire*: A modified version of the Edinburgh [35] and Waterloo [36] handedness questionnaires were given to all participants at the end of the block building task. This version included questions on hand preference for 22 different tasks. Participants had to rate which hand they prefer to use for each task on a scale +2 (right always) +1 (right usually), 0 (equal), −1 (left usually) and −2 (left always). Each response was scored as 2, 1, −1, or −2 and a total score was obtained by adding all values. Possible scores range from +44 for exclusive right-hand use to −44 for exclusive left-hand use. CB participants were also asked about their diagnosed visual condition, ability to read Braille, and ability to function independently (i.e. yes or no). This information is included in Table 1.

Block Building Task: A total of six models built with MEGA BLOKS (big blocks) andLEGO (small blocks) were used for the experiment. Three models were built using big blocks (ranging in size from 3.1 L×3.1 W×2.0 cm H to 6.3 L×3.1 W×2.0 cm H)

Table 1. Information pertaining to each CB and Late Blind participants' (initials included) visual condition, hand used to read Braille, and ability to function independently.

Participant	Visual Condition	Hand used for Braille	Functions independently?
1 BV	Congenital glaucoma	Both	Yes
2 CM	Bilateral Retinoblastoma	Both	Yes
3 WR	Optic nerve hypoplasia	Both	Yes
4 BD	Retinopathy of prematurity	Both	Yes
5 CM	Leber Congenital Amaurosis	Both	Yes
6 EC	Leber Congenital Amaurosis	Both	Yes
7 GE	Optic Atrophy	Both	Yes
8 LP	Retinopathy of prematurity	Right	Yes
9 RG	Optic Nerve Hypoplasia	Unknown	Partial*
10 NS	Retinitis pigmentosa	Unknown	Yes
11 WB	Retinitis pigmentosa	Left	Yes
12 MH	Leber Congenital Amaurosis	Both	Yes

*resides in an assisted living home.

and three using small blocks (ranging in size from <0.7 L×0.7 W×1.0 cm H to 6.3 L×1.5 W×1.0 cm H). Each model contained 10 blocks of various colours and shapes. Scattered on a table (122 L×122 W×74 cm H with a working space of 70 L×122 W×74 cm H) were all the blocks that made up the three models of each set (i.e. either 30 small blocks or 30 big blocks; see Figure 1A and 1B). The models were prepared ahead of time by the experimenter. The same six models were used with all participants. The same number of blocks were placed on the left and right side of the table. There was a fixed building plate (19L×19 cm W) located within arms' length of the participant. Additionally, there was an exact duplicate of this building plate in the front and center of the participant. The far plate had the model to be replicated attached to it, and the near plate was used for the construction of the new model.

Procedures. Participants were seated in front of the table facing the middle of the display that contained either "big blocks" or "small blocks". Participants were notified that for the next three models they would be building with big *or* small blocks. In other words, participants were never presented with a table that contained small and big blocks at the same time. After the participant was comfortably seated, they were instructed to replicate the model as quickly and accurately as possible from the blocks given on the table. No other instruction was given. All participants were blindfolded prior to and during the task. Therefore, they were only able to use their sense of touch to identify the model and blocks. Once the model was replicated, both models were removed from the table and a new model was given. No blocks were replaced after each model was completed. Six models were built in total. Starting block size (small or big) was counterbalanced among participants. The task was recorded on a JVC HD Everio video recorder approximately 160 cm away from the individual with a clear view of the tabletop, building blocks, and participants' hands.

Data Analysis. All recorded videos were analyzed offline. Each grasp was recorded as a left or right hand grasp in the participants' ipsilateral or contralateral space. The total number of grasps was calculated to determine a percent for right-hand use (number of right grasps/total number of grasps X 100). The time in which it took participants to construct each model was recorded on a stopwatch and reported in seconds. Therefore, the dependent variables included percentage of overall right-hand use, percentage of hand use in contralateral space (contralateral grasps), and the time in seconds that it took participants to complete the models. Data were assessed and no violations for homogeneity of variance and normality were found prior to analysis. Partial Eta Squared values were used to show effect size (ES). Data were analyzed using SPSS Statistics 18.0 for Windows (SPSS Inc., Chicago, IL, USA).

Results (Experiment One)

Handedness questionnaire. All participants self-reported as right-handers and this was confirmed by the handedness questionnaire. Congenitally Blind participants: Given that not all 22 questions applied to the CB participants, their scores were normalized to the traditional scale for this questionnaire (−44 to + 44) regardless of how many questions they answered. To normalize the scores, we took the participant's total score (e.g. 25) divided by the total number of questions that participant answered (e.g. 19) and this value was then multiplied by 22, which is the total number of possible questions that could have been answered (and the total number of questions all of the VU individuals answered). On average, CB participants received an overall average score of 33.8 (±1.0 SE; range +28 to +41.9) points out of a total possible score of −44/+44. VU-Matched controls: VU-Matched controls participants answered all 22 questions, and received an overall average score of 31.6 (±2.0 SE range +17 to + 40) points out of a total possible score of −44/+44. An independent samples t-test revealed that there was no significant difference between the two groups (t (22) = 1.2; $p = 0.2$).

Hand use for grasping. Analysis using a 2 (object size) X 2 (group) repeated measures ANOVA was performed on the percentage of right-hand use for grasping during the task. Object size (big, small) was a within subject factor and group (CB, VU-Matched controls) a between subject factor. Overall, we found a main effect of object size (F (1, 22) = 26.2; $p<0.0001$, ES = 0.54). Participants used their right hand significantly more to grasp the big blocks (59.6±1.4%) compared to the small blocks (52.0±1.5%). There was also a main effect of group (F (1, 22) = 8.1; $p = 0.009$, ES = 0.26). Participants in the CB group used their right hands significantly more to grasp the blocks

(59.5±1.8%) than the VU-Matched controls (52.2±1.8%), regardless of object size. The interaction between group and size was not significant ($p = 0.42$). Both groups displayed the same pattern of hand preference for both big and small blocks. CB participants used their right hand 62.7±2.0% when grasping big blocks and 56.3±2.1% when grasping small blocks. VU-Matched controls used their right hand 56.6±2.0% when grasping big blocks, and 47.8±2.1% when grasping small blocks (see Figure 2A).

Contralateral grasps: Analysis using a 2 (object size) X 2 (hand) X 2 (group) repeated measures ANOVA was performed on the percentage of contralateral grasps made during the task. Object size (big, small) and hand (right, left) were within factors and group (CB, VU-Matched controls) the between factor. Analyses did not show a significant effect of object size (F (1, 22) = 0.6; $p = 0.42$, ES = 0.02), therefore data were collapsed across this variable. A 2 (hand) X 2 (group) repeated measures ANOVA was performed on the percentage of contralateral grasps during the task. Hand (right, left) was a within subject factor and group (CB, VU-Matched controls) a between subject factor. There was no main effect of hand (F (1, 22) = 2.8; $p = 0.1$, ES = 0.11). There was no main effect of group ($p = 0.2$). However, the group by hand interaction was significant (F (1, 22) = 5.2; $p = 0.03$, ES = 0.19). Post hoc analysis (paired samples t-test) revealed that the CB group made significantly more right-handed grasps into left contralateral space (6.1±2.0%) than left-handed grasps into right contralateral space (1.6±0.5%; t (11) = 2.2; $p = 0.04$). This was not the case for the VU-Matched controls (2.4% versus 3.3%; t (11) = −0.6; $p = 0.55$).

Build times for models. Analysis using a 2 (object size) X 2 (group) repeated measures ANOVA was performed on the average time in seconds it took for participants to complete one model. Object size (big, small) was a within subject factor and group (CB, VU-Matched controls) a between subject factor. Overall, we found a main effect of object size (F (1, 22) = 14.2; $p = 0.001$, ES = 0.39). Participants were faster at completing one model made of big blocks (175.7±11.9s) compared to one model made of small blocks (213.0±14.2). There was no main effect of group (F (1, 22) = 0.0; $p = 0.53$, ES = 0.01). The interaction between size and group reached significance however (F (1, 22) = 4.1; $p = 0.05$). Post hoc analysis (paired samples t-test) revealed that VU-Matched controls were significantly faster at completing one model made of big blocks (173.2±12.6s) compared to one model made of small blocks (230.7±21.2s; t (11) = −3.7; $p = 0.003$). No such difference was found in the CB group, who completed one model made of big blocks in approximately the same time as one model made of small blocks (178.1±16.9s and 195.2±20.1s respectively; t (11) = −1.3; $p = 0.1$).

Discussion (Experiment One)

Although the majority of the participants were congenitally blind (n = 10), we recognize that two of them were late blind individuals. These individuals, however, reported suffering a lifetime of visual impairment, and had experienced total blindness for a significant number of years. Hand preference for grasping for these individuals was indistinguishable from that of CB individuals, and the results remained unaffected when the two participants are removed, thus they were included in the current study.

Overall the results yielded two interesting findings. First, CB participants preferred their right hand significantly more for grasping the blocks compared to the VU-Matched controls. Second, object size affected hand preference for grasping in both the CB and VU-Matched controls groups. Participants used the right hand more to grasp the big blocks when compared to the small blocks. This effect seen in haptically-guided grasping is opposite to what has previously been reported during visually-guided grasping. Thus, to contrast the effect that object size could have in haptically- versus visually-guided grasping, we tested a group of blindfolded young adult controls (VU-Blindfolded) and a group of sighted young adult controls (VU-Sighted). This last group was presented with the exact same task as the haptically-guided group but they completed the task using vision.

Experiment Two

Methods and Procedures

Participants. A priori power analysis suggested that with power at 0.95, effect size of 0.7, and statistical significance set at 0.05, the current study would require a total sample size of 16 participants (G*Power 3.1.9.2). A total of 24 participants were recruited for this experiment.

VU-Blindfolded participants: Twelve self-reported right-handers (4 males) from the University of Lethbridge, between the ages of 19 and 31, participated. VU-Sighted participants: Twelve self-

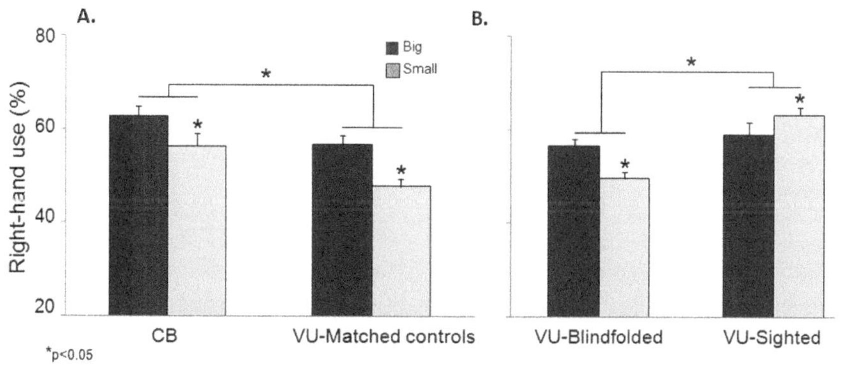

Figure 2. Hand use for grasping for big and small blocks in Experiment One (A). This graph demonstrates right-hand use as a function of object size for the two groups: CB and VU-Matched controls (Experiment One). The dark grey bars represent the big blocks. The light grey bars represent the small blocks. Note the significant difference between the CB and VU-Matched controls, as well as reduction in right-hand use for the small blocks seen in both groups. **Hand use for grasping for big and small blocks in Experiment Two (B).** This graph demonstrates right-hand use as a function of object size for the two groups: VU-Blindfolded and VU-Sighted groups (Experiment Two). The dark grey bars represent the big blocks. The light grey bars represent the small blocks. Note the significant difference between the VU-Sighted and VU-Blindfolded participants, as well as the opposite pattern of hand use exhibited for object size within the two groups.

reported right-handed individuals (4 males) from the University of Lethbridge, between the ages of 19 and 23, participated. The study was approved by the University of Lethbridge Human Subjects Research Committee (protocol #2011–22) and all participants gave written informed consent in accordance with the Declaration of Helsinki. Participants were naïve to the purposes of the study.

Apparatus and Stimuli. All the display material and equipment were the same as Experiment One.

Procedures. All procedures were identical to those in Experiment One, with one alteration: those in the VU-Sighted group did not wear a blindfold during the task. In turn, the task was haptically-guided (as in Experiment One) for the VU-Blindfolded group and visually-guided for the VU-Sighted group.

Data Analysis. Data analysis was the same as Experiment One. Bonferroni correction was applied to all multiple group comparisons.

Results (Experiment Two)

Handedness questionnaire. All participants self-reported as right-handers and this was confirmed by the handedness questionnaire. VU-Blindfolded: The average score was +30.4 (±1.7 SE; range +21 to +39) out of a total possible score of −44/+44. VU-Sighted: The average score was +32.2 (±1.9 SE; range +22 to +43) out of a total possible score of −44/+44. An independent samples t-test revealed that there was no significant difference between the two groups (t (22) = −0.7; p = 0.4).

Hand use for grasping. Analysis using a 2 (object size) X 2 (group) repeated measures ANOVA was performed on the percentage of right-hand use for grasping during the task. Object size (big, small) was a within subject factor and group (VU-Sighted, VU-Blindfolded) a between subject factor. There was no main effect of object size (F (1, 22) = 0.4; p = 0.52, ES = 0.01) but a main effect of group (F (1, 22) = 13.8; p = 0.001, ES = 0.38). Consistent with Stone and Gonzalez [12], blindfolded participants used their right hand significantly less for grasping (53.0±1.5%) than sighted individuals (61.1±1.5%), regardless of object size. A significant interaction between object size and group was found (F (1, 22) = 17.1; p<0.0001, ES = 0.43). Post hoc analysis (paired samples t-tests) revealed that, just as in Experiment One, VU-Blindfolded individuals used their right hand more to grasp big blocks (56.5±1.5%) compared to small blocks (49.6±1.2%; t (11) = 3.1; p = 0.009). However, VU-Sighted individuals used their right hand more to grasp small blocks (63.6±1.6%) compared to big blocks (58.6±2.5%; t (11) = −2.6; p = 0.02), as shown in Figure 2B. Noteworthy, the values of hand use for the VU-Blindfolded individuals were identical to those of the VU-Matched controls in Experiment One.

Contralateral grasps: Analysis using a 2 (object size) X 2 (hand) X 2 (group) repeated measures ANOVA was performed on the percentage of contralateral grasps made during the task. Object size (big, small) and hand (right, left) were within factors and group (VU-Blindfolded, VU-Sighted) the between factor. As in Experiment One, analyses did not show a significant effect of object size therefore data were collapsed across this variable (F (1, 22) = 2.8; p = 0.1, ES = 0.11). Therefore, a 2 (hand) X 2 (group) repeated measures ANOVA was performed on the percentage of contralateral grasps during the task. Hand (right, left) was a within subject factor and group (VU-Blindfolded, VU-Sighted) a between subject factor. There was a main effect of hand (F (1, 22) = 28.3; p<0.0001, ES = 0.56). Both groups made significantly more contralateral grasps with the right (6.2±0.9%) versus the left (0.9±0.3%) hand. There was a main effect of group (F (1, 22) = 49.0; p<0.0001, ES = 0.69). The VU-Sighted group made significantly more contralateral grasps than the VU-Blindfolded group (6.0% versus 1.1%, respectively). The group by hand interaction was also significant (F (1, 22) = 21.7; p<0.0001, ES = 0.49). Post hoc analysis (paired samples t-tests) revealed that the VU-Sighted group made significantly more right-handed grasps in the left contralateral space (10.9±1.8%) than left-handed grasps in the right contralateral space (0.8±0.3%; t (11) = 5.2; p<0.0001). This was not the case for the VU-Blindfolded group (1.5±.4% versus 0.8±0.3%; t (11) = 1.1; p = 0.2).

Build times for models. Given that the VU-Sighted group built the models substantially faster than the VU-Blindfolded group (likely due to visual availability; p<0.0001), the two groups were compared separately. A paired samples t-test revealed that VU-Sighted participants completed the task with the big blocks significantly faster than with the small blocks (t (11) = −3.8; p = 0.003). Participants completed one model made of big blocks in approximately 22.6±0.9s and one model made of small blocks in 25.7±1.2s. Similarly to the results of Experiment One, the VU-Blindfolded group completed one model made of big blocks significantly faster than one model made of small blocks (t (11) = −2.7; p = 0.01; Mean time = 128.3±9.2s and 153.6±15.4s for big and small blocks respectively).

Comparison between Experiment One and Experiment Two. We performed an analysis using a 2 (object size) X 4 (group) repeated measures ANOVA on the percentage of overall right-hand use for grasping. Object size (big, small) was a within subject factor and group (CB, VU-Matched controls, VU-Blindfolded, and VU-Sighted) a between subject factor. We found a main effect of size (F (1, 44) = 17.0; p<0.0001, ES = 0.28). Again, participants used the right hand more often to grasp big (58.6±1.0%), as opposed to small (54.3±0.9%) blocks. There was also a main effect of group (F (3, 44) = 7.1; p<0.0001, ES = 0.32). The CB group used their right hands significantly more for grasping than the VU-Blindfolded (p = 0.05) and the VU-Matched controls (p = 0.02). Interestingly, however, the CB group behaved similarly to the VU-Sighted group (p = 1.0). That is, both groups used their right hand to the same extent during the grasping task. Importantly, as depicted in Figure 3A, the VU-Matched controls and VU-Blindfolded groups differed from the VU-Sighted group (p = 0.003; p = 0.009, respectively). The VU-Matched controls and VU-Blindfolded group did not differ from each other (p = 1.0). The size by group interaction was also significant (F (3, 44) = 9.2; p<0.0001, ES = 0.38). Post hoc analysis (independent samples t-test) revealed that the VU-Sighted group used the right hand significantly more than the VU-Blindfolded (t (22) = −6.7; p< 0.0001), VU-Matched controls (t (22) = −6.9; p<0.0001), and CB (t (22) = −2.3; p = 0.03) groups when grasping small blocks. This was not the case for the big blocks, however (all comparisons p>0.1). This result reflects the different effect that object size poses on haptically- versus visually-guided grasping, particularly for small objects. In other words, small objects were more often picked up with the right hand during visually-guided, but less often during haptically-guided grasping. This is not surprising as we have previously shown less pronounced right-hand use for grasping big blocks [4,25].

Contralateral grasps: Analysis using a 2 (object size) X 2 (hand) X 4 (group) repeated measures ANOVA was performed on the percentage of contralateral grasps made during the task. Object size (big, small) and hand (right, left) were within factors and group (CB, VU-Matched controls, VU-Blindfolded, VU-Sighted) the between factor. Again, analyses did not show a significant effect of object size therefore data were collapsed across this variable (F (1,44) = 3.0; p = 0.1, ES = 0.05). Therefore, a 2 (hand) X 4 (group) repeated measures ANOVA was performed on the

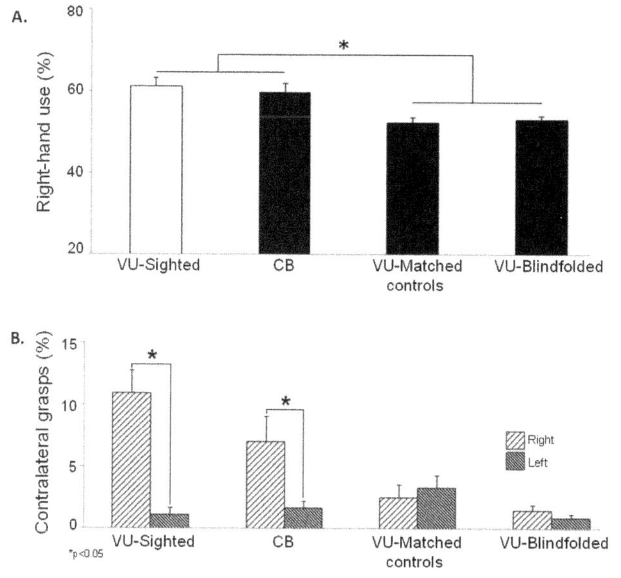

Figure 3. Overall hand use for grasping across all groups (A). This graph demonstrates overall right-hand use (across object size) in percentage for groups in Experiment One (CB, VU-Matched controls) and Experiment Two (VU-Sighted, VU-Blindfolded). White bars signify that the participants had vision for the duration of the task. Black bars signify that the participants had no vision (blind or blindfolded). Note that there is *no* significant different in right-hand use between VU-Sighted and CB participants, but these groups are different from the VU-Blindfolded and VU-Matched controls. **Hand use for contralateral grasps across all groups (B).** This graph demonstrates the average percentage of contralateral grasps made with the left and right hand for the VU-Sighted, CB, VU-Matched controls, and VU-Blindfolded groups. The spaced rightward diagonal bars represent the right hand and the compressed leftward diagonal bars represent the left hand. Note the significant difference in contralateral grasps made with each hand for the VU-Sighted and CB groups but not for the VU-Matched controls. Note also, that the VU-Sighted and CB groups behaved similarly.

percentage of contralateral grasps during the task. Hand (right, left) was a within subject factor and group (CB, VU-Matched controls, VU-Blindfolded, VU-Sighted) a between subject factor. There was a main effect of hand (F (1, 44) $= 20.1$; $p<0.0001$, ES $= 0.31$). Participants made significantly more right-handed grasps in the left contralateral space ($5.4 \pm 0.7\%$) compared to left-handed grasps in the right contralateral space ($1.7 \pm 0.3\%$). In other words, participants were more likely to reach across to the left contralateral space to grasp a block with the right hand compared to reaching into the right contralateral space to grasp a block with the left hand. There was a main effect of group (F (3, 44) $= 6.4$; $p = 0.001$, ES $= 0.30$). The VU-Sighted group made significantly more right-handed grasps in left contralateral space than the VU-Blindfolded ($p = 0.001$) and the VU-Matched controls ($p = 0.05$). No differences emerged between the VU-Sighted and CB groups ($p = 0.8$). The hand by group interaction was also significant (F (3, 44) $= 8.4$; $p<0.0001$, ES $= 0.36$). Post hoc analysis (paired samples t-tests) revealed that the VU-Sighted group made significantly more right-handed grasps in the left contralateral space ($10.9 \pm 1.8\%$) than left-handed grasps in the right contralateral space ($1.0 \pm 0.5\%$; t (11) $= 5.2$; $p<0.0001$). The CB also made significantly more right-handed grasps in the left contralateral space ($6.1 \pm 2.0\%$) than left-handed grasps in the right contralateral space ($1.6 \pm 0.5\%$; t (11) $= 2.2$; $p = 0.04$). However, this was not the case for the VU-Matched controls ($2.4 \pm 1.0\%$ versus $3.3 \pm 0.9\%$; t (11) $= -0.6$; $p = 0.55$) nor for the VU-Blindfolded group (1.5 ± 1.5 versus $0.8 \pm 1.2\%$; t (11) $= 1.1$; $p = 0.27$; see Figure 3B). Furthermore, independent samples t-test revealed that the VU-Matched controls made significantly more left-handed grasps in the right contralateral space than the VU-Blindfolded (3.3% versus 0.8%; $t(22) = 2.4$; $p = 0.02$). All remaining comparisons between hand and group were not significant. To emphasize, independent samples t-test results showed no significant difference in percentage of right-handed grasps completed in the left contralateral space between the CB and the VU-Sighted group (t (22) $= -1.4$) $p>0.1$). Thus, in terms of grasping in contralateral space, the CB group displayed similar behaviour to the VU-Sighted group.

General Discussion

The present study had two main goals: first, to document hand preference for grasping in a congenitally blind (CB) population and second, to investigate how object properties, specifically object size, would influence hand preference during haptically-guided grasping. CB and visually unimpaired (VU: Sighted and Blindfolded/Matched controls) individuals were asked to replicate 3D models using small or large blocks scattered on a tabletop. Results showed that CB individuals exhibit a right-hand preference for grasping, and this preference was significantly greater than the VU-Matched controls and VU-Blindfolded group. Furthermore, this right-hand preference in CB individuals was not different from the VU-Sighted group, which was further confirmed by the analysis of contralateral grasps. These results suggest that, regardless of visual experience, hand preference for gasping is lateralized to the right hand. A second finding was the influence that object size exerted on hand preference. Consistent with previous studies [4,25] VU-Sighted participants used their right hand more often to grasp the small, as opposed to the big blocks. However, when blindfolded, VU participants demonstrated the opposite pattern: they preferred their right hand to grasp the big, versus the small, blocks. This result was also seen in the CB participants. Overall, these findings suggest first, a left-hemisphere specialization for grasping regardless of lifetime visual *or* haptic experience; and second, that object properties such as size pose different demands on visually- versus haptically-guided grasping.

Studies exploring hand use in blind individuals have focused on haptically-guided tasks such as reading Braille [37–39] or identifying: geometrical shapes [2,40], tactile pictures [41–43], or spatial targets [44]. These studies have highlighted the ability, and in some cases, the advantage that CB individuals exhibit over VU participants during tactile recognition tasks. In some studies, this advantage was specific to one hand. For example, when CB participants were asked to read Braille they were more proficient when using their left hand [37]. Another study showed that when sorting different objects, CB individuals were faster with their left hand than VU participants were with either hand [16]. None of these studies however, specifically investigated hand preference for grasping in CB adults. In the present investigation, we document CB individuals' right-hand preference for grasping. Interestingly, this right-hand preference was similar to that of sighted individuals when using vision. A previous study has shown a reduction of right-hand use during haptically-guided grasping in VU individuals [12] which was replicated in the current study. CB participants however, used their right hand to the same extent as the sighted VU participants. In fact, the analysis of contralateral grasps confirmed that CB behave virtually identical to VU-Sighted individuals in terms of hand use. When reaching across the midline, both groups showed a marked right-hand preference over the left for grasping the blocks. These results suggest that the mechanisms of hand preference for grasping develop *independently* of visual experience. In an investigation of hand preference and ability in CB children, Ittyerah suggests that hand preference might not be determined by vision [17]. Furthermore, based on 39 neuroimaging studies, Ricciardi et al. [45] argue that brain functional organization is to a large extent independent from visual experience. For example, sighted and CB individuals were asked to tactically recognize different objects (bottles, shoes, and masks of faces) while brain activation was measured through functional MRI [46]. The results showed that category-relative object activation in occipito-temporal areas (ventral stream), was similar for sighted and CB individuals. Likewise, overlapping activation patterns in the dorsal stream have been shown during kinaesthetically guided hand movements in both sighted and CB individuals [47]. Our results of hand use during grasping are in line with these previous studies in that CB individuals behaved virtually identical to sighted individuals.

Another finding of the present investigation was the effect that object size exerted on hand preference during grasping. Studies have shown that the kinematics of prehensile movements are contingent upon object size. Movement time, peak velocity and grip apertures all respond to changes in object size. For instance, the larger the object to be grasped, the longer it takes to reach maximum grip aperture [26,48,49]. When reaching for smaller objects, individuals exhibit lower and earlier peak velocities and longer deceleration phases when compared to reaching for larger objects [50–53]. Interestingly, grip scaling in blind individuals is accurate and indistinguishable from sighted individuals when reaching for different sized objects [32]. These results illustrate how object size influences kinematics of reaching and grasping, even in the absence of vision. With respect to hand preference, previous investigations [4,25] have also highlighted the influence of object size and have shown that when grasping small objects, there is an increase in right-hand use. In the current investigation we replicated this finding for visually-guided grasping. Interestingly, during haptically-guided grasping, both CB and VU individuals used the right hand more often for grasping the large objects. This finding suggests that object characteristics affect patterns of hand use differently for haptically- versus visually-guided grasping.

We offer two non-mutually exclusive explanations for this phenomenon. First, it is possible that, as we have argued before [12], hand use during haptically-guided grasping could be influenced by the known advantage of this hand for haptic discrimination. Several studies have shown a left-hand advantage for object discrimination when guided by hapsis [1,18,54–61]. For instance, Benton et al. [54] applied tactile stimulation to the hands of individuals and asked them to identify the direction of the stimulus. Participants were significantly more accurate when the stimulation was applied to their left hand. In a series of experiments, Fagot and colleagues have demonstrated a left-hand superiority for recognizing shapes when given a discrimination task. Accordingly, they also found a left-hand advantage in terms of overall time the left hand explored the given objects for these tasks [56,62,63]. Fagot's results demonstrate that the left hand is better at encoding haptic information. Support for this evidence was provided via personal communication with the CB individuals in the present study. Upon reviewing the CB testimonials collected during and after our visit we encountered two statements that speak to this matter. When asking the participants if one hand was better for touch, one individual responded, "Well... I might look for more detail with the left". A second CB individual responded to the question similarly: "My left hand is more focused towards the two fingers, feeling the spatial [properties of the object], and I use my right hand to pick up [the object]." It appears then, that there is a division of labour between the hands when identifying (left hand) and grasping (right hand) an object that one cannot see.

The second possibility that could have contributed to the object size effect is the initial grasp formation. A previous study has shown facilitation of right-handed responses for pincer grasps (i.e. thumb and index finger) and facilitation of left-handed responses for power grasps [24]. Similarly, it has been shown that visually-guided grasps requiring more precision (pincer grasping) are more often executed with the right hand as opposed to grasps that require the whole hand (i.e. power grasps), even in left-handers [4,25,64]. In the current experiments we observed that all haptically-guided reaching movements (regardless of the block's size) exhibited an extension of all five fingers (see Figure 1C and 1D) resembling a power grasp (see [65] for similar results). It is possible that this power grasp formation, which favours left-handed grasps, affected the selection of hand use while grasping the small blocks. In fact, Overvliet et al. [66] found that individuals were better at localizing tactile stimuli when the fingers were spread apart (similar to a power grasp formation) compared to when they were close together. We speculate that the decrease in right-hand use seen for haptically-guided grasping stems in part from an increase of left-hand use during haptic discrimination, particularly for the small objects. Although this might not explain the increase in right-hand use seen when grasping the *big* blocks, it provides a preliminary explanation for change in hand use for grasping the small blocks. Furthermore, it remains unknown if these findings would persist in a population of left-handed individuals, which is a limitation of the current study. These possibilities warrant further investigation.

In conclusion, the results indicate that visual availability, but not visual experience, determines hand use in response to object size. Furthermore, the results suggest a left-hemisphere/right-hand specialization for grasping, regardless of visual experience.

Author Contributions

Conceived and designed the experiments: KDS CLRG. Performed the experiments: KDS CLRG. Analyzed the data: KDS CLRG. Contributed reagents/materials/analysis tools: KDS CLRG. Wrote the paper: KDS CLRG.

References

1. Tomlinson SP, Davis NJ, Morgan HM, Bracewell RM (2011) Hemispheric specialisation in haptic processing. Neuropsychologia 49: 2703–2710.
2. Withagen A, Kappers AM, Vervloed MP, Knoors H, Verhoeven L (2013) The use of exploratory procedures by blind and sighted adults and children. Atten Percept Psychophys.
3. Woods AT, Newell FN (2004) Visual, haptic and cross-modal recognition of objects and scenes. J Physiol Paris 98: 147–159.
4. Stone KD, Bryant DC, Gonzalez CL (2013) Hand use for grasping in a bimanual task: evidence for different roles? Exp Brain Res 224: 455–467.
5. Bishop DV, Ross VA, Daniels MS, Bright P (1996) The measurement of hand preference: a validation study comparing three groups of right-handers. Br J Psychol 87 (Pt 2): 269–285.
6. Bryden PJ, Roy EA (2006) Preferential reaching across regions of hemispace in adults and children. Dev Psychobiol 48: 121–132.
7. Calvert GA, Bishop DV (1998) Quantifying hand preference using a behavioural continuum. Laterality 3: 255–268.
8. Carlier M, Doyen AL, Lamard C (2006) Midline crossing: developmental trend from 3 to 10 years of age in a preferential card-reaching task. Brain Cogn 61: 255–261.

9. Gabbard C, Tapia M, Helbig CR (2003) Task complexity and limb selection in reaching. Int J Neurosci 113: 143–152.
10. Gonzalez CL, Whitwell RL, Morrissey B, Ganel T, Goodale MA (2007) Left handedness does not extend to visually guided precision grasping. Exp Brain Res 182: 275–279.
11. Sacrey LA, Karl JM, Whishaw IQ (2012) Development of rotational movements, hand shaping, and accuracy in advance and withdrawal for the reach-to-eat movement in human infants aged 6–12 months. Infant Behav Dev 35: 543–560.
12. Stone KD, Gonzalez CL (2014) Grasping with the eyes of your hands: Hapsis and vision modulate hand preference. Exp Brain Res 232: 385–393.
13. Thinus-Blanc C, Gaunet F (1997) Representation of space in blind persons: vision as a spatial sense? Psychol Bull 121: 20–42.
14. Caliskan E, Dane S (2009) Left-handedness in blind and sighted children. Laterality 14: 205–213.
15. Ittyerah M (1993) Hand preferences and hand ability in congenitally blind children. Q J Exp Psychol A 46: 35–50.
16. Ittyerah M (2000) Hand skill and hand preference in blind and sighted children. Laterality 5: 221–235.
17. Ittyerah M (2009) Hand Ability and Practice in Congenitally Blind Children. Journal of Developmental and Physical Disabilities 21: 329–344.
18. O'Boyle MW, Van Wyhe-Lawler F, Miller DA (1987) Recognition of letters traced in the right and left palms: evidence for a process-oriented tactile asymmetry. Brain Cogn 6: 474–494.
19. Kumar S (1977) Short term memory for a nonverbal tactual task after cerebral commissurotomy. Cortex 13: 55–61.
20. Harada T, Saito DN, Kashikura K, Sato T, Yonekura Y, et al. (2004) Asymmetrical neural substrates of tactile discrimination in humans: a functional magnetic resonance imaging study. J Neurosci 24: 7524–7530.
21. Cormier JM, Tremblay F (2013) Asymmetry in corticomotor facilitation revealed in right-handers in the context of haptic discrimination. Laterality 18: 365–383.
22. Benton AL, Varney NR, Hamsher KS (1978) Lateral differences in tactile directional perception. Neuropsychologia 16: 109–114.
23. Jeannerod M, Arbib MA, Rizzolatti G, Sakata H (1995) Grasping objects: The cortical mechanisms of visuomotor transfer. Trends in Neurosciences 18: 314–320.
24. Vainio L, Ellis R, Tucker M, Symes E (2006) Manual asymmetries in visually primed grasping. Exp Brain Res 173: 395–406.
25. Gonzalez CLR, Goodale MA (2009) Hand preference for precision grasping predicts language lateralization. Neuropsychologia 47: 3182–3189.
26. Jakobson LS, Goodale MA (1991) Factors affecting higher-order movement planning: a kinematic analysis of human prehension. Exp Brain Res 86: 199–208.
27. Rand MK, Lemay M, Squire LM, Shimansky YP, Stelmach GE (2007) Role of vision in aperture closure control during reach-to-grasp movements. Exp Brain Res 181: 447–460.
28. Jackson SR, Jackson GM, Rosicky J (1995) Are non-relevant objects represented in working memory? The effect of non-target objects on reach and grasp kinematics. Exp Brain Res 102: 519–530.
29. Pettypiece CE, Culham JC, Goodale MA (2009) Differential effects of delay upon visually and haptically guided grasping and perceptual judgments. Exp Brain Res 195: 473–479.
30. Schettino LF, Adamovich SV, Poizner H (2003) Effects of object shape and visual feedback on hand configuration during grasping. Exp Brain Res 151: 158–166.
31. Winges SA, Weber DJ, Santello M (2003) The role of vision on hand preshaping during reach to grasp. Exp Brain Res 152: 489–498.
32. Castiello U, Bennett KM, Mucignat C (1993) The reach to grasp movement of blind subjects. Exp Brain Res 96: 152–162.
33. Bennett KM, Mucignat C, Waterman C, Castiello U (1994) Vision and the reach to grasp movement. In: Bennett KM, Castiello U, editors. Insights into the reach to grasp movement. North-Holland: Elsevier Science B.V. 390.
34. Gabbard C, Helbig CR, Gentry V (2001) Lateralized effects on reaching by children. Dev Neuropsychol 19: 41–51.
35. Oldfield RC (1971) The assessment and analysis of handedness: the Edinburgh inventory. Neuropsychologia 9: 97–113.
36. Brown SG, Roy EA, Rohr LE, Bryden PJ (2006) Using hand performance measures to predict handedness. Laterality 11: 1–14.
37. Hermelin B, O'Connor N (1971) Functional asymmetry in the reading of Braille. Neuropsychologia 9: 431–435.
38. Grant AC, Thiagarajah MC, Sathian K (2000) Tactile perception in blind Braille readers: a psychophysical study of acuity and hyperacuity using gratings and dot patterns. Percept Psychophys 62: 301–312.
39. Millar S (1987) The perceptual "window" in two-handed braille: do the left and right hands process text simultaneously? Cortex 23: 111–122.
40. Theurel A, Frileux S, Hatwell Y, Gentaz E (2012) The haptic recognition of geometrical shapes in congenitally blind and blindfolded adolescents: is there a haptic prototype effect? PLoS One 7: e40251.
41. Theurel A, Witt A, Claudet P, Hatwell Y, Gentaz E (2013) Tactile picture recognition by early blind children: the effect of illustration technique. J Exp Psychol Appl 19: 233–240.
42. Heller MA, Calcaterra JA, Burson LL, Tyler LA (1996) Tactual picture identification by blind and sighted people: effects of providing categorical information. Percept Psychophys 58: 310–323.
43. Lederman SJ, Klatzky RL, Chataway C, Summers CD (1990) Visual mediation and the haptic recognition of two-dimensional pictures of common objects. Percept Psychophys 47: 54–64.
44. Collignon O, De Volder AG (2009) Further evidence that congenitally blind participants react faster to auditory and tactile spatial targets. Can J Exp Psychol 63: 287–293.
45. Ricciardi E, Bonino D, Pellegrini S, Pietrini P (2013) Mind the blind brain to understand the sighted one! Is there a supramodal cortical functional architecture? Neurosci Biobehav Rev.
46. Pietrini P, Furey ML, Ricciardi E, Gobbini MI, Wu WH, et al. (2004) Beyond sensory images: Object-based representation in the human ventral pathway. Proc Natl Acad Sci U S A 101: 5658–5663.
47. Fiehler K, Burke M, Bien S, Roder B, Rosler F (2009) The human dorsal action control system develops in the absence of vision. Cereb Cortex 19: 1–12.
48. Connolly JD, Goodale MA (1999) The role of visual feedback of hand position in the control of manual prehension. Exp Brain Res 125: 281–286.
49. Paulignan Y, Frak VG, Toni I, Jeannerod M (1997) Influence of object position and size on human prehension movements. Exp Brain Res 114: 226–234.
50. Heath M, Hodges NJ, Chua R, Elliott D (1998) On-line control of rapid aiming movements: Unexpected target perturbations and movement kinematics. Canadian Journal of Experimental Psychology 52: 163–173.
51. Kudoh N, Hattori M, Numata N, Maruyama K (1997) An analysis of spatiotemporal variability during prehension movements: effects of object size and distance. Exp Brain Res 117: 457–464.
52. Marteniuk RG, Leavitt JL, MacKenzie CL, Athenes S (1990) Functional relationships between grasp and transport components in a prehension task. Human Movement Science 9: 149–176.
53. Gentilucci M, Castiello U, Corradini ML, Scarpa M, Umilta C, et al. (1991) Influence of different types of grasping on the transport component of prehension movements. Neuropsychologia 29: 361–378.
54. Benton AL, Levin HS, Varney NR (1973) Tactile perception of direction in normal subjects. Implications for hemispheric cerebral dominance. Neurology 23: 1248–1250.
55. Dodds AG (1978) Hemispheric differences in tactuo-spatial processing. Neuropsychologia 16: 247–250.
56. Fagot J, Hopkins WD, Vauclair J (1993) Hand movements and hemispheric specialization in dichhaptic explorations. Perception 22: 847–853.
57. Milner B, Taylor L (1972) Right-hemisphere superiority in tactile pattern-recognition after cerebral commissurotomy: evidence for nonverbal memory. Neuropsychologia 10: 1–15.
58. Varney NR, Benton AL (1975) Tactile perception of direction in relation to handedness and familial handedness. Neuropsychologia 13: 449–454.
59. Squeri V, Sciutti A, Gori M, Masia L, Sandini G, et al. (2012) Two hands, one perception: how bimanual haptic information is combined by the brain. Journal of Neurophysiology 107: 544–550.
60. Heller MA, Joyner TD (1993) Mechanisms in the haptic horizontal-vertical illusion: evidence from sighted and blind subjects. Percept Psychophys 53: 422–428.
61. Riege WH, Metter EJ, Williams MV (1980) Age and hemispheric asymmetry in nonverbal tactual memory. Neuropsychologia 18: 707–710.
62. Fagot J, Lacreuse A, Vauclair J (1994) Hand-movement profiles in a tactual-tactual matching task: effects of spatial factors and laterality. Percept Psychophys 56: 347–355.
63. Fagot J, Lacreuse A, Vauclair J (1993) Haptic discrimination of nonsense shapes: hand exploratory strategies but not accuracy reveal laterality effects. Brain Cogn 21: 212–225.
64. Begliomini C, Nelini C, Caria A, Grodd W, Castiello U (2008) Cortical activations in humans grasp-related areas depend on hand used and handedness. PLoS One 3: e3388.
65. Karl JM, Schneider LR, Whishaw IQ (2013) Nonvisual learning of intrinsic object properties in a reaching task dissociates grasp from reach. Exp Brain Res 225: 465–477.
66. Overvliet KE, Anema HA, Brenner E, Dijkerman HC, Smeets JB (2011) Relative finger position influences whether you can localize tactile stimuli. Exp Brain Res 208: 245–255.

21

In Vitro and *In Vivo* Models of *Staphylococcus aureus* Endophthalmitis Implicate Specific Nutrients in Ocular Infection

Ama Sadaka[1,2,3], Kelli Palmer[1,2,3], Takashi Suzuki[1,2,3], Michael S. Gilmore[1,2,3]*

1 Departments of Ophthalmology, and Microbiology and Molecular Genetics, Harvard Medical School, Boston, Massachusetts, United States of America, **2** The Massachusetts Eye and Ear Infirmary, Boston, Massachusetts, United States of America, **3** Harvard Microbial Sciences Initiative, Cambridge, Massachusetts, United States of America

Abstract

Purpose: To define global transcriptional responses of *Staphylococcus aureus* and its *codY* mutant (CodY is a transcription regulator of virulence and metabolic genes in response to branched-chain amino acids) when growing in bovine aqueous (AH) and vitreous humor (VH) *in vitro*, and to investigate the impact of *codY* deletion on *S. aureus* virulence in a novel murine anterior chamber (AC) infection model.

Methods: For the *in vitro* model, differential transcriptomic gene expression of *S. aureus* and its *codY* mutant grown in chemically defined medium (CDM), AH, and VH was analyzed. Furthermore, the strains were inoculated into the AC of mice. Changes in bacterial growth, electroretinography and inflammation scores were monitored.

Results: Bovine AH and VH provide sufficient nutrition for *S. aureus* growth *in vitro*. Transcriptome analysis identified 72 unique open reading frames differentially regulated ≥10-fold between CDM, AH, and VH. In the AC model, we found comparable growth of the *codY* mutant and wild type strains *in vivo*. Average inflammation scores and retinal function were significantly worse for *codY* mutant-infected eyes at 24 h post-infection.

Conclusion: Our *in vitro* bovine AH and VH models identified likely nutrient sources for *S. aureus* in the ocular milieu. The *in vivo* model suggests that control of branched-chain amino acid availability has therapeutic potential in limiting *S. aureus* endophthalmitis severity.

Editor: José A. Lemos, University of Rochester Medical Center, United States of America

Funding: This project has been funded in part by NIH/NEI grant EY008289. KP was supported by NIH fellowship EY020734. The funders had no role in study design, data collection and analysis, decision to publish, or preparation of the manuscript.

Competing Interests: The authors have declared that no competing interests exist.

* Email: michael_gilmore@meei.harvard.edu

Introduction

Staphylococcus aureus is a commensal bacterium on the skin and mucosa, but is also a leading cause of infections in humans. When opportunistic pathogens infect sterile sites, they adapt, proliferate in the host, and exhibit virulence. The host becomes the sole source for nutrients. For many gram-positive bacteria, CodY provides an important regulatory link between nutrient availability and virulence factor production [1]. CodY controls expression of virulence and metabolic genes in response to the availability of branched-chain amino acids (BCAA) and GTP through Agr, a global regulator of the staphylococcal virulon [2]. In the presence of GTP and/or BCAA, CodY shows a higher affinity for its DNA targets, while in the absence of nutrients, there is a decrease in the GTP and BCAA levels causing decreased affinity of CodY to the DNA and thus induction of its regulon. In *S. aureus*, CodY regulates its regulon either indirectly via the quorum sensing regulator Agr or independent of the Agr system and through its direct binding to its DNA targets [2]. In general, CodY-regulated genes trigger adaptation to starvation [2–9] as well as play a role in virulence of pathogenic bacteria [3,4,10].

The human eye as well as eyes of animals like rabbits and mice possess sterile anterior and posterior compartments, which contain aqueous and vitreous humor, respectively. Infectious endophthalmitis [inflammation within the eye) is a complication of penetrating trauma to the eye and intraocular procedures such as cataract surgery that can lead to blindness [11–14]. The visual prognosis following infection depends greatly on the virulence of the causative organism, visual acuity at presentation, and the efficacy of antimicrobial treatment [15]. *S. aureus* is the second most common cause of acute postoperative infection following intraocular surgeries and is also associated with significant visual loss [15]. Given the presence of BCAA in human aqueous and vitreous humors [16,17] and the findings that CodY controls directly and indirectly *S. aureus* virulence genes such as *hla* and *agr* [1,2] which contribute to virulence in animal models of endophthalmitis [18,19], CodY may play a role in regulating *S. aureus* virulence during endophthalmitis.

S. aureus growth and virulence in animal models of endophthalmitis has been assessed, most frequently by intravitreal (posterior chamber) injection [18,19]. *S. aureus* strains grow *in vivo* to different extents, depending on the strain used and the inoculation site (anterior versus posterior compartments) [20,21]. For example, following injection into the anterior chamber, Balzli, et al. found that among 9 *S. aureus* isolates injected into the anterior chamber of rabbit eyes, only one strain, UMCR1, grew [20]. Wu, et al. [21] and Kowalski, et al. [22] found that *S. aureus* grew in the anterior chamber of rabbits, and used that model to test antibiotic efficacies. Several other studies have found that *S. aureus* can grow to high densities in the vitreous, and studied the contribution of toxins, the global virulence regulators Agr and Sar [18,23], and other cell wall components to pathogenesis. *S. aureus* clearly survives in the human eye, given that *S. aureus* can be recovered from the aqueous and vitreous humors of patients who develop endophthalmitis [24]. It is unknown what nutrient sources *S. aureus* utilizes during infection of the human eye. In this study, we use aqueous and vitreous fluids extracted from commercially-obtained bovine eyes as *ex vivo* endophthalmitis models for *S. aureus*, and define global transcriptional responses of *S. aureus* to growth in these media. Our goal was to identify genes that are consistently and highly differentially regulated by *S. aureus* during growth in pooled bovine AH and VH samples. We additionally interrogate the impact of *codY* deletion on *S. aureus* gene expression during growth in these media, as well as its impact on *S. aureus* virulence in a novel murine anterior chamber (AC) infection model.

Materials and Methods

Strains and growth media

S. aureus strains used are listed in Table 1. *S. aureus* was routinely cultured in brain heart infusion (BHI) or on BHI agar. All cultures were incubated at 37°C. For microarray experiments, *S. aureus* were grown in chemically defined Socransky's medium [25] supplemented with 20 mM glucose (referred to here as CDM), or bovine aqueous or vitreous humor (AH and VH, respectively). CDM contains 76 μM leucine, 85 μM valine, and 76 μM isoleucine. Bacterial growth was assessed by monitoring optical density at 600 nm (OD_{600}) using a Biotech Synergy 2 microplate reader or by serial dilution and plating on BHI agar to obtain colony forming units per milliliter (CFU/mL).

Bovine AH and VH collection

AH and VH were extracted from commercially available bovine eyes (Sierra for Medical Science, Whittier, CA) and pooled as described previously [26]. Typical volumes of AH and VH recovered per bovine eye were 0.5–1 mL and 3–4 mL, respectively. AH was filter-sterilized with a 0.45 μm HT Tuffryn membrane sterile acrodisc syringe filter (Pall Life Sciences, Batavia, IL). VH was filter-sterilized with a 0.45 μm PES sterile filter (Whatman, Clifton, NJ). Sterile AH and VH were stored at −80°C until use. For microarray experiments, aspirates were pooled to a total of 40 mL achieve adequate volume.

Microarray analysis

S. aureus strains were struck from freezer stock onto BHI agar and incubated overnight. Colonies were used to inoculate CDM, AH or VH broth cultures, which were incubated overnight and then used to inoculate new CDM, AH and VH broth cultures to an initial OD_{600} of 0.02–0.03. Bacteria were harvested for microarray analysis and semi-quantitative RT-PCR analyses during exponential growth, at an OD_{600} of 0.4–0.5 for CDM and 0.15–0.2 for AH and VH. Cells were stabilized with RNAProtect (Qiagen) and RNA was extracted using the RNA Bee reagent (TelTest, Inc.) per the manufacturer's instructions. Absence of DNA contamination was verified by PCR using primers targeting the 16S rRNA gene (For, 5′-AAC TCT GTT ATT AGG GAA GAA C-3′; Rev, 5′-CCA CCT TCC TCC GGT TTG TCA CC-3′). cDNA synthesis, fragmentation, biotin labeling and hybridization to Affymetrix *S. aureus* GeneChips were performed as previously described [27]. Hybridization and scanning of GeneChips were performed at the University of Iowa DNA Core. Microarray experiments were performed in duplicate. Affymetrix GeneChip data was analyzed with GeneChip Operating Software (GCOS version 1.4). Probe sets with statistically significant change calls (increased or decreased; $p \leq 0.05$) between control and test conditions were considered for further analysis, and fold change cut-offs were applied as described in the text. Microarray data have been deposited in ArrayExpress under accession numbers E-MTAB-2928.

For the Affymetrix *S. aureus* GeneChip, probe set IDs (for example, sa_c10261s8939_a_at) are used instead of gene names or ORF designations. To convert probe set IDs to genomic loci, we downloaded target DNA sequences corresponding to differentially expressed probe sets from the NetAffx Analysis Center (www.affymetrix.com/analysis/index.affx). Target sequences were compared to available *S. aureus* sequences in GenBank using NCBI BLAST (http://blast.ncbi.nlm.nih.gov). Transcription unit and metabolic pathway predictions were obtained from the BioCyc *Staphylococcus aureus* COL database (http://biocyc.org/organism-summary?object=SAUR93062). Where appropriate, predicted protein products of differentially expressed genes were analyzed for putative functions using NCBI protein BLAST and Pfam 26.0 (http://pfam.janelia.org). Subcellular localization of proteins was predicted using PSORTb version 3.0 (http://www.psort.org/).

Semiquantitative RT-PCR

Semiquantitative reverse transcription (RT)-PCR was performed using Superscript II reverse transcriptase as outlined by the manufacturer (Invitrogen). *S. aureus* RNA was used to make cDNA with priming by random hexamers. cDNA was purified

Table 1. Bacterial strains used in this study.

S. aureus strain	Description	Reference/source
SA564	Clinical isolate	[48]
CDM7	SA564 Δ*codY*::*ermC*	[29]
MS7	SA564 Δ*codY*::*ermC* pTL6936-*codY*	[29]

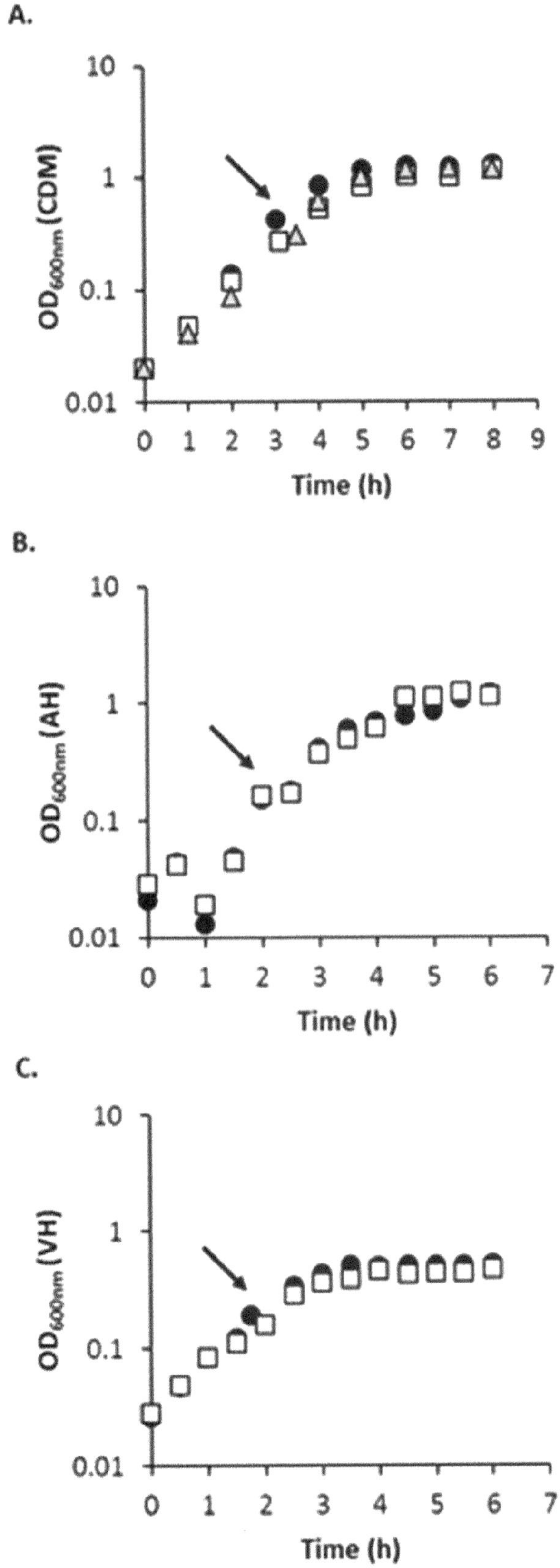

Figure 1. *S. aureus* growth in CDM, AH and VH. *S. aureus* SA564 (black circles), CDM7 (white squares), and MS7 (grey triangles) were grown in CDM, AH, or VH, as described in the text. Growth was monitored by optical density at 600 nm ($OD_{600\ nm}$). Representative growth curves are shown. Arrows indicate time points where microarray sampling occurred.

with the QIAquick PCR Purification kit (Qiagen). Five ng of the resulting purified cDNA was used as template in a 25 µl standard PCR reaction with Taq polymerase (New England Biolabs). For visualization, 5 µl of the PCR reaction was analyzed using agarose gel electrophoresis with ethidium bromide. The housekeeping gene *clpX* was used as a control for gene expression. Expression of *tst*, *cidA* and *nanA* was evaluated. Those genes were chosen based on their significant differential regulation across media (*nanA* was 54.8 in AH vs DM; *cidA* was 12.8 in VH vs DM; *tst* was 15.2 in AH vs DM). An independent set of pooled fluids was used for this experiment.

Murine AC infection model

Female C57BL/6J mice were obtained from the Charles River Laboratory (Boston, MA). All animals were treated according to the guidelines of the Association for Research in Vision and Ophthalmology Resolution on the Use of Animals in Research. The protocol was approved by Massachusetts Eye and Ear Infirmary's Institutional Animal Care and Use Committee (IACUC). Mice were anesthetized by intraperitoneal injection of ketamine (62.5 mg/kg) and xylazine (12.5 mg/kg). Animals were euthanized at the appropriate time points by CO_2 asphyxiation.

S. aureus colonies obtained after growth on BHI agar were cultured overnight in BHI broth and subcultured 1:500 with fresh BHI broth and grown to an $OD_{600\ nm}$ of 0.4–0.8, pelleted by centrifugation at 10,000 rpm, and washed twice with PBS. The ACs of the right eyes of 6–8-week-old female mice were inoculated with 1 µL of *S. aureus* culture using 35 gauge needle on a nanofil syringe (World Precision Instruments, Inc.), just anterior to the limbus without touching the iris. For *S. aureus* MS7, 2 mM isopropyl β-D-1-thiogalactopyranoside (IPTG) was added to subcultures and included in PBS washes. The left eyes were left untreated and served as internal controls for electroretinography (ERG). Experiments were performed at least in duplicate with a minimum of 3 animals per experimental group. Animals were given water with 12 mM IPTG for one week prior to infection with *S. aureus* MS7. Quantification of in vivo bacterial growth, slitlamp examination and ERG were performed as described previously [28]. Briefly, intraocular inflammation was graded using the following criteria: 0, normal; 1, small amount of fibrin on the pupil; 2, iris partially covered with fibrin and/or hypopyon; 3, iris covered with fibrin and/or hypopyon; 4, pupil not visible. The retinal function in the infected eye was measured using ERG and was defined as the ratio of the b-wave (measured from the trough of the a-wave to the peak of the b-wave) amplitude of the experimentally treated eye to that of the contralateral untreated eye, times 100.

Histological analysis

Enucleated eyes were fixed in buffered formalin solution and histological analysis was performed by Excalibur Pathology Inc. (Oklahoma City, OK). Pathology slides were examined for signs and extent of inflammation in the different compartments of the eye, and disruption in retinal architecture.

Statistical analysis

Normality tests were performed on all data sets. The data were analyzed with an unpaired t-test if the distribution was Gaussian, or with the nonparametric Mann-Whitney test if the data were not normally distributed. $P \leq 0.05$ was set as the basis for rejection of

Table 2. Transcriptomes of AH- and VH-grown *S. aureus* SA564.

ORF/intergenic region[a]	Gene[a]	Description of gene or queried region	AH vs DM Fold change[b]	VH vs DM Fold change[c]	VH vs AH Fold change[d]
Genes putatively involved in nutrient transport or metabolism					
SACOL0154	*aldA1*	Aldehyde dehydrogenase	13.2 (3.3)	*5.0 (1.1)*	
SACOL0173	*ipdC*	Indole-3-pyruvate decarboxylase	12.1 (2.2)	12.1 (1.3)	
SACOL0176		Conserved hypothetical protein	42.2 (1.1)	*3.9 (1.3)*	−10.9 (1.3)
SACOL0177	*murQ*	Glucokinase regulator-related protein	27.4 (1.2)		−11.5 (1.2)
SACOL0178[e]		PTS system, IIBC components	21.1 (1.2)		*−8.3 (1.3)*
SACOL0179		Phosphosugar-binding transcriptional regulator, RpiR family	12.1 (1.2)		*−6.2 (1.5)*
SACOL0192		Maltose ABC transporter, ATP-binding protein, putative	21.5 (1.5)		*−6.5 (1.6)*
SACOL0193		Maltose ABC transporter, maltose-binding protein, putative	14.4 (1.3)	*3.4 (1.2)*	*−4.2 (1.4)*
SACOL0194		Maltose ABC transporter permease protein	11.1 (1.5)	*3.3 (1.4)*	*−3.7 (1.4)*
SACOL0195		Maltose ABC transporter permease protein	13.9 (1.5)	*3.7 (1.4)*	*−3.4 (1.5)*
SACOL0196		Oxidoreductase, Gfo/Idh/MocA family	12.6 (1.5)	*3.3 (1.3)*	*−3.9 (1.5)*
SACOL0197		Oxidoreductase, Gfo/Idh/MocA family	10.2 (1.4)	*3.2 (1.1)*	*−3.2 (1.4)*
SACOL0198		Conserved hypothetical protein	10.7 (1.4)	*3.1 (1.3)*	*−3.1 (1.2)*
SACOL0200[e]		Phosphoglycerate transporter family protein	44.5 (1.4)		−27.9 (1.6)
SACOL0204	*pflB*	Formate acetyltransferase	16.0 (2.7)		*−4.4 (2.0)*
SACOL0205	*pflA*	Pyruvate formate-lyase-activating enzyme	11.5 (2.5)	*4.3 (1.8)*	
SACOL0215		Propionate CoA-transferase, putative		10.7 (1.4)	
SACOL0308[e]	(*yeiC*)	Carbohydrate kinase, PfkB family	54.8 (1.5)		−40.1 (1.8)
SACOL0309	(*yeiN*)	Conserved hypothetical protein	45.3 (1.6)		−38.7 (1.7)
SACOL0310	(*yeiM*)	Nucleoside permease NupC, putative	28.3 (2.1)		−32.0 (1.7)
SACOL0311	*nanT*	Sodium:solute symporter family protein	38.1 (1.7)		−13.2 (1.7)
SACOL0312	*nanA*	N-acetylneuraminate lyase	54.8 (1.7)	*3.5 (1.3)*	−14.4 (1.7)
SACOL0400	(*ulaA*)	Transport protein SgaT, putative	13.7 (1.4)		−12.6 (1.4)
SACOL0401	(*ulaB*)	Conserved hypothetical protein	20.7 (1.4)		−16.0 (1.5)
SACOL0402	(*ulaC*)	PTS system, IIA component	29.3 (1.4)		−23.8 (1.4)
SACOL0403		Transcriptional antiterminator, BglG family	28.3 (1.4)		−28.3 (1.6)
ig_SACOL0913		Intergenic region downstream of SACOL0913	−15.2 (1.9)	*−6.3 (2.4)*	
SACOL0960	*rocD2*	Ornithine aminotransferase	10.0 (2.0)	*3.5 (1.2)*	
SACOL1360		Aspartate kinase	10.6 (5.9)	*6.0 (1.3)*	
SACOL1734	*gapA2*	Glyceraldehyde-3-phosphate dehydrogenase	10.4 (4.9)		*−6.8 (4.9)*
SACOL1784	*acuA*	Acetoin utilization protein AcuA	13.7 (3.6)		
SACOL1785		Acetoin utilization protein AcuC	10.6 (3.2)		
SACOL1816	*putA*	Proline dehydrogenase	21.1 (1.7)	*3.7 (1.4)*	*−5.4 (1.7)*
SACOL2163		Conserved hypothetical protein	11.7 (1.4)	*7.2 (1.5)*	
SACOL2247		Hypothetical protein	−19.7 (7)		
SACOL2356		ABC transporter, ATP-binding protein			−10.0 (2.7)
SACOL2357		ABC transporter, permease protein			−10.6 (2.9)
SACOL2403		ABC transporter, substrate binding protein	*−6.7 (1.5)*	−15.7 (1.5)	
SACOL2415	*gpm*	Phosphoglycerate mutase	10.9 (1.7)	12.1 (1.6)	
SACOL2427	*bioA*	Adenosylmethionine-8-amino-7-oxononanoate aminotransferase	*8.3 (3.5)*	13.9 (1.5)	
SACOL2428	*bioD*	Dethiobiotin synthase	16.0 (3.9)	24.3 (1.7)	
SACOL2441		Amino acid permease	10.6 (4.4)	*3.9 (1.7)*	
SACOL2527		Fructose-1,6-bisphosphatase, putative	11.3 (2)	*6.7 (1.2)*	

Table 2. Cont.

ORF/intergenic region[a]	Gene[a]	Description of gene or queried region	AH vs DM Fold change[b]	VH vs DM Fold change[c]	VH vs AH Fold change[d]
Putative or confirmed virulence and biofilm factors					
SACOL0247	*lrgA*	Holin-like protein LrgA	*7.0 (3.8)*		−14.4 (4.0)
SACOL0248	*lrgB*	LrgB protein	*6.3 (4.1)*		−11.1 (3.8)
SACOL1187		Antibacterial protein (phenol soluble modulin)	10.4 (2.5)		*−6.5 (1.8)*
SACOL2509	*fnbB*	Fibronectin binding protein B		−13.0 (1.3)	
SACOL2554_1	*cidA*	LrgA family protein		12.8 (1.4)	34.9 (1.4)
SACOL2652	*clfB* (rev comp)	Queries 97 nt region complementary to the 5′ end of *clfB* (clumping factor B)	−30.4 (1.2)	*−6.4 (2.0)*	
SACOL2694	*geh*	Lipase	19.4 (1.4)	*3.7 (1.3)*	*−4.4 (1.5)*
SA1817[f]	*sec3*	Enterotoxin type C3	10.9 (3.0)		*−6.9 (2.4)*
SA1819[f]	*tst*	Toxic shock syndrome toxin-1	15.2 (5.5)		*−8.3 (5.7)*
Probable prophage or genomic island genes of unknown significance					
SACOL0325[g]		Prophage L54a, antirepressor, putative	−23.8 (2.2)	*−9.9 (2.0)*	
SACOL0326[g]		Hypothetical protein	−26.4 (2.4)	−15.7 (2.2)	
SAOUHSC_02028 [e]		φETA ORF57-like protein	−22.6 (1.9)	−25.5 (1.4)	
SAOUHSC_02078		φPV83 orf 10-like protein	−20.0 (2.0)	−10.4 (1.8)	
SAOUHSC_02206		Hypothetical phage protein	−10.4 (1.6)	*−9.5 (1.6)*	
SAV0859[h]		Hypothetical protein	−17.1 (1.7)	*−8.0 (2.3)*	
ig_SAV0860[h]		Intergenic region downstream of SAV0860	−14.2 (1.8)	−10.7 (1.9)	
SAV0905[h]		Similar to φETA ORF57-like protein	−22.6 (1.9)	−25.5 (1.4)	
SAV1985[i]		Hypothetical protein	−17.4 (1.9)	−11.5 (2.0)	

[a] ORFs were identified by BLAST analysis of Affymetrix array target sequences, as described in the materials and methods. If a corresponding ORF was identified in *S. aureus* COL, that strain's ORF identifiers were used as default. SACOL####, *S. aureus* COL (GenBank accession number CP000046.1); SAV####, *S. aureus* Mu50 (BA000017.4); SA####, *S. aureus* N315 (BA000018.3); SAOUHSC_####, *S. aureus* NCTC 8325 (CP000253.1). Vertical lines indicate genes computationally predicted to be in the same transcriptional unit. Gene names in brackets were assigned in this study using data shown in Table S1.
[b] Fold change in expression of genes during *S. aureus* SA564 growth in AH as compared to growth in glucose-supplemented CDM; a positive number indicates an up-regulation of the gene during growth in AH. Standard deviation is shown in parentheses. Fold changes ≥3 and <10 are shown and italicized.
[c] Fold change in expression of genes during *S. aureus* SA564 growth in VH as compared to growth in glucose-supplemented CDM; a positive number indicates an up-regulation of the gene during growth in VH. Standard deviation is shown in parentheses. Fold changes ≥3 and <10 are shown and italicized.
[d] Fold change in expression of genes during *S. aureus* SA564 growth in VH as compared to growth in AH; a positive number indicates an up-regulation of the gene during growth in VH. Standard deviation is shown in parentheses. Fold changes ≥3 and <10 are shown and italicized.
[e] At least two differentially expressed probe sets were assigned to these ORFs. Data for all probe sets are shown in Table S1.
[f] On genomic island *v*SA4 [48].
[g] On φCOL [48].
[h] On φSa1 [48].
[i] On φSa3 [48].

the null hypothesis. The statistical analysis was conducted with the aid of the Harvard Catalyst Biostatistical Consulting Program.

Results

S. aureus SA564 *in vitro* growth in bovine AH and VH

S. aureus SA564 is a clinical isolate that was previously used to evaluate a role for *codY* in *S. aureus* virulence regulation [29]. As a first step in understanding *S. aureus* physiology and metabolism during endophthalmitis, we evaluated *S. aureus* SA564 growth in pooled AH and VH harvested from commercially obtained bovine eyes. *S. aureus* SA564 was also grown in Sokransky's medium, a buffered, defined medium supplying amino acids, vitamins, nucleobases, metals, and other growth factors [25], supplemented with 20 mM glucose as a carbon source. For the purposes of this manuscript, Sokransky's medium with 20 mM glucose is referred to as CDM. Representative growth curves for *S. aureus* SA564 as assessed by $OD_{600\ nm}$ are shown in Fig. 1. These data demonstrate that CDM, pooled bovine AH, and pooled bovine VH support *in vitro* growth of *S. aureus* SA564. We reproducibly observed a clumping phenotype early in *S. aureus in vitro* AH growth, resulting in reduced cell density measurements obtained by $OD_{600\ nm}$, as shown in Fig. 1. Also of note, one pooled AH sample did not support robust *S. aureus in vitro* growth (data not shown), possibly as a result of antimicrobials such as antibiotics or inflammatory factors present in one or more individual AH samples. We were unable to obtain additional information from the vendor about the health and history of cows used in this study.

Transcriptome analysis of AH- and VH-grown *S. aureus* SA564

We used Affymetrix GeneChips to examine gene expression of *S. aureus* SA564 during growth in bovine AH and VH, using CDM-grown SA564 as a control. Cells were harvested for microarray analysis during exponential growth; representative time points are indicated by arrows in Fig. 1. Microarrays were

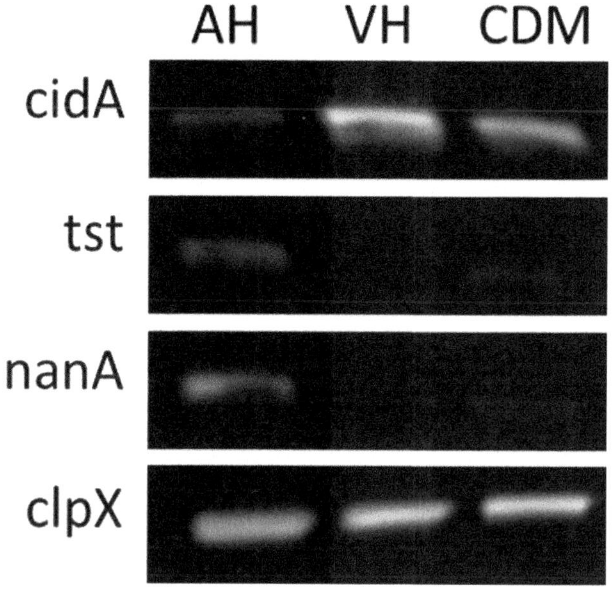

Figure 2. Semi-quantitative RT-PCR. Differential expression of *tst*, *nanA* and *cidA* in AH, VH and CDM. *clpX* was used as a constitutively expressed control gene.

performed in duplicate for each growth condition. The *S. aureus* GeneChip was designed using genome sequence from the *S. aureus* strains N315, Mu50, NCTC 8325, and COL, and queries over 3300 ORFs and intergenic regions [30]. Genome sequence data are not available for *S. aureus* SA564. For transcriptome experiments with wild-type SA564 and its isogenic *codY* mutant CDM7 (discussed further below), we obtained statistically significant hybridization over the background for an average of 64.8% of probe sets (range, 57–71.8% over 12 chips), corresponding to ~3763 probe sets queried.

We performed three comparative analyses of wild-type *S. aureus* SA564 transcriptomes. AH-grown cells compared to CDM-grown cells (to model growth of *S. aureus* in the anterior chamber), VH-grown cells compared to CDM-grown cells (to model growth of *S. aureus* in the posterior chamber), and VH-grown cells compared to AH-grown cells (to model transcriptional changes potentially occurring after translocation of *S. aureus* from the anterior to posterior chambers). A fold change cut-off of 10 was used to consider the most highly differentially regulated genes in each condition. For the *S. aureus* GeneChip, probe set IDs (for example, sa_c10261s8939_a_at) are used instead of gene names or ORF assignments. To convert differentially expressed probe set IDs to meaningful *S. aureus* genomic loci, we compared target DNA sequences corresponding to differentially expressed probe sets to *S. aureus* sequences in GenBank (see Materials and Methods).

A total of 78 unique probe sets corresponding to 72 ORFs, regulatory RNAs and intergenic regions were differentially regulated at least 10-fold across the three comparisons (Table 2 and Table S1). Table S1 is an expanded version of Table 2 showing probe set IDs, BLAST hit distribution among *S. aureus* COL, Mu50, N315, and NCTC 8325 genomes, and fold change data for every gene shown in Table 2, irrespective of meeting the fold change cut-off of 10. Fold changes ≥3 and <10 are also shown in Table 2 and are italicized. Two probe sets identified as being differentially regulated in the VH versus CDM analysis, sa_i7808d_x_at and sa_i9119u10r_x_at, query similar sequence at non-syntenic regions of multiple *S. aureus* genomes and could not be assigned to a single genomic locus (Table S1). Eleven of the differentially expressed probe sets identified for the two comparisons using CDM-grown cells as controls had high standard deviations (Table S1). Further investigation of the CDM control arrays revealed that those 11 probe sets were themselves differentially expressed between the two CDM controls (Table S1). Data for those 11 probe sets are shown only in Table S1. No other potential conflicts were detected in the control CDM arrays.

The differentially expressed genes identified by our microarray analysis can be divided into three categories: (1) genes putatively involved in transport or metabolism of nutrients; (2) putative or confirmed virulence and/or biofilm factors; and (3) probable prophage or genomic island genes of unknown significance. Perhaps not surprisingly, most differentially expressed genes in the analysis were assigned to the first category.

Several putative transcriptional units are highly up-regulated during growth in AH as compared to CDM, and are also down-regulated during VH growth compared to AH, suggesting that the corresponding carbon substrates may be specific to or more abundant in AH. These include SACOL0308-0310, putatively involved in pseudouridine transport and catabolism; SACOL0311-0312, encoding an operon required for sialic acid catabolism in *S. aureus* [30]; and SACOL0400-0403, putatively involved in ascorbate uptake. In addition to these genes, SACOL0176-0179, SACOL0192-0195, and SACOL0200 are upregulated during growth in AH, and each appear to involved in the uptake of and transcriptional response to sugars or phosphosugars (Table S1).

We additionally identified genes putatively involved in lysine biosynthesis from aspartate (SACOL1360, *bioA*, *bioD*) and gluconeogenesis (*gpm*, SACOL2527) as being up-regulated during growth in both AH and VH as compared to CDM, suggesting that their regulation is specific to growth in ocular fluids. Another gene putatively involved in gluconeogenesis, *gapA2*, was also differentially regulated, but its up-regulation was specific to AH growth.

We also observed differential regulation of a set of putative prophage and/or genomic island genes (Table 2). Interestingly, all of these genes were down-regulated in both AH and VH relative to growth in CDM, suggesting that increased expression of these genes is CDM-specific. The significance of this is unknown. Additionally, because genome sequence is not available for SA564 and thus the extent of its accessory genome is unknown, we cannot exclude the possibility of AH- and/or VH-specific differential regulation of prophage, plasmid and island genes that are not represented on the *S. aureus* Affymetrix chip.

Our microarray analysis was verified using semiquantitative RT-PCR to verify expression of a few genes discussed including *tst*, *cidA* and *nanA* (Figure 2). A more intense signal was observed for *tst* and *nanA* from AH samples when compared to CDM, and *cidA* signal was more intense in VH when compared to CDM. The results are consistent with the differential regulation of those genes in our microarray analysis.

The *S. aureus* SA564 *codY* mutant in CDM, AH, and VH

We speculated that *codY* might have a role in ocular infections given the presence of leucine, isoleucine and valine in human AH and VH [16,17,31,32] and given the possibility that those substrates might become depleted during *in vivo S. aureus* growth. We first explored the effect of *codY* deletion on SA564 transcriptional responses to CDM, bovine AH and bovine VH, using the previously described SA564 *codY*-mutant strain, CDM7 [29]. Using GeneChip analysis, we identified 130 probe sets as being differentially expressed ≥5-fold, corresponding to 125

Table 3. Genes differentially expressed by the *S. aureus* SA564 *codY* mutant during growth in CDM, AH and VH.

ORF[a]	Gene	Description of gene or queried region	DM Fold change[b]	AH Fold change[b]	VH Fold change[b]
SA1817	*sec3*	Enterotoxin type C3	6.7 (1.2)		
SACOL0136	*cap5A*	Capsular polysaccharide biosynthesis protein Cap5A	8.0 (1.6)		
SACOL0138	*cap5C*	Capsular polysaccharide biosynthesis protein Cap5C	6.2 (1.9)		
SACOL0185		Peptide ABC transporter permease	53.8 (1.3)	6.5 (1.9)	11.5 (1.2)
SACOL0186		Peptide ABC transporter permease	31.5 (1.2)	5.9 (1.9)	10.9 (1.1)
SACOL0187		RGD-containing lipoprotein	29.3 (1.3)		11.9 (1.1)
SACOL0188	*ggt*	γ-glutamyltranspeptidase	13.0 (1.2)		7.1 (1.1)
SACOL0214		Long-chain-fatty-acid-CoA ligase			6.3 (2.4)
SACOL0215		Propionate CoA-transferase			8.4 (1.5)
SACOL0222	*ldh1*	L-lactate dehydrogenase	7.9 (2.2)		
SACOL0267		Hypothetical protein	7.2 (1.0)		
SACOL0270		Staphyloxanthin biosynthesis protein	6.5 (1.4)		
SACOL0271		Hypothetical protein	5.3 (1.1)		
SACOL0274		Hypothetical protein	5.0 (3.2)		
SACOL0308[c]		Carbohydrate kinase (3′ region)		−7.2 (1.7)	
SACOL0309		Hypothetical protein		−6.8 (1.7)	
SACOL0310		Nucleoside permease NupC		−7.2 (2.0)	
SACOL0427		Hypothetical protein	7.5 (1.1)		
SACOL0428	*metE*	5-methyltetrahydropteroyltriglutamate/homocysteine S-methyltransferase	19.7 (1.2)		9.2 (1.6)
SACOL0429		Bifunctional homocysteine S-methyltransferase/5,10-methylenetetrahydrofolate reductase	28.3 (1.2)		11.5 (1.4)
SACOL0430		Trans-sulfuration enzyme family protein	36.1 (1.1)		12.8 (1.1)
SACOL0431		Trans-sulfuration enzyme family protein	30.9 (1.1)		10.4 (1.1)
SACOL0431 rev comp		Reverse complement of interior 105 nt region of SACOL0431	11.1 (1.4)		
ig_SACOL0431-2		121 nt region upstream of SACOL0431	12.3 (1.7)		
SACOL0480		Hypothetical protein	9.7 (1.2)		
SACOL0502		Cysteine synthase/cystathionine beta-synthase	7.6 (2.0)		
SACOL0503[c]	*metB*	Cystathionine γ-synthase	7.1 (2.0)		
SACOL0504		ABC transporter ATP-binding protein	30.4 (2.1)		
SACOL0505		ABC transporter permease	29.3 (2.4)		
SACOL0506		ABC transporter substrate-binding protein	18.4 (1.5)		
SACOL0514	*gltB*	Glutamate synthase	23.4 (1.3)		12.1 (1.5)
SACOL0515	*gltD*	Glutamate synthase, small subunit	15.7 (1.3)		9.8 (1.2)
ig_SACOL0701-2 rev comp		Reverse complement of intergenic region between SACOL0701-2; 5′ 106 nt overlap RsaD sRNA from Geissmann, et al. 2009 Nucleic Acids Res	20.4 (2.1)	5.4 (1.4)	9.2 (1.4)
SACOL0796		Iron compound ABC transporter permease	−5.5 (2.3)		
SACOL0797		Iron compound ABC transporter permease	−5.8 (2.0)		
SACOL0798		Iron compound ABC transporter ATP-binding protein	−6.0 (2.3)		
SACOL0815		Ribosomal subunit interface protein	5.5 (1.7)		
SACOL0860	*nuc*	Thermonuclease precursor	9.2 (1.2)		5.3 (1.3)
SACOL0991	*oppB*	Oligopeptide ABC transport permease	10.7 (1.3)		
SACOL0992	*oppC*	Oligopeptide ABC transporter permease	11.5 (1.4)		
SACOL0993	*oppD*	Oligopeptide ABC transporter ATP-binding protein	8.3 (1.3)		
SACOL0994	*oppF*	Oligopeptide ABC transporter ATP-binding protein	7.9 (1.2)		
SACOL0995		Oligopeptide ABC transporter oligopeptide-binding protein	8.3 (1.2)		
SACOL1018		Sodium:alanine symporter family protein	21.9 (1.2)	9.9 (3.4)	15.7 (1.7)

Table 3. Cont.

ORF[a]	Gene	Description of gene or queried region	DM Fold change[b]	AH Fold change[b]	VH Fold change[b]
ig_SACOL1018-9		Intergenic region between SACOL1018 and SACOL1019		12.3 (1.7)	21.9 (3.7)
SACOL1019		Hypothetical protein	6.1 (1.1)		
SACOL1033		Hypothetical protein	8.9 (1.5)		
SACOL1038		Membrane protein	9.5 (1.2)	6.3 (2.1)	12.3 (1.3)
SACOL1039		Hypothetical protein	7.0 (1.2)	5.6 (1.6)	13.0 (1.5)
SACOL1040		ABC transporter ATP-binding protein	9.4 (1.5)	7.6 (2.0)	8.4 (1.6)
SACOL1186		Antibacterial protein (phenol soluble modulin)	6.8 (2.6)		
SACOL1187		Antibacterial protein (phenol soluble modulin)	6.8 (2.4)		
SACOL1272[c]	*codY*	Transcriptional repressor CodY	−789.6 (1.1)	−652.6 (1.4)	−197.4 (1.5)
SACOL1360		Aspartate kinase	30.4 (1.3)		
SACOL1362	*hom*	Homoserine dehydrogenase	16.3 (1.3)		
SACOL1363	*thrC*	Threonine synthase	17.5 (1.4)		
SACOL1364	*thrB*	Homoserine kinase	14.9 (1.3)		
SACOL1368	*katA*	Catalase	5.3 (1.7)		
SACOL1403	*trpE*	Anthranilate synthase component I	6.0 (1.4)		
SACOL1404	*trpG*	Anthranilate synthase component II	6.4 (1.5)		
SACOL1405	*trpD*	Anthranilate phosphoribosyltransferase	8.6 (1.6)		6.5 (1.1)
SACOL1406	*trpC*	Indole-3-glycerol-phosphage synthase	13.7 (1.5)		7.7 (1.2)
SACOL1407	*trpF*	N-(5′-phosphoribosyl)anthranilate isomerase	21.9 (1.5)		10.0 (1.3)
SACOL1408	*trpB*	Tryptophan synthase subunit β	18.4 (1.7)		6.7 (1.2)
SACOL1409	*trpA*	tryptophan synthase subunit α	6.1 (1.4)		
SACOL1428	*lysC*	Aspartate kinase	10.9 (1.7)		
SACOL1429	*asd*	Aspartate semialdehyde dehydrogenase	14.2 (1.4)		
SACOL1430	*dapA*	Dihydrodipicolinate synthase	13.5 (1.2)		
SACOL1431	*dapB*	Dihydrodipicolinate reductase	14.4 (1.2)		
SACOL1432	*dapD*	2,3,4,5-tetrahydropyridine-2,6-dicarboxylate N-succinyltransferase	13.0 (1.1)		
ig_SACOL1432-3		Intergenic region between *dapD* and SACOL1433	26.4 (1.8)		
SACOL1433		M20/M25/M40 family peptidase	9.2 (1.3)		
SACOL1434		Alanine racemase	9.2 (1.2)		
SACOL1449	*sucA*	2-oxoglutarate dehydrogenase E1 component	5.2 (1.1)		
SACOL1772		Class V aminotransferase	24.3 (1.2)	5.4 (2.9)	13.7 (1.2)
SACOL1773	*serA*	D-3-phosphoglycerate dehydrogenase	21.5 (1.3)		11.9 (1.2)
SACOL2003	*hlb*	Queries 170 nt (positions 19–188) in 5′ region of *hlb* (phospholipase C)	5.6 (1.3)		
SACOL2021-2	RNAIII	3′ 345 nt of RNAIII; probes region downstream of δ-hemolysin gene	12.1 (3.2)		
SACOL2022	*hld*	δ-hemolysin	10.4 (3.8)		
SACOL2031		Ammonium transporter family protein	11.1 (1.3)	5.0 (1.9)	5.6 (1.2)
ig_SACOL2041-2		Intergenic region upstream of SACOL2042 *ilvD* (*ilvD* promoter region)	23.4 (4.3)		
SACOL2042	*ilvD*	Dihydroxy-acid dehydratase	48.5 (1.4)	11.3 (5.4)	26.4 (1.4)
SACOL2043	*ilvB*	Acetolactate synthase large subunit	80.2 (1.2)		39.4 (1.2)
SACOL2044		Acetolactate synthase 1 regulatory subunit	157.6 (1.7)	8.6 (3.1)	85.9 (1.4)
ig_SACOL2044-5		Intergenic region between SACOL2044 and *ilvC*			33.7 (1.3)
SACOL2045	*ilvC*	Ketol-acid reductoisomerase	100.4 (1.3)	5.3 (2.2)	61.8 (1.3)
SACOL2046	*leuA*	2-isopropylmalate synthase	109.5 (1.2)		64.0 (1.3)
SACOL2047	*leuB*	3-isopropylmalate dehydrogenase	89.0 (1.3)	5.2 (2.3)	64.0 (1.4)

Table 3. Cont.

ORF[a]	Gene	Description of gene or queried region	DM Fold change[b]	AH Fold change[b]	VH Fold change[b]
SACOL2048	*leuC*	Isopropylmalate isomerase large subunit	95.3 (1.2)		62.9 (1.4)
SACOL2049	*leuD*	Isopropylmalate isomerase small subunit	107.6 (1.2)	5.2 (1.7)	76.1 (1.2)
SACOL2050	*ilvA2*	Threonine dehydratase	78.8 (1.2)	5.2 (1.9)	41.5 (1.2)
SACOL2314		Sodium/bile acid symporter family protein	7.7 (1.1)		
SACOL2403		ABC transporter substrate-binding protein	−5.5 (1.4)		
SACOL2554.1		LrgA family protein			−5.0 (1.5)
SACOL2585		Hypothetical protein	20.0 (1.2)	7.7 (2.8)	10.2 (1.5)
ig_SACOL2585-4		Intergenic region downstream of SACOL2585	6.1 (1.1)		
SACOL2619		Amino acid permease	19.0 (1.2)	6.6 (2.9)	9.2 (1.7)
SACOL2620		4-aminobutyrate aminotransferase	29.3 (1.3)	9.0 (3.6)	16.0 (1.5)
ig_SACOL2620-1		Intergenic region upstream of SACOL2620	34.3 (1.3)	7.9 (3.4)	20.4 (2.1)
SACOL2627	*betA*	Choline dehydrogenase	5.0 (2.4)		
SACOL2628	*betB*	Betaine aldehyde dehydrogenase	5.4 (2.4)		
SACOL2641	*gpxA2*	Glutathione peroxidase	6.4 (1.4)		
ig_SACOL2641-2		Intergenic region between SACOL2642 and *gpxA2* (SACOL2641)	8.3 (1.6)		
ig_SACOL2641-2 rev comp		Reverse complement of intergenic region between SACOL2642 and *gpxA2*	6.5 (1.8)		
SACOL2659	*aur*	Zinc metalloproteinase aureolysin	12.3 (1.6)	5.1 (1.4)	9.2 (1.5)
SACOL2689	*icaA*	N-glycosyltransferase	6.7 (1.1)		
SACOL2690	*icaD*	Intercellular adhesion protein D	7.5 (1.3)		
ig_SACOL2695-6		Intergenic region between SACOL2696 (*hisI*) and SACOL2695	18.7 (1.5)		6.0 (1.5)
SACOL2696	*hisI*	Bifunctional phosphoribosyl-AMP cyclohydrolase/phosphoribosyl-ATP	14.7 (1.2)		11.5 (1.3)
SACOL2697	*hisF*	Imidazole glycerol phosphate synthase subunit HisF	16.6 (1.2)		12.3 (1.2)
SACOL2698	*hisA*	1-(5-phosphoribosyl)-5-((5-phosphoribosylamino)methylideneamino) imidazole-4-carboxamide isomerase	16.9 (1.2)		18.4 (1.4)
SACOL2699	*hisH*	Imidazole glycerol phosphate synthase subunit HisH	20.7 (1.1)		14.9 (1.5)
SACOL2700	*hisB*	Imidazoleglycerol-phosphate dehydratase	22.2 (1.0)		13.9 (1.2)
SACOL2701		Histidinol-phosphate aminotransferase	24.2 (1.1)		16.9 (1.2)
SACOL2702	*hisD*	Histidinol dehydrogenase	24.3 (1.1)		14.9 (1.1)
SACOL2703	*hisG*	ATP phosphoribosyltransferase catalytic subunit	27.9 (1.1)		11.5 (1.2)
SACOL2704	*hisZ*	ATP phosphoribosyltransferase regulatory subunit	23.0 (1.1)		16.9 (1.1)
ig_SACOL2704-5		Intergenic region between SACOL2705-4	11.7 (1.9)		8.7 (1.5)
SACOL2705		Hypothetical protein	13.9 (1.3)		10.9 (1.1)
ig_SACOL2705-6		Intergenic region between SACOL2706-5		6.1 (1.8)	
SACOL2706		Hypothetical protein	18.7 (1.1)		19.4 (1.5)
SACOL2707		Cobalt transport family protein	20.0 (1.2)		16.9 (1.3)
SACOL2708		ABC transporter ATP-binding protein	30.4 (1.3)		19.7 (1.1)
SACOL2709		Hypothetical protein	31.5 (1.5)		13.5 (1.3)
SACOL2710		Hypothetical protein	59.7 (1.3)	8.6 (3.6)	24.7 (1.3)

[a] ORFs were identified by BLAST analysis of Affymetrix array target sequences, as described in the materials and methods. If a corresponding ORF was identified in *S. aureus* COL, that strain's ORF identifiers were used as default. SACOL####, *S. aureus* COL (GenBank accession number CP000046.1); SAV####, *S. aureus* Mu50 (BA000017.4); SA####, *S. aureus* N315 (BA000018.3); SAOUHSC_####, *S. aureus* NCTC 8325 (CP000253.1).
[b] Fold change in expression of genes by *S. aureus* CDM7 as compared to the wild-type strain during growth in the indicated medium; a positive number indicates an up-regulation of the gene by the *codY* mutant. Standard deviation is shown in parentheses.
[c] At least two differentially expressed probe sets were assigned to these ORFs. Data for all probes sets are shown in Table S2.

Table 4. *S. aureus* SA564, CDM7 and MS7 *in vivo* growth yields.

SA564		CDM7		MS7	
Inoculum (CFU)	**24 h (CFU)[a]**	**Inoculum (CFU)**	**24 h (CFU)[a]**	**Inoculum (CFU)**	**24 h (CFU)[a]**
5.5×10^3	4.0×10^2	8.3×10^3	1.0×10^2	1.2×10^4	ND[b]
	7.0×10^3		9.0×10^2		1.0×10^2
	2.0×10^4		1.1×10^3		1.0×10^2
	2.6×10^4		1.2×10^4		3.0×10^2
	3.7×10^5		1.9×10^5		2.3×10^3
	5.5×10^5		6.0×10^5		2.4×10^5
	2.3×10^6		1.3×10^6		
6.0×10^3	1.0×10^3	5.0×10^3	1.0×10^2	3.0×10^3	ND
	3.9×10^3		2.7×10^3		ND
	1.3×10^6		7.8×10^3		2.0×10^2
			7.3×10^4		3.0×10^2
					6.0×10^2
					1.2×10^3
					3.1×10^3

[a] Number of CFU recovered per homogenized eye is shown. Each entry represents one eye.
[b] ND, Not detected. The limit of detection for these experiments was 1×10^2 CFU.

ORFs, regulatory RNAs and intergenic regions (Table 3 and Table S2).

Genes differentially regulated by the *S. aureus* SA564 *codY* mutant as compared to the wild-type strain during exponential growth in CDM are similar to those previously identified for *S. aureus* Newman (1) and *S. aureus* UAMS-1 (2) *codY* mutants during exponential growth in a chemically defined medium and tryptic soy broth, respectively (Table S2). As for Newman and UAMS-1, *codY* inactivation in SA564 results in an up-regulation of amino acid metabolic and virulence genes including BCAA metabolism (*ilvDBC, leuABCD, ilvA*), hemolysins (*hlb, hld*), and phenol-soluble modulins (SACOL1186, SACOL1187). As expected based on previous studies on CodY regulation in SA564 [29], we observed up-regulation of *icaA*, RNAIII and *hld*. We also identified expression of an enterotoxin, capsular polysaccharide biosynthesis proteins, metalloproteinase aureolysin and others as being affected by *codY* deletion. All other genes are shown in Table 3. Interestingly, of 117 ORFs, regulatory RNAs and intergenic regions identified as being differentially regulated in CDM when comparing *S. aureus codY*-mutant to SA564, all but one (SA1817, the enterotoxin gene) are core to the four *S. aureus* strains used to generate the GeneChip (Table S2) [33]. However, it is possible that as yet unknown *S. aureus* SA564-specific genes are under CodY control.

Of the 117 ORFs, regulatory RNAs and intergenic regions identified as being differentially regulated in the SA564 *codY* mutant relative to the wild-type strain during growth in CDM, 55 of those were also identified as being differentially regulated during growth in VH (Table 3 and Table S2). Of the 117, only 23 were identified as being differentially regulated during growth in AH. We were curious as to why this expression pattern was observed in AH, and whether it could be explained by a relief of CodY repression occurring during growth in AH at the cell density chosen for our microarray experiments. To explore this further, we returned to the microarray analysis of the SA564 wild-type strain grown in AH, as compared to CDM. Expression data for all differentially expressed genes for the SA564 *codY* mutant during growth in CDM were extracted from each of the four SA564 AH versus CDM analyses (Table S2). Analysis of these data revealed that genes previously identified as being under CodY control [1,2,5,29] were de-repressed in one AH sample (AH2), but not the other (AH1), relative to CDM (Table S2), most likely as a result of BCAA becoming depleted from the pooled AH2 sample. Speculatively, these data suggest that, *in vivo* in the anterior chamber, where BCAA are present [16,31], CodY repression may limit virulence of *S. aureus* during early stages of infection when cell densities are likely to be low. Future studies that track BCAA concentrations and expression of CodY-regulated genes in *ex vivo* AH samples over the course of *S. aureus* growth could be used to explore this further.

We additionally observed AH-specific up-regulation of *lrgAB* and VH-specific up-regulation of *cidA*. *lrgAB* and *cidA* are involved in coordination of cell death and autolysis, in addition to their role in biofilm development through the release of genomic DNA that becomes a structural component of the biofilm matrix. Note that *lrgAB* expression varied between the two AH gene expression experiments, with low albeit significant up-regulation observed during growth in one AH sample (1.4–2.6 fold up-regulated compared to CDM controls), and comparatively higher up-regulation during growth in another AH sample (17.1–27.8-fold up-regulated compared to CDM controls).

codY deletion enhances *S. aureus* virulence in a murine AC infection model

To assess a potential role for CodY in endophthalmitis, we began by examining the potential for intraocular growth of *S. aureus* after injection into the murine AC. Approximately 5×10^3 CFU of *S. aureus* SA564 or *codY*-mutant were injected into the murine AC, and bacterial growth was assessed after 24 h by extraction and homogenization of the entire eye (Table 4). In all cases, viable *S. aureus* were recovered (SA564 range, 4×10^2–$2.3\text{-}10^6$ CFU; *codY* mutant range, 1×10^2–1.3×10^6 CFU). Average *in vivo* growth yields of SA564 and CDM7 were similar (4.6×10^5 CFU for SA564; 2×10^5 CFU for CDM7). Thus, after introduction

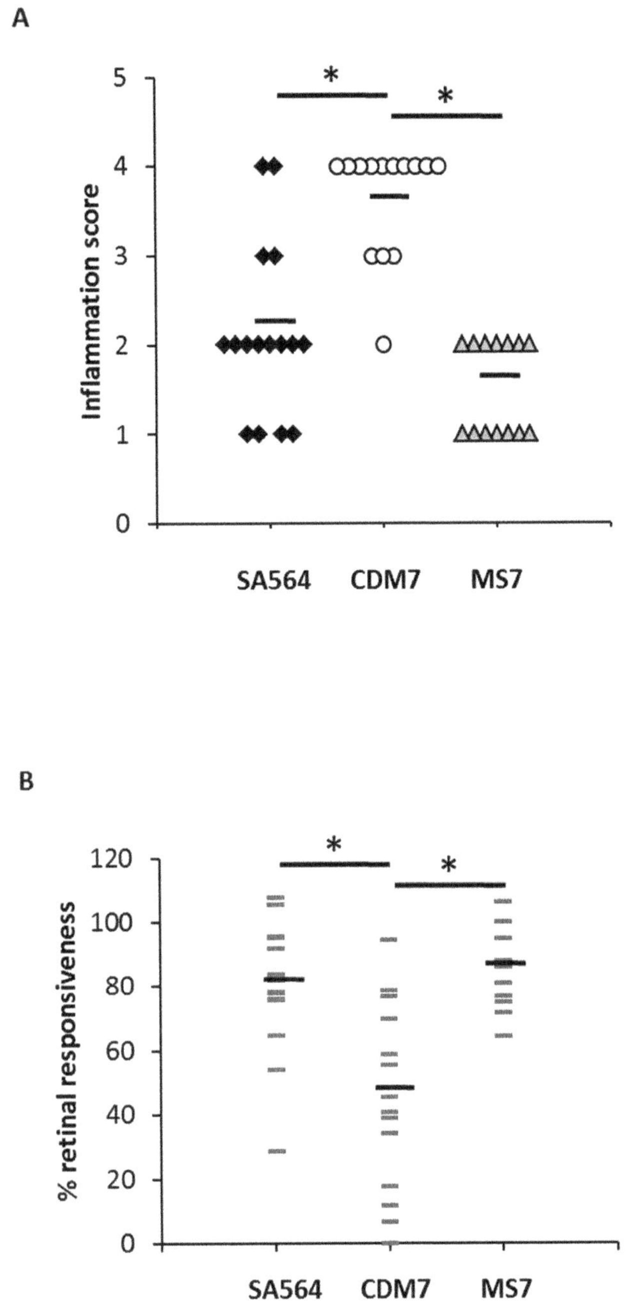

Figure 3. Inflammation and retinal responsiveness in *S. aureus* infected eyes. Inflammation scores (A) and % retinal responsiveness (B) for murine eyes infected with SA564, CDM7, or MS7, assessed 24 h post-inoculation. Average values are indicated by heavy black horizontal lines. *, $p \leq 0.001$, Mann-Whitney test.

into the anterior chamber, the murine eye was a permissive environment for the survival of each strain. Because the entire eye was homogenized for these experiments, it is unknown whether growth occurred in the anterior chamber, the posterior chamber, or both.

We next assessed the impact of *codY* on inflammation (Fig. 3A) and retinal responsiveness (Fig. 3B) at 24 h after infection. The distribution of inflammation scores were significantly different for eyes infected with the two strains ($p<0.001$; one-tailed Wilcoxon rank-sum test), with a higher average inflammation score for the *codY* mutant (3.6 versus 2.1) (Fig. 3A). Average retinal responsiveness was lower for eyes inoculated with the *codY* mutant (45% of control versus 80% of control), and the distribution of percent retinal responsiveness values was significantly different between eyes infected with the *codY* mutant and those infected with SA564 ($p = 0.001$, one-tailed Wilcoxon rank-sum test) (Fig. 3B). Representative histology images are shown in Fig. 4. As seen in the figure, the eye infected with the *codY* mutant shows more inflammation in the cornea, anterior chamber, and vitreous, as well as disruption of retinal architecture. Collectively, these data suggest that CodY regulation of its target genes limits *S. aureus* disease in the murine anterior chamber infection model.

Similar experiments were performed using previously described MS7, *codY* complemented strain [29]. In this vector, *codY* expression is under the control of a leaky IPTG-inducible promoter (P_{SPAC}) [29]. *codY* expression from pTL6936 appears to be leaky, as partial complementation was observed for an *S. aureus* UAMS-1 *codY* mutant in the absence of IPTG [34]. We observed increased retinal responsiveness and decreased inflammation as assessed by slitlamp for murine eyes inoculated with 10^3–10^4 CFU MS7, compared to SA564 and CDM7 (Fig. 4A–B), suggesting that *in vivo* complementation of the *codY* occurred. However, decreased *in vivo* growth yields were observed for MS7 compared to SA564 and CDM7 (Table 4; range, <100–2.5×10^5 CFU; average, 1.9×10^4 CFU). Thus it is unknown whether the increased retinal responsiveness and decreased inflammation observed for MS7 were due to complementation of the *codY* lesion or to an *in vivo* growth defect of this strain. MS7 does not have an *in vitro* growth defect relative to CDM7 as assessed by growth in CDM; the average doubling time of MS7 is 49.0 ± 0.5 min, compared to 50.7 ± 0.3 min for CDM7 (Fig. 1).

Discussion

CodY controls expression of virulence and metabolic genes in response to branched-chain amino acids (BCAA) and GTP. This makes it an important regulatory link between nutrient availability and virulence factor production [1]. However, little is known about its contribution to virulence *in vitro* and *in vivo* in the ocular milieu.

AH is a complex mixture of electrolytes, organic solutes, growth factors, cytokines, and proteins including BCAA that provide the metabolic requirements to the avascular tissues of the anterior segment. It is produced from the non-pigmented ciliary body epithelium through simple diffusion as well as active transport of ions and solutes and exits the anterior chamber mainly via the trabecular meshwork. The volume of human AH in the anterior chamber generally turns over once every 100 minutes replenishing nutrients that have been taken up by avascular ocular tissues and carries away metabolic wastes [16,17,31].

In this study, we demonstrated that bovine AH and VH provide adequate nutrition for growth of *S. aureus* SA564, and result in differential gene expression when compared to each other, and to a defined medium. While our *in vitro* bovine AH and VH models lack the nutritional replenishment and immune response that would be characteristic of *in vivo* growth environments, the models are useful in that they allow for the identification of nutrients that *S. aureus* specifically detects and responds to in the ocular milieu, in particular, sialic acid, ascorbate, and pseudouridine.

Pseudouridine is a nucleoside present in RNAs of humans and other animals [32]. It has been detected in tRNAs of the bovine lens [34]. SACOL0308, SACOL0309, and SACOL0310 share protein sequence homology and conserved protein domains with

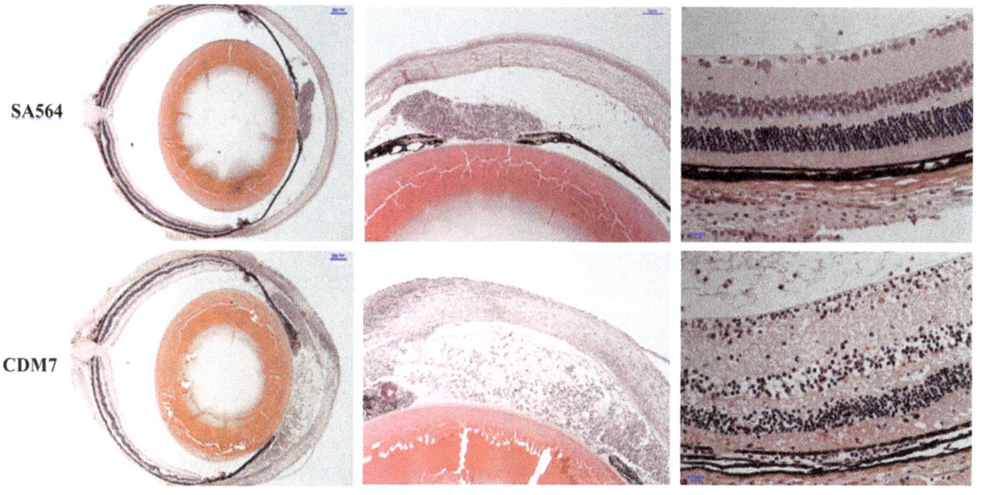

Figure 4. Histology images. Representative histology images of *S. aureus* SA564- and CDM7-infected eyes at 24 h post-inoculation. Retinal responsiveness values for the infected eyes shown were 95.9% (SA564) and 11.9% (CDM7). Panels shown, from top to bottom, are the whole eye, the AC, and the retina.

the YeiC, YeiN, and YeiM proteins, respectively, of *Escherichia coli* (Table S1) [35]. YeiC is a pseudouridine kinase, and YeiN is a pseudouridine-5′-phosphate glycosidase. Together, YeiC and YeiN comprise a pathway for the catabolism of pseudouridine to uracil and ribose-5-phosphate [35]. YeiM is a predicted nucleoside transporter and may be involved in uptake of pseudouridine from the environment. It is possible that *S. aureus* SA564 catabolizes pseudouridine for energy (via ribose-5-phosphate), and/or for uracil scavenging in AH.

N-acetylneuraminate, another highly upregulated gene in AH, is the primary sialic acid moiety present in mammalian tissues, and sialic acid modification of human cell surfaces is used as a "self versus non-self" signal to the immune system, allowing for discrimination of cell types, among other functions of sialic acids [36]. In the eye, sialic acid is distributed in all structures, including cornea, sclera, AH, trabecular meshwork, lens, VH and retina, and its concentration seems to increase with aging [37]. SACOL0312 and SACOL0311 encode a putative sodium:solute symporter protein (NanT) and N-acetylneuraminate lyase (NanA), respectively. NanA converts N-acetylneuraminate to N-acetylmannosamine and pyruvate [38]. Recently, it was shown that *nanA* and *nanT* are co-transcribed in *S. aureus* strain AH1263 [30]. Further, *nanA* and *nanT* are required for *S. aureus* growth with sialic acid [30]. Our microarray results suggest that *S. aureus* SA564 transports and catabolizes sialic acid during growth in bovine AH.

Ascorbate (vitamin C) is abundant in the eye and present at much higher concentrations than in the plasma [39]. It is actively transported by the iris-ciliary body into the AH and serves as an antioxidant to protect the eye against light-induced free radical damage [40]. SACOL0400-SACOL0403 encode a putative ascorbate uptake transport system (*ulaABC*) and a predicted transcriptional antiterminator (Table 2 and Table S1). In *E. coli*, the PTS-like UlaABC system (alternatively named SgaTBA) transports ascorbate with concomitant phosphorylation, trapping ascorbate-6-phosphate in the cell [41]. *S. aureus* may transport ascorbate to prevent Fenton reaction damage occurring as a result of extracellular iron reduction by ascorbate under aerobic conditions [42].

Several virulence factors were specifically up-regulated during growth in AH, including an enterotoxin (*sec3*), the toxic shock syndrome toxin (*tst*), and a phenol soluble modulin (Table 2). The toxic shock syndrome toxin and the SEC enterotoxin are superantigens that are important in infections such as infective endocarditis and pneumonia [43–45]. Immunization against those exotoxins was found to protect against those serious illnesses [44,46]. Phenol soluble modulins have also been found in animal models to have an essential role in bacteremia and skin infections [47]. The AH-specific up-regulation of these factors may facilitate translocation of *S. aureus* or *S. aureus*-produced factors into the posterior chamber and/or retinal damage during *S. aureus* endophthalmitis.

As for the analysis of the *codY* mutant, our microarray results demonstrate that *codY* deletion impacts expression of metabolic and virulence genes in *S. aureus* SA564. However, genes affected by *codY* were not consistent across the two pooled AH samples used here, suggesting that BCAA became depleted from one of the samples. These data indicate that, *in vivo* in the AC, where BCAA are present and replenished by AH turnover continuously, CodY repression may limit virulence of *S. aureus* during early stages of infection when cell densities are likely to be low. Consistent with this proposal, deletion of *codY* enhanced virulence of *S. aureus* in a murine AC infection model, as assessed by retinal function measurements, degree of inflammation in the eye, and histological assessments of ocular tissue damage. The microarray results suggest a role for enterotoxin (*sec3*), the toxic shock syndrome toxin (*tst*), and a phenol soluble modulin in endophthalmitis progression. Collectively, these data suggest that CodY repression of its target genes limits *S. aureus* disease in the murine AC infection model.

In conclusion, we used novel *in vitro* and *in vivo* infection models to characterize the behavior of *S. aureus* during endophthalmitis, one a nutritional model utilizing bovine ocular fluids as media for *S. aureus* growth *ex vivo*, and one an *in vivo* infection model evaluating endophthalmitis progression after *S. aureus* injection into the murine AC. We identified metabolic pathways that may be important for *S. aureus* endophthalmitis, specifically sialic acid, ascorbate, and pseudouridine metabolism. We are now directly assessing the roles of these pathways in the pathogenesis of *S. aureus* endophthalmitis. We additionally identified several virulence factors whose expression was activated by growth in ocular fluids, suggesting that transcriptional regulation of these genes is influenced by specific nutrients present in the eye. Our *in vivo* endophthalmitis model, a murine AC infection model, revealed a link between the BCAA-responsive transcriptional regulator CodY and experimental endophthalmitis progression. More specifically, relief of CodY repression of its target genes (by deletion of *codY*) enhanced *S. aureus* pathogenesis in the murine eye. Interestingly, this result suggests that it may be possible to use BCAA to mitigate *S. aureus* endophthalmitis progression by supplementing BCAA in eye drops postoperatively or by adding BCAA to the infusion solution that goes through the eye during intraocular surgery.

Supporting Information

Table S1 An expanded version of Table 2 with probe set IDs, BLAST hit distribution among *S. aureus* COL, Mu50, N315, and NCTC 8325 genomes, and fold change data for every gene shown in Table 2, irrespective of meeting the fold change cut-off of 10.

Table S2 Expression data for all differentially expressed genes for the SA564 and SA564 *codY* mutant during growth in CDM versus AH.

Author Contributions

Conceived and designed the experiments: AS KP TS MG. Performed the experiments: AS KP TS MG. Analyzed the data: AS KP TS MG. Contributed reagents/materials/analysis tools: AS KP TS MG. Contributed to the writing of the manuscript: AS KP TS MG.

References

1. Pohl K, Francois P, Stenz L, Schlink F, Geiger T, et al. (2009) CodY in Staphylococcus aureus: a regulatory link between metabolism and virulence gene expression. J Bacteriol 191: 2953–2963.
2. Majerczyk CD, Dunman PM, Luong TT, Lee CY, Sadykov MR, et al. (2010) Direct targets of CodY in Staphylococcus aureus. J Bacteriol 192: 2861–2877.
3. Geiger T, Goerke C, Fritz M, Schafer T, Ohlsen K, et al. (2010) Role of the (p)ppGpp synthase RSH, a RelA/SpoT homolog, in stringent response and virulence of Staphylococcus aureus. Infect Immun 78: 1873–1883.
4. Bennett HJ, Pearce DM, Glenn S, Taylor CM, Kuhn M, et al. (2007) Characterization of relA and codY mutants of Listeria monocytogenes: identification of the CodY regulon and its role in virulence. Mol Microbiol 63: 1453–1467.
5. Sonenshein AL (2005) CodY, a global regulator of stationary phase and virulence in Gram-positive bacteria. Curr Opin Microbiol 8: 203–207.
6. Guedon E, Serror P, Ehrlich SD, Renault P, Delorme C (2001) Pleiotropic transcriptional repressor CodY senses the intracellular pool of branched-chain amino acids in Lactococcus lactis. Mol Microbiol 40: 1227–1239.
7. den Hengst CD, Groeneveld M, Kuipers OP, Kok J (2006) Identification and functional characterization of the Lactococcus lactis CodY-regulated branched-chain amino acid permease BcaP (CtrA). J Bacteriol 188: 3280–3289.
8. Levdikov VM, Blagova E, Colledge VL, Lebedev AA, Williamson DC, et al. (2009) Structural rearrangement accompanying ligand binding in the GAF domain of CodY from Bacillus subtilis. J Mol Biol 390: 1007–1018.
9. Levdikov VM, Blagova E, Joseph P, Sonenshein AL, Wilkinson AJ (2006) The structure of CodY, a GTP- and isoleucine-responsive regulator of stationary phase and virulence in gram-positive bacteria. J Biol Chem 281: 11366–11373.
10. Slack FJ, Serror P, Joyce E, Sonenshein AL (1995) A gene required for nutritional repression of the Bacillus subtilis dipeptide permease operon. Mol Microbiol 15: 689–702.
11. Wu PC, Kuo HK, Li M, Lai IC, Fang PC, et al. (2006) Nosocomial postoperative endophthalmitis: a 14-year review. Graefes Arch Clin Exp Ophthalmol 244: 920–929.
12. Endophthalmitis Study Group ESoC, Refractive S (2007) Prophylaxis of postoperative endophthalmitis following cataract surgery: results of the ESCRS multicenter study and identification of risk factors. J Cataract Refract Surg 33: 978–988.
13. Andreoli CM, Andreoli MT, Kloek CE, Ahuero AE, Vavvas D, et al. (2009) Low rate of endophthalmitis in a large series of open globe injuries. Am J Ophthalmol 147: 601–608 e602.
14. Jonas JB, Knorr HL, Budde WM (2000) Prognostic factors in ocular injuries caused by intraocular or retrobulbar foreign bodies. Ophthalmology 107: 823–828.
15. Hanscom T (1996) The Endophthalmitis Vitrectomy Study. Arch Ophthalmol 114: 1029–1030; author reply 1028–1029.
16. Durham DG, Dickinson JC, Hamilton PB (1971) Ion-exchange chromatography of free amino acids in human intraocular fluids. Clin Chem 17: 285–289.
17. Nakatsukasa M, Sotozono C, Shimbo K, Ono N, Miyano H, et al. (2011) Amino Acid profiles in human tear fluids analyzed by high-performance liquid chromatography and electrospray ionization tandem mass spectrometry. Am J Ophthalmol 151: 799–808 e791.
18. Booth MC, Atkuri RV, Nanda SK, Iandolo JJ, Gilmore MS (1995) Accessory gene regulator controls Staphylococcus aureus virulence in endophthalmitis. Invest Ophthalmol Vis Sci 36: 1828–1836.
19. Callegan MC, Engelbert M, Parke DW, 2nd, Jett BD, Gilmore MS (2002) Bacterial endophthalmitis: epidemiology, therapeutics, and bacterium-host interactions. Clin Microbiol Rev 15: 111–124.
20. Balzli CL, Bartell J, Dajcs JJ, McCormick CC, Caballero AR, et al. (2010) A highly virulent Staphylococcus aureus: rabbit anterior chamber infection, characterization, and genetic analysis. Invest Ophthalmol Vis Sci 51: 5114–5120.
21. Wu X, Chen H, Jiang H, Xu Y, Liu T, et al. (2012) Prophylactic effect of topical fluoroquinolones in a rabbit model of Staphylococcus aureus endophthalmitis. J Ocul Pharmacol Ther 28: 186–193.
22. Kowalski RP, Romanowski EG, Mah FS, Sasaki H, Fukuda M, et al. (2008) A comparison of moxifloxacin and levofloxacin topical prophylaxis in a fluoroquinolone-resistant Staphylococcus aureus rabbit model. Jpn J Ophthalmol 52: 211–216.
23. Booth MC, Cheung AL, Hatter KL, Jett BD, Callegan MC, et al. (1997) Staphylococcal accessory regulator (sar) in conjunction with agr contributes to Staphylococcus aureus virulence in endophthalmitis. Infect Immun 65: 1550–1556.
24. Labit CM, Claeys GW, Verbraeken HE, Verschraegen GL (2001) Methicillin resistance of bacteria isolated from vitreous fluid from patients undergoing vitrectomy. Eur J Ophthalmol 11: 160–165.
25. Socransky SS, Dzink JL, Smith CM (1985) Chemically defined medium for oral microorganisms. J Clin Microbiol 22: 303–305.
26. Suzuki T, Campbell J, Swoboda JG, Walker S, Gilmore MS (2011) Role of wall teichoic acids in Staphylococcus aureus endophthalmitis. Invest Ophthalmol Vis Sci 52: 3187–3192.
27. Palmer KL, Mashburn LM, Singh PK, Whiteley M (2005) Cystic fibrosis sputum supports growth and cues key aspects of Pseudomonas aeruginosa physiology. J Bacteriol 187: 5267–5277.
28. Suzuki T, Wada T, Kozai S, Ike Y, Gilmore MS, et al. (2008) Contribution of secreted proteases to the pathogenesis of postoperative Enterococcus faecalis endophthalmitis. J Cataract Refract Surg 34: 1776–1784.
29. Majerczyk CD, Sadykov MR, Luong TT, Lee C, Somerville GA, et al. (2008) Staphylococcus aureus CodY negatively regulates virulence gene expression. J Bacteriol 190: 2257–2265.
30. Olson ME, King JM, Yahr TL, Horswill AR (2013) Sialic acid catabolism in Staphylococcus aureus. J Bacteriol 195: 1779–1788.
31. WM H (1992) Adler's Physiology of the Eye.
32. Bertram KM, Bula DV, Pulido JS, Shippy SA, Gautam S, et al. (2008) Amino-acid levels in subretinal and vitreous fluid of patients with retinal detachment. Eye (Lond) 22: 582–589.
33. Affymetrix I. GeneChip Made-to-Order Array Program Data Sheet: Affymetrix, Inc.
34. Ortwerth BJ, Yonuschot GR, Heidlege JF, Chu-Der OM, Juarez D, et al. (1975) Induction of a new species of phenylalanine transfer RNA during lens cell differentiation. Exp Eye Res 20: 417–426.
35. Preumont A, Snoussi K, Stroobant V, Collet JF, Van Schaftingen E (2008) Molecular identification of pseudouridine-metabolizing enzymes. J Biol Chem 283: 25238–25246.
36. Varki A, Gagneux P (2012) Multifarious roles of sialic acids in immunity. Ann N Y Acad Sci 1253: 16–36.
37. Haddad HM (1962) Sialic acids in human eyes. Relationship to lens aging and retinal pathology. Arch Ophthalmol 67: 459–463.
38. Vimr ER, Kalivoda KA, Deszo EL, Steenbergen SM (2004) Diversity of microbial sialic acid metabolism. Microbiol Mol Biol Rev 68: 132–153.
39. Johnsen H, Ringvold A, Blika S (1985) Ascorbic acid determination in serum and aqueous humour by high-performance liquid chromatography. Acta Ophthalmol (Copenh) 63: 31–34.
40. Tso MO, Woodford BJ, Lam KW (1984) Distribution of ascorbate in normal primate retina and after photic injury: a biochemical, morphological correlated study. Curr Eye Res 3: 181–191.
41. Zhang Z, Aboulwafa M, Smith MH, Saier MH, Jr. (2003) The ascorbate transporter of Escherichia coli. J Bacteriol 185: 2243–2250.
42. Campos E, Montella C, Garces F, Baldoma L, Aguilar J, et al. (2007) Aerobic L-ascorbate metabolism and associated oxidative stress in Escherichia coli. Microbiology 153: 3399–3408.

43. Pragman AA, Yarwood JM, Tripp TJ, Schlievert PM (2004) Characterization of virulence factor regulation by SrrAB, a two-component system in Staphylococcus aureus. J Bacteriol 186: 2430–2438.
44. Mattis DM, Spaulding AR, Chuang-Smith ON, Sundberg EJ, Schlievert PM, et al. (2013) Engineering a soluble high-affinity receptor domain that neutralizes staphylococcal enterotoxin C in rabbit models of disease. Protein Eng Des Sel 26: 133–142.
45. Strandberg KL, Rotschafer JH, Vetter SM, Buonpane RA, Kranz DM, et al. (2010) Staphylococcal superantigens cause lethal pulmonary disease in rabbits. J Infect Dis 202: 1690–1697.
46. Spaulding AR, Lin YC, Merriman JA, Brosnahan AJ, Peterson ML, et al. (2012) Immunity to Staphylococcus aureus secreted proteins protects rabbits from serious illnesses. Vaccine 30: 5099–5109.
47. Wang R, Braughton KR, Kretschmer D, Bach TH, Queck SY, et al. (2007) Identification of novel cytolytic peptides as key virulence determinants for community-associated MRSA. Nat Med 13: 1510–1514.
48. Gill SR, Fouts DE, Archer GL, Mongodin EF, Deboy RT, et al. (2005) Insights on evolution of virulence and resistance from the complete genome analysis of an early methicillin-resistant Staphylococcus aureus strain and a biofilm-producing methicillin-resistant Staphylococcus epidermidis strain. J Bacteriol 187: 2426–2438.

Assessment of Choroidal Thickness in Healthy and Glaucomatous Eyes Using Swept Source Optical Coherence Tomography

Chunwei Zhang[1,2], Andrew J. Tatham[1], Felipe A. Medeiros[1], Linda M. Zangwill[1], Zhiyong Yang[1], Robert N. Weinreb[1]*

1 Hamilton Glaucoma Center and Department of Ophthalmology, University of California San Diego, San Diego, California, United States of America, **2** Department of Ophthalmology, the First Affiliated Hospital, Harbin Medical University, Harbin, China

Abstract

Purpose: To evaluate choroidal thickness (CT) in healthy and glaucomatous eyes using Swept Source Optical Coherence Tomography (SS-OCT).

Methods: A cross-sectional observational study of 216 eyes of 140 subjects with glaucoma and 106 eyes of 67 healthy subjects enrolled in the Diagnostic Innovations in Glaucoma Study. CT was assessed from wide-field (12×9 mm) SS-OCT scans. The association between CT and potential confounding variables including age, gender, axial length, intraocular pressure, central corneal thickness and ocular perfusion pressure was examined using univariable and multivariable regression analyses.

Results: Overall CT was thinner in glaucomatous eyes with a mean (± standard deviation) of 157.7±48.5 μm in glaucoma compared to 179.9±36.1 μm in healthy eyes ($P<0.001$). The choroid was thinner in both the peripapillary and macular regions in glaucoma compared to controls. Mean peripapillary CT was 154.1±44.1 μm and 134.0±56.9 μm ($P<0.001$) and macular CT 199.3±46.1 μm and 176.2±57.5 μm ($P<0.001$) for healthy and glaucomatous eyes respectively. However, older age ($P<0.001$) and longer axial length ($P<0.001$) were also associated with thinner choroid and when differences in age and axial length between glaucomatous and healthy subjects were accounted for, glaucoma was not significantly associated with CT. There was also no association between glaucoma severity and CT.

Conclusions: Glaucoma was not associated with CT measured using SS-OCT; however, older age and longer axial length were associated with thinner choroid so should be considered when interpreting CT measurements.

Editor: Andreas Wedrich, Medical University Graz, Austria

Funding: The study was supported in part by National Institutes of Health/National Eye Institute grants EY021818 (to FAM), EY11008 (to LMZ), EY14267 (to LMZ), Cover Letter EY019869 (to LMZ), core grant P30EY022589 (http://www.nei.nih.gov/index.asp) and an unrestricted grant from Research to Prevent Blindness (http://www.rpbusa.org/rpb/). The study was funded in part by participant retention incentive grants in the form of glaucoma medication at no cost from Alcon Laboratories, Allergan, Pfizer, and Santen. The funders had no role in study design, data collection and analysis, decision to publish, or preparation of the manuscript.

Competing Interests: We wish to disclose the following competing interests: Chunwei Zhang: None. Andrew J. Tatham: Research Support; Heidelberg Engineering, GmbH. Felipe A. Medeiros: Funding; Alcon Laboratories, Bausch & Lomb, Carl Zeiss Meditec, Heidelberg Engineering, GmbH, Merck, Allergan, Sensimed, Topcon, Reichert, National Eye Institute. Research Support: Alcon Laboratories, Allergan, Carl Zeiss Meditec, Reichert, Consultant: Allergan, Carl-Zeiss Meditec, Novartis. Linda M. Zangwill: Funding; Carl Zeiss Meditec, Heidelberg Engineering, GmbH, Optovue, Topcon Medical Systems, Nidek. Zhiyong Yang: None. Robert N. Weinreb: Funding; Aerie, Carl Zeiss Meditec, Genentech, Heidelberg Engineering GmbH, National Eye Institute, Nidek, Novartis, Optovue, Quark, Topcon. Consultant; Alcon, Allergan, Bausch & Lomb, Carl Zeiss Meditec, Sensimed, Topcon.

* Email: rweinreb@ucsd.edu

Introduction

Glaucoma is characterized by progressive damage to retinal ganglion cells leading to optic nerve head (ONH) morphological changes, thinning of the retinal nerve fiber layer and loss of visual field [1]. The underlying mechanism of damage is incompletely understood, but is likely multifactorial [2]. Raised intraocular pressure (IOP) is a major risk factor [3–6]. It also has been proposed that the microcirculation and vascular perfusion can contribute to the health of the optic nerve. As choroidal derived vasculature perfuses the prelaminar area of the ONH [7], there is interest in the role of the choroid in the pathogenesis of glaucoma [8].

Initial histological studies supported an association between choroidal morphology and glaucoma, with several reports of thinner choroid in glaucomatous compared to non-glaucomatous eyes [9–11]. Reduced thickness was thought to be due to loss of the innermost choroidal vasculature and it was suggested that choroidal thinning might be associated with choroidal insufficiency which could contribute to glaucomatous retinal ganglion cell damage. However, further evidence is needed to support or refute this theory, particularly as histological studies have limitations due to fixation methods and delays between death and fixation that may induce artifacts. Also, previous histological studies were limited to small numbers of patients and did not control for other factors now known to influence choroidal thickness (CT) including age and axial length [9,12,13].

It is now possible to obtain in vivo images of the choroid using enhanced depth imaging optical coherence tomography (EDI-OCT), a modified version of spectral domain OCT (SD-OCT) [14]. Enhanced depth imaging has been used to examine macular CT in healthy and glaucomatous eyes, with most studies finding no significant difference [15–18]. However, although enhanced depth imaging allows visualization of the choroid, the choroidal-scleral boundary may be difficult to discern. Furthermore, as choroidal segmentation software is not readily available, the assessment of CT has often relied on manual measurements at localized points [19–20]. Recently, a new generation of high-penetration OCT devices has been introduced with the potential to improve assessment of the choroid [21]. These Fourier-domain OCT devices are based on an alternative approach to image acquisition, known as Swept Source OCT (SS-OCT). SS-OCT devices use a tunable laser (i.e., one whose wavelength of operation can be altered in a controlled manner) and photodetectors instead of the silicone-based, line-scan, charge-coupled device camera used in SD-OCT systems. These innovations reduce light scatter by the retinal pigment epithelium and therefore enable better visualization of deeper ocular structures including the choroid. Previous studies have shown the potential of using SS-OCT for choroidal imaging [22] especially given the availability of software for segmentation of multiple retinal layers and the choroid [23]. SS-OCT also provides the capability of a wide field 12×9 mm scan enabling simultaneous imaging of the macula and ONH and measurement of CT over a larger area than previously possible in a single scan. Peripapillary and macular CT can therefore be calculated from a single scan.

The aim of the present study was to use SS-OCT to assess CT in healthy and glaucomatous eyes. We also assessed the effect of factors including age, gender, race, axial length, retinal nerve fiber layer (RNFL) thickness, mean deviation (MD), intraocular pressure (IOP), blood pressure (BP) and ocular perfusion pressure (OPP) on choroidal thickness.

Methods

This was a cross-sectional observational study of participants from the Diagnostic Innovations in Glaucoma Study (DIGS) at the University of California San Diego (UCSD). The DIGS is a prospective longitudinal study designed to evaluate optic nerve structure and visual function in glaucoma. Informed consent was obtained from all participants, and the institutional review board and human subjects committee at UCSD prospectively approved all methods. All study methods adhered to the tenets of the Declaration of Helsinki for research involving human subjects and the study was conducted in accordance with the regulations of the Health Insurance Portability and Accountability Act.

Methodological details have been described in detail previously [24]. At each visit during follow-up, subjects underwent a comprehensive ophthalmologic examination including review of medical history, BP, best-corrected visual acuity, slit-lamp biomicroscopy, IOP measurement, gonioscopy, dilated fundoscopic examination, stereoscopic optic disc photography, and standard automated perimetry (SAP) using the Swedish Interactive Threshold Algorithm (Standard 24-2). Central corneal thickness (CCT) was measured with ultrasound Pachymetry (DGH Technology Inc, Exton, PA) and axial length measurement using the IOL Master (Carl Zeiss Meditec, Dublin, CA) was also performed. Diastolic and systolic ocular perfusion pressure was calculated as diastolic or systolic BP minus IOP respectively. Objective measurements of choroidal and RNFL thickness were obtained using the swept source Deep Range Imaging OCT (DRI-OCT-1 Atlantis, Topcon, Inc., Tokyo, Japan). The study included only subjects with open angles on gonioscopy. Subjects were excluded if they presented with a best-corrected visual acuity less than 20/40, spherical refraction outside ±5.0 diopters or cylinder correction outside 3.0 diopters, or any other ocular or systemic disease that could affect the optic nerve or visual field.

The study included 322 eyes of 207 participants, including 106 healthy and 216 glaucomatous eyes. Eyes were classified as glaucoma if they had repeatable (≥2 consecutive) abnormal SAP test results or progressive glaucomatous changes on masked grading of optic disc stereophotographs. Healthy subjects were recruited from the general population through advertisements and from the staff and employees of the University of California San Diego. Healthy eyes had IOP≤21 mmHg, with no history of increased IOP and a normal SAP result.

Standard Automated Perimetry

SAP was performed using the Humphrey Field Analyzer II (Carl Zeiss Meditec, Dublin, CA, USA) and the 24-2 Swedish interactive threshold algorithm (SITA Standard 24-2, Carl Zeiss Meditec, Inc., Dublin, CA, USA). All visual fields were evaluated by the UCSD Visual Field Assessment Center (VisFACT) [25]. Visual fields with more than 33% fixation losses or false-negative errors, or more than 15% false-positive errors, were excluded. The only exception was the inclusion of visual fields with false-negative errors of more than 33% when the field showed advanced disease (worse than −12 dB). SAP tests were defined as normal if the MD and pattern standard deviation was within 95% normal confidence limits and the Glaucoma Hemifield Test (GHT) was also within normal limits. An abnormal SAP test was defined as a visual field with a pattern standard deviation with $P<0.05$ and/or a GHT outside normal limits.

Optic Disc Stereophotographs

Simultaneous stereoscopic optic disc photography (Kowa Nonmyd WX3D, software version VK27E, Kowa Company Ltd., Tokyo, Japan) was performed for all subjects and digital stereoscopic images were reviewed with a stereoscopic viewer (Screen-VU stereoscope, PS Mfg., Portland, Oregon, USA) by two or more experienced graders. Each grader was masked to the subject's identity and to the other test results. Details of the methodology employed to grade optic disc photographs at the UCSD Optic Disc Reading Center have been provided elsewhere [24,26].

Deep Range Imaging Optical Coherence Tomography

CT was assessed from images acquired using DRI-OCT, which is a new Swept Source OCT, currently not available commercially in the United States. The DRI-OCT acquires 100,000 A-scans per second and provides an axial resolution in tissue of 8 mm. DRI-OCT has a center wavelength of 1,050 nm and a sweeping range of approximately 100 nm, compared to the 850 nm wavelength of SDOCT [23,27]. For the present study, all eyes were imaged using

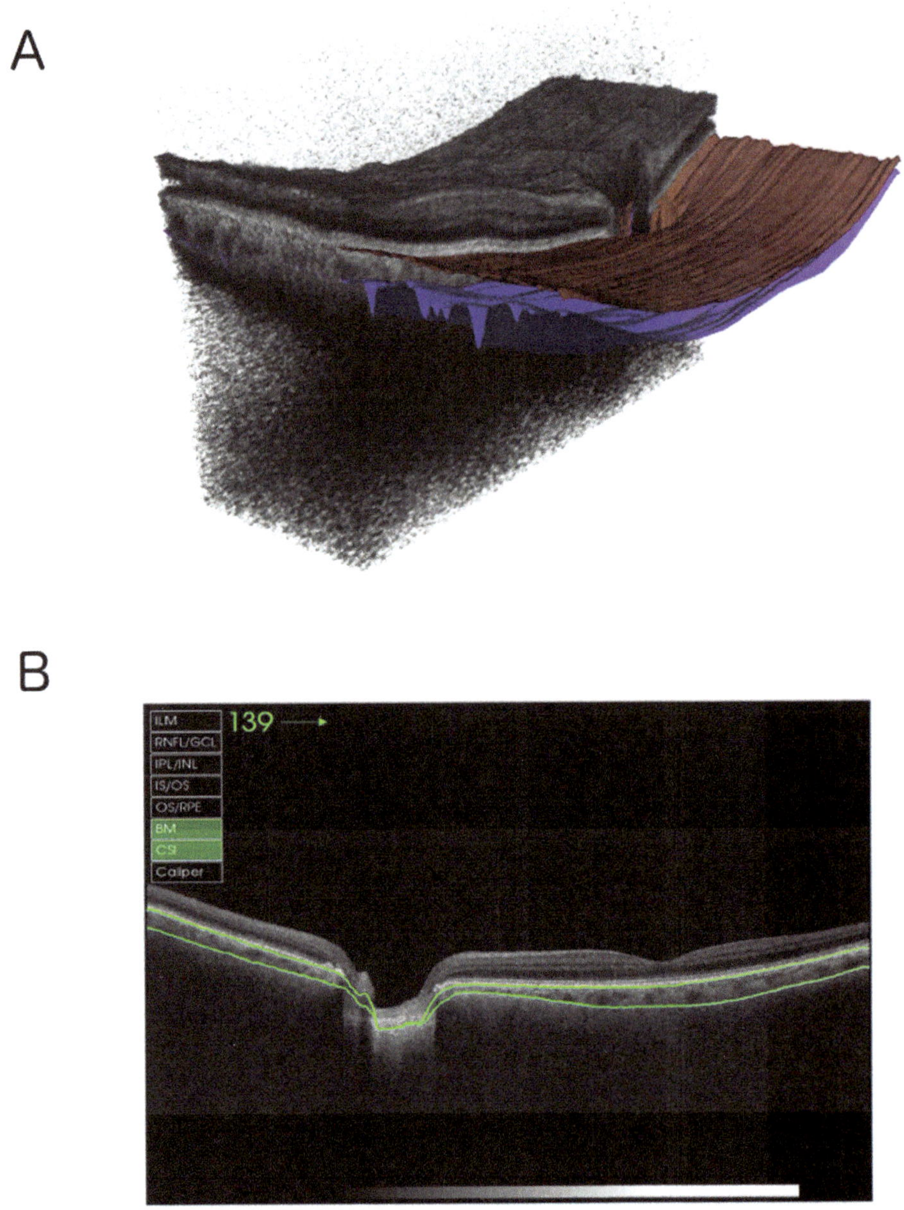

Figure 1. Partial 3-dimensional image of a 12×9 mm scan obtained with DRI-OCT using the instrument's cropping function and showing segmentation of the choroid (A). Horizontal B scan showing a segmented choroid with thickness measured between the two green demarcated lines (B).

the wide field 12×9 mm raster scan setting with the scan centered on the posterior pole. It was therefore possible to obtain images of the macular and ONH region in a single scan. The 12×9 mm scan comprises 256 B-scans, each comprising 512 A-scans for a total of 131,072 axial scans/volume. The total acquisition time was 1.3 seconds per 12×9 mm scan.

DRI-OCT segmentation software (version 9.11, Topcon, Inc., Tokyo, Japan) was used to identify the limits of the choroid and determine CT throughout the 12×9 mm scan. Data was exported using the manufacturer's OCT-Batch (version 9.1.10) utility. The quality of each scan and accuracy of the segmentation algorithm were reviewed by an experienced examiner and poor quality images (quality score <50, clipped or poorly focused scans) were excluded.

Scans with segmentation failures and motion artifacts were also excluded.

Figure 1 shows an example of a 3-dimensional SS-OCT scan with the segmented borders of the choroid delineated. The SS-OCT software calculates the average CT for each 1 mm^2 grid square of the 12×9 mm scan and allows this date to be displayed and exported. Therefore for each eye the average CT in a total of 108 locations was calculated (Figure 2). The mean CT in 20 central 1 mm×1 mm squares was calculated to represent the macular CT (Figure 3). The peripapillary CT was estimated as the mean CT of 20 1 mm×1 mm squares in the region of the optic

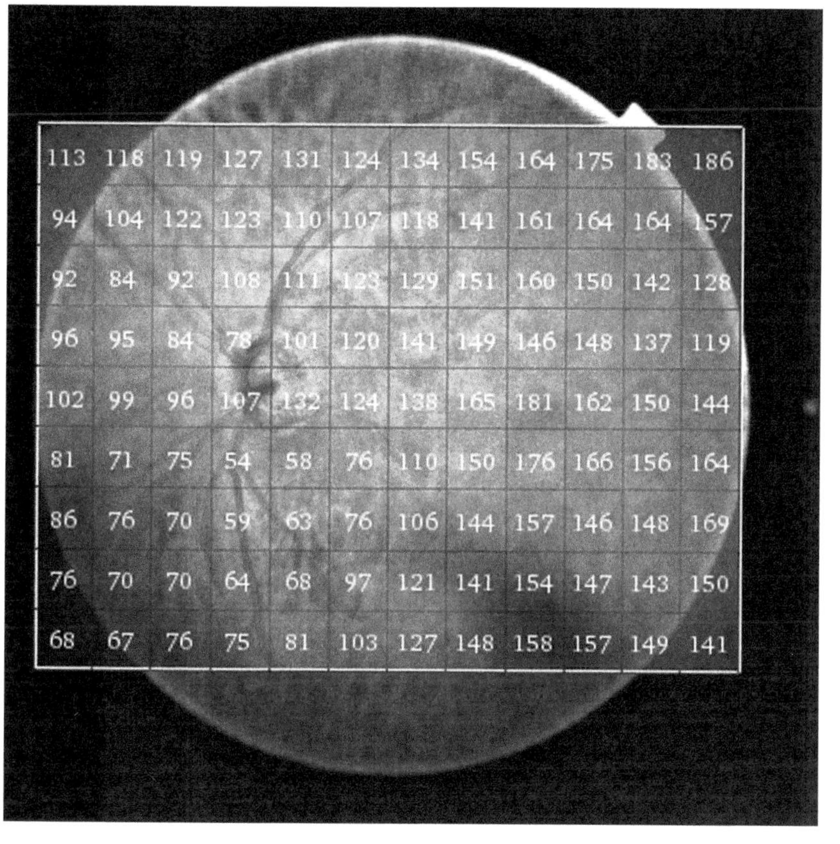

Figure 2. Example of a 12×9 mm DRI-OCT image of a glaucomatous eye included in the study. The numbers correspond to the average choroidal thickness (in μm) for each of the 108 1 mm^2 regions of the scan.

disc. The total CT was calculated as the mean CT for all sectors in the 12×9 mm^2 scan. Segmentation software was also used to calculate the average RNFL thickness over the total 12×9 mm^2 area from the wide field SS-OCT scan. The data for this study is deposited in Table S1.

Statistical Analysis

Normality assumption was assessed by inspection of histograms and using Shapiro-Wilk tests. Student *t*-tests were used for group comparison for normally distributed variables and Wilcoxon rank-sum test for continuous non-normally distributed variables. The association between CT and parameters including age, axial length, CCT, ocular perfusion pressure, MD, RNFL thickness, gender and ancestry was assessed using scatter plots and univariate linear regression in healthy and glaucomatous eyes. Observations from two eyes of the same subject are likely to be correlated, which can lead to underestimation of true variance. A between-cluster variance estimator was therefore used to account for correlations between eyes of the same subject and calculate robust variance estimates in univariate and multivariable analyses [28]. Variables from univariate analysis with a significance of 0.2 or smaller were examined in multivariable models with total CT as the dependent variable. The analysis was repeated for peripapillary and macular CT. The relationship between CT and glaucoma, and between CT and SAP MD, was examined in the multivariable model accounting for the covariables associated with CT. All statistical analyses were performed with commercially available software (Stata version 13; StataCorp, College Station, TX).

Results

The study included 265 glaucomatous eyes from 187 patients and 125 healthy eyes from 84 subjects. 10 eyes with poor quality scans (quality score <50 or poorly focused scans) and 58 eyes with scans with segmentation failures and motion artifacts were excluded. This left a total of 216 glaucomatous eyes from 140 patients and 106 healthy eyes from 67 subjects.

The demographic and clinical characteristics of those included in the study are summarized in Table 1. Subjects with glaucoma were significantly older than healthy subjects ($P<0.001$). Those with glaucoma had a mean age of 71.8±10.2 years compared to 61.2±11.9 years in healthy subjects. The mean total CT in glaucomatous eyes was 157.7±48.5 μm, which was significantly thinner than in healthy eyes 179.9±36.1 μm ($P<0.001$) (Table 1 and Figure 4). Peripapillary and macular CT were also significantly thinner in glaucomatous subjects. The mean peripapillary choroidal thickness was 154.1±44.1 μm in healthy subjects compared to only 134.0±56. 9 μm in those with glaucoma ($P<0.001$). The mean macular CT was 199.3±46.1 μm in healthy subjects compared to only 176.2±57.5 μm in those with glaucoma ($P<0.001$) (Table 1 and Figure 4). For both glaucomatous and healthy eyes, CT was largest in the macular region. Eyes with glaucoma had longer axial length ($P=0.039$), worse SAP MD ($P<0.001$), thinner RNFL thickness ($P<0.001$) and higher systolic OPP ($P=0.001$) than healthy eyes (Table 1). The distribution of SAP MD and IOP for healthy and glaucomatous eyes is shown in Figures 5A and 5B. Subjects with glaucoma also had higher systolic BP ($P<0.001$) than healthy subjects. CCT and IOP were

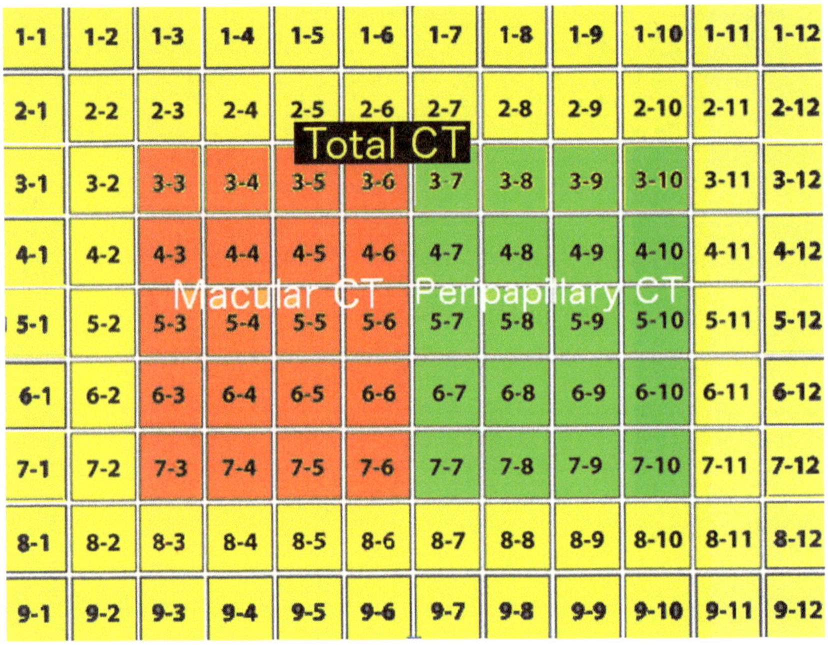

Figure 3. Example of the analysis map for the right eye used in the study. The figure shows the 12×9 mm scan divided into 1 mm^2 sectors. The areas used for the calculation of macular choroidal thickness (red), peripapillary choroidal thickness (green) and total choroidal thickness (yellow, red and green) are shown. The numbers represent the row and column co-ordinates for each sector.

not significantly different between groups (P = 0.392 and P = 0.195 respectively).

The relationship between total CT and variables including age, gender, ancestry, axial length, systolic and diastolic OPP, and CCT was examined in healthy subjects. Scatter plots suggested a tendency for total CT to be lower in older subjects and those with longer axial length (Figures 6A and 6B). Univariable linear regression analyses also indicated longer axial length (P = 0.027) and older age (P = 0.039) to be associated with thinner total CT in healthy eyes (Table 2). Other variables including gender, ancestry, OPP and CCT were not significant. In the multivariable analysis, axial length (P = 0.008) and age (P = 0.007) remained significantly

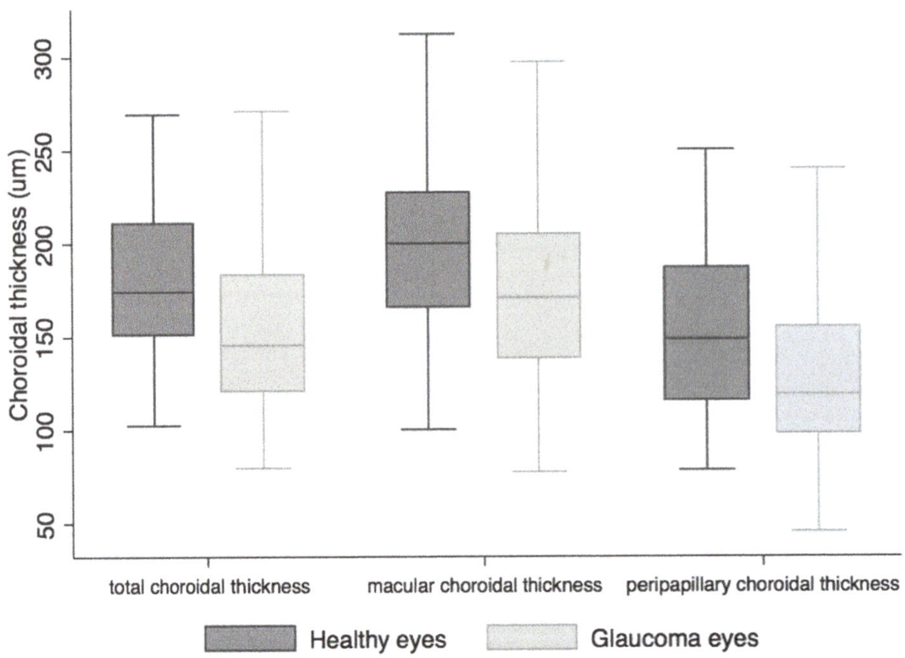

Figure 4. Boxplot illustrating the distribution of total, macular and peripapillary choroidal thickness values in glaucomatous and healthy eyes.

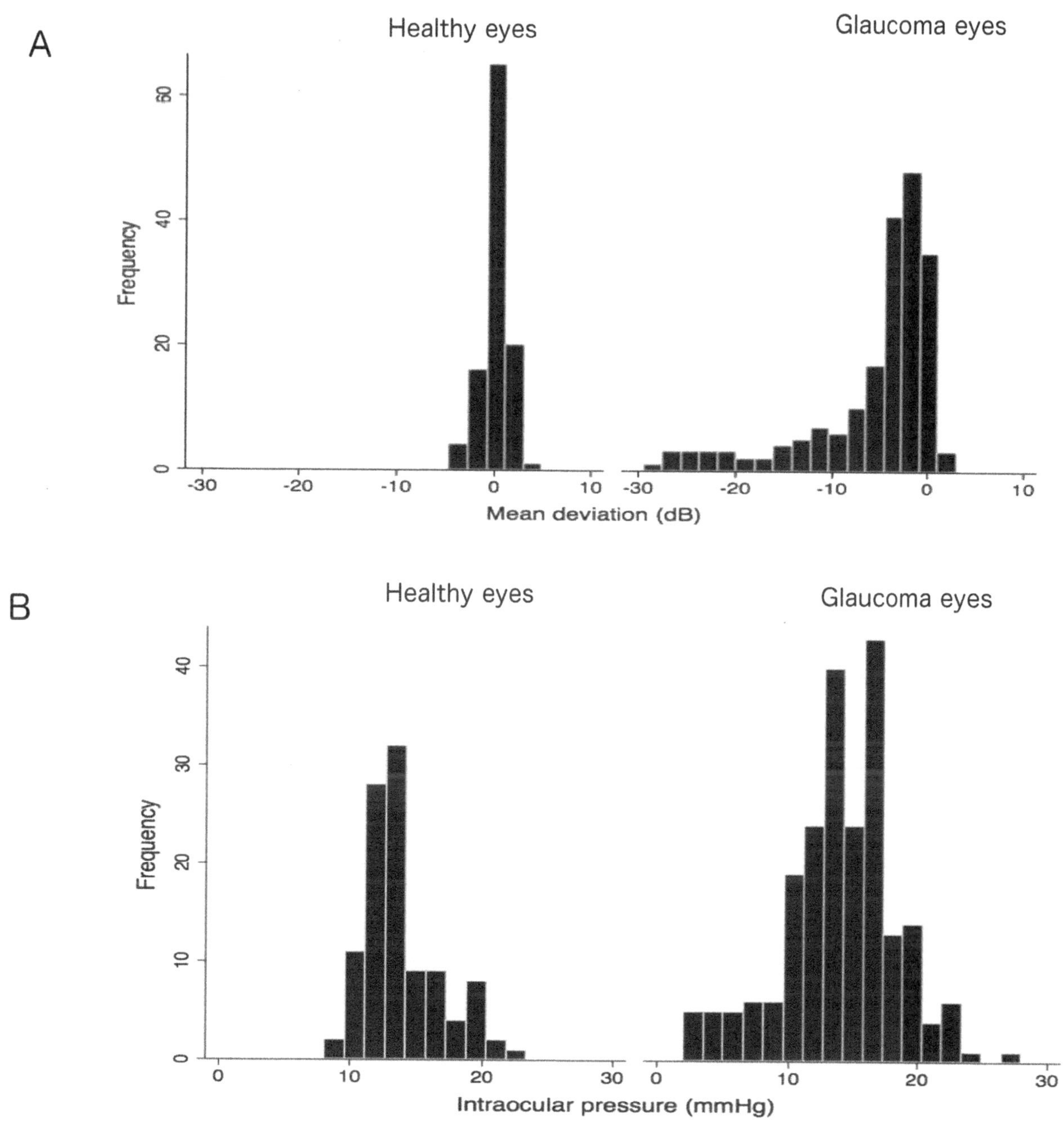

Figure 5. Distribution of standard automated perimetry (SAP) mean deviation (decibels) in healthy and glaucomatous eyes (A). Distribution of intraocular pressure (mmHg) in healthy and glaucomatous eyes (B).

associated with total CT in healthy subjects. Each decade of increasing age was associated with a 8.6 μm decrease in total CT and each 1 mm longer axial length, a 12.7 μm decrease in total CT in healthy eyes (Table 3). In addition, age was significantly associated with peripapillary CT ($P = 0.038$), and axial length was significantly associated with peripapillary CT ($P = 0.001$) in healthy eyes. In contrast, macular CT was not significantly associated with age ($P = 0.064$) and axial length ($P = 0.078$) in healthy eyes in the multivariable models (Table 3).

A similar analysis was performed using glaucomatous and healthy eyes and for macular and peripapillary CT. Age and axial length were associated with thinner total, peripapillary and macular CT (Table 4). In univariable models thinner RNFL thickness was also associated with thinner total, peripapillary and macular CT ($P<0.001$ for all comparisons) (Table 4). Variables with $P<0.2$ in the univariable analyses were examined using multivariable models (Table 5). Age and axial length remained significantly associated with total, peripapillary and macular CT. Once age and axial length were corrected for, the presence or absence of glaucoma had no significant relationship on total ($P = 0.216$), peripapillary ($P = 0.417$) or macular CT ($P = 0.330$) (Table 5). Similar multivariable models were constructed to examine the relationship between RNFL thickness, age, axial length and CT. RNFL thickness was not significant in the total CT (coefficient $= 0.03$, 95% CI: -0.01 to 0.06, $P = 0.107$) analyses.

Table 1. Demographic and ocular characteristics of healthy and glaucomatous subjects included in the study.

	Healthy (n = 106 eyes, 67 subjects)	Glaucoma (n = 216 eyes, 140 subjects)	P-value
Age (years)	61.21±11.89	71.82±10.19	<0.001
Sex (female)	69 (65%)	98 (45%)	0.001*
Ancestry			
European	31 (46%)	94 (67%)	0.004 *
African	31 (46%)	33 (24%)	
Other	5 (8%)	13 (9%)	
Axial length (mm)	23.87±1.00	24.13±1.25	0.039
CCT (μm)	547.36 ± 45.21	543.12 ± 39.84	0.392†
Systolic BP (mmHg)	129.15±14.35	136.84±15.96	<0.001
Diastolic BP (mmHg)	77.26±10.33	75.27±9.47	0.183
IOP (mmHg)	13.94±2.79	14.02±4.33	0.195
Systolic OPP (mmHg)	115.21±14.53	122.82±15.90	0.001
Diastolic OPP (mmHg)	63.32±10.20	61.25±9.75	0.140
SAP MD (dB)	0.13±1.30	−5.25±6.29	<0.001
RNFL thickness (μm)	57.37±7.35	41.25±11.23	<0.001
Total CT (μm)	179.90±36.05	157.70±48.54	<0.001
Peripapillary CT (μm)	154.12±44.11	133.99±56.89	<0.001
Macular CT (μm)	199.30±46.10	176.15±57.54	<0.001
CT – inferior (μm)	169.33±38.54	150.96±49.44	<0.001
CT – superior (μm)	190.05±37.59	164.45±51.23	<0.001

Mean ± standard deviation and Wilcoxon rank sum test unless specified otherwise. *Fisher's exact test.
†Student t-test. Abbreviations: CCT = Central corneal thickness; BP = blood pressure; IOP = intraocular pressure; OPP = ocular perfusion pressure; SAP = standard automated perimetry; MD = mean deviation; RNFL = retinal nerve fiber layer; CT = choroidal thickness.
Where appropriate P-values were adjusted for correlations between eyes of the same subject using a between-cluster variance estimator.

Discussion

In the present study SS-OCT was used to measure CT in healthy and glaucomatous eyes. The wide-field SS-OCT scan allowed imaging of the macular and peripapillary regions in a single scan, and over a wider area than previously studied. Although we found an association between glaucoma and thinner choroid in the univariable analysis, any association disappeared after adjusting for differences in age and axial length between groups. Older age and longer axial length were both associated with thinner choroid, suggesting that the apparent association between glaucoma and thinner choroid was in fact due to the confounding effect of age and axial length. Accounting for age and axial length, there was also no significant relationship between glaucoma and thickness of the macular or peripapillary choroid.

We also examined the relationship between CT and markers of glaucoma severity, however there was no significant association between SAP MD and total, macular or papillary CT. Thinner RNFL was associated with thinner choroid in univariable analyses (Table 4), however, RNFL thickness was not significant in the multivariable analyses, accounting for age and axial length. The likely explanation for this is that, similarly to choroidal thickness, RNFL thickness decreases with age and is also thinner in eyes with large axial length [29–32].

These findings are in agreement with previous studies using EDI-OCT suggesting that in vivo measurements of CT are not significantly different in patients with open angle glaucoma compared to controls [15,16,18,33,34]. However, our study goes further as most previous studies have only examined the thickness of the choroid in the macular region and have not used SS-OCT technology or employed a wide-field scanning technique to image a greater choroidal area.

Due to the proximity of the peripapillary choroid to the ONH, one might suppose that peripapillary CT would be a better measure of the blood supply to the ONH and therefore of more relevance to glaucoma. There is some evidence that peripapillary CT might be important in specific subtypes of glaucoma [35–36]. For example, Roberts and colleagues found peripapillary CT was 25 to 30% thinner in those with sclerotic glaucomatous disc damage than in patients with focal and diffuse optic disc damage or healthy controls [35]. However several other studies have not detected an association between glaucoma and peripapillary CT [9,37,38]. In a study of eyes with glaucoma without history of raised IOP, Hirooka and colleagues suggested that the portion of the macular choroid closest to the ONH may be thinner in those with glaucoma [35]. There was also correlation between CT in this region and SAP MD. To investigate this possibility in our sample, we calculated CT in the zone between the macula and ONH (measured as the average CT in the 20 squares in region 3–5 to 3–8×7–5 to 7–8 in Figure 3) but found no association between CT and glaucoma or between CT in this region and SAP MD. However, our sample was not selected to include only eyes with normal intraocular pressure.

The current study has provided useful information about the normal choroid. The results indicate that CT is largest at the macula and decreases towards the peripapillary region. The macular choroid was typically 29% thicker than the peripapillary choroid in healthy subjects. The finding that CT is greatest near the macula is consistent with previous studies, however, overall the CT measurements in this study were slightly thinner than those

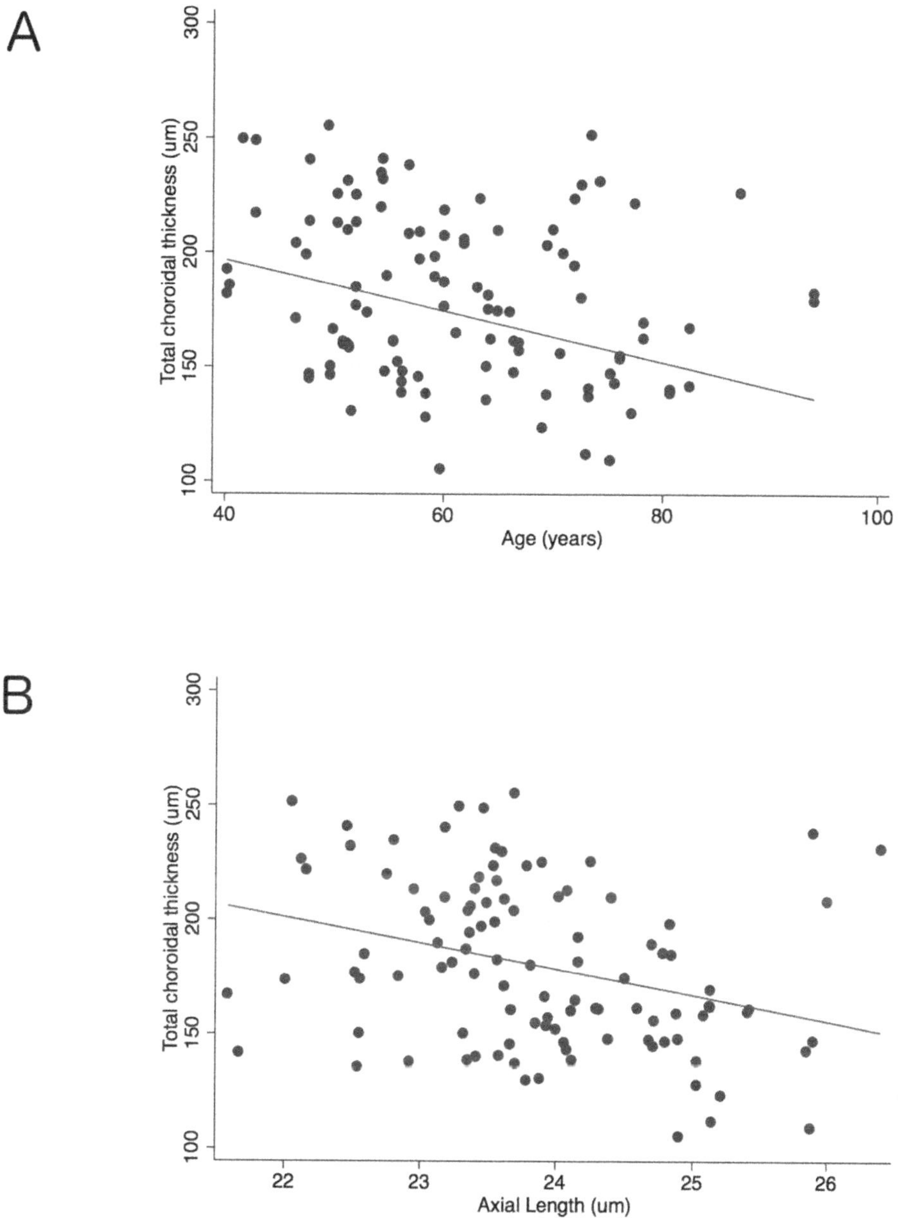

Figure 6. Scatter plots showing the relationship between total choroidal thickness and age in healthy eyes ($R^2 = 0.057$, Slope: −0.72 μm/year, $P = 0.039$) (A) and the relationship between axial length and total choroidal thickness in healthy eyes ($R^2 = 0.099$, Slope: −11.36 μm/year $P = 0.027$) (B).

previously reported using both SS-OCT and EDI OCT [14,20,21,39]. For example, two recent studies, which used SS-OCT to examine CT in healthy subjects, found average subfoveal CT to be approximately 270 to 280 μm. In comparison, using EDI-OCT subfoveal CT using SD-OCT was 263 μm to 273 μm [40,41]. These results suggest that EDI-OCT and SS-OCT produce similar CT measurements. The thinner choroid noticed in the present study is likely to be due to differences in patient characteristics between the studies. Another possible explanation is that previous studies relied on manual segmentation and measured a few points along the choroid rather than the large area measured in the present study.

Previous studies have shown an association between thinner choroid and older age, longer axial length, thicker CCT, and lower ocular perfusion pressure [13,15,21,42–44]. We found thinner CT was associated with longer axial length and older age, however, there was no significant relationship between CT and gender, ancestry, systolic or diastolic OPP, or CCT. In healthy eyes total CT was inversely proportional to age with an approximate 9 μm decrease in CT with each decade. This is slightly smaller than the 16 to 31 μm per decade decrease in macular CT previously reported in studies using EDI-OCT but could be explained by the thinner overall CT in the present study [15,16,20,29,45]. In multivariable models, accounting for axial length, we found a similar relationship between age and peripapillary CT (9.0 μm decrease per decade) and macular CT (7.8 μm decrease per decade) (Table 3). In healthy eyes the total CT also decreased by almost 13 μm for each 1 mm increase in

Table 2. Results of the univariable regression analyses evaluating the association between choroidal thickness and clinical variables in healthy eyes.

	Total Choroidal Thickness		Peripapillary Choroidal Thickness		Macular Choroidal Thickness	
	Coefficient (95% CI)	**P- value**	**Coefficient (95% CI)**	**P-value**	**Coefficient (95% CI)**	**P-value**
Age (years)	−0.72	0.039	−0.72	0.14	−0.67	0.124
	(−1.41 to 0.04)		(−1.66 to 0.23)		(−1.52 to 0.19)	
Gender	4.35	0.620	8.37	0.457	6.25	0.537
	(−13.08 to 21.78)		(−13.99 to 30.72)		(−13.85 to 26.35)	
Ancestry	0.99	0.911	9.54	0.381	−16.23	0.136
	(−16.68 to 18.66)		(−12.04 to 31.11)		(−37.71 to 5.25)	
Axial length (mm)	−11.36	0.027	−15.01	0.007	−8.96	0.133
	(−21.38 to −1.35)		(−25.74 to −4.27)		(−20.71 to 2.80)	
Systolic OPP (mmHg)	−0.248	0.441	−0.24	0.546	−0.47	0.129
	(−0.89 to 0.39)		(−1.04 to 0.56)		(−1.08 to 0.14)	
Diastolic OPP (mmHg)	−0.31	0.478	−0.21	0.704	−0.80	0.105
	(−1.17 to 0.55)		(−1.33 to 0.90)		(−1.77 to 0.17)	
CCT (μm)	0.03	0.770	−0.02	0.865	0.04	0.664
	(−0.15 to 0.21)		(−0.25 to 0.21)		(−0.16 to 0.24)	
Systolic BP (mmHg)	−0.37	0.245	−0.26	0.509	−0.509	0.147
	(−1.01 to 0.26)		(−1.05 to 0.53)		(−1.20 to 0.18)	
Diastolic BP (mmHg)	−0.48	0.256	−0.18	0.730	−0.81	0.08
	(−1.31 to 0.35)		(−1.20 to 0.85)		(−1.73 to −0.11)	
IOP (mmHg)	−1.00	0.512	0.50	0.791	−0.58	0.761
	(−4.04 to 2.03)		(−3.26 to 4.27)		(−4.36 to 3.20)	

Abbreviations: OPP = ocular perfusion pressure; CCT = central corneal thickness; BP = blood pressure; IOP= intraocular pressure.

axial length, compared to a decrease in peripapillary CT of 16.4 μm, and a decrease in macular CT of 10.2 μm, for similar increases in axial length. Similar results were found in the analyses including all eyes (Table 3).

Interestingly, we found the regression coefficient between age and choroidal thickness was smaller in healthy subjects compared to those with glaucoma (−0.72 (95% CI = −1.41 to 0.04) versus −1.03 (95% CI = −1.65 to −0.40). This indicates that the relationship between older age and thinner choroid may be steeper in glaucomatous eyes than controls, or in other words, there may be a greater decrease in CT with aging in those with glaucoma compared to controls. Although the confidence intervals overlap,

Table 3. Results of multivariable analysis for total, macular and peripapillary choroidal thickness in healthy eyes including variables from univariable analysis with P<0.2.

Characteristic	Coefficient	95% CI	P-value
Total CT			
Constant (μm)	537.24	314.75 to 759.74	<0.001
Age (per decade older)	−8.62	−14.76 to −2.48	0.007
Axial length (per 1 mm longer)	−12.70	−21.91 to −3.49	0.008
Peripapillary CT			
Constant (μm)	600.23	364.16 to 836.30	<0.001
Age (per decade older)	−8.96	−17.41 to −0.50	0.038
Axial length (per 1 mm longer)	−16.39	−26.26 to −6.52	0.001
Macular CT			
Constant (μm)	553.95	284.00 to 823.89	<0.001
Age (per decade older)	−7.76	−15.98 to −0.46	0.064
Axial length (per 1 mm longer)	−10.16	−21.50 to 1.18	0.078

Abbreviations: CT = choroidal thickness.

Table 4. Results of univariable regression analyses evaluating the association between choroidal thickness (total, peripapillary and macular) and demographic and clinical characteristics in healthy and glaucomatous eyes.

	Total Choroidal Thickness		Peripapillary Choroidal Thickness		Macular Choroidal Thickness	
	Coefficient (95% CI)	P- Value	Coefficient (95% CI)	P-value	Coefficient (95% CI)	P-value
Age (years)	−1.12	<0.001	−0.98	0.003	−1.21	<0.001
	(−1.66 to −0.57)		(−1.61 to −0.35)		(−1.87 to −0.54)	
Gender	−14.76	0.021	−13.33	0.071	−12.82	0.071
	(−27.27 to −2.24)		(−27.83 to 1.17)		(−27.79 to 2.16)	
Ancestry	12.05	0.081	18.72	0.02	0.23	0.976
	(−1.52 to 25.63)		(2.94 to 34.50)		(−15.47 to 15.00)	
Axial length (mm)	−12.25	<0.001	−14.33	<0.001	−12.34	<0.001
	(−17.51 to −6.99)		(−20.27 to 8.40)		(−18.36 to −6.32)	
Systolic OPP (mmHg)	−0.23	0.259	−0.21	0.349	−0.16	0.493
	(−0.63 to 0.17)		(−0.66 to 0.24)		(−0.61 to 0.30)	
Diastolic OPP (mmHg)	0.39	0.188	0.24	0.493	0.37	0.302
	(−0.19 to 0.96)		(−0.44 to 0.92)		(−0.34 to 1.08)	
CCT (µm)	0	0.956	−0.04	0.666	0.02	0.865
	(−0.15 to 0.15)		(−0.21 to 0.14)		(−0.16 to 0.19)	
RNFL thickness (µm)	1.10	<0.001	1.19	<0.001	1.14	<0.001
	(0.63 to 1.56)		(0.65 to 1.71)		(0.58 to 1.70)	
SAP MD (dB)	0.62	0.402	0.49	0.543	0.81	0.366
	(−0.83 to 2.06)		(−1.09 to 2.06)		(−0.95 to 2.57)	
Glaucoma	−22.20	<0.001	−20.14	0.005	−23.15	0.001
	(−33.74 to −10.65)		(−34.01 to −6.26)		(−37.15 to −9.14)	

Abbreviations: OPP = ocular perfusion pressure; CCT = Central corneal thickness; RNFL = retinal nerve fiber layer; SAP = standard automated perimetry; MD = mean deviation.

Table 5. Results of multivariable analysis including variables from univariable analysis with P<0.2 for healthy and glaucomatous eyes.

Characteristic	Coefficient	95% CI	P-value
Total CT			
Constant (µm)	548.70	428.38 to 669.02	<0.001
Age (per decade older)	−10.78	−16.19 to −5.34	<0.001
Axial length (mm)	−12.69	−17.64 to −7.73	<0.001
Glaucoma (yes)	−7.45	−19.29 to 4.38	0.216
Peripapillary CT			
Constant (µm)	566.52	414.95 to 690.83	<0.001
Age (per decade older)	−9.80	−1.61 to −0.35	0.003
Axial length (mm)	−14.76	−20.54 to −9.00	<0.001
Glaucoma (yes)	−5.89	−20.16 to 8.36	0.417
Macular CT			
Constant (µm)	577.86	436.63 to 719.08	<0.001
Age (per decade older)	−11.74	−18.52 to −4.96	0.001
Axial length (mm)	−12.85	−18.56 to −7.14	<0.001
Glaucoma (yes)	−7.33	−22.14 to 7.47	0.330

Abbreviations: CT= choroidal thickness.

indicating the differences in slopes of change in CT did not reach statistical significance; it raises the possibility that there may be an interaction between glaucoma, aging and changes in choroidal thickness over time. It would be interesting to evaluate this possible interaction in a longitudinal study, using age-matched glaucomatous and healthy subjects.

There were limitations to the present study. 68 of 390 eyes (17.4%) were excluded due to poor scan quality or segmentation failures, which potentially could have introduced bias. For example, it is possible that eyes with thicker choroid may have been more difficult to image due to deeper penetration needed. However, it was important to have a rigorous quality control to ensure included scans were accurate and significant bias seems unlikely as the proportion of glaucomatous and healthy eyes excluded was similar (49 of 265 (18.5%) versus 19 of 125 (15.2%) respectively). A further potential limitation of this study was that patients with glaucoma were already receiving treatment, For this reason, the study had limited ability to evaluate the association between IOP and CT and IOPs as shown from the observation that IOPs were not significantly different between glaucomatous and healthy eyes (Table 1 and Figure 5B). It is possible that CT may be different in untreated subjects, with higher IOPs. Using CT measurements obtained with radiofrequency, Cristini and colleagues found glaucomatous eyes with elevated IOP (30 to 45 mmHg) had 20% greater CT than healthy eyes [46]. Using EDI-OCT, Usui and colleagues found increased CT with IOP reduction following trabeculectomy [47]. In contrast, it has also been observed that in eyes with acute primary angle closure, a reduction in CT may occur following successful reduction in IOP [48]. Choroidal thinning has also been found to accompany acute increases in IOP induced by darkroom prone provocation testing in those with suspected primary angle closure [50]. It was proposed that raised IOP might induce choroidal thinning secondary to an IOP-induced reduction in choroidal blood flow [51,52]. A further limitation of our study is we did not regulate patients fluid intake prior to testing. This is a potential problem as hydration status is likely to influence CT, with an increase in CT reported after water drinking. In future studies it may be important to regulate subjects' fluid intake prior to imaging [49]. We did not investigate choroidal blood flow. Although the majority of total ocular blood volume and flow (~80–90%) is derived from the choroidal vascular, a causal relationship between measurements of ocular blood flow and glaucoma progression has not been established [53]. In addition, we estimated the macular and peripapillary CT using the grid pattern provided by the SS-OCT software which was centered on the fovea. Although during scanning the SS-OCT device uses a fixation target to center the grid on the fovea, it is possible that the macular and peripapillary CT measurements may not have been obtained at the same location relative to the macula and optic disc in every patient. For this reason we reviewed each scan and included only those passing the quality control process described in the methods.

In conclusion, this study has shown that SS-OCT is a useful tool for evaluation of CT. Using cross-sectional data we have demonstrated a relationship between increasing age, longer axial length and thinner choroid. However, when differences in age and axial length between glaucomatous and healthy subjects were accounted for there was no association between glaucoma and CT. Although we found no relationship between glaucoma and CT, prior studies have indicated an association between glaucoma and both impaired choroidal circulation and decreased blood flow to the ONH [52,54–55]. It may be that CT is a poor marker of functional integrity of the choroid, particularly as the choroid has an extravascular space that could explain much thickness variability. Further studies that explore the relationship between CT and choroidal blood flow may provide further insight into the potential role of the choroid in glaucoma.

Supporting Information

Table S1 Choroidal thickness dataset. The dataset contains data for all 216 glaucomatous eyes and 106 healthy eyes included in the study.

Author Contributions

Conceived and designed the experiments: CZ AJT FAM LMZ ZY RNW. Performed the experiments: CZ. Analyzed the data: CZ AJT FAM ZY RNW. Wrote the paper: ZA AJT FAM LMZ RNW.

References

1. Weinreb RN, Aung T, Medeiros FA (2014) The pathophysiology and treatment of glaucoma: a review. JAMA 311: 1901–1911.
2. Fechtner RD, Weinreb RN (1994) Mechanisms of optic nerve damage in primary open angle glaucoma. Survey of Ophthalmology 39: 23–42.
3. Goldberg I (2003) Relationship between intraocular pressure and preservation of visual field in glaucoma. Survey of Ophthalmology 48 Suppl 1: S3–7.
4. Shetgar AC, Mulimani MB (2013) The central corneal thickness in normal tension glaucoma, primary open angle glaucoma and ocular hypertension. Journal of clinical and diagnostic research 6: 1063–1067.
5. Lee J, Kong M, Kim J, Kee C (2013) Comparison of visual field progression between relatively low and high intraocular pressure groups in normal tension glaucoma patients. J Glaucoma, in press.
6. Hayamizu F, Yamazaki Y (2013) Effects of optic disc size on progression of visual field defects in normal-tension glaucoma. Nihon Ganka Gakkai Zasshi 117: 609–615.
7. Hayreh SS (1969) Blood supply of the optic nerve head and its role in optic atrophy, glaucoma, and oedema of the optic disc. Br J Ophthalmol 53: 721–748.
8. Banitt M (2013) The choroid in glaucoma. Curr Opin Ophthalmol 24: 125–129.
9. Yin ZQ, Vaegan, Millar TJ, Beaumont P, Sarks S (1997) Widespread choroidal insufficiency in primary open-angle glaucoma. J Glaucoma 6: 23–32.
10. Kubota T, Jonas JB, Naumann GO (1993) Decreased choroidal thickness in eyes with secondary angle closure glaucoma. An aetiological factor for deep retinal changes in glaucoma? Br J Ophthalmol 77: 430–432.
11. Francois J, Neetens A (1964) Vascularity of the eye and optic nerve in glaucoma. Arch Ophthalmol 71: 219–225.
12. Spraul CW, Lang GE, Lang GK, Grossniklaus HE (2002) Morphometric changes of the choriocapillaris and the choroidal vasculature in eyes with advanced glaucomatous changes. Vision Res 42: 923–932.
13. Arora KS, Jefferys JL, Maul EA, Quigley HA (2012) The choroid is thicker in angle closure than in open angle and control eyes. Investigative ophthalmology & visual science 53: 7813–8.
14. Spaide RF, Koizumi H, Pozonni MC (2008) Enhanced depth imaging spectral-domain optical coherence tomography. Am J Ophthalmol 146: 496–500.
15. Maul EA, Friedman DS, Chang DS, Boland MV, Ramulu PY, et al. (2011) Choroidal thickness measured by spectral domain optical coherence tomography: Factors affecting thickness in glaucoma patients. Ophthalmology 118: 1571–1579.
16. Mwanza JC, Hochberg JT, Banitt MR, Feuer WJ, Budenz DL (2011) Lack of association between glaucoma and macular choroidal thickness measured with enhanced depth-imaging optical coherence tomography. Investigative ophthalmology & visual science 52: 3430–3435.
17. McCourt EA, Cadena BC, Barnett CJ, Ciardella AP, Mandava N, et al (2010) Measurement of subfoveal choroidal thickness using spectral domain optical coherence tomography. Ophthalmic Surg Lasers Imaging 41: S28–33.
18. Rhew JY, Kim YT, Choi KR (2014) Measurement of subfoveal choroidal thickness in normal-tension glaucoma in korean patients. J Glaucoma 23: 46–49.
19. Marco Pellegrini, Carol L. Shields, Sruthi Arepalli, Jerry A. Shields (2014) Choroidal Melanocytosis Evaluation with Enhanced Depth Imaging Optical Coherence Tomography. Ophthalmology 121: 257–261.
20. Ron Margolis, Richard F. Spaide (2009) A Pilot Study of Enhanced Depth Imaging Optical Coherence Tomography of the Choroid in Normal Eyes. Am J Ophthalmol 147: 811–815.

21. Ikuno Y, Kawaguchi K, Nouchi T, Yasuno Y (2010) Choroidal thickness in healthy japanese subjects. Investigative ophthalmology & visual science 51: 2173–2176.
22. Mansouri K, Medeiros FA, Tatham AJ, Marchase N, Weinreb RN (2014) Evaluation of retinal and choroidal thickness by swept-source optical coherence tomography: Repeatability and assessment of artifacts. Am J Ophthalmol 13: 1–35.
23. Hirata M, Tsujikawa A, Matsumoto A, Hangai M, Ooto S, et al. (2011) Macular choroidal thickness and volume in normal subjects measured by swept-source optical coherence tomography. Investigative ophthalmology & visual science 52: 4971–4978.
24. Sample PA, Girkin CA, Zangwill LM, Jain S, Racette L et al. (2009) The african descent and glaucoma evaluation study (ADAGES): Design and baseline data. Arch Ophthalmol 127: 1136–1145.
25. Racette L, Liebmann JM, Girkin CA, Zangwill LM, Jain S, et al. (2010) African descent and glaucoma evaluation study (ADAGES): III. Ancestry differences in visual function in healthy eyes. Arch Ophthalmol 128: 551–559.
26. Medeiros FA, Zangwill LM, Bowd C, Sample PA, Weinreb RN (2005) Use of progressive glaucomatous optic disk change as the reference standard for evaluation of diagnostic tests in glaucoma. Am J Ophthalmol 139: 1010–1018.
27. Yasuno Y, Hong Y, Makita S, Yamanari M, Akiba M, et al. (2007) In vivo high-contrast imaging of deep posterior eye by 1-microm swept source optical coherence tomography and scattering optical coherence angiography. Opt Express 15: 6121–39.
28. Williams RL (2000) A note on robust variance estimation for cluster-correlated data. Biometrics 56: 645–646.
29. Parikh RS, Parikh SR, Sekhar GC, Prabakaran S, Babu JG, et al. (2007) Normal age-related decay of retinal nerve fiber layer thickness. Ophthalmology 114: 921–926.
30. Alasil T, Wang K, Keane PA, Lee H, Baniasadi N, et al. (2013) Analysis of normal retinal nerve fiber layer thickness by age, sex, and race using spectral domain optical coherence tomography. J Glaucoma 22: 532–541.
31. Cheung CY, Chen D, Wong TY, Tham YC, Wu R, et al. (2011) Determinants of quantitative optic nerve measurements using spectral domain optical coherence tomography in a population-based sample of non-glaucomatous subjects. Investigative ophthalmology & visual science 52: 9629–9635.
32. Knight OJ, Girkin CA, Budenz DL, Durbin MK, Feuer WJ (2012) Cirrus OCT Normative Database Study Group. Effect of race, age, and axial length on optic nerve head parameters and retinal nerve fiber layer thickness measured by cirrus HD-OCT. Arch Ophthalmol 130: 312–318.
33. Mwanza JC, Sayyad FE, Budenz DL (2012) Choroidal thickness in unilateral advanced glaucoma. Investigative ophthalmology & visual science 53: 6695–6701.
34. Fénolland JR, Giraud JM, Maÿ F, Mouinga A, Seck S, et al. (2011) Enhanced depth imaging of the choroid in open-angle glaucoma: A preliminary study. J Fr Ophtalmol 34: 313–317.
35. Roberts KF, Artes PH, O'Leary N, Reis AS, Sharpe GP, et al. (2012) Peripapillary choroidal thickness in healthy controls and patients with focal, diffuse, and sclerotic glaucomatous optic disc damage. Arch Ophthalmol 130: 980–986.
36. Hirooka K, Fujiwara A, Shiragami C, Baba T, Shiraga F (2012) Relationship between progression of visual field damage and choroidal thickness in eyes with normal-tension glaucoma. Clin Experiment Ophthalmol 40: 576–82.
37. Ehrlich JR, Peterson J, Parlitsis G, Kay KY, Kiss S, et al. (2011) Peripapillary choroidal thickness in glaucoma measured with optical coherence tomography. Exp Eye Res 2011;92: 189–194.
38. Li L, Bian A, Zhou Q, Mao J (2013) Peripapillary choroidal thickness in both eyes of glaucoma patients with unilateral visual field loss. Am J Ophthalmol 156: 1277–1284.
39. Manjunath V, Taha M, Fujimoto JG, Duker JS (2010) Choroidal thickness in normal eyes measured using cirrus HD optical coherence tomography. Am J Ophthalmol 150: 325–329.e1.
40. Matsuo Y, Sakamoto T, Yamashita T, Tomita M, Shirasawa M, et al. (2013) Comparisons of choroidal thickness of normal eyes obtained by two different spectral-domain OCT instruments and one swept-source OCT instrument. Investigative ophthalmology & visual science 54: 7630–7636.
41. Park HY, Shin HY, Park CK (2014) Imaging the posterior segment of the eye using swept-source optical coherence tomography in myopic glaucoma eyes: Comparison with enhanced-depth imaging. Am J Ophthalmol 157: 550–557.
42. Esmaeelpour M, Povazay B, Hermann B, Hofer B, Kajic V, et al. (2010) Three-dimensional 1060-nm OCT: Choroidal thickness maps in normal subjects and improved posterior segment visualization in cataract patients. Investigative ophthalmology & visual science 51: 5260–5266.
43. Fujiwara T, Imamura Y, Margolis R, Slakter JS, Spaide RF (2009) Enhanced depth imaging optical coherence tomography of the choroid in highly myopic eyes. Am J Ophthalmol 148: 445–450.
44. Ikuno Y, Tano Y (2009) Retinal and choroidal biometry in highly myopic eyes with spectral-domain optical coherence tomography. Investigative ophthalmology & visual science 50: 3876–3880.
45. Fujiwara A, Shiragami C, Shirakata Y, Manabe S, Izumibata S, et al. (2012) Enhanced depth imaging spectral-domain optical coherence tomography of subfoveal choroidal thickness in normal japanese eyes. Jpn J Ophthalmol 56: 230–235.
46. Cristini G, Cennamo G, Daponte P (1991) Choroidal thickness in primary glaucoma. Ophthalmologica 202: 81–85.
47. Usui S, Ikuno Y, Uematsu S, Morimoto Y, Yasuno Y, et al. (2013) Changes in axial length and choroidal thickness after intraocular pressure reduction resulting from trabeculectomy. Clin Ophthalmol 7: 1155–1161.
48. Wang W, Zhou M, Huang W, Chen S, Ding X, et al. (2013) Does acute primary angle-closure cause an increased choroidal thickness? Investigative ophthalmology & visual science 54: 3538–3545.
49. Mansouri K, Medeiros FA, Marchase N, Tatham AJ, Auerbach D, et al. (2013) Assessment of choroidal thickness and volume during the water drinking test by swept-source optical coherence tomography. Ophthalmology 120: 2508–2516.
50. Hata M, Hirose F, Oishi A, Hirami Y, Kurimoto Y (2012) Changes in choroidal thickness and optical axial length accompanying intraocular pressure increase. Jpn J Ophthalmol 56: 564–568.
51. Kiel JW, Van Heuven WA (1995) Ocular perfusion pressure and choroidal blood flow in the rabbit. Investigative ophthalmology & visual science 36: 579–85.
52. Grunwald JE, Piltz J, Hariprasad SM, DuPont J (1998) Optic nerve and choroidal circulation in glaucoma. Investigative ophthalmology & visual science 39: 2329–2336.
53. Weinreb RN, Harris A (2009) Ocular blood flow in glaucoma. Amsterdam: the Netherlands: Kugler Publications. 155–159 p.
54. Galassi F, Sodi A, Ucci F, Renieri G, Pieri B, et al. (2003) Ocular hemodynamics and glaucoma prognosis: A color doppler imaging study. Arch Ophthalmol 121: 1711–1715.
55. Nicolela MT, Hnik P, Drance SM (1996) Scanning laser doppler flowmeter study of retinal and optic disk blood flow in glaucomatous patients. Am J Ophthalmol 122: 775–783.

23

Diabetes, Glucose Metabolism, and Glaucoma: The 2005–2008 National Health and Nutrition Examination Survey

Di Zhao[1,¶], Juhee Cho[2,¶], Myung Hun Kim[3]*, David Friedman[4], Eliseo Guallar[1]

1 Department of Epidemiology and Welch Center for Prevention, Epidemiology, and Clinical Research, Johns Hopkins University Bloomberg School of Public Health, Baltimore, Maryland, United States of America, 2 Department of Health Sciences and Technology, Samsung Advanced Institute for Health Sciences and Technology, Sungkyunkwan University, Seoul, Korea, 3 Saevit Eye Hospital, Goyang, Gyeonggi-do, Korea, 4 Department of Ophthalmology, Johns Hopkins University School of Medicine, Baltimore, Maryland, United States of America

Abstract

Background: Diabetes may affect vascular autoregulation of the retina and optic nerve and may be associated with an increased risk of glaucoma,but the association of prediabetes, insulin resistance, markers of glucose metabolismwith glaucoma has not beenevaluated in general population samples.

Objective: To examine the relation between diabetes, pre-diabetes, metabolic syndrome and its components and the levels of fasting glucose, HbA1c and HOMA-IR with the prevalence of glaucoma in the general U.S. population.

Methods: Cross-sectional study of 3,299 adult men and women from the 2005–2008 National Health and NutritionExamination Survey (NHANES). The presence of diabetes, prediabetes, the metabolic syndrome and its individual components and biomarkers of glucose metabolisms were based on standardized questionnaire and physical exam data and laboratory tests. The history of glaucoma was assessed through questionnaire during the home interview.

Results: Diabetes was strongly associated with prevalent glaucoma.In fully adjusted models, the odds ratiofor glaucoma comparing participants with diabetes with participants in the reference group with neither pre-diabetes nor diabetes was 2.12 (95% CI: 1.23, 3.67). The corresponding odd ratio comparing participants with pre-diabetes to those in the reference group was 1.01 (95% CI: 0.57, 1.82). Patients with 5 or more years of diabetes duration hadan OR for glaucoma of 3.90 (95% CI: 1.63, 9.32) compared with patients with <5 years of diabetes duration. We also found a hockey-stick shaped associations between biomarkers of glucose metabolisms and the prevalence of glaucoma.

Conclusions: Diabetes was associated with higher risk of glaucoma. Participants without diabetes but at the higher levels of fasting glucose, fasting insulin, HbA1c and HOMA-IR spectrum may also be at greater risk of glaucoma.

Editor: Sanjoy Bhattacharya, Bascom Palmer Eye Institute, University of Miami School of Medicine;, United States of America

Funding: The authors have no support or funding to report.

Competing Interests: The authors have declared that no competing interests exist.

* Email: philip.mhkim@gmail.com

¶ DZ and JC are co-first authors on this work.

Introduction

Diabetes is a common chronic disease worldwide with a dramatic increase in incidence in recent decades [1]. Diabetes is associated with a variety of ocular complications, including retinopathy, cataracts, uveitis and neovascularization [2]. Several studies also suggested that diabetes may be associated with an increased risk of glaucoma [3–5].A meta-analysis of 12 studies published prior to 2004 found a pooled odds ratio for primary open angle glaucoma (POAG) comparing participants with diabetes to those without diabetes of 1.50 (95% confidence interval [CI] 1.16–1.93) [6], but there was significant heterogeneity and many studies reported non-significant associations [7–11] or negative point estimates [12–15].

Other abnormalities of glucose metabolism, including pre-diabetes, metabolic syndrome, insulin resistance, and elevated fasting glucose or hemoglobin A1c (HbA1c), may also be associated with glaucoma risk, but few studies have examined this issue, with conflicting results [16–19].The objective of this study was thus to examine the relation between diabetes, pre-diabetes, metabolic syndrome, and markers of glucose metabolism with the prevalence of glaucoma in the U.S. populationaged 40 years and older using data from the 2005–2008 National Health and Nutrition Examination Survey (NHANES).

Research Design and Methods

Study population

The National Health and Nutrition Examination Survey (NHANES) is a nationally representative study of the non-institutionalized US population, obtained by using a stratified multistage probability design with planned oversampling of certain age and minority groups. NHANES is conducted by the National Center of Health Statistics of the Centers for Disease Control and Prevention [20]. Information on glaucoma prevalence was only available in the 2005–2008 survey waves, and fasting glucose and insulin levels were only assessed in participants who were examined in the morning session. Therefore, we restricted our analysis to NHANES 2005–2008 participants 40 years of age or older who were examined in the morning session (N = 3,299). We then excluded 255 participants whose duration of fasting was < 8 h (if they didn't have a prior diagnosis of diabetes), 17 participants who had missing information regarding glaucoma in the questionnaire, and 1 participant with missing data in all exposure variables of interest. The final analysis was based on3,026 participants (1,501 men and 1,525 women).

The 2005–2008 NHANES study protocols were approved by the Institutional Review Board of the National Center for Health Statistics. Written informed consent was obtained from all participants.

Measurements

NHANES included a standardized questionnaire administered at home by a trained interviewer and a detailed physical examination at a mobile examination center. Self-reported glaucoma status was ascertained via the question "Have you ever been told by an eye doctor that you have glaucoma, sometimes called high pressure in your eyes?" Demographic information, education, smoking history, physical activity levels, alcohol consumption, medication use, health history, and age of diabetes onset were also determined by self-report. Leisure-time physical activities were coded and classified according to the rate of energy expenditure (<7.5, 7.5 to <15, and ≥15 metabolic equivalent hours per week) to correspond with cut points in the 2008 US federal physical activity guidelines [21] and the 2010 World Health Organization (WHO) guidelines. [22] Height, weight, and blood pressure were measured at the mobile examination center using standard procedures by trained health technicians [23,24]. Body mass index (BMI) was calculated as weight in kilograms divided by height in meters squared.

The average (SD) Fasting time was 12.3 (2.6) hours. Fasting blood samples were centrifuged and plasma was separated within 30 minutes from blood collection. Plasma glucose was analyzed using the hexokinase method in a Roche/Hitachi 911 (Roche Diagnostics, 9115 Hague Road, Indianapolis, IN) and a Roche Modular P chemistry analyzer (Roche Diagnostics, 9115 Hague Road, Indianapolis, IN) in 2005–2006 and 2007–2008, respectively [25]. Fasting insulin was analyzed using Merocodia Insulin ELISA kits [20]. HbA1cwas measured using high-performance liquid chromatography on an A1c 2.2 Plus Glycohemoglobin Analyzer (Tosoh Medics, Inc., San Francisco, Ca) in 2005–2006 and on an A1c G7 HPLC Glycohemoglobin Analyzer (Tosoh Medics, Inc., San Francisco, Ca) in 2007–2008 [26].

Diabetes was defined as a fasting plasma glucose level ≥ 126 mg/dL, an HbA1c level ≥6.5%, a self-reported diagnosis of diabetes (excluding gestational diabetes mellitus), or a self-report of current insulin or diabetes medication use. Pre-diabetes was defined in participants without diabetes as a fasting plasma glucose level between 100 mg/dL and 126 mg/dL, an HbA1c level between 5.7 and 6.5%, or a self-report of a diagnosis of borderline diabetes. Additional analyses were conducted defining diabetes and pre-diabetes using fasting plasma glucose or HbA1 ccriteria separately. Diabetes duration was calculated as the age at interview minus the age at the first time that the participant was told to have diabetes.

Metabolic syndrome components were defined as detailed in the Adult Treatment Panel (ATP) III report [27]: 1) waist circumference ≥102 cm in men and ≥88 cm in women; 2) fasting triglycerides ≥150 mg/dL; 3) HDL cholesterol <40 mg/dL in men and <50 mg/dL in women; 4) blood pressure ≥130/85 mm Hg; and 5) fasting glucose ≥110 mg/dL or use of antidiabetic medication. Persons with at least 3 of these characteristics were defined as having metabolic syndrome. We also calculated the homeostatic model assessment of insulin resistance (HOMA-IR) as fasting glucose (mg/dl) x fasting Insulin (uU/mL)/405 and defined insulin resistance as HOMA-IR >2.6 [28].

Statistical analysis

All statistical analyses were performed using NHANES weights and *svy* commands in STATA (version 12; Stata Corp., College Station, TX) to account for the complex multistage probability sampling design. Analyses of fasting glucose, fasting insulin, HOMA-IR, and HbA1 clevels were restricted to participants not taking insulin or antidiabetic medications (N = 2,509). Fasting glucose, fasting insulin, HOMA-IR, and HbA1 clevels were categorized into quartiles based on the weighted population distribution.

We used multivariable logistic regression models to calculate odds ratios (OR) and 95% CI for the prevalence of glaucoma associated with glucose metabolism variables. Diabetes and pre-diabetes were included as exposures in the same model, and we fitted separate models for diabetes duration, metabolic syndrome and each its components, insulin resistance, fasting glucose, fasting insulin, HOMA-IR, and HbA1c. For each exposure, we used 3 models with progressive degrees of adjustment. Initial models were crude and then we adjusted for age, sex (male, female) and race/ethnicity (non-Hispanic, white, non-Hispanic black, Mexican American, and other). Finally, fully adjusted models further included education (< high school, high school, > high school), smoking (never, former, current), average physical activity level (low, medium, vigorous), alcohol drinking (<1 drink/week, 1 to < 3 drinks/week, ≥3 drinks/week) and BMI (continuous).

For dose-response analyses of the associations of fasting glucose, fasting insulin, HOMA-IR, and HbA1c levels with the prevalence of glaucoma, we calculated OR and 95% CI comparing quartiles 2–4 with the first quartile in categorical analyses, as well as OR and 95% CI comparing the 80th to the 20th percentiles of markers of glucose metabolism modeled as log-transformed continuous variables. In addition, we used restricted cubic spline models with knots at the 10th, 50th and 90th percentiles of the distribution of fasting glucose, fasting insulin, HOMA-IR, and HbA1c concentrations to provide a smooth yet flexible description of the shape of dose-response relationship. Tests for non-linear trends computed by log likelihood ratio tests comparing nested models with and without non-linear spline terms.

Results

The study population had a weighted mean (SE) age of 57.0(0.4) years (**Table 1**). The prevalence of diabetes, pre-diabetes, metabolic syndrome, and insulin resistance were 17.1, 49.0, 32.1, and 43.4%, respectively, and the prevalence of glaucoma was 4.2% (95% CI 3.3–5.3%). The average duration of diabetes was

Table 1. Characteristics of study participants by glaucoma status.*

		Glaucoma		p-value†
	Overall N = 3,026	No N = 2,835	Yes N = 191	
Age, year	57.0 (0.4)	56.5 (0.4)	68.7 (1.5)	<0.001
Female, %	53.2 (1.2)	53.2 (1.1)	52.3 (4.9)	0.87
Race, %				0.009
Mexican American	5.6 (0.8)	5.7 (0.8)	4.5 (1.6)	
NonHispanic white	76.2 (2.1)	76.4 (2.1)	71.6 (4.8)	
NonHispanic black	10.2 (1.4)	9.8 (1.4)	17.8 (3.7)	
Others	8.0 (1.1)	8.1 (1.1)	6.2 (2.5)	
Education, %				0.005
<High school	18.5 (1.2)	18.0 (1.1)	29.0 (5)	
High school	27.0 (1.3)	26.9 (1.3)	30.6 (5.2)	
>High school	54.5 (2.1)	55.1 (2.1)	40.4 (4.9)	
Waist circumference, cm	100.3 (0.4)	100.2 (0.4)	103 (1.3)	0.04
Systolic blood pressure, mm Hg	126.9 (0.5)	126.4 (0.5)	136.3 (2.2)	<0.001
Diastolic blood pressure, mm Hg	70.7 (0.4)	70.9 (0.4)	65.7 (1.7)	0.005
Body mass index, kg/m^2	29.0 (0.1)	29.0 (0.1)	29.7 (0.5)	0.15
Insulin, uU/mL‡	11.2 (0.3)	11.2 (0.3)	11.9 (1.1)	0.54
Serum fasting glucose, mg/dL‡	103.5 (0.7)	103.4 (0.7)	108.6 (2.0)	0.01
HDL, mg/dL	55.5 (0.3)	55.5 (0.3)	55.4 (1.5)	0.97
Triglycerides, mg/dL	146.0 (2.7)	145.6 (2.7)	154.0 (12.7)	0.52
HbA1c, %‡	5.5 (0.02)	5.5 (0.02)	5.7 (0.08)	0.01
HOMA-IR‡	3.0 (0.1)	3.0 (0.1)	3.3 (0.4)	0.40

*Data are means (SEs) or percentages (SEs).
†P value for homogeneity of means or proportions comparing participants with to those without glaucoma.
‡Values are based on the subsample of participants not taking insulin or medication for diabetes (N = 2,409).

11.8 years. Participants with prevalent glaucoma were more likely to be older, non-Hispanic black, less educated, and had higher waist circumference, blood pressure, fasting glucose and HbA1c levels (**Table 1**) and to have a significantly higher prevalence of diabetes, elevated blood pressure, and elevated fasting glucose (**Table 2**).

The prevalence of glaucoma in participants with diabetes, with pre-diabetes, and without diabetes or pre-diabetes was 9.5, 3.5, and 2.6%, respectively (P<0.001).In age-, sex-, and race/ethnicity-adjusted models, the OR for glaucoma comparing participants with diabetes to those without diabetes or pre-diabetes was 2.09 (95% CI 1.11 to 3.92) (**Table 3**). The corresponding OR

Table 2. Prevalence of glucose metabolism abnormalities by glaucoma status.*

		Glaucoma		p-value†
	Overall N = 3,026	No N = 2,835	Yes N = 191	
Diabetes, %	17.1 (0.9)	16.1 (0.9)	38.8 (4.1)	<0.001
Prediabetes, %	49.0 (1.4)	49.4 (1.4)	40.4 (3.7)	0.34
Insulin resistance, %	43.4 (1.5)	43.1 (1.5)	49.8 (4.7)	0.13
Metabolic syndrome, %	32.1 (1.2)	31.7 (1.2)	41.1 (5.4)	0.06
Elevated waist circumference, %	60.3 (1.4)	60.0 (1.4)	66.4 (4.1)	0.14
Elevated blood pressure, %	42.1 (1.1)	41.1 (1.1)	63.3 (4.1)	<0.001
Elevated triglyceride, %	33.7 (0.9)	33.7 (1.0)	33.6 (5.5)	0.98
Reduced HDL, %	24.0 (0.8)	24.2 (0.8)	18.0 (3.9)	0.17
Elevated fasting glucose, %	28.8 (1.4)	28.2 (1.4)	43.3 (3.7)	<0.001
Duration of diabetes, years	11.7 (0.6)	11.3 (0.6)	15.2 (1.8)	0.04

*Data are percentages or means (SEs).
†P value for homogeneity of means or proportions comparing participants with to those without glaucoma.

in fully adjusted models was 1.80 (95% CI 0.93 to 3.47). The association of diabetes with glaucoma prevalence was stronger when the definition of diabetes was based on either fasting glucose or HbA1c levels only, with ORs of 2.12 (95% CI 1.23 to 3.67) and 2.10 (95% CI 1.19 to 3.71), respectively. The fully adjusted OR (95% CI) for glaucoma comparing participants with pre-diabetes to those without diabetes or pre-diabetes was 0.88 (95% CI 0.45 to 1.75). Diabetes duration was also significantly associated with glaucoma. Among participants with diabetes, the multivariable-adjusted OR for glaucoma comparing participants with a duration of disease ≥5 years to those with a duration of disease <5 years was3.90 (95% CI 1.63 to 9.32).

The prevalence of glaucoma in patients with and without metabolic syndrome was 5.3 and 3.6%, respectively ($P = 0.06$). The OR for glaucoma comparing participants with to those without metabolic syndrome was 1.30 (95% CI 0.83 to 2.03) in age-, sex-, and race/ethnicity-adjusted models and 1.13 (95% CI 0.60 to 2.16) in fully adjusted models (**Table 3**). In fully adjusted models, none of the individual components of the metabolic syndrome or the presence of insulin resistance were significantly associated with the prevalence of glaucoma (**Table 3**).

In dose-response models with glucose biomarkers modeled as continuous variables or categorized in quartiles, the prevalence of glaucoma increased with increasing biomarker levels but the trends were only statistically significant for fasting glucose (**Table 4**). In fully adjusted models, the OR for glaucoma comparing the fourth to the first quartiles of fasting glucose, insulin, HOMA-IR, and HbA1C were 1.20 (95% CI 0.67 to 2.13; P trend 0.27), 1.22 (95% CI 0.54 to 2.75; P trend 0.75), 1.37 (95% CI 0.57 to 3.27; P trend 0.19) and 1.55 (95% CI 0.59 to 4.08; P trend 0.48), respectively. In spline models, however, the dose-response relationships between markers of glucose metabolism and the prevalence of glaucoma were hockey-stick shaped for insulin, HOMA-IR, and HbA1C and J-shaped for fasting glucose (**Figure 1**).The P values for the non-linear spline terms in the restricted cubic models were significant for all glucose biomarkers ($p<0.001$ for all).

Discussion

In a large sample representative of the general US population, the prevalence of glaucoma was higher in participants with diabetes compared to those with no glucose abnormality, even after controlling for multiple potential confounders. Pre-diabetes and the metabolic syndrome and its components were not consistently associated with the prevalence of glaucoma. However, markers of glucose metabolism showed significant non-linear associations with glaucoma prevalence, including hockey-stick shaped associations for fasting insulin, HbA1c and HOMA-IR, and a J-shaped association for fasting glucose. These non-linear relationships suggest threshold effects for the association of glucose metabolism markers and glaucoma.

The association between diabetes and glaucoma has been evaluated in many studies [9,13–15,17,29,30]. An increased risk of glaucoma in persons with diabetes compared to those who did not have diabetes was also observed in the Beaver Dam Eye study, the Blue Mountains Eye study, the Los Angeles Latino Eye Study and several other population-based studies [3,5,16,19,31–35], but some well-known cohorts did not show statistically significant associations [9,14,17]. The discrepancy with these studies may be attributed to study population, sample size, methods to assess diabetes or glaucoma, or drop-out rates. The Baltimore Eye

Table 3. Odds ratio and 95% CIs for the presence of glaucoma.

	Crude model	Model 1[†]	Model 2[‡]
Diabetes			
HbA1c or fasting glucose*	3.99 (2.05, 7.76)	2.09 (1.11, 3.92)	1.80 (0.93, 3.47)
Fasting glucose only[§]	3.83 (2.24, 6.55)	2.28 (1.37, 3.81)	2.12 (1.23, 3.67)
HbA1c only[†]	4.52 (2.65, 7.68)	2.65 (1.49, 4.71)	2.10 (1.19, 3.71)
Prediabetes			
HbA1c or fasting glucose*	1.36 (0.72, 2.56)	0.96 (0.52, 1.75)	0.88 (0.45, 1.75)
Fasting glucose only[§]	1.23 (0.75, 2.02)	1.02 (0.63, 1.66)	1.01 (0.57, 1.82)
HbA1c only[†]	2.63 (1.53, 4.51)	1.72 (0.98, 3.05)	1.57 (0.85, 2.92)
Metabolic syndrome	1.50 (0.98, 2.29)	1.30 (0.83, 2.03)	1.13 (0.60, 2.16)
Elevated waist circumference	1.31 (0.91, 1.90)	1.19 (0.81, 1.75)	0.89 (0.55, 1.45)
Elevated blood pressure	2.47 (1.71, 3.56)	1.38 (0.97, 1.97)	1.39 (0.92, 2.09)
Elevated triglyceride	0.99 (0.59, 1.68)	1.09 (0.65, 1.81)	0.90 (0.52, 1.57)
Reduced HDL	0.69 (0.40, 1.18)	0.83 (0.47, 1.47)	0.73 (0.35, 1.52)
Elevated fasting glucose	1.95 (1.40, 2.70)	1.35 (1.00, 1.83)	1.29 (0.85, 1.95)
Diabetes duration >5 years	2.48 (1.06, 5.76)	2.20 (1.02, 4.73)	3.90 (1.63, 9.32)
Insulin resistance[||]	1.19 (0.78, 1.81)	1.22 (0.78, 1.90)	1.14 (0.64, 2.01)

[†]Adjusted for age, gender, and ethnicity.
[‡]Further adjusted for smoking, physical activity, alcohol intake, education, and BMI.
*Diabetes defined as self-report, HbA1c ≥6.5%, fasting glucose ≥126 mg/dL, or taking diabetic medications.Pre-diabetes defined as self-report, HbA1c ≥5.7% to < 6.5%, or fasting glucose ≥100 mg/dL to <126 mg/dL.
[§]Diabetes defined as self-report, HbA1c ≥6.5%, or taking diabetic medications. Pre-diabetes defined as self-report or HbA1c ≥5.7% to <6.5%.
[†]Diabetes defined as self-report, fasting glucose ≥126 mg/dL or taking diabetic medications. Pre-diabetes defined as self-report or fasting glucose ≥100 mg/dL to < 126 mg/dL.
[||]Values are based on the subsample of participants not taking insulin or medication for diabetes.

Table 4. Association between markers of glucose metabolism and the presence of glaucoma*

	Odds ratio for glaucoma					P value for quadratic trend
	80th vs. 20th	Quartile 1	Quartile 2	Quartile 3	Quartile 4	
Fasting glucose						
Crude Model	1.37 (1.13, 1.64)	1.00 (reference)	0.71 (0.37, 1.34)	1.06 (0.55, 2.06)	1.56 (0.96, 2.56)	0.02
Model 1†	1.22 (0.97, 1.54)	1.00 (reference)	0.67 (0.35, 1.29)	0.98 (0.51, 1.88)	1.05 (0.64, 1.72)	0.47
Model 2‡	1.30 (1.00, 1.68)	1.00 (reference)	0.67 (0.34, 1.34)	1.08 (0.47, 2.47)	1.20 (0.67, 2.13)	0.26
Fasting Insulin						
Crude Model	1.06 (0.65, 1.73)	1.00 (reference)	1.00 (0.55, 1.81)	0.96 (0.44, 2.06)	1.14 (0.61, 2.15)	0.83
Model 1†	1.16 (0.67, 2.01)	1.00 (reference)	1.02 (0.54, 1.90)	0.97 (0.44, 2.11)	1.32 (0.70, 2.49)	0.54
Model 2‡	1.13 (0.53, 2.41)	1.00 (reference)	0.92 (0.43, 1.98)	0.80 (0.30, 2.14)	1.22 (0.54, 2.75)	0.56
HOMA-IR						
Crude Model	1.16 (0.70, 1.92)	1.00 (reference)	0.67 (0.34, 1.35)	1.36 (0.67, 2.76)	1.15 (0.61, 2.17)	0.24
Model 1†	1.21 (0.70, 2.11)	1.00 (reference)	0.68 (0.34, 1.39)	1.39 (0.71, 2.71)	1.22 (0.64, 2.34)	0.17
Model 2‡	1.25 (0.57, 2.72)	1.00 (reference)	0.61 (0.28, 1.34)	1.27 (0.53, 3.05)	1.37 (0.57, 3.27)	0.22
HbA1C						
Crude Model	1.43 (1.16, 1.77)	1.00 (reference)	1.43 (0.62, 3.31)	2.35 (0.95, 5.85)	3.91 (1.75, 8.71)	0.003
Model 1†	1.23 (0.94, 1.60)	1.00 (reference)	1.10 (0.48, 2.51)	1.60 (0.61, 4.21)	1.86 (0.80, 4.28)	0.21
Model 2‡	1.15 (0.85, 1.55)	1.00 (reference)	0.96 (0.38, 2.40)	1.51 (0.53, 4.30)	1.55 (0.59, 4.08)	0.32

*Conducted in people not taking diabetes medications.
†Adjusted for age, gender, and ethnicity.
‡Further adjusted for smoking, physical activity, alcohol intake, education, and BMI.

Survey was primarily composed of African Americans and used self-report to define diabetes [9].The Rotterdam Study used a prospective cohort design, but had few participants with diabetes and a high drop-out rate, so that the results were based only on 5 incident cases of glaucoma among 264 participants with diabetes [14].The Singapore Malay Eye Study used random serum glucose measurements instead of fasting glucose to define diabetes, which may result in substantial underdiagnosis, and had also limited power to identify an association between diabetes and glaucoma [17]. In spite of these negative studies, the majority of the epidemiological evidence points to an increased prevalence of glaucoma in patients with diabetes.

Few studies have evaluated the association between metabolic syndrome or glucose metabolism biomarkers and glaucoma, with conflicting results [16–19]. In the Singapore Malay Eye Study, participants with metabolic syndrome had a lower prevalence of

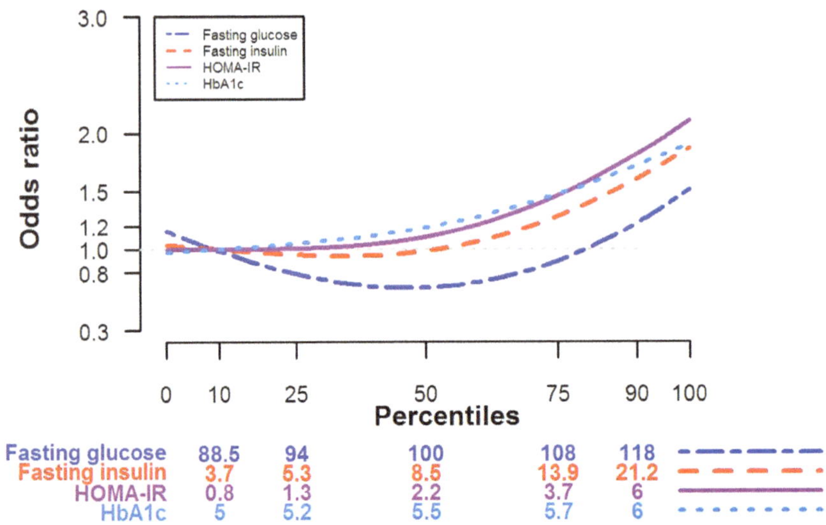

Figure 1. Adjusted odds ratio for glaucoma by levels of markers of glucose metabolism. Adjusted odds ratios were estimated using restricted cubic splines with knots at the 10th, 50th, and 90th percentiles of the distribution of each marker of glucose metabolism. The reference value (odds ratio = 1) was set at the 10th percentile of each parameter. Odds ratios were adjusted for age, sex, race, education, smoking status, physical activity, alcohol consumption, and body mass index (see text for details).

glaucoma [17], while the number of metabolic syndrome components was positively associated with the hazard of open-angle glaucoma in a US cohort [19]. As for HbA1c and glucose, the Singapore Malay Eye Study showed an elevated but non-significant trend while a case-control study in Europe showed a significantly positive association between increased HbA1c levels and glaucoma [16]. In our study, the association between glucose metabolism biomarkers and the prevalence of glaucoma was non-linear and affected only to participants in the higher half of the distribution of glucose metabolism parameters. These findings suggest that a certain degree of impairment in glucose metabolism is needed before glaucoma appears as a complication of insulin resistance.

In addition to the level of glucose metabolism biomarkers, the duration of the metabolic abnormalities may also be important in determining glaucoma risk. We found that duration of diabetes was significantly associated with an increased prevalence of glaucoma, but we did not have information on the duration of the elevations in glucose metabolism biomarkers or on their trajectories over time. Additional research is needed to confirm these thresholds and to understand the increase in glaucoma risk with increasing duration in glucose metabolism abnormalities.

Several biological mechanisms could explain an increased risk of glaucoma in patients with diabetes. Diabetes may induce structural and functional abnormalities to the small blood vessels feeding the optic nerve, resulting in damage to the optic nerve and the retinal nerve fiber layer [36]. Besides the vascular implications, diabetes may also exacerbate glaucomatous optic neuropathy by increasing the susceptibility of retinal ganglion cells to apoptosis due to elevated intraocular pressure (IOP) [37]. This mechanism may also explain progressive optic nerve injury and neuronal damage with a longer duration of diabetes. Furthermore, diabetic retinopathy may also compromise the glial and neuronal elements, impair retinal function and metabolism, and result in accelerated degeneration of retinal inner neurons [38].

The potential mechanisms underlying the association between glucose metabolism abnormalities and the prevalence of glaucoma in subjects without diabetes are unclear. The presence of the metabolic syndrome and elevated levels of glucose, HOMA IR and glycosylated hemoglobin may be associated with increased levels of IOP, a key causal factor for glaucoma [31,39–44]. Hyperglycemia increased fibronectin production in the bovine trabecular meshwork, which may increase the resistance to aqueous humor outflow and lead to elevated IOP [45]. Moreover, hyperglycemia could induce apoptosis in retinal neuronal cells through the hexosamine biosynthetic pathway [46]. Additionally, hyperglycemia-induced oxidative stress and advanced glycation end products may increase apoptotic death in retinal neurons [47,48].

Several limitations need to be considered in the interpretation of our findings. First, the cross-sectional nature of this study limited our ability to establish the causality of the observed associations. Second, while we used high quality laboratory methods and fasting plasma samples to assess glucose metabolism status, the prevalence of glaucoma was assessed by self-report without an ophthalmologic exam. Although the prevalence of glaucoma in NHANES was similar to that reported in other US studies [49], the lack of a clinical assessment of glaucoma may have resulted in under-diagnosis and recall bias. Previous studies of the validity of self-report of glaucoma have shown low sensitivity and very high specificity when compared to eye examinations, and substantial agreement when compared to medical records [50,51]. Additional studies with high quality measurements of both glucose metabolism parameters and glaucoma status are needed to confirm our findings. Third, the increased prevalence of glaucoma in patients with diabetes and in those with longer duration of diabetes may have been overestimated because of more frequent ophthalmology visits in persons with compared to those without diabetes. We did not have information on the frequency of eye examinations in study participants, but other studies suggested that this type of surveillance bias could not completely account for the positive association between diabetes and glaucoma risk [5,31]. In the Blue Mountains Eye study, most cases of glaucoma had been diagnosed before the diabetes diagnosis [5], and the Nurses' Health Study also showed that the prospective association between diabetes and glaucoma was unaltered when adjusting for factors related with the number of eye examinations [31]. In spite of these limitations, the large sample size, the standardization and rigorous quality control procedures of NHANES, and the generalizability of the findings to the general US population are important strengths that add to the relevance of our findings.

Glaucoma has a long latency period, in which glaucomatous optic nerve damage is ongoing but remains asymptomatic until later stages. Since vision loss is irreversible, screening and early detection of glaucoma is important in persons with diabetes, given the increased risk for glaucoma and the high frequency coexistence of other mechanisms for vision loss. The adherence to regular ophthalmological exams should be emphasized in diabetic patients, especially among those with long duration of diabetes, regardless of age. Our results also indicate that ophthalmologist referral may be considered for adults without diabetes but with elevated levels of glucose biomarkers.

In conclusion, data from NHANES 2005–2008, a large sample representative of the general US population, showed a higher prevalence of glaucoma in patients with diabetes, particularly in those with longer duration of disease, as well as an increased prevalence of glaucoma with increasing levels of glucose metabolism abnormalities in participants in the higher end of the distribution of glucose metabolism parameters. The mechanisms underlying these associations and the impact of the duration of glucose abnormalities on glaucoma risk need to be established in future studies. Our results support the recommendation that patients with diabetes, as well as those with elevated levels of glucose metabolism parameters, undergo regular ophthalmological exams to monitor for the onset or progression of glaucoma.

Author Contributions

Conceived and designed the experiments: MK EG. Analyzed the data: DZ JC. Wrote the paper: DZ JC. Interpretation of data and reviewed and edited the manuscript: EG DF MK. Supervision of data analysis: EG.

References

1. Wild S, Roglic G, Green A, Sicree R, King H (2004) Global prevalence of diabetes: estimates for the year 2000 and projections for 2030. Diabetes Care 27: 1047–1053.
2. Stanga PE, Boyd SR, Hamilton AM (1999) Ocular manifestations of diabetes mellitus. CurrOpinOphthalmol 10: 483–489.
3. Klein BE, Klein R, Jensen SC (1994) Open-angle glaucoma and older-onset diabetes. The Beaver Dam Eye Study. Ophthalmology 101: 1173–1177.
4. Dielemans I, de Jong PT, Stolk R, Vingerling JR, Grobbee DE, et al. (1996) Primary open-angle glaucoma, intraocular pressure, and diabetes mellitus in the general elderly population. The Rotterdam Study. Ophthalmology 103: 1271–1275.
5. Mitchell P, Smith W, Chey T, Healey PR (1997) Open-angle glaucoma and diabetes: the Blue Mountains eye study, Australia. Ophthalmology 104: 712–718.

6. Bonovas S, Peponis V, Filioussi K (2004) Diabetes mellitus as a risk factor for primary open-angle glaucoma: a meta-analysis. Diabet Med 21: 609–614. doi:10.1111/j.1464-5491.2004.01173.x.
7. Kaimbo DK, Buntinx F, Missotten L (2001) Risk factors for open-angle glaucoma: a case-control study. J ClinEpidemiol 54: 166–171.
8. KaimboWaKaimbo D, Missotten L (1997) Risk factors for open-angle glaucoma in 260 black subjects in Congo. Bull SocBelgeOphtalmol 267: 29–34.
9. Tielsch JM, Katz J, Sommer A, Quigley HA, Javitt JC (1995) Hypertension, perfusion pressure, and primary open-angle glaucoma. A population-based assessment. Arch Ophthalmol 113: 216–221.
10. Leske MC, Connell AMS, Wu S-Y, Hyman LG, Schachat AP, et al. (1995) Risk Factors for Open-angle Glaucoma: The Barbados Eye Study. Arch Ophthalmol 113: 918–924. doi:10.1001/archopht.1995.01100070092031.
11. Quigley HA, West SK, Rodriguez J, Munoz B, Klein R, et al. (2001) The prevalence of glaucoma in a population-based study of Hispanic subjects: Proyecto VER. Arch Ophthalmol 119: 1819–1826.
12. Charliat G, Jolly D, Blanchard F (1994) Genetic risk factor in primary open-angle glaucoma: a case-control study. Ophthalmic Epidemiol 1: 131–138.
13. Jonas JB, Gründler AE (1998) Prevalence of diabetes mellitus and arterial hypertension in primary and secondary open-angle glaucomas. Graefes Arch ClinExpOphthalmol 236: 202–206.
14. De Voogd S, Ikram MK, Wolfs RCW, Jansonius NM, Witteman JCM, et al. (2006) Is diabetes mellitus a risk factor for open-angle glaucoma? The Rotterdam Study. Ophthalmology 113: 1827–1831. doi:10.1016/j.ophtha.2006.03.063.
15. Howard DL, Kim MM, Hartnett ME (2011) Predicting glaucoma diagnosis in an elderly sample: revisiting the established populations for epidemiologic studies of the elderly. J Natl Med Assoc 103: 332–341.
16. Welinder LG, Riis AH, Knudsen LL, Thomsen RW (2009) Diabetes, glycemic control and risk of medical glaucoma treatment: A population-based case-control study. ClinEpidemiol 1: 125–131.
17. Tan GS, Wong TY, Fong C-W, Aung T (2009) Diabetes, metabolic abnormalities, and glaucoma. Arch Ophthalmol 127: 1354–1361.
18. Elisaf M, Kitsos G, Bairaktari E, Kalaitzidis R, Kalogeropoulos C, et al. (2001) Metabolic abnormalities in patients with primary open-angle glaucoma. ActaOphthalmolScand 79: 129–132.
19. Newman-Casey PA, Talwar N, Nan B, Musch DC, Stein JD (2011) The relationship between components of metabolic syndrome and open-angle glaucoma. Ophthalmology 118: 1318–1326. doi:10.1016/j.ophtha.2010.11.022.
20. Centers for Disease Control and Prevention. National Health and Nutrition Examination Survey: questionnaires, datasets, and related documentation (n.d.). Available: http://www.cdc.gov/nchs/nhanes/nhanes_questionnaires.htm. Accessed 26 March 2013.
21. Physical Activity Guidelines for Americans (n.d.). Available: http://www.health.gov/paguidelines/guidelines/. Accessed 6 July 2013.
22. WHO | Global recommendations on physical activity for health (n.d.). WHO. Available: http://www.who.int/dietphysicalactivity/publications/9789241599979/en/. Accessed 6 July 2013.
23. Centers for Disease Control and Prevention. 2005–2006 National Health and Nutrition Examination Survey: survey operations manuals, brochures, consent documents (n.d.). Available: http://www.cdc.gov/nchs/nhanes/nhanes2005-2006/current_nhanes_05_06.htm. Accessed 26 March 2013.
24. Centers for Disease Control and Prevention. 2007–2008 National Health and Nutrition Examination Survey: survey operations manuals, brochures, consent documents (n.d.). Available: http://www.cdc.gov/nchs/nhanes/nhanes2007-2008/current_nhanes_07_08.htm. Accessed 26 March 2013.
25. NHANES 2007–2008: Plasma Fasting Glucose and Insulin Data Documentation, Codebook, and Frequencies (n.d.). Available: http://www.cdc.gov/nchs/nhanes/nhanes2007-2008/Glu_E.htm. Accessed 26 March 2013.
26. NHANES 2007–2008: Glycohemoglobin Data Documentation, Codebook, and Frequencies (n.d.). Available: http://www.cdc.gov/nchs/nhanes/nhanes2007-2008/GHB_E.htm. Accessed 7 July 2013.
27. Third Report of the National Cholesterol Education Program (NCEP) Expert Panel on Detection, Evaluation, and Treatment of High Blood Cholesterol in Adults (Adult Treatment Panel III) final report (2002). Circulation 106: 3143–3421.
28. Ascaso JF, Pardo S, Real JT, Lorente RI, Priego A, et al. (2003) Diagnosing Insulin Resistance by Simple Quantitative Methods in Subjects With Normal Glucose Metabolism. Dia Care 26: 3320–3325. doi:10.2337/diacare.26.12.3320.
29. Uhm KB, Shin DH (1992) Glaucoma risk factors in primary open-angle glaucoma patients compared to ocular hypertensives and control subjects. Korean J Ophthalmol 6: 91–99.
30. Orzalesi N, Rossetti L, Omboni S (2007) Vascular risk factors in glaucoma: the results of a national survey. Graefes Arch ClinExpOphthalmol 245: 795–802. doi:10.1007/s00417-006-0457-5.
31. Pasquale LR, Kang JH, Manson JE, Willett WC, Rosner BA, et al. (2006) Prospective Study of Type 2 Diabetes Mellitus and Risk of Primary Open-Angle Glaucoma in Women. Ophthalmology 113: 1081–1086. doi:10.1016/j.ophtha.2006.01.066.
32. Chopra V, Varma R, Francis BA, Wu J, Torres M, et al. (2008) Type 2 Diabetes Mellitus and the Risk of Open-angle Glaucoma: The Los Angeles Latino Eye Study. Ophthalmology 115: 227–232.e1. doi:10.1016/j.ophtha.2007.04.049.
33. Graw J, Welzl G, Ahmad N, Klopp N, Heier M, et al. (2011) The KORA Eye Study: a population-based study on eye diseases in Southern Germany (KORA F4). Invest Ophthalmol Vis Sci 52: 7778–7786. doi:10.1167/iovs.10-7113.
34. Ellis JD, Evans JM, Ruta DA, Baines PS, Leese G, et al. (2000) Glaucoma incidence in an unselected cohort of diabetic patients: is diabetes mellitus a risk factor for glaucoma? DARTS/MEMO collaboration. Diabetes Audit and Research in Tayside Study. Medicines Monitoring Unit. Br J Ophthalmol 84: 1218–1224.
35. Wise LA, Rosenberg L, Radin RG, Mattox C, Yang EB, et al. (2011) A prospective study of diabetes, lifestyle factors, and glaucoma among African-American women. Ann Epidemiol 21: 430–439. doi:10.1016/j.annepidem.2011.03.006.
36. Szaflik JP, Rusin P, Zaleska-Zmijewska A, Kowalski M, Majsterek I, et al. (2010) Reactive oxygen species promote localized DNA damage in glaucoma-iris tissues of elderly patients vulnerable to diabetic injury. Mutat Res 697: 19–23. doi:10.1016/j.mrgentox.2010.02.003.
37. Kanamori A, Nakamura M, Mukuno H, Maeda H, Negi A (2004) Diabetes has an additive effect on neural apoptosis in rat retina with chronically elevated intraocular pressure. Curr Eye Res 28: 47–54. doi:10.1076/ceyr.28.1.47.23487.
38. Nakamura M, Kanamori A, Negi A (2005) Diabetes mellitus as a risk factor for glaucomatous optic neuropathy. Ophthalmologica 219: 1–10. doi:10.1159/000081775.
39. Oh SW, Lee S, Park C, Kim DJ (2005) Elevated intraocular pressure is associated with insulin resistance and metabolic syndrome. Diabetes Metab Res Rev 21: 434–440. doi:10.1002/dmrr.529.
40. Chen H-Y, Lai S-W (2005) Relation between intraocular pressure and systemic health parameters in Taiwan. South Med J 98: 28–32.
41. Xu L, Xie XW, Wang YX, Jonas JB (2009) Ocular and systemic factors associated with diabetes mellitus in the adult population in rural and urban China. The Beijing Eye Study. Eye (Lond) 23: 676–682. doi:10.1038/sj.eye.6703104.
42. Chang YC, Lin J-W, Wang LC, Chen HM, Hwang JJ, et al. (2010) Association of intraocular pressure with the metabolic syndrome and novel cardiometabolic risk factors. Eye (Lond) 24: 1037–1043.
43. Lin C-P, Lin Y-S, Wu S-C, Ko Y-S (2012) Age- and gender-specific association between intraocular pressure and metabolic variables in a Taiwanese population. Eur J Intern Med 23: 76–82. doi:10.1016/j.ejim.2011.06.002.
44. Park S, Lee E-H, Jargal G, Paek D, Cho S (2010) The distribution of intraocular pressure and its association with metabolic syndrome in a community. J Prev Med Public Health 43: 125–130.
45. Sato T, Roy S (2002) Effect of high glucose on fibronectin expression and cell proliferation in trabecular meshwork cells. Invest Ophthalmol Vis Sci 43: 170–175.
46. Nakamura M, Barber AJ, Antonetti DA, LaNoue KF, Robinson KA, et al. (2001) Excessive hexosamines block the neuroprotective effect of insulin and induce apoptosis in retinal neurons. J BiolChem 276: 43748–43755. doi:10.1074/jbc.M108594200.
47. King GL, Brownlee M (1996) The cellular and molecular mechanisms of diabetic complications. EndocrinolMetabClin North Am 25: 255–270.
48. Van Dam PS (2002) Oxidative stress and diabetic neuropathy: pathophysiological mechanisms and treatment perspectives. Diabetes Metab Res Rev 18: 176–184. doi:10.1002/dmrr.287.
49. Leske MC (2007) Open-angle glaucoma – an epidemiologic overview. Ophthalmic Epidemiol 14: 166–172. doi:10.1080/09286580701501931.
50. Patty L, Wu C, Torres M, Azen S, Varma R, et al. (2012) Validity of self-reported eye disease and treatment in a population-based study: the Los Angeles Latino Eye Study. Ophthalmology 119: 1725–1730. doi:10.1016/j.ophtha.2012.02.029.
51. MacLennan PA, McGwin G, Searcey K, Owsley C (2013) Medical record validation of self-reported eye diseases and eye care utilization among older adults. Curr Eye Res 38: 1–8. doi:10.3109/02713683.2012.733054.

Permissions

All chapters in this book were first published in PLOS ONE, by The Public Library of Science; hereby published with permission under the Creative Commons Attribution License or equivalent. Every chapter published in this book has been scrutinized by our experts. Their significance has been extensively debated. The topics covered herein carry significant findings which will fuel the growth of the discipline. They may even be implemented as practical applications or may be referred to as a beginning point for another development.

The contributors of this book come from diverse backgrounds, making this book a truly international effort. This book will bring forth new frontiers with its revolutionizing research information and detailed analysis of the nascent developments around the world.

We would like to thank all the contributing authors for lending their expertise to make the book truly unique. They have played a crucial role in the development of this book. Without their invaluable contributions this book wouldn't have been possible. They have made vital efforts to compile up to date information on the varied aspects of this subject to make this book a valuable addition to the collection of many professionals and students.

This book was conceptualized with the vision of imparting up-to-date information and advanced data in this field. To ensure the same, a matchless editorial board was set up. Every individual on the board went through rigorous rounds of assessment to prove their worth. After which they invested a large part of their time researching and compiling the most relevant data for our readers.

The editorial board has been involved in producing this book since its inception. They have spent rigorous hours researching and exploring the diverse topics which have resulted in the successful publishing of this book. They have passed on their knowledge of decades through this book. To expedite this challenging task, the publisher supported the team at every step. A small team of assistant editors was also appointed to further simplify the editing procedure and attain best results for the readers.

Apart from the editorial board, the designing team has also invested a significant amount of their time in understanding the subject and creating the most relevant covers. They scrutinized every image to scout for the most suitable representation of the subject and create an appropriate cover for the book.

The publishing team has been an ardent support to the editorial, designing and production team. Their endless efforts to recruit the best for this project, has resulted in the accomplishment of this book. They are a veteran in the field of academics and their pool of knowledge is as vast as their experience in printing. Their expertise and guidance has proved useful at every step. Their uncompromising quality standards have made this book an exceptional effort. Their encouragement from time to time has been an inspiration for everyone.

The publisher and the editorial board hope that this book will prove to be a valuable piece of knowledge for researchers, students, practitioners and scholars across the globe.

List of Contributors

Fabiane Frota da Rocha Morgado and Maria da Consolação Gomes Cunha Fernandes Tavares
Department of Physical Education, University of Campinas, Campinas, São Paulo, Brazil

Angela Nogueira Neves Betanho Campana
Sagrado Coração University, Bauru, São Paulo, Brazil

Ramani Soundararajan, Timothy M. Stearns, Jeremy R. Charette, Wanda L. Hicks, Gayle B. Collin, Jürgen K. Naggert, Mark P. Krebs and Patsy M. Nishina
The Jackson Laboratory, Bar Harbor, Maine, United States of America

Jungyeon Won
National Disaster Management Institute, Seoul, Korea

Francisco Cavas-Martínez, Daniel G. Fernández-Pacheco, José Nieto
Martínez and Francisco J. Fernández Cañavate
Department of Graphical Expression, Technical University of Cartagena, Cartagena, Spain

Ernesto De la Cruz-Sánchez
Department of Physical Activity and Sport, University of Murcia, Murcia, Spain

Alfredo Vega-Estrada, Ana B. Plaza-Puche and Jorge L. Alió
Vissum Corporación Oftalmológica, Alicante, Spain

Stefan Markun, Elisabeth Brändle and Thomas Rosemann
Institute of General Practice and Health Service Research, University of Zurich, University Hospital of Zurich, Zurich, Switzerland

Avraham Dishy
Department of Ophthalmology, Cantonal Hospital Aarau, Aarau, Switzerland

Anja Frei
Institute of General Practice and Health Service Research, University of Zurich, University Hospital of Zurich, Zurich, Switzerland
Institute of Social and Preventive Medicine, University of Zurich, Zurich, Switzerland

Lung-Chang Chien
Division of Biostatistics, University of Texas School of Public Health at San Antonio Regional Campus, San Antonio, Texas, United States of America

Yi-Jen Lien and Hwa-Lung Yu
Department of Bioenvironmental Systems Engineering, National Taiwan University, Taipei, Taiwan

Chiang-Hsin Yang
Department of Health Care Management, National Taipei University of Nursing and Health Sciences, Taipei, Taiwan

Masahiro Miyake, Kenji Yamashiro, Yumiko Akagi-Kurashige, Akio Oishi, Akitaka Tsujikawa, Masanori Hangai and Nagahisa Yoshimura
Department of Ophthalmology and Visual Sciences, Kyoto University Graduate School of Medicine, Kyoto, Japan

Shahid Husain, Yasir Abdul, Sudha Singh, Anis Ahmad and Mahvash Husain
Hewitt Laboratory of the Ola B. Williams Glaucoma Center, Department of Ophthalmology, Storm Eye Institute, Medical University of South Carolina, Charleston, South Carolina, United States of America

Masakazu Akahori and Takeshi Iwata
Division of Molecular and Cellular Biology, National Institute of Sensory Organs, National Hospital Organization Tokyo Medical Center, Tokyo, Japan

Yuri Surgeev
National Eye Institute, National Institutes of Health, Bethesda, MD, United States of America

Kazutoshi Yoshitake and Kazuho Ikeo
Laboratory of DNA Data Analysis, National Institute of Genetics, Shizuoka, Japan

Masaaki Kuniyoshi
RIKEN Center for Life Science Technologies, Division of Genomic Technologies, Life Science Accelerator Technology Group, Transcriptome Technology Team, Yokohama, Japan

Takaaki Hayashi
Department of Ophthalmology, The Jikei University School of Medicine, Tokyo, Japan

Mineo Kondo
Department of Ophthalmology, Mie University Graduate School of Medicine, Tsu, Japan

Shinji Ueno
Department of Ophthalmology, Nagoya University Graduate School of Medicine, Nagoya, Japan

Kazushige Tsunoda
Laboratory of Visual Physiology, National Institute of Sensory Organs, Tokyo, Japan

Kei Shinoda
Department of Ophthalmology, Teikyo University School of Medicine, Tokyo, Japan

Kazuki Kuniyoshi
Department of Ophthalmology, Kinki University Faculty of Medicine, Osaka, Japan

Yohinori Tsurusaki and Naomichi Matsumoto
Department of Human Genetics, Yokohama City University, Yokohama, Japan

Satoshi Katagiri
Division of Molecular and Cellular Biology, National Institute of Sensory Organs, National Hospital Organization Tokyo Medical Center, Tokyo, Japan
Department of Ophthalmology, The Jikei University School of Medicine, Tokyo, Japan

M. Ali Behzadian
Vascular Biology Center, Georgia Regents University, Augusta, Georgia, United States of America

Jutamas Suwanpradid
Vascular Biology Center, Georgia Regents University, Augusta, Georgia, United States of America
Culver Vision Discovery Institute, Georgia Regents University, Augusta, Georgia, United States of America

R. William Caldwell
Culver Vision Discovery Institute, Georgia Regents University, Augusta, Georgia, United States of America
Department of Pharmacology and Toxicology, Department of Cellular Biology & Anatomy, Georgia Regents University, Augusta, Georgia, United States of America

Ruth B. Caldwell
Culver Vision Discovery Institute, Georgia Regents University, Augusta, Georgia, United States of America
Vascular Biology Center, Georgia Regents University, Augusta, Georgia, United States of America
Charlie Norwood VA Medical Center, Augusta, Georgia, United States of America

Modesto Rojas
Culver Vision Discovery Institute, Georgia Regents University, Augusta, Georgia, United States of America
Vascular Biology Center, Georgia Regents University, Augusta, Georgia, United States of America
Department of Pharmacology and Toxicology, Department of Cellular Biology & Anatomy, Georgia Regents University, Augusta, Georgia, United States of America

Yingyan Ma, Haiyun Liu, Lin Bai, Xun Xu and Xi Zhang
Department of Ophthalmology, Shanghai First People's Hospital, Shanghai Jiao Tong University, Shanghai, China

Xiaohua Ying and Xiaocheng Xu
School of Public Health, Fudan University, Shanghai, China

Haidong Zou
Department of Ophthalmology, Shanghai First People's Hospital, Shanghai Jiao Tong University, Shanghai, China
Shanghai Eye Disease Prevention & Treatment Center, Shanghai, China

Ponnalagu Murugeswari and Veerappan Muthukkaruppan
Department of Immunology and Cell Biology, Aravind Medical Research Foundation, Dr.G.Venkataswamy Eye Research Institute, Madurai, India

Dhananjay Shukla, Ramasamy Kim and Perumalsamy Namperumalsamy
Vitreous and Retina Service, Aravind Eye Care System, Madurai, India

Alan W. Stitt
Centre for Experimental Medicine, Queens University, Belfast, United Kingdom

Leonardo Murgiano, Vidhya Jagannathan and Cord Drögemüller
Institute of Genetics, Vetsuisse Faculty, University of Bern, Bern, Switzerland

Valerio Calderoni
Bovine practitioner, Fontanelice, Italy

Monika Joechler and Arcangelo Gentile
Department of Veterinary Medical Sciences, University of Bologna, Ozzano dell'Emilia, Italy

Shunsuke Nakakura, Minami Yamamoto, Etsuko Terao, Toshihiko Nagasawa and Hitoshi Tabuchi
Department of Ophthalmology, Saneikai Tsukazaki Hospital, Himeji, Japan

Yoshiaki Kiuchi
Department of Ophthalmology and Visual Sciences, Graduate School of Biomedical Sciences, Hiroshima University, Hiroshima, Japan

Huanhuan Cheng
Department of Ophthalmology, The Third Affiliated Hospital of Sun Yat-sen University, Guangzhou, China

Yong Ding
Department of Ophthalmology, The First Affiliated Hospital of Jinan University, Guangzhou, China

Rongjie Yu
Bio-engineering Institute of Jinan University, Jinan University, Guangzhou, China

Jiansu Chen
Department of Ophthalmology, Medical College, Jinan University, Guangzhou, China

Chunyun Wu
Department of Parasitology, Medical College, Jinan University, Guangzhou, China

Ian J. Saldanha, Kay Dickersin, Xue Wang and Tianjing Li
Department of Epidemiology, Johns Hopkins Bloomberg School of Public Health, Baltimore, Maryland, United States of America

Heli Nordgren
Production Animal Section, Finnish Food Safety Authority (Evira), Seinäjoki, Finland

Paula M. Kinnunen, Antti Sukura and Udo Hetzel
Department of Veterinary Biosciences, Faculty of Veterinary Medicine, University of Helsinki, Helsinki, Finland

Ilkka Kivistö
Department of Virology, Haartman institute, University of Helsinki, Helsinki, Finland

Mirja Raunio-Saarnisto
Seinäjoki Laboratory Section, Finnish Food Safety Authority (Evira), Seinäjoki, Finland

Anna-Maria Moisander-Jylhä and Johanna Korpela
Finnish Fur Breeders Association (FFBA), Vantaa and Vaasa, Finland

Ulla-Maija Kokkonen
Section for Poultry, Wild and Laboratory Animals, Finnish Food Safety Authority (Evira), Helsinki, Finland

Kirsi Aaltonen and Tarja Sironen
Department of Veterinary Biosciences, Faculty of Veterinary Medicine, University of Helsinki, Helsinki, Finland
Department of Virology, Haartman institute, University of Helsinki, Helsinki, Finland

Olli Vapalahti
Department of Veterinary Biosciences, Faculty of Veterinary Medicine, University of Helsinki, Helsinki, Finland
Department of Virology, Haartman institute, University of Helsinki, Helsinki, Finland
Department of Virology and Immunology, HUSLAB, Hospital district of Helsinki and Uusimaa, Helsinki, Finland

Pia Lundgren, Ann Hellström and Chatarina Löfqvist
Institute of Neuroscience and Physiology, Sahlgrenska Academy at University of Gothenburg, Gothenburg, Sweden

Eva M. Andersson
Department of Occupational and Environmental Medicine, Sahlgrenska Academy at University of Gothenburg, Gothenburg, Sweden

Ingrid Hansen Pupp and David ley
Department of Pediatrics, Institute of Clinical Sciences, Lund University and Skane University Hospital, Lund, Sweden

Gerd Holmström
Department of Neuroscience, Ophthalmology, Uppsala University, Uppsala, Sweden

Aimon Niklasson
Department of Pediatrics, Institute of Clinical Sciences, Sahlgrenska Academy at University of Gothenburg, Gothenburg, Sweden

Lois E. H. Smith and Carolyn Wu
Department of Ophthalmology, Boston Children's Hospital, Harvard Medical School, Boston, Massachusetts, United States of America

Anna Kistner
Institute of Neuroscience and Physiology, Sahlgrenska Academy at University of Gothenburg, Gothenburg, Sweden
Institution of Molecular Medicine and Surgery, Karolinska Institutet, Stockholm, Sweden

Dong Ming
Department of Biomedical Engineering, Tianjin University, Tianjin, China

Benjamin Blankertz
Neurotechnology Group, Berlin Institute of Technology, Berlin, Germany

Xingwei An
Department of Biomedical Engineering, Tianjin University, Tianjin, China
Neurotechnology Group, Berlin Institute of Technology, Berlin, Germany

Johannes Höhne
Neurotechnology Group, Berlin Institute of Technology, Berlin, Germany
Machine Learning Group, Berlin Institute of Technology, Berlin, Germany

Wei Wang and Xiulan Zhang
Zhongshan Ophthalmic Center, State Key Laboratory of Ophthalmology, Sun Yat-Sen University, Guangzhou, People's Republic of China

Kayla D. Stones and Claudia L. R. Gonzalez
The Brain in Action Laboratory, Department of Kinesiology, University of Lethbridge, Lethbridge, Alberta, Canada

Ama Sadaka, Kelli Palmer, Takashi Suzuki and Michael S. Gilmore
Departments of Ophthalmology, and Microbiology and Molecular Genetics, Harvard Medical School, Boston, Massachusetts, United States of America
The Massachusetts Eye and Ear Infirmary, Boston, Massachusetts, United States of America
Harvard Microbial Sciences Initiative, Cambridge, Massachusetts, United States of America

Andrew J. Tatham, Felipe A. Medeiros, Linda M. Zangwill, Zhiyong Yang and
Robert N. Weinreb
Hamilton Glaucoma Center and Department of Ophthalmology, University of California San Diego, San Diego, California, United States of America

Chunwei Zhang
Hamilton Glaucoma Center and Department of Ophthalmology, University of California San Diego, San Diego, California, United States of America
Department of Ophthalmology, the First Affiliated Hospital, Harbin Medical University, Harbin, China

Di Zhao and Eliseo Guallar
Department of Epidemiology and Welch Center for Prevention, Epidemiology, and Clinical Research, Johns Hopkins University Bloomberg School of Public Health, Baltimore, Maryland, United States of America

Juhee Cho
Department of Health Sciences and Technology, Samsung Advanced Institute for Health Sciences and Technology, Sungkyunkwan University, Seoul, Korea

Myung Hun Kim
Saevit Eye Hospital, Goyang, Gyeonggi-do, Korea

David Friedman
Department of Ophthalmology, Johns Hopkins University School of Medicine, Baltimore, Maryland, United States of America

Index

A
Aminoguanidine, 62-63, 66, 71
Anesthesia, 23, 89, 92-93
Angiogenesis, 82-83, 90-91, 100, 103, 105, 107, 163
Antiangiogenic Therapy, 40, 42
Asian Dust Storms, 43, 45, 47, 49, 51-52
Asthma, 36, 39, 43-44, 52

B
Blindness, 1-5, 7-9, 53, 62, 73, 76, 79-80, 93, 99, 108, 156, 178, 180, 189, 194, 208
Blood Circulation, 62, 128
Blood Pressure, 118, 125, 209, 214, 216, 221-223
Blood Vessels, 35, 82-84, 225
Bronchopulmonary Dysplasia, 156, 162

C
Cardiovascular Diseases, 43, 48
Cataract, 4, 33-34, 54, 93, 99, 108-117, 121, 138-144, 194, 206, 219
Cataract Surgery, 34, 54, 93, 99, 121, 194, 206
Cell Death, 35, 67, 71, 83-86, 90-91, 127, 130, 133, 137, 203
Chorioretinal Atrophy, 53, 56, 58-59, 61
Choroidal Thickness, 118-126, 208-209, 211-219
Chromosome, 78-79, 108-111, 115-116
Chronic Care Model, 35, 37, 39-41
Chronic Disease, 41, 108, 220
Chronic Illness, 35-36, 40-42
Ciliary Body Epithelium, 204
Conjunctivitis, 43-52, 148, 151-152, 154
Corneal Topography, 23-24, 34
Coronary Artery Disease, 36, 38-39, 41
Curvature, 23-24, 28-29, 33, 53-55, 57-61

D
Depression, 1, 8-9, 35-36, 39, 41-42
Diabetic Retinopathy, 36, 38-39, 91, 99-107, 127, 136-138, 141-142, 144

E
Eating Disorders, 1
Endothelial Cells, 82-85, 87, 90, 100, 102-103, 105, 107
Eye Diseases, 43, 51, 93, 226
Eye Irritation, 43
Eye Lens, 108, 114

F
Fungal Spores, 43, 51

G
Genetic Disorders, 162
Glaucomatous Injury, 62-71

H
Health Care, 9, 35, 41, 43, 93, 99, 146
Hyperammonemia, 82-83
Hyperoxia, 82-91
Hypertension, 36, 39, 71, 93, 121, 178, 180-182, 218, 226

I
Intraocular Pressure, 62-63, 65, 71, 109, 121, 127, 137-138, 140-141, 144, 208-209, 213-214, 216, 218-219, 225-226

K
Keratoconus, 23-26, 29-34

M
Magnetic Resonance Imaging, 61, 193
Microphthalmia, 10-11, 19-22
Myopia, 10-11, 21-22, 53, 59-61, 93, 125

N
Neovascularizations, 36
Night Blindness, 76, 79
Nitric Oxide, 62-63, 65-69, 71-72, 82-84, 89-91
Nitric Oxide Synthase, 62-63, 68, 71-72, 82, 91
Nitrotyrosine, 62, 65, 67-68, 71, 82, 84-85, 88-89

O
Ocular Blood Flow, 118, 218-219
Ocular Disease, 10, 117
Ocular Surgery, 54, 101
Optic Nerve, 4, 62, 65, 67-71, 89, 121, 124-127, 130, 188, 208-209, 218-220, 225
Optic Nerve Head, 62, 68, 71, 124, 126, 208, 218
Optic Neuropathy, 53, 62, 68, 71, 225-226
Optical Coherence Tomography, 33, 36, 53-54, 61, 118-119, 121, 125-126, 208-209, 218-219
Osteoarthritis, 35, 40, 42
Outer Segments, 10, 20-22
Oxygen-induced Retinopathy, 82, 89-91

P
Pacap, 127-129, 131-137
Peroxynitrite, 71-72, 82-86, 90
Photoreceptor, 10, 13, 17-22, 134, 136
Photoreceptor Degeneration, 10, 17, 20, 22
Pneumonia, 43, 48, 52, 149, 151, 205
Posterior Corneal Surfaces, 23-24, 28-29, 32-33
Psychological Health, 1, 8

R
Ranibizumab, 37, 42, 100, 102-103, 105, 107, 178-185
Reactive Oxygen Species, 82, 127, 135, 137, 226
Refractive Surgery, 23, 33
Respiratory Disease, 43, 52
Retinal Degeneration, 10-11, 13-14, 17, 19-22, 68, 78-81, 128, 134-137
Retinal Detachments, 55, 58, 99
Retinal Ganglion Cells, 62, 66-67, 71-72, 127, 136-137, 225
Retinal Pigment Epithelium, 10, 16, 22, 60, 85, 122, 209
Retinal Structure, 53, 83
Retinitis Pigmentosa, 4, 10, 16, 21-22, 73-74, 79, 81, 188
Retinoschisis, 55-61
Rrd Surgery, 92-98

S
Sas-eb, 1-5, 7-9
Scanning Laser Ophthalmoscope, 54
Sirius Topographer, 23-25, 27
Staphyloma, 53-55, 57-61

U
Ultrasonography, 23

V
Vascular Endothelial Cells, 87
Vascular Injury, 67, 82-83, 86-88
Visual Function, 35-36, 42, 98, 132-133, 209, 219
Visual Impairment, 2-9, 36, 93, 99, 189
Visual Loss, 36, 39, 59, 99-100
Vitreous Surgery, 92-94, 96-98